D1561086

Gene Therapy for Neurological Disorders

Gene Therapy for Neurological Disorders

edited by

Pedro R. Lowenstein

*Board of Governors' Gene Therapeutics Research Institute,
Cedars-Sinai Medical Center, and Departments of Medicine, and
Medical and Molecular Pharmacology, David Geffen School of Medicine,
University of California, Los Angeles, California, U.S.A.*

Maria G. Castro

*Board of Governors' Gene Therapeutics Research Institute,
Cedars-Sinai Medical Center, and Departments of Medicine, and
Medical and Molecular Pharmacology, David Geffen School of Medicine,
University of California, Los Angeles, California, U.S.A.*

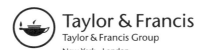

Taylor & Francis
Taylor & Francis Group
New York London

Taylor & Francis an imprint of the
Taylor & Francis Group, an informa business

Published in 2006 by
Taylor & Francis Group
270 Madison Avenue
New York, NY 10016

International Standard Book Number-10: 0-8247-2847-5 (Hardcover)
International Standard Book Number-13: 978-0-8247-2847-2 (Hardcover)
Library of Congress Card Number 2006040381

This book contains information obtained from authentic and highly regarded sources. Reprinted material is quoted with permission, and sources are indicated. A wide variety of references are listed. Reasonable efforts have been made to publish reliable data and information, but the author and the publisher cannot assume responsibility for the validity of all materials or for the consequences of their use.

Library of Congress Cataloging-in-Publication Data

Gene therapy for neurological disorders / edited by Pedro R. Lowenstein, Maria G. Castro.
   p. ; cm.
  Includes bibliographical references and index.
  ISBN-13: 978-0-8247-2847-2 (hardcover : alk. paper)
  ISBN-10: 0-8247-2847-5 (hardcover : alk. paper)
  1. Nervous System--Diseases--Gene therapy. I. Lowenstein, P.R. (Pedro R.) II. Castro, Maria G.
  [DNLM: 1. Nervous System Diseases--therapy. 2. Gene Therapy--methods. 3. Genetic Vectors. WL 140 G3273 2006]

RC350.G45G454 2006
616.8'0442--dc22   2006040381

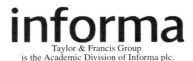

Taylor & Francis Group
is the Academic Division of Informa plc.

**Visit the Taylor & Francis Web site at
http://www.taylorandfrancis.com**

Dedication

I dedicate this book to my husband, Pedro, for being my inspiration and love during the past 20 years of my life; to my son, Elijah, for his irreverence, his joy of life and his bright light; to my parents, Nestor and Piru, for having taught me my way in life; and to my mentors and all the people that worked with me over the years for their zest for scientific discoveries, their drive and their passion. Thank you all from the bottom of my heart.

Dr. Maria G. Castro

I wish to dedicate this book to my life partner of the last 20 years for being that—a partner providing life and sustenance during the light and the dark years; to my son, Elijah, for showing me the joy of snowboarding, skateboarding, and even the appreciation of American football; and to many friends, advisors, coaches, and other gurus (you all know you are forever inscribed in my heart even if you'll never read this book), who have kept the candles burning during the Dark Ages.

Dr. Pedro R. Lowenstein

Foreword

The promise of Gene Therapy offers the cure of fatal genetic diseases to interceding in the progression of deadly acquired diseases. Rarely does come along a technology with such wide potential and applicability that can influence nearly every aspect of human health. No wonder, expectations are high and consequently any disappointments are also magnified. Truth as usual lies in the middle. The early practitioners of gene therapy underestimated the obstacles that lay in the path of safe and efficient gene delivery. Progress has been slow and successes few and far in-between. The drum beats of demise of gene therapy grow louder.

Some time ago in a series of editorials for *Molecular Therapy* I defined a scientist as a seeker of truth, someone who with determination and hope builds hypothesis to be sustained by experimentation. I also argued that science is a passion and an obsession, a hobby, not a profession. Fortunately a large group of dedicated and accomplished scientists have continued to explore safer, novel and more efficient ways of gene delivery. They have found ways to deal with the immunological problems, lower expression levels, sustained production of the therapeutic entity and ability to generate large amounts of delivery vehicles. The progress is incremental but important to set the stage for sustained success. More importantly gene therapy approaches are being developed to tackle specific problems and diseases.

Two veteran gene therapy advocates and practitioners, Maria G. Castro and Pedro R. Lowenstein of Cedars-Sinai Medical Center in Los Angeles, California have put together an excellent collection of sixteen articles detailing the gene therapy approaches dealing solely with neurological diseases. Not surprisingly, the editors have specifically selected procedures, diseases, and vectors that are most likely to intervene in neurological impairments. The editors have further emphasized those technologies that are currently being considered closest to the bedside. After a hiatus during which the field reconsidered the ways forward, clinical trials are again on the rise (see the interesting data in Figure 1 in the Preface!), especially for the treatment of neurological diseases. This is not surprising, since neurological therapeutics continues to lag behind the treatment of diseases of other bodily systems. Gene therapy offers an unique opportunity in the intervention of neurological diseases.

This edited book describes novel approaches to preparing viral vectors that are now completely devoid of any viral proteins, new therapeutic targets for chronic brain neurodegenerations, and the treatment of brain tumors described from the perspective of novel treatment developments, or the implementation of large clinical trials. Significantly, encouraging results from clinical trials for brain cancer are moving again into Phase III trials, the final measuring stick by which success in the clinical arena will be measured.

Maria and Pedro deserve our thanks for this timely effort to bring forward the progress made in the field of gene therapy in neurological disorders. More importantly this books offers valuable information for new investigators joining the field of gene therapy of central nervous system. I hope that you, the reader will find this book useful and enjoyable to read.

Inder Verma, PhD, The Salk Research Institute for Biological Sciences, La Jolla, CA.

Preface

"Auch Gedanken fallen manchmal unreif vom Baum"
"Thoughts can also sometimes be unripe when falling from the tree"

Ludwig Wittgenstein

It is difficult to know whether the apple that fell onto Newton's head was ripe or not; the fact is that it kindled Sir Isaac into action. Whether ideas are truly ripe or not at the time of their fall from the tree is only determined a posteriori. Thus, one of the important aspects that gene therapy has launched is new therapeutic approaches to the treatment of disease.

As illustrated in Figure 1, from humble beginnings in the early 1980s, gene therapy has progressed to establish professional societies throughout the world, specialty journals, international conferences, clinical trials, and the recent first commercialization of gene therapy in China in 2005 (1). As originally promised, cures of heretofore incurable diseases have come to pass: bubble boys have been able to leave their sterile bubbles and receive without fears the germ laden embraces of their parents (2). However, eating from the tree of knowledge has its price, and gene therapy, in spite of its successes, has fallen short of the magic bullet approach expected.

The side effects of this new therapeutic approach, which is part of the larger field of pharmacology, have thrown the news reporters into disarray. Society has found it difficult to balance the reports of new cures for so far untreatable diseases with the fact that the new therapies also can have side effects. We all would like to eat from the tree of knowledge without being banned from paradise. As the Bible has taught for generations, this is impossible in faith, as it is in science. The compromise must be to eat of the tree of knowledge (i.e., developing new therapeutic approaches), knowing, predicting, and being prepared for the fact that side effects will be part of the price to pay for the therapeutic advances.

Scientists, clinicians, clinical investigators, and other professionals have responded, as suggested by Orkin and Motulsky in 1996 (3), by returning to the lab benches to continue developing and expanding the rather simple, powerful, even once revolutionary idea of clinical gene therapy. This book provides the reader with an overview of some of the latest achievements in this field, results from the Orkin and Motulsky "return to the bench" injunction!

From the recognition of some of the most challenging limitations of gene therapy, i.e., the immune responses against viral vectors and transgenes, to novel developments, and

The evolution of gene therapy: the bench to bedside years (1983-2005)

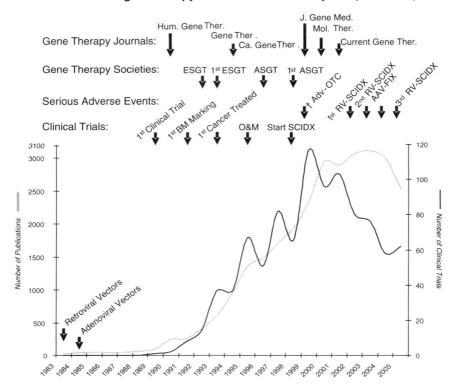

Figure 1   This figure illustrates the yearly number of publications that mention "gene therapy" from the PubMed database, compared with the number of clinical gene therapy trials, taken from the Journal of Gene Medicine database and the clinical trials reports of the ORDA of the NIH. Above the figure, we have indicated the start of the first and significant clinical trials, the most serious adverse effects detected in those trials. In addition, we have shown the appearance of International Gene Therapy Societies, and the most important journals in the field. The first clinical trials in gene therapy were those performed by Malcolm Brenner and collaborators in Memphis on bone marrow marking, and the treatment of ADA-deficiency. O&M indicates the publication of the Orkin and Motulsky report (3) on the status of gene therapy that recommended a return to the basic science of gene therapy; and SCIDX is the trial done by Alain Fischer and collaborators in Paris, accepted as the first ever conclusive "cure" achieved by gene therapy (9). †Adv-OTC indicates the death of J. Gelsinger during the clinical trial for ornithine transcarbamylase deficiency at the University of Pennsylvania (10). 1st, 2nd, and 3rd RVSCIDX indicate the time that leukemia was diagnosed in each of the affected patients treated for SCID-X in Paris (11–14). AAV-FIX indicates the description of the loss of transgene expression and transient hepatitis in one patient treated with AAV-FIX for hemophilia in the trial led by Kay and High in Stanford and Philadelphia (4). *Abbreviations:* ORDA, office of recombinant ONA activities; NIH, national institutes of health; SCIDX, X-linked severe combined immuodeficiency.

clinical applications, the editors have worked hard to provide a picture as comprehensive as possible on the current developments of gene therapies for brain diseases. The book chapters review the latest developments in the construction and production of vectors to contain large transgenic constructs, such as the novel HSV-1 derived amplicons and iBAC vectors (Chapter 2, by Epstein, Chapter 5, by Lawler et al.) and high-capacity, helper-dependent adenoviral vectors (discussed in Chapter 1, by Zirger et al. and Chapter 13, by Castro et al.), or the replication-competent viral vectors, as well as the uses of vectors to treat brain tumors, chronic neurodegenerations such as Parkinson's (Chapter 9, by Torres et al.) and Alzheimer's disease, and the challenge of chronic pain, a particularly felicitous application of herpes simplex virus1 (HSV-1) derived vectors (Chapter 10, by Mata et al.). Also, the use of vaccination strategies to treat brain tumors (Chapter 14, by Wheeler and Black), and potentially Alzheimer's disease is described (Chapter 11, by Bowers and Federoff), and how this can be implemented using viral vectors, is presented in various chapters.

Since commissioning the initial chapters for this book, stem cells broke the sound barrier in the field of the neurosciences and, as basic knowledge, moved forward—so did the potential of their clinical applications. Even if stem cells have the great potential for replacing populations of highly differentiated cells, such as brain cells, the challenge remains to guide their differentiation. And the easiest manner of doing so is indeed the use of viral vectors to express specific factors to guide the differentiation of stem cells in predetermined directions. This is discussed in detail in many chapters throughout the book, but is central to Chapter 6 by Cortes and Breakefield.

The immune response has two sides. On the one hand it presents us with the most challenging topic in the field, having been most likely the cause of the failure of a number of clinical trials (Chapter 1, by Zirger et al.), while the therapeutic use of the immune system to actually treat disease, whether to eradicate brain tumors (Chapters 13, 14) or treat neurodegeneration (Chapter 11). Although most discussions on the immune system and gene therapy have compared challenges and positive effects, a more recent discussion involves the potential of utilizing immunosuppression to thwart early immune responses to allow viral vectors such as adeno-associated viral vectors (AAV), novel high-capacity adenoviruses, or heres simplex virus1 (HSV-1)-derived amplicons to deliver their therapeutic genomes to target cells without being attacked by the immune system (4). Finally, the potential of utilizing gene therapy to treat autoimmune brain diseases, a future challenge for neurological gene therapy, is discussed in Chapter 12, by Larocque et al.

Other developments, such as non-viral vectors that may take advantage of applications for which only short-term gene therapy may be the therapeutic target are discussed in Chapter 8, by Medina-Kauwe, and the potential targeting of astrocytes to treat brain diseases, is given in depth treatment in Chapter 7 by Imura and Sofroniew.

In the long run, gene therapy for brain diseases will be judged by its clinical results, and it is thus that the book ends with the clinical experience of Pulkkanen and Yla-Herttuala in Chapter 16. This group has performed some of the best designed clinical trials in gene therapy, including relevant comparative controls to judge the efficacy of their new therapies. Other clinical trials for neurodegenerative diseases such as Parkinson's disease (Chapter 7) or Alzheimer's disease (Chapter 8) have been tested or will be tested in Phase I clinical trials, but the recent nature of these studies, and their current plans for expansion to larger, controlled trials, is eagerly expected. It is also expected that recent developments of siRNA techniques to develop experimental gene therapies for dominantly inherited diseases, or the use of gene transfer into neonatal brains for the treatment of recessive lysosomal disorders such as Batten's disease and others, will be soon entering advanced clinical trials. The fact that this book is not able to cover all possible areas of neurological gene therapy is a recognition of how much the field has grown during the last ten years, as to truly stun anyone who has not followed the field closely during these years.

We expect this book to provide a current illustration of the reviewed fields, and the expectation to leave the reader asking for more, in the hope that future books will have to be dedicated solely to clinical trials in gene therapy for the treatment of neurological disorders.

For those of us in the field, we expect to enroll you readers in the excitement and privilege of further developing the possibility of establishing true molecular medicine as an essential addition to the modern armamentarium of the clinician and surgeon in the 21st century.

"Welche seltsame Stellungsnahme der Wissenschafter: 'Das wissen wir noch nicht; aber es läßt sich wissen, und es ist nur eine Frage der Zeit, so wird man es wissen!' Als ob es sich von selbst verstünde."

"What a strange position that of the scientist: 'We still don't know this; but it is knowable, and it is only a question of time, until we will know it!' As if this would be obvious."

Ludwig Wittgenstein

Pedro R. Lowenstein
Maria G. Castro

REFERENCES

1. Wilson JM, Gendicine: the first commercial gene therapy product. Hum Gene Ther 2005; 16:1014–1015.
2. Fox JL, Orkin-Motulsky panel calls for gene therapy basic research. Gene Ther 1996; 3 p. pre-1.
3. Fischer A, Le Deist F, Hacein-Bey-Abina S, et al. Severe combined immuno-deficiency. A model disease for molecular immunology and therapy. Immunol Rev 2005; 203:98–109.
4. Cavazzana-Calvo M, Hacein-Bey S, de Saint Basile G, et al. Gene therapy of human severe combined immunodeficiency (SCID)-X1 disease. Science 2000; 288:669–672.
5. Raper SE, Chirmule N, Lee FS, et al. Fatal systemic inflammatory response syndrome in a ornithine transcarbamylase deficient patient following adenoviral gene transfer. Mol Genet Metab 2003; 80:148–158.
6. Lowenstein PR. The case for immunosuppression in clinical gene transfer. Mol Ther 2005; 12:185–186.
7. Chiocca, EA, Abbed KM, Tatter S, et al. A phase I open-label, dose-escalation, multi-institutional trial of injection with an E1B-Attenuated adenovirus, ONYX-015, into the peritumoral region of recurrent malignant gliomas, in the adjuvant setting. Mol Ther 2004; 10:958–966
8. Immonen A, Vapalahti M, Tyynela K, et al. AdvHSV-tk gene therapy with intra-venous ganciclovri improves survival in human malignant glioma: a randomised, controlled study. Molecular Therapy Available Online 2004.
9. Fischer A, Abina SH, Thrasher A, von Kalle C, Cavazzana-Calvo M. LMO2 and gene therapy for severe combined immunodeficiency. N Engl J Med 2004; 350:2526–2527; author reply 2526–2527

10. Fisher KJ, Jooss K, Alston J, et al. Recombinant adeno-associated virus for muscle directed gene therapy. Nat Med 1997; 3:306–312.

11. Hacein-Bey-Abina S, von Kalle C, Schmidt M, et al. A serious adverse event after successful gene therapy for X-linked severe combined immunodeficiency. N Engl J Med 2003; 348:255–256

12. Hacein-Bey-Abina S, Von Kalle C, Schmidt M, et al. LMO2-associated clonal T cell proliferation in two patients after gene therapy for SCID-X1. Science 2003; 302:415–419.

13. During MJ, Kaplitt MG, Stern MB, Eidelberg D. Subthalamic GAD gene transfer in Parkinson disease patients who are candidates for deep brain stimulation. Hum Gene Ther 2001; 12:1589–1591

14. Tuszynski MH, Thal L, Pay M, et al. A phase 1 clinical trial of nerve growth factor gene therapy for Alzheimer disease. Nat Med 2005; 11:551–555.

Acknowledgments

We gratefully acknowledge the dedicated, painstaking efforts of our Assistant Editor, Mr. Kurt Kroeger, for the editing, assembly and production of this book.

Work from our Institute described in this book was funded by the National Institute of Neurological Disorders & Stroke (NINDS), grant # 1RO1 NS44556.01, by NIDDK, grant # 1 RO3 25 TW006273-01 to M.G.C., by NINDS grants # 1 RO1 NS42893; U54 4 NS04-5309 and R21 NS47298 to P.R.L.; The Linda Tallen & David Paul Kane Annual Fellowship in Cancer Research; and The Board of Governors at Cedars-Sinai Medical Center. We wish to thank Dr. Shlomo Melmed for his academic leadership and Mr. Richard Katzman and Dr. David Meyer for their support.

We also thank Carlos Barcia-Gonzalez for the skillful production of the cover image.

Contents

Contributors

Carlos Barcia-Gonzalez   Gene Therapeutics Research Institute, Cedars-Sinai Medical Center, and Departments of Medicine, and Medical and Molecular Pharmacology, David Geffen School of Medicine, University of California Los Angeles, Los Angeles, California, U.S.A.

Josée Bergeron   Gene Therapeutics Research Institute, Cedars-Sinai Medical Center, and Departments of Medicine, and Medical and Molecular Pharmacology, David Geffen School of Medicine, University of California Los Angeles, Los Angeles, California, U.S.A.

Keith L. Black   Maxine Dunite Neurosurgical Institute, Cedars-Sinai Medical Center, Los Angeles, California, U.S.A.

William J. Bowers   Department of Neurology, Center for Aging and Developmental Biology, University of Rochester School of Medicine and Dentistry, Rochester, New York, U.S.A.

Xandra O. Breakefield   Departments of Neurology and Radiology, Massachusetts General Hospital, Charlestown and Program in Neuroscience, Harvard Medical School, Boston, Massachusetts, U.S.A.

Marianela Candolfi   Gene Therapeutics Research Institute, Cedars-Sinai Medical Center, and Departments of Medicine, and Medical and Molecular Pharmacology, David Geffen School of Medicine, University of California Los Angeles, Los Angeles, California, U.S.A.

Maria G. Castro   Gene Therapeutics Research Institute, Cedars-Sinai Medical Center, and Departments of Medicine, and Medical and Molecular Pharmacology, David Geffen School of Medicine, University of California Los Angeles, Los Angeles, California, U.S.A.

E. Antonio Chiocca   The Dardinger Laboratory for Neuro-oncology and Neurosciences, Department of Neurological Surgery, The Ohio State University Medical Center, Columbus, Ohio, U.S.A.

Maria L. Cortes   Departments of Neurology and Radiology, Massachusetts General Hospital, Charlestown and Program in Neuroscience, Harvard Medical School, Boston, Massachusetts, U.S.A.

David T. Curiel   Med-Division of Human Gene Therapy, University of Alabama at Birmingham, Birmingham, Alabama, U.S.A.

James F. Curtin   Gene Therapeutics Research Institute, Cedars-Sinai Medical Center, and Departments of Medicine, and Medical and Molecular Pharmacology, David Geffen School of Medicine, University of California Los Angeles, Los Angeles, California, U.S.A.

Peter Czer   Gene Therapeutics Research Institute, Cedars-Sinai Medical Center, and Departments of Medicine, and Medical and Molecular Pharmacology, David Geffen School of Medicine, University of California Los Angeles, Los Angeles, California, U.S.A.

S. B. Dunnett   The Brain Repair Group, School of Biosciences, Cardiff University, Cardiff, U.K.

Alberto L. Epstein   Centre de Génétique Moléculaire et Cellulaire, CNRS, Université Claude Bernard, Villeurbanne, France

Tamer Fakhouri   Gene Therapeutics Research Institute, Cedars-Sinai Medical Center, and Departments of Medicine, and Medical and Molecular Pharmacology, David Geffen School of Medicine, University of California Los Angeles, Los Angeles, California, U.S.A.

Howard J. Federoff   Departments of Neurology, Microbiology and Immunology, Center for Aging and Developmental Biology, University of Rochester School of Medicine and Dentistry, Rochester, New York, U.S.A.

David J. Fink   Department of Neurology, University of Michigan and Neurology Service, Ann Arbor VA Healthcare System, Ann Arbor, Michigan, U.S.A.

Juan Fueyo   Department of Neuro-Oncology, University of Texas M. D. Anderson Cancer Center, Houston, Texas, U.S.A.

Fred H. Gage   The Salk Institute for Biological Studies, La Jolla, California, U.S.A.

Joseph C. Glorioso   Department of Molecular Genetics and Biochemistry, University of Pittsburgh, Pittsburgh, Pennsylvania, U.S.A.

Candelaria Gomez-Manzano   Department of Neuro-Oncology, University of Texas M. D. Anderson Cancer Center, Houston, Texas, U.S.A.

Sarah Honig   Gene Therapeutics Research Institute, Cedars-Sinai Medical Center, and Departments of Medicine, and Medical and Molecular Pharmacology, David Geffen School of Medicine, University of California Los Angeles, Los Angeles, California, U.S.A.

Joanna Howarth   Henry Wellcome Laboratories for Integrative Neuroscience and Endocrinology, University of Bristol, Bristol, U.K.

Tetsuya Imura   Department of Neurobiology and Brain Research Institute, UCLA School of Medicine, University of California, Los Angeles, California, U.S.A.

and Department of Pathology and Applied Neurobiology, Graduate School of Medical Science, Kyoto Prefectural University of Medicine, Kawaramachi-Hirokoji, Kamigyo-ku, Kyoto, Japan

Hong Jiang   Department of Neuro-Oncology, University of Texas M. D. Anderson Cancer Center, Houston, Texas, U.S.A.

Stephen Johnson   Gene Therapeutics Research Institute, Cedars-Sinai Medical Center, and Departments of Medicine, and Medical and Molecular Pharmacology, David Geffen School of Medicine, University of California Los Angeles, Los Angeles, California, U.S.A.

Terry Kang   Gene Therapeutics Research Institute, Cedars-Sinai Medical Center, and Departments of Medicine, and Medical and Molecular Pharmacology, David Geffen School of Medicine, University of California Los Angeles, Los Angeles, California, U.S.A.

Brian K. Kaspar   Department of Gene Therapy and Neuromuscular Research, Columbus Children's Research Institute and Department of Pediatrics, The Ohio State University, Columbus, Ohio, U.S.A.

Stephen Kelly   Henry Wellcome Laboratories for Integrative Neuroscience and Endocrinology, University of Bristol, Bristol, U.K.

Gwendalyn D. King   Gene Therapeutics Research Institute, Cedars-Sinai Medical Center, and Departments of Medicine, and Medical and Molecular Pharmacology, David Geffen School of Medicine, University of California Los Angeles, Los Angeles, California, U.S.A.

Kurt Kroeger   Gene Therapeutics Research Institute, Cedars-Sinai Medical Center, and Departments of Medicine, and Medical and Molecular Pharmacology, David Geffen School of Medicine, University of California Los Angeles, Los Angeles, California, U.S.A.

William Kuoy   Gene Therapeutics Research Institute, Cedars-Sinai Medical Center, and Departments of Medicine, and Medical and Molecular Pharmacology, David Geffen School of Medicine, University of California Los Angeles, Los Angeles, California, U.S.A.

Frederick F. Lang   Department of Neurosurgery, University of Texas M. D. Anderson Cancer Center, Houston, Texas, U.S.A.

Daniel Larocque   Gene Therapeutics Research Institute, Cedars-Sinai Medical Center, and Departments of Medicine, and Medical and Molecular Pharmacology, David Geffen School of Medicine, University of California Los Angeles, Los Angeles, California, U.S.A.

Sean E. Lawler   The Dardinger Laboratory for Neuro-oncology and Neurosciences, Department of Neurological Surgery, The Ohio State University Medical Center, Columbus, Ohio, U.S.A.

Chunyan Liu   Gene Therapeutics Research Institute, Cedars-Sinai Medical Center, and Departments of Medicine, and Medical and Molecular Pharmacology,

David Geffen School of Medicine, University of California Los Angeles, Los Angeles, California, U.S.A.

Pedro R. Lowenstein   Gene Therapeutics Research Institute, Cedars-Sinai Medical Center, and Departments of Medicine, and Medical and Molecular Pharmacology, David Geffen School of Medicine, University of California Los Angeles, Los Angeles, California, U.S.A.

Marina Mata   Department of Neurology, University of Michigan and Neurology Service, Ann Arbor VA Healthcare System, Ann Arbor, Michigan, U.S.A.

Frank McCormick   Cancer Center/Cancer Research Institute, University of California at San Francisco, San Francisco, California, U.S.A.

Lali K. Medina-Kauwe   Gene Therapeutics Research Institute, Cedars-Sinai Medical Center, Los Angeles, California, U.S.A.

C. Monville   The Brain Repair Group, School of Biosciences, Cardiff University, Cardiff, U.K.

A. K. M. Ghulam Muhammad   Gene Therapeutics Research Institute, Cedars-Sinai Medical Center, and Departments of Medicine, and Medical and Molecular Pharmacology, David Geffen School of Medicine, University of California Los Angeles, Los Angeles, California, U.S.A.

Kalevi J. Pulkkanen   Department of Molecular Medicine, A. I. Virtanen Institute, University of Kuopio and Department of Oncology, Kuopio University Hospital, Kuopio, Finland

Mariana Puntel   Gene Therapeutics Research Institute, Cedars-Sinai Medical Center, and Departments of Medicine, and Medical and Molecular Pharmacology, David Geffen School of Medicine, University of California Los Angeles, Los Angeles, California, U.S.A.

Yoshinaga Saeki   The Dardinger Laboratory for Neuro-oncology and Neurosciences, Department of Neurological Surgery, The Ohio State University Medical Center, Columbus, Ohio, U.S.A.

Sandra A. Sciascia   Gene Therapeutics Research Institute, Cedars-Sinai Medical Center, and Departments of Medicine, and Medical and Molecular Pharmacology, David Geffen School of Medicine, University of California Los Angeles, Los Angeles, California, U.S.A.

Michael V. Sofroniew   Department of Neurobiology and Brain Research Institute, UCLA School of Medicine, University of California Los Angeles, Los Angeles, California, U.S.A.

E. M. Torres   The Brain Repair Group, School of Biosciences, Cardiff University, Cardiff, U.K.

James B. Uney   Henry Wellcome Laboratories for Integrative Neuroscience and Endocrinology, University of Bristol, Bristol, U.K.

Richard Wade-Martins   The Wellcome Trust Centre for Human Genetics, University of Oxford, Oxford, U.K.

Christopher J. Wheeler   Maxine Dunite Neurosurgical Institute, Cedars-Sinai Medical Center, Los Angeles, California, U.S.A.

Weidong Xiong   Gene Therapeutics Research Institute, Cedars-Sinai Medical Center, and Departments of Medicine, and Medical and Molecular Pharmacology, David Geffen School of Medicine, University of California Los Angeles, Los Angeles, California, U.S.A.

Seppo Yla-Herttuala   Department of Molecular Medicine, A. I. Virtanen Institute, University of Kuopio and Department of Medicine and Gene Therapy Unit, Kuopio University Hospital, Kuopio, Finland

W. K. Alfred Yung   Department of Neuro-Oncology, University of Texas M. D. Anderson Cancer Center, Houston, Texas, U.S.A.

Jeffrey Zirger   Gene Therapeutics Research Institute, Cedars-Sinai Medical Center, and Departments of Medicine, and Medical and Molecular Pharmacology, David Geffen School of Medicine, University of California Los Angeles, Los Angeles, California, U.S.A.

1

Immune Responses to Viral Vectors: Implications for Neurological Gene Therapy

Jeffrey Zirger, Carlos Barcia-Gonzalez, Mariana Puntel, Kurt Kroeger, Weidong Xiong, Terry Kang, Tamer Fakhouri, A. K. M. Ghulam Muhammad, Chunyan Liu, Josée Bergeron, Stephen Johnson, Maria G. Castro, and Pedro R. Lowenstein
Gene Therapeutics Research Institute, Cedars-Sinai Medical Center, and Departments of Medicine, and Medical and Molecular Pharmacology, David Geffen School of Medicine, University of California Los Angeles, Los Angeles, California, U.S.A.

INTRODUCTION

Gene therapy presents a new approach to alter the consequences of defective gene expression and to utilize nucleic acids as therapeutic tools. Over the course of the last decade there have been many new techniques developed for the transfer of therapeutic genes into cells, derived from the modified viruses, or artificial non-viral liposome-based approaches. Non-viral methods have advanced much in the last few years; however, its efficiency remains below that achieved by virus-derived methods. Viral-derived gene transfer vectors have become reliable tools for gene transfer.

Many of the vectors used as vehicles in gene therapy, including the retrovirus, lentivirus, adeno-associated virus, and herpes simplex virus are derived from pathogenic viruses from humans as well as other species (1). Each vector system has its particular target tissue. For transduction of continually dividing bone marrow cells, a retroviral or lentiviral vector ought to be used, while for the transduction of terminally differentiated muscle or brain cells, adenoviral and AAV-derived vectors are ideal. Lentivirus-derived vectors can transduce both dividing and non-dividing cells, thus making this system a choice for the transduction of most organ systems. However, the derivation of these vectors from pathogenic viruses such as HIV raises concerns on its acceptance by human patients.

Thus, in the absence of one single ideal vector, each vector system has its particular target niche. The parent virus, the size of transgenic constructs that can be inserted into different vectors, their intrinsic ease or difficulty of production, their capacity to infect, express in dividing or non-dividing target cells, all contribute to the choice of vector.

Adenoviral vectors have been shown to provide reliable, efficient, and high level of expression, following gene transfer into different tissues and organs. Adenoviruses do not cause major lethal diseases, but are effectively neutralized by the humoral and cellular host immune system. This review will focus on the immune response to adenoviral vectors used in the context of gene therapy for the treatment of brain diseases. Immune responses elicited against the other viral vectors used in gene therapy applications will be discussed elsewhere in this volume.

IMMUNE RESPONSES TO RECOMBINANT ADENOVIRAL VECTORS

Adenoviral Vectors

The main advantages of adenoviral vectors are their ability to transduce both dividing and non-dividing cells, their strong expression from an episomal locus without need to integrate the vector genome into host DNA, their ability to produce high titers of vectors, the production of high levels of transgene expression in a large variety of cells, and their capacity to encode up to 30 kbp of transgenic sequence in the newer generation of high-capacity adenoviral vectors. Adenoviruses are non-enveloped viruses that contain a 36 kb double-stranded DNA genome. Although roughly 50 different serotypes of adenovirus have been identified, serotypes 2 and 5 have been most extensively studied for use in gene therapy applications. The wild type adenoviral genome contains short, inverted terminal repeats (ITR) at both the $5'$ and $3'$ ends that are required for viral DNA replication; the exact sequences from the wild type adenovirus genome depend on the type of vector employed.

Replication-defective adenoviral vectors can be divided into several groups. Briefly, first generation vectors are deleted in the E1 region rendering them unable to replicate in host cells in the absence of E1a. These vectors can also have deletions in the E3 region to increase cloning capacity. Second and third generation adenovirus vectors contain additional deletions in the E2 or E4 regions to increase safety, reduce toxicity, and expand cloning capacity (2). The latest generation of high-capacity, helper-dependent (HC-Ad) or "gutless" adenoviral vectors have been deleted of the entire viral coding region, only retaining the inverted ITRs (necessary for replication) and the packaging signal (3). These new helper-dependent adenovirus vectors have been shown to increase the efficiency of transduction, reduce the immunogenicity and vector toxicity, and extend the length of transgene expression in various target tissues, such as the liver and brain.

Vectors can be administered systemically or directly into tissues or tumors. If injected into the bloodstream they will encounter cells and antibodies of the immune system and trigger the earliest inflammatory responses. Direct injections into tissues or tumors may avoid the initial interaction with circulating antibodies and monocytes. Entry of gene therapy vectors into target cells is the first step in viral infection towards transduction. It can also represent the initial triggering of cellular host inflammatory and immune responses, depending on the cell type infected.

Adenovirus binding to the cell surface and cell entry has been examined in detail (4). The adenovirus initially attaches to the cell via interaction between the fiber knob protein of the adenovirus and the coxsackievirus-adenovirus receptor (CAR) (5). Internalization is then mediated by an interaction between an arginine-glycine-aspartic acid (RGD) motif on penton base capsid proteins of the adenovirus and α_v integrins on cells, followed by entry of the virus into the cell by endocytosis that utilizes clathrin-coated vesicles (6,7). There are also less well understood interactions between fiber protein and heparin sulphate proteoglycans present on cellular membranes. The interaction of the adenovirus with the cell membrane has also been found to activate various cell signaling pathways; activation of pathways is cell-type dependent. Examples include the phophoinositide-3-OH kinase

(PI-3K) and Raf/mitogen-activated protein kinase (MAPK) pathways (4). Following binding, vectors are internalized into endosomes from which adenoviral vectors escape to the cytoplasm through a pH-dependent change in adenoviral penton base and an interaction with the $\alpha_v\beta_5$ integrins (8–10). Adenovirus particles then travel to the nucleus via microtubules where the viral genome crosses the nuclear pore and enters the nucleus (10). Transcription under control of the adenoviral early (E1–E5) and late (L1–L3) genes of the viral genome is then initiated.

Classical adenovirology studies determined that in the absence of E1a, the genome would not replicate. In those experiments, low multiplicity infections had naturally been used. To achieve high-level gene expression with gene therapy vectors, however, higher vector loads are used, between 100–1000 vector particles per cell, a value that can increase further in vivo. In these circumstances, expression is detected from the remaining transcriptional cassettes present in all vector systems, apart from the HC-Adv. Thus, although not predicted by classical experiments, the use of high MOI infection causes adenoviral expression of proteins that can be toxic, inflammatory, or provide antigenic epitopes to the immune system.

Innate Immune Response

One of the many challenges that face the successful use of adenoviral vectors in gene therapy is the inflammation and immune responses that are generated following vector administration. As stated, viral infection with wild type virus is a complex process that requires virus entry and the subsequent replication of genetic material, production of viral gene products, and the assembly and release of new viral particles. The function of the host immune system is thus tuned to detect and eliminate infectious pathogens. For gene therapy applications the inflammatory and immune response will vary depending on the virus dose, site of administration, type of vector used, and transgene being delivered.

The innate immune response is the earliest line of defense generated by the host. Although the pathways to trigger innate immune responses are pathogen dependent, once it has been triggered it results in a standard set of consequences designed in general to prevent the entry of micro-organisms into tissues or, once they have gained entry, eliminate them prior to the occurrence of disease. Following injection of recombinant adenoviral vectors carrying therapeutic transgenes, the innate immune response is seen to be activated very rapidly (i.e., within minutes to hours). Thus the innate immune response represents the first line of defense against viral infection.

One of the initial aspects in the recognition of foreign infectious agents is performed by antigen presenting cells (APCs). Examples of APCs include the dendritic cells (DCs) and macrophages that are located in many different tissues throughout the body. These cells demonstrate a high level of phagocytic activity that allows for the capture of foreign antigens for further processing (11). Although this recognition is non-specific, the ability of the APC to recognize foreign antigen is the first in a sequence of events that leads to the eventual activation of effector T and B cells (12). Importantly, DCs are the main cells responsible for carrying antigenic epitopes from the infecting organisms to the lymph nodes where these antigens will be presented to naïve T lymphocytes to prime the adaptive immune response. Thus, DCs are the link that coordinate the translation of non-specific innate inflammatory responses to the adaptive antigen specific immune responses, based on recombination and selection of specific effector T cells.

Other important components of the innate immune system include granulocytes, neutrophils, natural killer (NK) cells, and natural killer T (NKT) cells, in addition to the macrophages and DCs. All these cell types are rapidly recruited to the site of viral infection, and participate in antiviral responses directly, by killing infected cells and producing antiviral cytokines, as well as indirectly, by the production of chemokines that act to recruit other immune cells into infected tissues. Later, these cytokines and chemokines can also be involved in the activation of the adaptive immune response (13). Interaction of viral vectors with receptors on cell surfaces leads to the stimulation of intracellular signaling pathways including activation of NF-kB (14), AT-2/c-Jun (Paludan et al. 2001), interferon regulatory factors (IRFs) (15), and MAP kinases (16). The final end point of these pathways is the production of inflammatory cytokines, such as IFNα/β, IFNγ IL-6 and IL-12 (17–19), as well as the production of a variety of chemokines, including RANTES, IP-10, and the MIP and MCP families of molecules (20–23). The production of antiviral cytokines and chemokines provide many functions as a major defense mechanism for the body against viral infection, and can act to decrease transcription of transgenes contained in vectors used for gene therapy (24,25).

In the case of the adenovirus, it has been shown that several of the innate immune mechanisms mentioned above play a significant role in the very early clearance of the virus. Studies that utilized systemic administration of vectors to organs such as the liver and lungs demonstrated that inflammation resulted in elimination of transgene expression and was mediated by macrophages, activation of NK cells and production of cytokines including TNFα and IFNγ (26–28). Adenovirus-induced activation of NF-kB, also stimulates a key regulator of the innate antiviral immune response (29).

The immune response to the injection of adenoviral vectors into the Central Nervous System (CNS) differs greatly from the response seen following injection into peripheral organ systems. Several factors, including the presence of a blood brain barrier (BBB), a lack of lymphatic capillaries, the absence of DCs from the naïve non-inflamed brain, and a low level constitutive expression of major histocompatibility complex (MHC) expression have caused the brain to be considered a relatively immune-privileged organ. Thus, comparison of immune responses in the brain versus those seen in peripheral organs is difficult, and has generally been misunderstood. Following systemic injection of adenovirus, immune responses result in the complete elimination of both vector and transgene expression in 2–3 wk (30). In the CNS, expression of transgenes can be sustained for much longer periods of time as compared to that seen in peripheral organs, as studies performed by Byrnes, Wood and Charlton (31–36), Zermansky et al. (37) and Thomas et al. (38) have demonstrated that expression of transgene from adenoviral vectors can be detected for up to 6–13 mo in the absence of systemic immunization against adenovirus. However, long-term expression in the CNS depends on the dose of vector injected. Injection of doses above the threshold of 1×10^8 iu causes a massive activation of the innate immune response in the brain that will completely eliminate transgene expression and cause a brain lesion, even in the absence of the priming of the systemic immune response (Fig. 1) (39).

Although the immune-privileged status of the CNS acts to limit the amount of immune cells that are able to gain access to the brain, the brain cells themselves initiate an innate immune response. Injection of first-generation adenovirus vectors and HC-Ads into the brain results in the stimulation of a rapid local inflammatory reaction. This early response is characterized by recruitment of macrophages and non-antigen specific lymphocytes, increased expression of MHC class I antigens and activation of local microglia and astrocytes are all found proximal to the site of infection (31). This response can first be detected at vector doses above 1×10^6 to 1×10^7 iu. The existence of a threshold for adenoviral vector-mediated gene therapy has recently been established at 1×10^8 iu. Injections below this threshold result in cytokine and cellular-mediated inflammation that is acute, transient, and attenuated

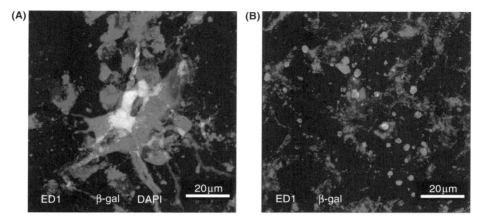

Figure 1 (*See color insert*) Innate immune responses. Injection of 1×10^8 iu of RAd36 into the rat brain. (**A**) Macrophages/microglia immunoreactive for ED1 (*in red*) contact β-gal expressing cells (*green*). (**B**) Presence of β-gal immunoreactivity within macrophages/microglia have phagocytosed dead transduced brain cells.

within 30 days, and which does not clear transgene expression from the brain. Injection of vectors above this 1×10^8 iu threshold results in increased cytotoxicity, irreversible inflammation, elimination of transgene expression, and the loss of neurons and glia (40).

Various experiments have been conducted to determine whether gene expression from the viral vectors is necessary to generate an immune response against adenovirus. To this end, studies were undertaken that utilized adenoviral vectors that could not express genes from their genomes, either due to psoralen/UV inactivation or because capsids were unable to package vector genomes. Even though all these vectors cause the same inflammation when injected into the brain (38), systemic injection of psoralen/UV inactivated vectors did prime a systemic immune response detectable as CTLs (41), while injection of similar vectors in rats did not prime a systemic immune response that could abolish transgene expression from the brain, suggesting that in rats psoralen/UV inactivated vectors in mice did not prime a systemic immune response (39). Thus, whether genome expression is needed to prime systemic anti-adenoviral immune responses remains to be determined. Importantly, however, work by Samulski et al. (42,43) demonstrated by gene expression microarrays that the number of genes whose expression is altered following infection of target cells is substantially reduced when infection proceeds with adenovirus virions devoid of genomes, compared to those containing vector genomes.

Adaptive Immune Response

The second, later, long-term immune response that is generated against an invading pathogen is the adaptive immune response. The kinetics of this response are slower than those of the innate immune system, occurring on the order of days to weeks, rather than hours in the case of the innate immune response. The need to select those T cells that express the correct T-cell receptor (TCR) that matches the antigenic epitopes displayed on DCs and their subsequent clonal expansion explains the delay in detecting the peak of the adaptive immune response. The adaptive immune response is further divided into cell-mediated or humoral responses.

Cell-Mediated Immune Response

Cellular effector T cells provide a specific, long-term, memory response to the antigen, compared to the response acheived by the innate immune system. Activated T lymphocytes recognize foreign antigenic epitopes displayed by MHC molecules on the surface of infected cells. T cells, through specific interactions with their antigens, can either secrete cytokines, such as IFN-γ, or TNFα, or kill target cells through mechanisms that utilize the proteins perforin, and/or Fas-Ligand.

Administration of adenoviral vectors induces adaptive immune responses in hosts that have been shown to occur by 5–7 days after virus administration (44). Administration of adenoviral vectors alone are sufficient to stimulate adaptive responses, because they induce both the innate as well as the adaptive immune responses. Antigens that do not stimulate innate immune responses, rely on other agents to stimulate the innate immune activations, such as CpG islands present on plasmids, LPS, or Freund's adjuvant, amongst various stimulators.

In peripheral organs, such as the liver and lung, it has been determined by deletion studies that both CD8$^+$ and CD4$^+$ T cells, restricted to MHC class I and II, respectively, play an important role in the anti-adenoviral vector response (45,46). One of the predominant effector cells involved in the eventual elimination of virus from the host are the CD8$^+$ cytotoxic T cells (CTLs) (45). Following infection with wild type adenovirus, the immunodominant epitopes recognized by the immune system reside in E1a and E1b proteins. Given that adenoviral vectors do not express these proteins, it was unclear what the immunodominant peptides would be.

It has now been determined that immunodominant peptides present within the viral capsid, e.g., within the fiber protein, contain immunodominant peptides recognized by the immune system following infection with adenoviral vectors. Eventhough the adenoviral vectors cannot replicate within non-human cells, we described before that due to the high MOI used to transduce cells, transcriptional cassettes from the wild type genome would still be expressed. Thus, following infection with an early generation vector these antigens will be present within the viral capsid and produced in transduced cells. Following infection with an HC-Adv vector, the antigenic epitopes will only be present within the vector capsid, and thus, only be available to the immune system while the vector is uncoating. Once uncoating has been finalized, there will be no more antigenic epitopes produced from an HC-Adv genome. Potential immune responses to the transgene, however, could continue to be recognized, even when expressed from an HC-Ad.

Adenovirus-specific CTL recognition does not require de novo gene expression, and the capsid proteins of adenoviral vectors complexed with MHC class I molecules can serve as targets for CTL recognition and induction of antiviral CTL responses (31,41,47). ^{51}Cr release assays have also shown that CTLs can be generated against the therapeutic transgene contained in viral vectors in mice immunized with a lacZ-expressing adenovirus (48). Immune responses against transgenes will of course be more difficult to address; however, in the treatment of diabetes and hemophilia, a percentage of patients are known to develop blocking immune responses, while continuing to respond to higher doses of therapeutic proteins. The interactions between the immune responses, and effective gene therapies during clinical trials, will have to be addressed individually. Methods to induce tolerance both in the treatment of diabetes and hemophilia, as well as for the treatment of organ transplantation have been developed and could be adapted to gene therapy. Even if

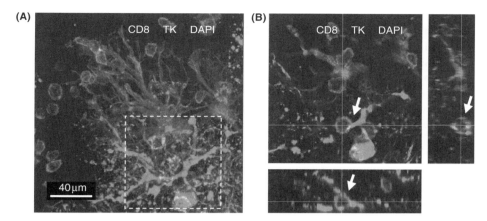

Figure 2 (*See color insert*) Adaptive immune responses. Presence of CD8$^+$T cells within the brain parenchyma of a systemically immunized rat, following the injection into the brain of RAd-TK. (**A**) Triple labelling with CD8 (*red*), Thymidine kinase positive cells (*green*) and nuclei (DAPI *blue*). Note the presence of CD8 positive cells in the striatum of a rat injected intracranially with RAdTK and immunized intradermally with RAdHPRT, and sacrificed 14 days after the immunization. (**A**) CD8 cells usually were close to TK positive brain cells. (**B**) We could detect frequent contacts between CD8 cells and TK positive cells (*arrows*). The analysis of the contacts can be observed in 0.5 μm thick optical layers examined by confocal microscopy, illustrated by the views from the x and y axes as shown in **B**. *Abbreviation*: TK, thymidine kinase.

gene therapy has been somewhat reluctant in utilizing short term, transient immune-suppression regimes at the start of the therapies, their potential in making clinical trials safer is starting to be appreciated.

Studies in a variety of immunodeficient mice have demonstrated the central role of the adaptive immune response in eliminating transgene expression (44–46,49–53). Yang et al. (44) first postulated direct killing of transduced hepatocytes by CTLs, potentially through apoptotic mechanisms. However, direct in situ demonstration of the killing of target cells by CD8$^+$ in vivo has been elusive. Thus, recent work on the clearing of hepatitis B virus from the liver in a transgenic model by Guidotti and Chisari (13), has provided strong evidence that CD8$^+$ CTLs, through the secretion of IFN γ, inhibit viral genome replication with only limited toxicity to liver cells. Therefore, the precise cellular and immune mechanism for inhibition of transgene expression in the brain remains to be determined (Fig. 2).

Despite low basal MHC class I and II expression in the brain, inflammation increases their expression—a necessary step to allow immune cell infiltration of the brain. Studies in the brain by Byrnes et al. (33) have shown that the early innate inflammation can be reduced following depletion of CD4$^+$ and CD8$^+$ T cells, and that brain lymphocytes following injection of adenoviral vectors in the brain are mainly CD8$^+$ T cells in sensitized animals, whereas in unprimed animals CD4$^+$ T cells dominate (54). In contrast to what is seen in other organs, however, transgene expression levels in the brain remain largely unaltered in the presence of these presumably antigen non specific T lymphocytes that enter the brain during the early innate inflammatory responses (35). This suggests that the mechanism underlying persistent transgene expression is due to an ineffective T-cell mediated response in the brain, which results in a response that is unable to clear vector or transgene product from the naïve brain (32,36,55,56). This is thought to be due to the lack of a functional DC system present in the naïve brain (56), although once brain inflammation occurs, various populations of DCs have been shown to be present within the brain parenchyma (56–69).

Because it is believed that a large portion of the human population has at some point in time been exposed to adenovirus, it is important to determine whether adenoviral vectors used as gene transfer systems are able to produce stable and long-term expression of transgene in the presence of a systemic immune challenge. Upon injection of first generation adenoviral vector into brain parenchyma only, a local inflammatory response is elicited. This localized inflammation is a non-specific response characterized by influx of T cells, macrophages, and other cells of the innate immune system and is only found to be present for one month after vector administration. Furthermore, this inflammatory response does not result in elimination of transgene expression (31,32,36). As previously discussed, the inability to mount a response that eliminates transgene expression may be the result of the failure of the brain to produce an effective antigen-specific T-cell response against the injected adenoviral vector (31,32,36).

Activation of antiviral T cells by previous exposure or peripheral immunization with adenovirus results in the infiltration of T lymphocytes into the brain parenchyma, activation of other immune effectors such as macrophages and microglia, and finally the elimination of adenoviral-mediated transgene expression (32,70). Further, recent experiments from our laboratory [Zirger et al. submitted, 2005] have demonstrated that the systemic immune response is dependent on both sets of $CD4^+$ and $CD8^+$ T cells, IFNγ and perforin, and leads to the phagocytosis and cell death of at least a significant number of transduced cells. Even though our data strongly suggest the existence of cell death during the adaptive immune response mediated elimination of transgene expression from the brain, the exact percentage of elimination that proceeds by cell death versus that resulting from functional inhibition of transgene expression from the vectors, remains to be fully explored (Fig. 3). These experiments highlight one of the major limitations for the use of first generation E1 deleted vectors for gene therapy (Fig. 2), and one of the major limitations for the use of viral vectors since immune responses against virions and transgenes have been detected when utilizing AAV and lentiviral vectors (71,72).

As stated earlier, the development of second- and third-generation vectors as well as HC-Ads or "gutless" adenoviral vectors, which have the entire viral genome deleted, has generated newer gene transfer systems that are less immunogenic, but more importantly do not express those proteins that provide the antigenic epitopes targeted by the immune system. Recent studies have shown that unlike the effect that is seen with first-generation vectors, the HC-Ad vectors are able to achieve long-term expression of transgene in the brain following the induction of a systemic anti-adenoviral immune response (38). These results have shown for the first time that stable transduction and gene expression from adenoviral vectors is possible in the brain even after peripheral immune challenge results in the generation of a systemic anti-adenoviral immune response.

The potential immunogenicity of therapeutic transgenes encoded by adenoviral vectors used for gene therapy is another area that requires intensive study in order for gene therapy to become a realization. Although most of the work on the immune response to adenoviral vectors is focused on the viral capsid or the viral proteins that are produced, studies have shown that the transgene encoded by viral vectors may play a role in mediation by the immune system. It has been previously shown that following adenoviral vector-mediated delivery of the same therapeutic transgene from different species into mouse muscle, immune responses are directed against only the foreign (human) transgene-encoded proteins but not the murine (self) protein, and that long-term expression can be attained following a single injection of the vector containing the gene for the self protein (73). It has

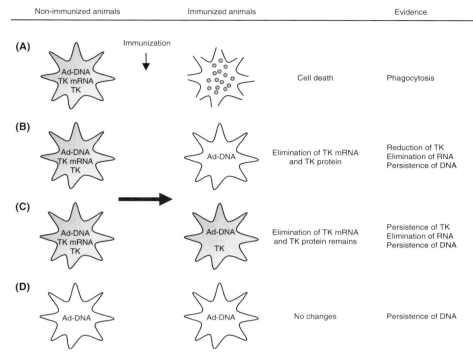

Figure 3 (*See color insert*) Hypothetical model to explain the loss of transgene expression from the CNS following the systemic immunization against adenovirus. We hypothesize that there are 4 possible mechanisms that lead to the loss of transgene expression. (**A**) The immune system induces cell death of a population of transduced cells. (**B**) The immune system selectively reduces or eliminates the expression of TK mRNA, leading to loss of TK protein, without inducing cell death. (**C**) The immune system reduces or eliminates the TK mRNA but TK protein remains. (**D**) Some cells are infected but the transgene is not expressed. The immunization does not induce any change in these cells, but the presence of Ad genome contributes to any molecular quantification of the presence of Ad genomes in the brain. Which are the most important mechanisms that account for the elimination of transgene from the brain remain to be elucidated. *Abbreviations*: CNS, central nervous system; TK, thymidine kinase.

also been determined that although it is the CTL response directed against viral antigens that are responsible for transgene elimination, CTL responses can also be generated against the β-galactosidase transgene. In preparation for clinical trials, the immunogenicity of both the vector and the transgene will need to be considered. This may not impose limitations on clinical trials needing short-term transgene expression; however, in those where long-term expression is needed, immune responses against the transgene could be decisive. In this case, application of various immune-suppressive, or even tolerazing regimes, as have been developed for the treatment of patients suffering from diabetes or hemophilia and who developed immune responses against the therapeutic protein will need to be considered.

Humoral Immune Response

Although it is cellular immunity, including the recruitment of macrophages and T lymphocytes into the brain, that is believed to be the chief mechanism resulting in the removal of virus-infected cells and elimination of transgene expression from adenoviral vectors, recent evidence has also shown that the humoral arm of the adaptive immune response may also play a role. Upon injection of first-generation E1-deleted adenovirus vectors into the brain, it has been shown that circulating antibodies against both the adenovirus vector and transgene product can be detected in serum. These studies detected anti-adenovirus antibodies in the serum by 2 days after injection with a peak at day 30 as well as the presence of CD4$^+$ T cells and B cells in the brain (34). The kinetics of the humoral response also differs greatly from those seen in the cellular immune response.

It is of extreme importance in the context of gene therapy to understand whether transgene expression is able to elicit an immune response. Previous studies have detected the presence of antibodies against transgene in serum when adenoviral vectors were injected intravenously (74). Similarly, infusion of lacZ-expressing adenovirus leads to the production of β-galactosidase-specific antibodies (48). Results from Kajiwara et al. (34) have also shown antibody production against transgene when adenovirus vectors were injected the brain. Antibodies to the β-galactosidase transgene were detected at 30 days post-injection. Generation of antibodies to adenovirus injection into the brain occurs much slower than when injected peripherally, where antibodies can be detected between 7 and 15 days.

Re-administration of adenoviral vectors may be a treatment paradigm for some gene therapy applications. Repeat administration of adenoviral vectors as gene transfer systems in the periphery results in the loss of transgene expression due to the presence of neutralizing antibodies. However, the presence of neutralizing antibodies was not detected in serum after injection into the brain (34). Because it is the neutralizing antibodies that act to sequester virus and prevent subsequent adenoviral infection, their absence in these studies provides preliminary evidence that repeated administration of adenoviral vectors as gene transfer vehicles may be possible.

To achieve repeat administration, the vector serotype could be exchanged for the follow up injections or transient immune-suppression during the first week post-infection could be considered. Either method can work experimentally and in patients, and these are currently being optimized.

FUTURE DIRECTIONS

Viral vectors currently represent the best available vehicles for efficient gene transfer. Considerable gains in the field of gene therapy have been made in recent decades, however, the remaining immunogenic properties of these vectors is a major drawback to the use of adenoviral vectors in clinical procedures. Currently the use of adenoviral vectors for gene therapy applications could lead to inflammation, transgene elimination, and local damage in cases where subjects may have been previously exposed to adenovirus or could be infected in the future. This inflammation would occur not only at the site of virus injection but also in synaptically linked brain regions (35).

Despite these potential problems, great advances have been made for the use of adenoviral vectors as gene transfer vectors. The creation of newer adenoviral gene transfer systems and the production of gene-deleted and "gutless" vectors that are less immunogenic will have a great impact on the field.

Immunosuppression has been shown to enhance the expression of transgenes from adenoviral vectors in the periphery (75), and development of new immunosuppressive therapies could lead to control of the inflammatory response. Co-administration of several E1/E3a-deleted adenoviral vectors encoding YTS 191 (anti-CD4), YTS 169 (anti-CD8), and TIB 213 (anti-CD11a) have also proven to be very efficient in blocking both cellular and humoral immune reactions (76). Alternatively, the use of different adenoviral serotypes that may escape recognition by the immune system is another option that is currently being explored (77,78).

Early interest in adenoviral gene therapy has been tempered following the realization that the immune system can mount an effective response after administration, as was evidenced in the first clinical trials using adenoviral vectors where even the lower doses caused an acute decrease in platelet function, e.g., the initial stages that at higher doses led to full blown disseminated intravascular coagulation. Much of the current work in the field of adenoviral-mediated gene therapy is focused on the development of increasingly less immunogenic vector systems. Although it is important that future work using viral vectors as gene transfer systems produce vectors that are able to target specific populations of cells and express therapeutic levels of transgene, it is also important to recognize that the actions of the host immune system play an enormous role in both of these aspects of gene therapy. Therefore, the molecular nature of both the innate and adaptive immune responses to adenoviral vectors must continue to be examined. Elucidation of all aspects of the immune response in the context of gene therapy and understanding of its mechanisms are paramount before the application of gene therapy can become a clinical success.

ACKNOWLEDGMENTS

Gene therapy projects for neurological diseases are funded by the National Institutes of Health/National Institute of Neurological Disorders & Satoke Grant 1R01 NS44556.01, National Institute of Diabetes and Digestive and Kidney Diseases 1 RO3 TW006273-01 to M.G.C.; National Institutes of Health/National Institute of Neurological Disorders & Stroke Grant 1 RO1 NS 42893.01, U54 NS045309-01, and 1R21 NS04729-01 and Bram and Elaine Goldsmith Chair In Gene Therapeutics to P.R.L.; and the Linda Tallen & David Paul Kane Annual Fellowship to M.G.C. and P.R.L. We also thank the generous funding our Institute receives from the Board of Governors at Cedars Sinai Medical Center. We thank the support and academic leadership of S. Melmed, and R. Katzman, and D. Meyer for their superb administrative and organizational support.

REFERENCES

1. Kay MA, Glorioso JC, Naldini L. Viral vectors for gene therapy: the art of turning infectious agents into vehicles of therapeutics. Nat Med 2001; 7:33–40.
2. Lusky M, Christ M, Rittner K, et al. In vitro and in vivo biology of recombinant adenovirus vectors with E1, E1/E2A, or E1/E4 deleted. J Virol 1998; 72:2022–2032.
3. Morsy MA, Caskey CT. Expanded-capacity adenoviral vectors—the helper-dependent vectors. Mol Med Today 1999; 5:18–24.
4. Russell WC. Update on adenovirus and its vectors. J Gen Virol 2000; 81:2573–2604.
5. Bergelson JM, Cunningham JA, Droguett G, et al. Isolation of a common receptor for Coxsackie B viruses and adenoviruses 2 and 5. Science 1997; 275:1320–1323.
6. Wickham TJ, Mathias P, Cheresh DA, Nemerow GR. Integrins alpha v beta 3 and alpha v beta 5 promote adenovirus internalization but not virus attachment. Cell 1993; 73:309–319.
7. Li E, Brown SL, Stupack DG, Puente XS, Cheresh DA, Nemerow GR. Integrin alpha(v)beta1 is an adenovirus coreceptor. J Virol 2001; 75:5405–5409.

8. Wang K, Guan T, Cheresh DA, Nemerow GR. Regulation of adenovirus membrane penetration by the cytoplasmic tail of integrin beta5. J Virol 2000; 74:2731–2739.

9. Wickham TJ, Filardo EJ, Cheresh DA, Nemerow GR. Integrin alpha v beta 5 selectively promotes adenovirus mediated cell membrane permeabilization. J Cell Biol 1994; 127:257–264.

10. Greber UF, Suomalainen M, Stidwill RP, Boucke K, Ebersold MW, Helenius A. The role of the nuclear pore complex in adenovirus DNA entry. EMBO J 1997; 16:5998–6007.

11. Banchereau J, Steinman RM. Dendritic cells and the control of immunity. Nature 1998; 392:245–252.

12. Jooss K, Chirmule N. Immunity to adenovirus and adeno-associated viral vectors: implications for gene therapy. Gene Ther 2003; 10:955–963.

13. Guidotti LG, Chisari FV. Noncytolytic control of viral infections by the innate and adaptive immune response. Annu Rev Immunol 2001; 19:65–91.

14. Alexopoulou L, Holt AC, Medzhitov R, Flavell RA. Recognition of double-stranded RNA and activation of NF-kappaB by toll-like receptor 3. Nature 2001; 413:732–738.

15. Paludan SR, Ellermann-Eriksen S, Kruys V, Mogensen SC. Expression of TNF-alpha by herpes simplex virus-infected macrophages is regulated by a dual mechanism: transcriptional regulation by NF-kappa B and activating transcription factor 2/Jun and translational regulation through the AU-rich region of the 3' untranslated region. J Immunol 2001; 167:2202–2208.

16. Sato M, Suemori H, Hata N, et al. Distinct and essential roles of transcription factors IRF-3 and IRF-7 in response to viruses for IFN-alpha/beta gene induction. Immunity 2000; 13:539–548.

17. Dong C, Davis RJ, Flavell RA. MAP kinases in the immune response. Annu Rev Immunol 2002; 20:55–72.

18. Higginbotham JN, Seth P, Blaese RM, Ramsey WJ. The release of inflammatory cytokines from human peripheral blood mononuclear cells in vitro following exposure to adenovirus variants and capsid. Hum Gene Ther 2002; 13:129–141.

19. Malmgaard L, Salazar-Mather TP, Lewis CA, Biron CA. Promotion of alpha/beta interferon induction during in vivo viral infection through alpha/beta interferon receptor/STAT1 system-dependent and -independent pathways. J Virol 2002; 76:4520–4525.

20. Schnell MA, Zhang Y, Tazelaar J, et al. Activation of innate immunity in nonhuman primates following intraportal administration of adenoviral vectors. Mol Ther 2001; 3:708–722.

21. Muruve DA, Barnes MJ, Stillman IE, Libermann TA. Adenoviral gene therapy leads to rapid induction of multiple chemokines and acute neutrophil-dependent hepatic injury in vivo. Hum Gene Ther 1999; 10:965–976.

22. Bowen GP, Borgland SL, Lam M, Libermann TA, Wong NC, Muruve DA. Adenovirus vector-induced inflammation: capsid-dependent induction of the C-C chemokine RANTES requires NF-kappa B. Hum Gene Ther 2002; 13:367–379.

23. Tibbles LA, Spurrell JC, Bowen GP, et al. Activation of p38 and ERK signaling during adenovirus vector cell entry lead to expression of the C-X-C chemokine IP-10. J Virol 2002; 76:1559–1568.

24. Borgland SL, Bowen GP, Wong NC, Libermann TA, Muruve DA. Adenovirus vector-induced expression of the C-X-C chemokine IP-10 is mediated through capsid-dependent activation of NF-kappaB. J Virol 2000; 74:3941–3947.

25. Sung RS, Qin L, Bromberg JS. TNFalpha and IFNgamma induced by innate anti-adenoviral immune responses inhibit adenovirus-mediated transgene expression. Mol Ther 2001; 3:757–767.

26. Qin L, Ding Y, Pahud DR, Chang E, Imperiale MJ, Bromberg JS. Promoter attenuation in gene therapy: interferon-gamma and tumor necrosis factor-alpha inhibit transgene expression. Hum Gene Ther 1997; 8:2019–2029.

27. Peng Y, Trevejo J, Zhou J, et al. Inhibition of tumor necrosis factor alpha by an adenovirus-encoded soluble fusion protein extends transgene expression in the liver and lung. J Virol 1999; 73:5098–5109.

28. Worgall S, Singh R, Leopold PL, et al. Selective expansion of alveolar macrophages in vivo by adenovirus-mediated transfer of the murine granulocyte-macrophage colony-stimulating factor cDNA. Blood 1999; 93:655–666.

29. Worgall S, Wolff G, Falck-Pedersen E, Crystal RG. Innate immune mechanisms dominate elimination of adenoviral vectors following in vivo administration. Hum Gene Ther 1997; 8:37–44.

30. Lieber A, He CY, Meuse L, Himeda C, Wilson C, Kay MA. Inhibition of NF-kappaB activation in combination with bcl-2 expression allows for persistence of first-generation adenovirus vectors in the mouse liver. J Virol 1998; 72:9267–9277.

31. Elkon KB, Liu CC, Gall JG, et al. Tumor necrosis factor alpha plays a central role in immune-mediated clearance of adenoviral vectors. Proc Natl Acad Sci USA 1997; 94:9814–9819.

32. Byrnes AP, Rusby JE, Wood MJ, Charlton HM. Adenovirus gene transfer causes inflammation in the brain. Neuroscience 1995; 66:1015–1024.

33. Byrnes AP, Wood MJ, Charlton HM. Role of T cells in inflammation caused by adenovirus vectors in the brain. Gene Ther 1996; 3:644–651.

34. Byrnes AP, MacLaren RE, Charlton HM. Immunological instability of persistent adenovirus vectors in the brain: peripheral exposure to vector leads to renewed inflammation, reduced gene expression, and demyelination. J Neurosci 1996; 16:3045–3055.

35. Kajiwara K, Byrnes AP, Ohmoto Y, Charlton HM, Wood MJ, Wood KJ. Humoral immune responses to adenovirus vectors in the brain. J Neuroimmunol 2000; 103:8–15.

36. Wood MJ, Charlton HM, Wood KJ, Kajiwara K, Byrnes AP. Immune responses to adenovirus vectors in the nervous system. Trends Neurosci 1996; 19:497–501.

37. Kajiwara K, Byrnes AP, Charlton HM, Wood MJ, Wood KJ. Immune responses to adenoviral vectors during gene transfer in the brain. Hum Gene Ther 1997; 8:253–265.

38. Zermansky AJ, Bolognani F, Stone D, et al. Towards global and long-term neurological gene therapy: unexpected transgene dependent, high-level, and widespread distribution of HSV-1 thymidine kinase throughout the CNS. Mol Ther 2001; 4:490–498.

39. Thomas CE, Abordo-Adesida E, Maleniak TC, Stone D, Gerdes G, Lowenstein PR. Gene transfer into rat brain using adenoviral vectors. In: Gerfen JN, McKay R, Rogawski MA, Sibley DR, Skolnick P, eds. In: Current Protocols in Neuroscience, Vol. 4.23.1–4.23.40. New York, NY: John Wiley and Sons, 2000:4.23.21–24.23.40.

40. Thomas CE, Birkett D, Anozie I, Castro MG, Lowenstein PR. Acute direct adenoviral vector cytotoxicity and chronic, but not acute, inflammatory responses correlate with decreased vector-mediated transgene expression in the brain. Mol Ther 2001; 3:36–46.

41. Lowenstein PR. Immune responses to viral vectors for gene therapy. In: Lowenstein PR, ed. In: Gene Ther, Vol. 10, 2003:933–998.

42. Kafri T, Morgan D, Krahl T, Sarvetnick N, Sherman L, Verma I. Cellular immune response to adenoviral vector infected cells does not require de novo viral gene expression: implications for gene therapy. Proc Natl Acad Sci USA 1998; 95:11377–11382.

43. Stilwell JL, Samulski RJ. Role of viral vectors and virion shells in cellular gene expression. Mol Ther 2004; 9:337–346.

44. Stilwell JL, McCarty DM, Negishi A, Superfine R, Samulski RJ. Development and characterization of novel empty adenovirus capsids and their impact on cellular gene expression. J Virol 2003; 77:12881–12885.

45. Yang Y, Ertl HC, Wilson JM. MHC class I-restricted cytotoxic T lymphocytes to viral antigens destroy hepatocytes in mice infected with E1-deleted recombinant adenoviruses. Immunity 1994; 1:433–442.

46. Yang Y, Nunes FA, Berencsi K, Furth EE, Gonczol E, Wilson JM. Cellular immunity to viral antigens limits E1-deleted adenoviruses for gene therapy. Proc Natl Acad Sci USA 1994; 91:4407–4411.

47. Yang Y, Li Q, Ertl HC, Wilson JM. Cellular and humoral immune responses to viral antigens create barriers to lung-directed gene therapy with recombinant adenoviruses. J Virol 1995; 69:2004–2015.

48. Molinier-Frenkel V, Gahery-Segard H, Mehtali M, et al. Immune response to recombinant adenovirus in humans: capsid components from viral input are targets for vector-specific cytotoxic T lymphocytes. J Virol 2000; 74:7678–7682.

49. Yang Y, Jooss KU, Su Q, Ertl HC, Wilson JM. Immune responses to viral antigens versus transgene product in the elimination of recombinant adenovirus-infected hepatocytes in vivo. Gene Ther 1996; 3:137–144.

50. Barr D, Tubb J, Ferguson D, et al. Strain related variations in adenovirally mediated transgene expression from mouse hepatocytes in vivo: comparisons between immunocompetent and immunodeficient inbred strains. Gene Ther 1995; 2:151–155.

51. Dai Y, Schwarz EM, Gu D, Zhang WW, Sarvetnick N, Verma IM. Cellular and humoral immune responses to adenoviral vectors containing factor IX gene: tolerization of factor IX and vector antigens allows for long-term expression. Proc Natl Acad Sci USA 1995; 92:1401–1405.

52. Yang Y, Wilson JM. Clearance of adenovirus-infected hepatocytes by MHC class I-restricted CD4+ CTLs in vivo. J Immunol 1995; 155:2564–2570.

53. Yang Y, Trinchieri G, Wilson JM. Recombinant IL-12 prevents formation of blocking IgA antibodies to recombinant adenovirus and allows repeated gene therapy to mouse lung. Nat Med 1995; 1:890–893.

54. Zsengeller ZK, Wert SE, Hull WM, et al. Persistence of replication-deficient adenovirus-mediated gene transfer in lungs of immune-deficient (nu/nu) mice. Hum Gene Ther 1995; 6:457–467.

55. Ohmoto Y, Wood MJ, Charlton HM, Kajiwara K, Perry VH, Wood KJ. Variation in the immune response to adenoviral vectors in the brain: influence of mouse strain, environmental conditions and priming. Gene Ther 1999; 6:471–481.

56. Wood MJA, Byrnes AP, McMenamin M, et al. In: ??? PRaE, Lowenstein LW, eds. Immune responses to viruses: practical implications for the use of viruses as vectors for experimental and clinical gene therapy. New York, NY: John Wiley and Sons Ltd., 1996.

57. Lowenstein PR. Immunology of viral-vector-mediated gene transfer into the brain: an evolutionary and developmental perspective. Trends Immunol 2002; 23:23–30.

58. Fischer HG, Bonifas U, Reichmann G. Phenotype and functions of brain dendritic cells emerging during chronic infection of mice with Toxoplasma gondii. J Immunol 2000; 164:4826–4834.

59. Fischer HG, Bielinsky AK. Antigen presentation function of brain-derived dendriform cells depends on astrocyte help. Int Immunol 1999; 11:1265–1274.

60. Santambrogio L, Belyanskaya SL, Fischer FR, et al. Developmental plasticity of CNS microglia. Proc Natl Acad Sci USA 2001; 98:6295–6300.

61. Fischer HG, Reichmann G. Brain dendritic cells and macrophages/microglia in central nervous system inflammation. J Immunol 2001; 166:2717–2726.

62. Matyszak MK, Perry VH. The potential role of dendritic cells in immune-mediated inflammatory diseases in the central nervous system. Neuroscience 1996; 74:599–608.

63. Carson MJ, Reilly CR, Sutcliffe JG, Lo D. Disproportionate recruitment of CD8+ T cells into the central nervous system by professional antigen-presenting cells. Am J Pathol 1999; 154:481–494.

64. McMenamin PG. Distribution and phenotype of dendritic cells and resident tissue macrophages in the dura mater, leptomeninges, and choroid plexus of the rat brain as demonstrated in wholemount preparations. J Comp Neurol 1999; 405:553–562.

65. Stevenson PG, Austyn JM, Hawke S. Uncoupling of virus-induced inflammation and anti-viral immunity in the brain parenchyma. J Gen Virol 2002; 83:1735–1743.

66. Hart DN, Fabre JW. Demonstration and characterization of Ia-positive dendritic cells in the interstitial connective tissues of rat heart and other tissues, but not brain. J Exp Med 1981; 154:347–361.

67. Lowe J, MacLennan KA, Powe DG, Pound JD, Palmer JB. Microglial cells in human brain have phenotypic characteristics related to possible function as dendritic antigen presenting cells. J Pathol 1989; 159:143–149.

68. McMahon EJ, Bailey SL, Castenada CV, Waldner H, Miller SD. Epitope spreading initiates in the CNS in two mouse models of multiple sclerosis. Nat Med 2005; 11:335–339.
69. Greter M, Heppner FL, Lemos MP, et al. Dendritic cells permit immune invasion of the CNS in an animal model of multiple sclerosis. Nat Med 2005; 11:328–334.
70. Ponomarev ED, Shriver LP, Maresz K, Dittel BN. Microglial cell activation and proliferation precedes the onset of CNS autoimmunity. J Neurosci Res 2005; 81:374–389.
71. Thomas CE, Schiedner G, Kochanek S, Castro MG, Lowenstein PR. Peripheral infection with adenovirus causes unexpected long-term brain inflammation in animals injected intracranially with first-generation, but not with high-capacity, adenovirus vectors: toward realistic long-term neurological gene therapy for chronic diseases. Proc Natl Acad Sci USA 2000; 97:7482–7487.
72. Abordo-Adesida E, Follenzi A, Barcia C, et al. Stability of lentiviral vector-mediated transgene expression in the brain in the presence of systemic antivector immune responses. Hum Gene Ther 2005; 16:741–751.
73. Peden CS, Burger C, Muzyczka N, Mandel RJ. Circulating anti-wild-type adeno-associated virus type 2 (AAV2) antibodies inhibit recombinant AAV2 (rAAV2)-mediated, but not rAAV5-mediated, gene transfer in the brain. J Virol 2004; 78:6344–6359.
74. Tripathy SK, Black HB, Goldwasser E, Leiden JM. Immune responses to transgene-encoded proteins limit the stability of gene expression after injection of replication-defective adenovirus vectors. Nat Med 1996; 2:545–550.
75. Juillard V, Villefroy P, Godfrin D, Pavirani A, Venet A, Guillet JG. Long-term humoral and cellular immunity induced by a single immunization with replication-defective adenovirus recombinant vector. Eur J Immunol 1995; 25:3467–3473.
76. Kass-Eisler A, Falck-Pedersen E, Elfenbein DH, Alvira M, Buttrick PM, Leinwand LA. The impact of developmental stage, route of administration and the immune system on adenovirus-mediated gene transfer. Gene Ther 1994; 1:395–402.
77. Guerette B, Vilquin JT, Gingras M, Gravel C, Wood KJ, Tremblay JP. Prevention of immune reactions triggered by first-generation adenoviral vectors by monoclonal antibodies and CTLA4Ig. Hum Gene Ther 1996; 7:1455–1463.
78. Morral N, O'Neal W, Rice K, et al. Administration of helper-dependent adenoviral vectors and sequential delivery of different vector serotype for long-term liver-directed gene transfer in baboons. Proc Natl Acad Sci USA 1999; 96:12816–12821.
79. Parks R, Evelegh C, Graham F. Use of helper-dependent adenoviral vectors of alternative serotypes permits repeat vector administration. Gene Ther 1999; 6:1565–1573.

2

Gene Transfer to the Nerve System Using HSV-1-Derived Amplicon Vectors

Alberto L. Epstein

Centre de Génétique Moléculaire et Cellulaire, CNRS, Université Claude Bernard, Villeurbanne, France

INTRODUCTION

HSV-1 and Its Derived Vectors

Herpes simplex virus type 1 (HSV-1) is a major human pathogen whose lifestyle is based on a long-term dual interaction with the infected host. After initial infection and lytic replication at the body periphery, the virus enters the sensory neurons that innervate the epithelia and establishes a lifelong latent infection in sensory ganglia. Periodic reactivation from latency usually leads to the return of the virus to epithelial cells, where it produces secondary lytic infections resulting in mild illness symptoms, such as cold sores.

During lytic infection, the HSV-1 153-kilobase pairs (kbp) double-stranded DNA genome expresses more than 80 genes that are strictly temporarily regulated in a cascade fashion, giving rise to three phases of gene expression. The expression cascade, which is regulated mainly at the transcriptional level, begins with the expression of the immediate-early (IE) genes. The resulting IE gene products are regulatory proteins responsible for controlling viral gene expression during subsequent phases of the replication cycle and for inducing shutoff of cellular protein synthesis. Transcription of IE genes occurs in the absence of de novo viral protein synthesis and is highly stimulated by a virion protein known as VP16, which is a powerful transcription factor. The early (E) gene products that are synthesized next include enzymes that act to increase the pool of deoxynucleotides of the infected cells and replication proteins involved in viral DNA synthesis. The last set of genes expressed are the late (L) genes, which encode the structural proteins involved in the assembly of the capsid, the tegument, and the envelope of the virus particles. Some of these structural proteins play major regulatory roles in the next infectious cycle. Lytic viral replication results in the impairment of host macromolecular synthesis, the release of newly assembled viral progeny particles and the ultimate death of the host cell. During latency, the viral genome remains as a circular episome within the cell nuclei, and undergoes dramatic changes resulting in an almost complete silencing of transcription.

Only one region of the viral genome, known as the LAT locus, is actively transcribed during latency, resulting in the synthesis of non-messenger RNA molecules of unknown function, which accumulates in the nucleus of latently infected neurons (for a review on HSV-1 lytic and latent cycles see Ref. 1).

Three different types of vectors can be derived from HSV-1: recombinant attenuated vectors, recombinant defective vectors and amplicons, which are defective, helper-dependent vectors. The different kinds of vectors that derive from HSV-1 were conceived to take advantage of distinct biological properties of this virus. Recombinant HSV-1 vectors, either attenuated or defective, exploit several adaptations of HSV-1 to the nerve system, such as latency, the presence of powerful neuro-specific promoters, or the occurrence of viral genes controlling neuroinvasiveness or neurovirulence. The amplicon vectors allow exploiting the capacity of the virus capsid to accommodate more than 150 kbp of foreign DNA. This report will focus on recent technological and conceptual breakthroughs, as well as on the applications of amplicon vectors to the nerve system.

AMPLICONS

Technological Breakthroughs and State of the Art

Amplicon vectors (2) are HSV-1 particles identical to wild type HSV-1 from the structural, immunological, and host-range points of view, but they carry a DNA plasmid, named the amplicon plasmid, instead of the viral genome. An amplicon plasmid is a standard *E. coli* plasmid carrying one origin of replication (ori-S) and one packaging signal ("a") from HSV-1, in addition to the transgenic sequences of interest. The major interest of amplicons as gene transfer tools stems from the fact that they carry no virus genes and consequently do not induce synthesis of virus proteins. Therefore, these vectors are neither toxic for the infected cells nor pathogenic for the inoculated organisms. A second and major advantage that arises from the lack of virus genes is that most of the 153 kbp capacity of the HSV-1 particle can be used to accommodate very large foreign pieces of DNA. This is undoubtedly the most outstanding property of amplicons, as there is no other viral vector system available displaying the capacity to deliver such a large amount of foreign DNA to the nuclear environment of mammalian cells. In addition to possessing a larger delivering capacity, amplicons are safer than defective recombinant HSV-1 vectors, because the absence of virus genes in the amplicon genome strongly reduces the risk of reactivation, complementation or recombination with latent HSV-1 genomes. At the opposite, amplicons are considerably more difficult to prepare in high amounts than recombinant defective vectors. The possibility of using amplicons to transduce large amounts of foreign DNA to both quiescent and dividing cells appeared for a long-time as an unattainable dream. Some major recent improvements in amplicon technology have now brought these potentialities to reality.

Generation of Helper-Free Amplicon Vectors

Classically, amplicon vectors were prepared in cells transfected with the amplicon plasmid and superinfected with helper HSV-1. As the helper virus was generally a replication-defective mutant of HSV-1, the amplicon stocks were produced in transcomplementing cell lines (3). However, the use of HSV-1 as helper resulted in the production of helper-contaminated vector stocks. These particles, though defective, induced significant cytotoxicity and inflammatory responses, preventing their use in gene therapy of vaccination protocols. To overcome these obstacles, novel helper systems that produce essentially helper-free vector stocks, have been recently developed. One of these systems is based on the cotransfection of amplicon plasmids with bacterial artificial chromosomes (BACs) supplying the full set of transacting HSV-1 functions (4). The HSV-1 helper genome carried by the BAC does not contain the viral packaging signals and its size largely exceeds that of the wild type HSV-1 genome. As a consequence, these helper genomes cannot be packaged into newly assembled HSV-1 particles. Although the more recent version of these systems allows production of entirely helper-free amplicon stocks (5), the amount of amplicon vectors produced with this method is rather limited. Therefore, while this strategy is well suited for producing amplicons for fundamental research or for application in small animals, it appears hardly suitable for large-scale production of amplicon vectors, as required for vaccination or gene therapy approaches.

A very different helper system recently developed is based on the deletion, by Cre/loxP-based site-specific recombination, of the packaging signals of the helper virus in the cells that are producing the amplicons. This system uses as helper a novel recombinant HSV-1 (named HSV-1 LaLdeltaJ) that carries a unique and ectopic packaging "a" signal flanked by two loxP sites in parallel orientation (6). This virus is Cre-sensitive and cannot be packaged in Cre-expressing cells due to efficient deletion of the packaging signals. In addition, HSV-1 LaLdeltaJ lacks the gene encoding the essential protein ICP4. This helper virus is thus defective and can be produced only in ICP4 transcomplementing cells. Therefore, upon transfection of the amplicon plasmid to cells simultaneously expressing Cre and ICP4, infection with HSV-1 LaLdeltaJ helper virus generates amplicon stocks that are only marginally contaminated with defective helper particles. Since this system is based on infection, instead of transfection procedures, it allows serial passages of the vector stocks, and a two-step protocol has been set-up that allows us to prepare as many amplicons as required for a particular purpose (6–8). This system is consequently well suited for large-scale production of amplicon vectors.

Infectious Transfer of Very Large Foreign DNA

Thanks to their ability to transduce very large transgenic sequences, amplicons can be used to deliver complete genomic DNA loci or DNA sequences that regulate chromatin structure and function or subnuclear localisation. This may prove useful to design improved gene therapy vectors having advantages such as prolonged and tissue-specific expression, generation of multiple splice variants, or synthesis of the full set of proteins required to assemble complex structures as well as metabolic or signalling pathways.

The feasibility of transducing very large genomic sequences using amplicons has been recently demonstrated. Wade-Martins and colleagues have used amplicons to express a 115 kbp insert containing the complete human hypoxanthine phosphoribosyl transferase (HPRT) locus into a human HPRT-deficient fibroblast cell line (9). They have also used amplicons to deliver a 135 kbp fragment carrying the human, low-density lipoprotein receptor (LDLR) into human fibroblasts derived from patients with familial hypercho-lesterolemia (FH). The infectious LDLR locus was shown to express at physiological levels in these cells (9). Furthermore, the LDLR locus was maintained within a replicating episomal amplicon vector, carrying the Epstein-Barr virus latent replicon, composed of EBNA-1 and oriP sequences (10), and was expressed for 3 mo at physiological levels following infectious delivery to CHO cells. More recently, this group used amplicons to deliver a 132 kbp of genomic DNA comprising the CDKN2A/CDKN2B region, and demonstrated that this locus was correctly expressed, allowing the synthesis of three cell-cycle regulatory proteins that are expressed from overlapping genes, utilizing alternative splicing and promoter usage (11). These exciting experiments illustrate the outstanding potential of amplicons as genomic transfer vectors.

GENE TRANSFER TO NEURAL CELLS AND TISSUES USING AMPLICON VECTORS

Founder Studies

After the initial demonstration that they could be used to deliver foreign DNA (12), amplicons have been widely and successfully used to express genes of neurobiological, immunological, or virological interest in cultured cells or living organisms. Some 170 papers have been published reporting gene transfer using amplicons and about half of them concern the nerve system. This first section brings together some of the initial studies that have founded this field and established the conditions for amplicon transduction to cultured neurons, to organotypic cultures, and to the PNS and CNS of experimental animal models. The first of these studies (13) showed that beta-galactosidase could be expressed in rat cultured peripheral neurons from superior cervical ganglia (SCG) and dorsal root ganglia (DRG), using amplicons that had been prepared with a temperature-sensitive HSV-1 mutant (tsK) as helper. Further studies soon extended this observation to a variety of rat cultured neurons from spinal cord, cerebellum, thalamus, basal ganglia, hippocampus, occipital cortex, temporal cortex, frontal cortex, and striatum (14,15), or to cultured neurons or neuronal cell lines from other species, including mice, primates, and humans (16). In these works, transgenic expression was observed during at least two weeks after infection, with minor or no cell damage. Additional studies— then quickly and almost simultaneously— extended the use of amplicons to organotypic hippocampal slice cultures and acute hippocampal slices (17,18) and to adult rat peripheral and central nerve systems in vivo (19,20), while still other studies extended the application of amplicons to the expression of a variety of genes of neurobiological interest (21–25).

These earlier studies were based on amplicon stocks contaminated with helper particles. These stocks were toxic and elicited inflammatory responses, thus perturbing interpretation of results and precluding their use in experimental gene therapy protocols. Two studies performed during this period, using antibodies specific for amplicon or helper encoded proteins, demonstrated that high-level transgenic expression from amplicons could however be observed in cultured neurons that had escaped infection by helper particles (26) and that coinfection of cells with amplicon and helper particles could affect distribution and intensity of the transgenes encoded by the amplicon genome (27). While the helper systems then progressively improved, giving rise to stocks containing higher ratios of amplicon to helper particles, the first major technological breakthrough took place only with the generation of the first system that allowed to produce helper-free amplicon stocks (28). More efficient helper systems then progressively appeared, until the advent of the two above-described helper systems currently in use (5,6). It is of interest to note that while these helper-free systems have been described by many groups to be neither toxic nor pathogenic, and to elicit lower levels of inflammation than helper-contaminated vectors (29), the absence of helper particles in the stocks can result in lower intensities, cell type-dependence and even cell cycle-dependent transgene expression from the amplicon vector.

Other early studies focused on the identification of the promoters required to obtain strong, long-term, tissue specific, or controllable transgenic expression from amplicon vectors. Few works explored the use of viral (30) or inducible (31) promoters, while most studies tested cellular, neuron-specific cellular promoters. The rat preproenkephalin (PA) promoter was the first described to yield region-specific and long-term expression (32). Amplicons expressing beta-galactosidase under the control of this promoter induced a restricted pattern of protein expression, which followed previously observed patterns of endogenous PA expression in rat brains. The most studied of these promoters is the rat tyrosine hydroylase (TH) promoter. The first study reported that amplicons containing the rat TH promoter were able to direct cell-specific expression of beta-galactosidase expression in cultured rat peripheral neurons of SCG but not in the DRG (33). Further studies reported that TH promoter could be used to drive prolonged and specific transgenic expression in vivo in the substantia nigra and locus ceruleus ipsilateral to the caudate nucleus, where the vector had been inoculated (34,35), and that a TH-neurofilament chimeric promoter enhanced long-term expression in rat forebrain neurons (36). While the mouse neurofilament heavy subunit promoter supported specific, but not long-term, expression in neurons in the midbrain, striatum and hippocampus, the rat neuron enolase promoter and a rat voltage-gated sodium channel promoter supported only low levels of expression in the amplicon context (37). The most important recent breakthrough in this field is, however, the use of very large genomic regulatory sequences, as already described (9,38). Although such sequences have not been exploited yet in the context of neurons, it is likely that they will be the best in providing not only tissue-specific, but also physiological regulation of transgene expression, which is more relevant for gene therapy than strong or long-term expression.

APPLICATIONS

Most studies using amplicons for gene transfer to neural cells or tissues can be grouped in four major classes: protection against neurological insults, treatment of gliomas, treatment of Parkinson's disease (PD), and behavioral studies.

Protection Against Toxicity, Ischemias, and Other Neurological Insults

By far, the most frequent gene transfer studies using amplicon vectors are related to the protection of neurons and neural tissue against a variety of neurological insults. The works grouped in this section can be further subdivided into several classes according to the physiological actions accomplished by the delivered genes.

Neurotrophins

Delivery of nerve growth factor (NGF) using amplicons is able to prevent effects of axotomy on sympathetic cervical ganglia (SCG) (20). Axotomy of a SCG results in NGF deprivation, causing a decline in tyrosine hydroxylase (TH) activity, and it had been shown that continuous local application of NGF could prevent this decline. This effect could be obtained also by direct injection of amplicons expressing NGF in SCG, demonstrating that these vectors could be used to modify neuronal physiology in vivo and that expression of a critical gene product by neural cells that do not normally produce it has potential applications for gene therapy. In a subsequent study, exogenous NGF was shown to protect also against the neurotoxicity and nerve tissue destruction that resulted from gene delivery to the striatum using helper-contaminated amplicon vectors (39).

Amplicon transduction of brain-derived neurotrophic factor (BDNF) to explanted cultures prepared from spiral ganglia of the murine ear elicited robust neurite process outgrowth, comparable to exogenously added BDNF (40) and promoted neuronal survival by preventing spiral ganglion degeneration resulting from hair cell loss and neurotrophin

3-deprivation-induced apoptosis (41). In an attempt to better define the importance of individual members of the neurotrophin family, amplicons expressing NGF or BDNF were compared in a further study that addressed the role of these two neurotrophins for innervation of the chicken cochlea (42). Using dissociated cultures of avian cochlear neurons, amplicon-delivered BDNF promoted neuronal survival similar to the maximal level seen by exogenously added BDNF and exceeds its potency to produce neurite outgrowth, whereas no response was observed in cells infected with the NGF expressing amplicon. These experiments therefore confirmed the importance of BDNF as a mediator of neurotrophin signaling inside avian cochlear neurons.

Two further studies addressed the role of neurotrophin 3 (NT-3) in protection of spiral ganglion neurons (SGN) from cisplatin (DDP)-induced damage, a drug that causes destruction of hair cells and neurons in the auditory system. Transduction of cultured murine cochlear explants exposed to DDP with a helper-free amplicon that expressed a c-Myc-tagged NT-3 chimera, resulted in significantly greater numbers of surviving SGNs than those infected with control amplicons, demonstrating that amplicon-mediated NT-3 delivery could attenuate the ototoxic action of DDP on organotypic culture (43). By injecting the amplicon vectors directly into the cochlea of aged mice prior to DDP treatment, the same group subsequently demonstrated that amplicon-directed NT-3 overexpression could also attenuate the ototoxic actions of DDP in the peripheral auditory system (44).

A recent study demonstrated neuroprotection against ischemic injury by direct intracerebral administration of amplicons expressing glial cell-line-derived neurotrophic factor (GDNF). The vector was injected into the cerebral cortex prior of after unilateral occlusion of the middle cerebral artery. Pretreatment with the GDNF-amplicons significantly reduced motor deficits, as compared to control-treated animals, or to animals receiving the vector after the ischemic insult. Histological analyses performed 1 mo after stroke revealed a reduction in ischemic tissue loss, as well as less immunostaining for GFAP and caspase 3 in the pretreated animals (45).

Antiapoptotic, Antioxidant and Heat-Shock Proteins

Several studies addressed the role of Bcl-2 in protection against ischemias and other neurologic insults, with very consistent results. Thus, amplicons expressing Bcl-2 have been demonstrated to limit neuronal death in neocortical focal cerebral ischemia when administrated before tandem occlusion of the right middle cerebral artery and ipsilateral common carotid artery (46). Bcl-2 transduction also protected hippocampal neurons from transient global ischemia resulting from bilateral common carotid artery occlusion (47). Most interestingly, and more relevant for gene therapy, Bcl-2 expressing amplicons were shown also to be neuroprotective for striatal neurons when delivered after the onset of the ischemic insult (48). Amplicon-induced overexpression of Bcl-2 also protected hippocampal neurons after exposure to adriamycin, a potent oxygen radical generator, and enhanced survival of cultured neurons after exposure to glutamate and hypoglycemia (49). In addition to Bcl-2, other antiapoptotic proteins, like the viral proteins p35 and γ34.5, were found to significantly reduce hippocampal lesions caused by exocytotoxic insults such as kainic acid administration (50).

Amplicon-directed overexpression of heat shock protein HSP72 after induction of experimental stroke also protected striatal neurons from ischemic damage. Survival of striatal neurons was, however, significant only when HSP72-expressing vectors were administered no more than 2 hr after ischemic onset (51). In a further study, this team demonstrated that amplicon expressed HSP72 also protected the cornu ammonis 1 region of the hippocampus neurons from global ischemia and showed that this protection may be mediated in part by increased expression of Bcl-2 (52). Amplicon-induced overexpression of the antioxydant enzymes catalase (CAT) or glutathione peroxidase (GPX), both of which catalyze the degradation of oxygen peroxide, in primary hippocampal or cortical cultures, potently decreased the neurotoxicity induced by kainic acid, glutamate, sodium cyanide and oygen/glucose deprivation (53). Enhancement of neuronal protection from oxidative stress (H_2O_2) was also obtained in cultured primary neurons infected with amplicons expressing glutamic acid decarboxylase 67 (GAD67), a protection that was related to increased energy metabolism and involved the GABA shunt (54).

Proteins Affecting Neuronal Metabolism

Amplicon vectors overexpressing the rat brain glucose transporter (GT) gene enhance glucose uptake in hippocampal cultures and the hippocampus (24). These vectors can maintain neuronal metabolism and reduce the extent of neuron loss after a period of hypoglycemia. They also reduce kainic acid-induced seizure damage in the CA3 cell field, even when amplicons were delivered after onset of the seizure (55). Moreover, overexpression of GT from these amplicons was shown to protect cultured hippocampal, spinal cord, and septal neurons against various necrotic insults, including hypoglycemia, glutamate and 3-nitropropionic acid administration (56).

Increases in cytoplasmic Ca^{2+} concentration, due to overactivation of glutamate receptors, can lead to neuron death, and calcium-binding proteins (CaBP) are thought to be important in buffering intracellular calcium. Two members of the CaBP family have been tested for neuroprotection with apparent contradictory results. Whereas amplicons expressing calbindin D28K gene decreased hippocampal damage and increased neuronal survival following application of antimetabolite 3-acetylpyridine and kainic acid (57), expression of parvalbumin in cultured cortical neurons not only did not protected, but enhanced NMDA neurotoxicity, suggesting that ectopic expression of parvalbumin in cortical cultures may increase glutamate release, resulting in enhanced cell death (58).

Infection of Glioma-Derived Cell Lines and Experimental Gliomas

Several studies have used amplicons to explore different strategies to fight against gliomas. Breakefield and colleagues (59) delivered a chimeric fusion protein of GFP and the prodrug activating cytochrome CYP4B1, in an attempt to combine the advantages of a potent bioactivating suicide gene with a marker gene for living cells. Using this suicide gene strategy, this study showed that the chimeric protein retained the toxic features of the native CYP4B1 enzyme, while offering the possibility to analyze the distribution of the toxic transgene in experimental malignant gliomas.

A different approach was based on the expression of cytokines for enhancing vaccination therapy. Subcutaneous vaccination of mice with irradiated glioma cells that had been previously infected with amplicons expressing granulocyte-macrophage colony-stimulating factor (GM-CSF), proved effective in protecting animals subsequently challenged by intracerebral implantation of wild type tumor cells (60). Some 60% of animals survived for more than 80 days after implantation, similar to results obtained by vaccination using retrovirally-transduced glioma cells. However, amplicons have the advantage over retrovirally-transduced cells in that both dividing and non-dividing tumor cells can be efficiently infected.

A third strategy that has been explored is the use of amplicons expressing tumor necrosis factor-related apoptosis-inducing ligand (TRAIL), to induce apoptosis of tumor cells.

Using amplicons expressing either wild type TRAIL or the extracellular domain of TRAIL, together with a second transcription unit expressing Renilla luciferase to monitor infected cells, this study showed that both forms of TRAIL induced similar degrees of apoptosis in cultured human glioma cells (61). After direct amplicon injection into subcutaneous gliomas, TRAIL-treated gliomas regressed in size over a period of 4 wk, as compared to mock-injected gliomas, demonstrating the efficacy of amplicon-delivered TRAIL in treating these tumors in vivo.

Other works have attempted to improve transgenic delivery, stability or expression in glioma cells. Hybrid HSV-1/AAV amplicons could improve transgene expression by combining the high infectability and large transgene capacity of amplicons with the potential for episomal amplification and chromosomal integration of AAV vectors. In these hybrid amplicon vectors, a reporter transgenic unit (HCMV-lacZ) has been flanked by AAV inverted terminal repeats (ITR) sequences, and the stability of expression was analyzed in the presence or absence of AAV Rep protein (62). After infecting a human glioma cell line, the hybrid HSV-1/AAV vectors supported transgene retention and expression for over 2 wk, whereas control HSV-1 amplicons expressing the same reporter transcription unit lost the transgene after 10 days. Although expression appears to be somewhat longer in the presence of Rep, this protein seems to reduce intensity of expression, likely due to its cytotoxic effects. Interestingly, the level of transgene expression appeared to be independent of the 19q allelic status or the number of endogenous AAVS1 sequences, the locus where AAV genome preferentially integrates, in the various glioma cell lines studied (63). This is of particular interest because a significant proportion of human glioblastoma tumors are reported to have loss heterozygosity in this locus.

Also to improve transgenic delivery and killing activity for experimental gliomas, amplicon vectors have been used in combination with defective recombinant HSV-1 vectors. A replication-competent piggyback vector system, in which both elements of the system complement each other, allowed co-propagation of amplicon and recombinant HSV-1. Injection of this vector system into experimental gliomas followed by ganciclovir treatment, inhibited tumor growth via focal virus replication and pro-drug activation without systemic toxicity (64).

Lastly, a very interesting recent study describes the construction of amplicons whereby gene expression could be targeted to glial cells by placing transgene expression under the control of glial cell specific GFAP enhancer element, in a backbone amplicon genome whose expression is, in addition, controlled by cell cycle events (65). This work shows that when several cell cycle-specific regulatory elements (which affect expression of the cyclin A promoter) are incorporated together in a single amplicon genome, reporter gene (luciferase) activity is greatly enhanced and could be regulated in a cell cycle-dependent manner in a variety of cell lines. In this way, cell type-specific and cell cycle-dependent transgene expression could be demonstrated specifically in glioma-bearing animals.

Gene Therapy of Parkinson's Disease

Rather surprisingly, only few studies have addressed the use of amplicons for gene therapy of neurodegenerative or inherited genetic diseases affecting the nerve system, and most of these works focused on the study or treatment of experimental models of PD. A first study on this field showed that helper-contaminated amplicons expressing TH were able to induce long-term recovery in parkinsonian rats after vector inoculation into the partially denervated striatum of 6-hydroxydopamine-lesioned animals (66). In this study, efficient biochemical recovery, including increases in both striatal TH enzyme activity and in extracellular dopamine concentrations, was maintained for 1 yr after gene transfer. In a subsequent study, the same team demonstrated that infection of dissociated cultured rat striatal cells with amplicon vectors bearing a human TH cDNA, resulted in expression of TH RNA and TH immunoreactivity, and converted the infected striatal cells into L-DOPA-producing cells. Expression of TH and release of catecholamines were maintained for at least 1 wk after infection (67).

The modulation of motor behavior in nigrostriatal neurons was also examined by using amplicons expressing the catalytic domain of PKCbetaII (PKCdelta), a protein displaying constitutively active protein kinase activity with a substrate specificity similar to that of rat brain PKC. As demonstrated in cultured sympathetic neurons, expression of PKCdelta caused a long-lasting activation-dependent increase in neurotransmitter release. Microinjection in the rat brain of amplicons bearing PKCdelta under the control of TH promoter targeted expression to dopaminergic nigrostriatal neurons (68). Expression of this protein in a small percentage of nigrostriatal neurons was sufficient to produce a long-term change in apomorphine-induced rotational behavior, and this change was blocked by fluphenazine, a dopamine receptor antagonist. This study, therefore, enabled the demonstration that PKC pathways in nigrostriatal neurons modulate apomorphine-induced rotational behavior, and that altered dopaminergic transmission from nigrostriatal neurons appears to be the affected neuronal physiology responsible for the change in rotational behavior.

In a further study (69), correction of a rat model of PD was obtained by coexpression of TH and aromatic amino acid decarboxylase (AADC), using helper-free amplicon vectors and a modified neurofilament gene promoter that supported long-term expression in forebrain neurons. Coexpression of TH and AADC supported high-level behavioral correction of the 6-hydroxydopamine rat model of PD for 5 wk. Biochemical correction included increases of in extracellular dopamine and DOPAC concentration between 2 and 4 mo after gene transfer. Histological analyzes demonstrated neuronal-specific coexpression of TH and AADC at 4 days to 7 mo after gene transfer.

As it has been already quoted, a combination of critical elements from HSV-1 amplicons and AAV can be used to improve gene transfer to the brain. This mixed vector system was used for testing transduction efficiency and stability of GFP expression in primary neuronal cultures from rat ventral mesencephalon (70). The HSV-1/AAV hybrid vectors transduced the highest number of primary cultured neurons 2 days after infection, when compared to traditional HSV-1 amplicons, AAV or adenovirus (AdV) vectors, at the same multiplicity of infection. Only hybrid vectors containing the AAV Rep gene maintained the 2-day level of transgenic expression over 12 days in culture. The Rep containing vector was then tested for efficiency and safety in the brain, after inoculation into adult rat striatum. One month after injection, GFP expression was observed within the striatum and the substantia nigra, with efficacy similar or higher than classic amplicons. No immune response was observed using this system.

Behavioral Studies

A short but very interesting group of studies showed that gene delivering using amplicons could be successfully employed to modify behavioral traits in experimental models of memory, learning and anxiety. A first work demonstrated that amplicons mediating NGF expression in the hippocampus paralleled enhanced spatial learning in mice (71). This phenotype requires the integrity of the NGF-responsive septohippocampal pathway, and loss of a single NGF allele reduces levels of NGF and of NGF-regulated cholinergic neurotransmitter enzymes, resulting in spatial learning deficits. Amplicons were used to locally deliver NGF to the hippocampus of mice heterozygous (ngf $+/-$) or wild type (ngf $+/+$) at the NGF locus. Though transient increase in NGF levels and choline acetyltransferase activity was observed in both types of mice, spatial learning capability was improved only in the heterozygous (ngf $+/-$) mice. These results suggest that amplicon-expressed NGF can correct spatial learning deficits in subjects with baseline septohippocampal dysfunction.

To investigate the role of protein kinase C (PKC) pathways in hippocampal mediated learning, the catalytic domain of rat PKC betaII was amplicon-delivered into hippocampal dentate granule neurons (72). Interestingly, activation through amplicon infection of PKC pathways in a small percentage of dentate granule neurons was sufficient to enhance auditory discrimination reversal learning. Furthermore, this study showed that the affected neurons altered hippocampal physiology, as revealed by elevated glutamate NMDA receptor densities in specific areas of the hippocampus.

Amplicons expressing the NR1 subunit of the NMDA receptor, either in sense or antisense orientations, as well as GFP, were inoculated into the dorsal rat hippocampus of adult male rats, which were then trained for habituation to an open field and for inhibitory avoidance to a foot-shock (73,74). The animals injected with control amplicons expressing GFP, or with amplicons expressing NR1 protein showed no deficit in habituation to a new environment and achieved the criteria for a step-down avoidance of foot-shock. In contrast, animals injected with the vectors expressing the antisense NR1 sequences showed neither habituation nor appropriate performance in the inhibitory avoidance task, whereas there was no evidence for motor impairment or motivational disturbance. These results suggest that the impaired performance might be due to either retrograde amnesia or disability to record events. Transgenic GFP expression in brain was mainly observed in pyramidal cells of CA1, but also in CA3. These results therefore suggest the participation of NR1 subunit in habituation to a new environment, but also in recording events for the inhibitory avoidance tasks.

In the only study that did not address the hippocampus, amplicons were used to induce overexpression of the 5-HT(1B) receptor in rat dorsal raphe nucleus (DRN) (75). The 5-HT(1B) autoreceptors, which regulate serotonin release from DRN projections throughout forebrain, have been implicated in animal models of stress. The amplicons used in this study express an hemagglutinin-tagged form of this receptor and GFP, driven from a separate transcription unit, to assist in monitoring infection and expression. When injected stereotaxically into rat DRN, HA-5HT(1B) receptors were expressed in serotonergic neurons and translocated to the forebrain. Control animals received amplicons expressing GFP only. HA-5HT(1B) expression significantly reduced entrances into the central region of an open field arena after water-restraint stress, without altering overall locomotor activity, but not in the absence of stress exposure. HA-5HT(1B) expression also reduced entries into the open arms of the elevated plus maze after water restraint. Since these tests are sensitive to increases in anxiety-like behavior, these results suggest that overactivity of 5HT(1B) autoreceptors in DRN neurons may be an important mediator of pathological responses to stressful events.

CONCLUSION AND PERSPECTIVES

To summarize, amplicon vectors can be safely and efficiently used for gene transfer to cultured neural cells and nerve tissues of animal models and have proven useful for the genetic manipulation of the nerve system in very different experimental situations. Furthermore, the improvements in our ability to produce high amounts of relatively high-titre vectors, as well as the demonstration that amplicons can be effectively used to transduce very large genomic sequences, will certainly increase the interest on these vectors. However, amplicons have not yet reached the clinic. This is due, at least in part, to residual difficulties in preparing very large amounts of purified vectors with the required quality level. We also need more information regarding the intensity and the architecture of the innate and specific immune responses elicited by amplicons in the nerve system, as well as a better understanding of factors controlling vector stability and transgene expression from helper-free vectors in neurons and glial cells. Achieving these goals is the next dream that, we hope, will be brought into reality in the next years (76).

ACKNOWLEDGMENTS

ALE would like to acknowledge AFM (Association Française contre les Myopathies) and ARC (Association pour la Recherche sur le Cancer) for continuous support to his laboratory.

REFERENCES

1. Roizman B, Knipe DM. Herpes simplex viruses and their replication. In: Knipe DM, Howley PM, eds. Fields Virology Vol. 2. Philadelphia, PA: Lippincot, Williams and Wilkins, 2001: 2399–2460.
2. Spaete RR, Frenkel N. The herpes simplex virus amplicon: a new eucaryotic defective-virus cloning-amplifying vector. Cell 1982; 30:295–304.
3. Geller AI, Keyomarsi K, Bryan J, Pardee AB. An efficient deletion mutant packaging system for defective herpes simplex virus vectors; potential applications to human gene therapy and neuronal physiology. Proc Natl Acad Sci USA 1990; 87:8950–8954.
4. Saeki Y, Ichikawa T, Saeki A, et al. Herpes simplex virus type 1 DNA amplified as bacterial artificial chromosomes in Escherichia coli: rescue of replication-competent virus progeny and packaging of amplicon vectors. Hum Gene Ther 1998; 9:2787–2794.
5. Saeki Y, Fraefel C, Ichikawa T, Breakefield XO, Chiocca EA. Improved helper virus-free packaging system for HSV amplicon vectors using an ICP27-deleted, oversized HSV-1 DNA in bacterial artificial chromosome. Mol Ther 2001; 3:591–601.
6. Zaupa C, Revol-Guyot V, Epstein AL. Improved packaging system for generation of high-level non-cytotoxic HSV-1 amplicon vectors using Cre-loxP site-specific recombination to delete the packaging signals of defective helper genomes. Hum Gen Ther 2003; 14:1049–1063.
7. Logvinoff C, Epstein AL. Intracellular Cre-mediated deletion of the unique packaging signal carried by a herpes simplex virus type 1 recombinant and its relationship to the cleavage-packaging process. J Virol 2000; 74:8402–8412.
8. Logvinoff C, Epstein AL. A novel approach for herpes simplex virus type 1 amplicon production, using the Cre-loxP recombination system to remove helper virus. Hum Gen Ther 2001; 12:161–167.
9. Wade-Martins R, Smith ER, Tyminski E, Chiocca AE, Saeki Y. An infectious transfer and expression system for genomic DNA loci in human and mouse cells. Nat Biotechnol 2001; 19:1067–1070.
10. Wang S, Voss J-MH. A hybrid herpesvirus infectious vector based on Epstein-Barr virus and herpes simplex virus type 1 for gene transfer into human cells in vitro and in vivo. J Virol 1996; 70:8422–8430.

11. Inoue R, Moghaddam KA, Ranasinghe M, Saeki Y, Chiocca EA and Wade-Martins R. Infectious delivery of the 132 kb CDKN2A/CDKN2B genomic DNA region results in correctly spliced gene expression and growth suppression in glioma cells. Gene Ther advanced online publication 2004.

12. Kwong AD, Frenkel N. The herpes simplex virus amplicon IV. Efficient expression of a chimeric chicken ovalbumin gene amplified within defective virus genomes. Virology 1985; 142:421–425.

13. Geller AI, Breakefield XO. A defective HSV-1 vector expresses Escherichia coli beta-galactosidase in cultured peripheral neurons. Science 1988; 241:1667–1669.

14. Freese A, Geller AI. Infection of cultured striatal neurons with a defective HSV-1 vector: implications for gene therapy. NAR 1991; 19:7219–7223.

15. Geller AI, Freese A. Infection of cultured central nervous system neurons with a defective herpes simplex virus 1 vector results in stable expression of Escherichia coli beta-galactosidase. Proc Natl Acad Sci USA 1990; 87:1149–1153.

16. Geller AI. A system, using neural cell lines, to characterize HSV-1 vectors containing genes which affect neuronal physiology or neural promoters. J Neurosci Methods 1991; 36:91–103.

17. Bahr BA, Neve RL, Sharp J, Geller AI, Lynch G. Rapid and stable gene expression in hippocampal slice cultures from a defective HSV-1 vector. Brain Res Mol Brain Res 1994; 26:277–285.

18. Casaccia-Bonnefil P, Benedikz E, Shen H, et al. Localized gene transfer into organotypic hippocampal slice cultures and acute hippocampal slices. J Neurosci Methods 1993; 50:341–351.

19. Kaplitt MG, Pfaus J, Kleopoulos S, Hanlon B, Rabkin S, Pfaff D. Expression of a foreign gene in adult mammalian brain following in vivo transfer via a herpes simplex virus type 1 viral vector. Mol Cell Neurosci 1991; 2:320–330.

20. Federoff HJ, Geschwind MD, Geller AI, Kessler JA. Expression of nerve growth factor in vivo from a defective herpes simplex virus 1 vector prevents effects of axotomy on sympathetic ganglia. Proc Natl Acad Sci USA 1992; 89:1636–1640.

21. Battleman DS, Geller AI, Chao MV. HSV-1 vector-mediated gene transfer of the human nerve growth factor receptor p75hNGFR defines high affinity NGF binding. J Neurosci 1993; 13:941–951.

22. Bergold PJ, Casaccia-Bonnefil P, Zeng XL, Federoff HJ. Transsynaptic neuronal loss induced in hippocampal slice cultures by a herpes simplex virus vector expressing the GluR6 subunit of the kainate receptor. Proc Natl Acad Sci USA 1993; 90:6165–6169.

23. Geschwind MD, Kessler JA, Geller AI, Federoff HJ. Transfer of nerve growth factor gene into cell lines and cultured neurons using a defective herpes simplex virus vector. Brain Res Mol Brain Res 1994; 24:327–335.

24. Ho DY, Mocarski ES, Sapolsky RM. Altering central nervous system physiology with a defective herpes simplex virus vector expressing the glucose transporter gene. Proc Natl Acad Sci USA 1993; 90:3655–3659.

25. Neve RL, Ivins KJ, Benowitz LI, During MJ, Geller AI. Molecular analysis of the function of the neuronal growth-associated protein GAP-43 by genetic intervention. Mol Neurobiol 1991; 5:131–141.

26. Lowenstein PR, Fournel S, Bain D, et al. Herpes simplex virus 1 (HSV-1) helper co-infection affects the distribution of an amplicon encoded protein in glia. Neuroreport 1994; 5:1625–1630.

27. Lowenstein PR, Fournel S, Bain D, et al. Simultaneous detection of amplicon and HSV-1 helper encoded proteins reveals that neurons and astrocytoma cells do express amplicon-borne transgenes in the absence of virus immediate-early proteins. Brain Res Mol Brain Res 1995; 30:169–175.

28. Fraefel C, Song S, Lim F, et al. Helper virus-free transfer of herpes simplex virus type 1 plasmid vectors into neural cells. J Virol 1996; 70:7190–7197.

29. Olschowka JA, Bowers WJ, Hurley SD, Mastrangelo MA, Federoff HJ. Helper-free HSV-1 amplicons elicit a markedly less robust innate immune response in the CNS. Mol Ther 2003; 7:18–27.

30. Smith RL, Geller AI, Escudero KW, Wilcox CL. Long-term expression in sensory neurons in tissue culture from herpes simplex virus type 1 (HSV-1) promoters in an HSV-1-derived vector. J Virol 1995; 69:4593–4599.

31. Ho DY, McLaughlin JR, Sapolsky RM. Inducible gene expression from defective herpes simplex virus vectors using the tetracycline-responsive promoter system. Brain Res Mol Brain Res 1996; 41:200–209.

32. Kaplitt MG, Kwong AD, Kleopoulos S, Mobs CV, Rabkin SD, Pfaff DW. Preproenkephalin promoter yields region-specific and long-term expression in adult rat brain after direct in vivo gene transfer via a defective herpes simplex viral vector. Proc Natl Acad Sci USA 1994; 91:8979–8983.

33. Oh YJ, Moffat M, Wong S, Ullrey D, Geller AI, O'Malley KL. A herpes simplex virus-1 vector containing the rat tyrosine hydroxylase promoter directs cell type-specific expression of beta-galactosidase in cultured rat peripheral neurons. Brain Res Mol Brain Res 1996; 35:227–236.

34. Jin BK, Belloni M, Conti B, et al. Prolonged in vivo gene expression driven by a tyrosine hydroxylase promoter in a defective herpes simplex virus amplicon vector. Hum Gene Ther 1996; 7:2015–2024.

35. Song S, Wang Y, Bak SY, et al. An HSV-1 vector containing the rat tyrosine hydroxylase promoter enhances long-term and cell-type specific expression in the midbrain. J Neurochem 1997; 68:1792–1803.

36. Zhang GR, Wang X, Yang T, et al. A tyrosine hydroxylase-neurofilament chimeric promoter enhances long-term expression in rat forebrains neurons from helper virus-free HSV-1 vectors. Brain Res Mol Brain Res 2000; 84:17–31.

37. Wang Y, Lu L, Geller AI. Diverse stabilities of expression in the rat brain from different cellular promoters in a helper virus-free herpes simplex virus type 1 vector system. Hum Gene Ther 1999; 10:1763–1771.

38. Wade-Martins R, Saeki Y, Chiocca EA. Infectious delivery of a 135-kb LDLR genomic locus leads to regulated complementation of low-density lipoprotein receptor deficiency in human cells. Mol Ther 2003; 7:604–612.

39. Pakzaban P, Geller AI, Isacson O. Effect of exogenous nerve growth factor on neurotoxicity of and neuronal gene delivery by a herpes simplex amplicon vector in the rat brain. Hum Gene Ther 1994; 5:987–995.

40. Geschwind MD, Hartnick CJ, Liu W, Amat J, Van de Water TR, Federoff HJ. Defective HSV-1 vector expressing BDNF in auditory ganglia elicits neurite outgrowth: model for treatment of neuron loss following cochlear degeneration. Hum Gene Ther 1996; 7:173–182.

41. Staecker H, Gabaizadeh R, Federoff H, Van de Water TR. Brain-derived neurotrophic factor gene therapy prevents spiral ganglion degeneration after hair cell loss. Otolaryngol Head Neck Surg 1998; 119:7–13.

42. Garrido JJ, Alonso MT, Lim F, Carnicero E, Giraldez F, Shimmang T. Defining responsiveness of avian cochlear neurons to brain-derived neurotrophic factor and nerve growth factor by HSV-1 immediate-early gene transfer. J Neurochem 1998; 70:2336–2346.

43. Chen X, Frisina RD, Bowers WJ, Frisina DR, Federoff HJ. HSV amplicon-mediated Neurotrophin-3 expression protects murine spiral ganglion neurons from cisplatin-induced damage. Mol Ther 2001; 3:958–963.

44. Bowers WJ, Chen X, Guo H, Frisina DR, Federoff HJ, Frisina RD. Neurotrophin-3 transduction attenuates cisplatin spiral ganglion neuron ototoxicity in the cochlea. Mol Ther 2002; 6:12–18.

45. Harvey BK, Chang CF, Chiang YH, et al. HSV amplicon delivery of glial cell line-derived neurotrophic factor is neuroprotective against ischemic injury. Exp Neurol 2003; 183:47–55.

46. Linnik MD, Zahos P, Geschwind MD, Federoff HJ. Expression of bcl-2 from a defective herpes simples virus-1 vector limits neuronal death in focal cerebral ischemia. Stroke 1995; 26:1670–1675.

47. Antonawich FJ, Federoff HJ, Davis JN. BCL-2 transduction using a herpes simplex virus amplicon protects hippocampal neurons from transient global ischemia. Exp Neurol 1999; 156:130–137.

48. Lawrence MS, McLaughlin JR, Sun GH, et al. Herpes simplex viral vectors expressing Bcl-2 are neuroprotective when delivered after a stroke. J Cereb Flow Metab 1997; 17:740–744.

49. Lawrence MS, Ho DY, Steinberg GK, Sapolsky RM. Overexpression of Bcl-2 with herpes simplex virus vectors protects CNS neurons against neurological insults in vitro and in vivo. J Neurosci 1996; 16:486–496.

50. Roy M, Hom JJ, Sapolsy RM. HSV-mediated delivery of virally derived anti-apoptotic genes protects the rat hippocampus from damage following exocytotoxicity, but not metabolic disruption. Gene Ther 2002; 9:214–219.

51. Hoehn B, Ringer TM, Xu L, et al. Overexpression of HSP72 after induction of experimental stroke protects neurons from ischemic damage. J Cereb Blood Flow Metab 2001; 21:1303–1309.

52. Kelly S, Zhanf ZJ, Zhao H, et al. Gene transfer of HSP72 protects cornu ammonis 1 region of the hippocampus neurons from global ischemia: influence of Bcl-2. Ann Neurol 2002; 52:160–167.

53. Wang H, Cheng E, Brooke S, Chang P, Sapolsky R. Over-expression of antioxidant enzymes protects cultured hippocampal and cortical neurons from necrotic insults. J Neurochem 2003; 87:1527–1534.

54. Lamigeon C, Prod'Hon C, De Frias V, Michoudet C, Jacquemont B. Enhancement of neuronal protection from oxidative stress by glutamic acid decarboxylase delivery with a defective herpes simplex virus vector. Exp Neurol 2003; 184:381–392.

55. Lawrence MS, Ho DY, Dash R, Sapolsky RM. Herpes simplex virus vectors overexpressing the glucose transporter gene protects against seizure-induced neuron loss. Proc Natl Acad Sci USA 1995; 92:7247–7251.

56. Ho DY, Saydam TC, Fink SL, Lawrence MS, Sapolsky RM. Defective herpes simplex virus vectors expressing the rat brain glucose transporter protect cultured neurons from necrotic insults. J Neurochem 1995; 65:842–850.

57. Phillips RG, Meier TJ, Giuli LC, McLaughlin JR, Ho DY, Sapolsky RM. Calbindin D28K gene transfer via herpes simplex virus amplicon vector decreases hippocampal damage in vivo following neurotoxic insults. J Neurochem 1999; 73:1200–1205.

58. Hartley DM, Neve RL, Bryan J, et al. Expression of the calcium-binding protein parvalbumin, in cultured cortical neurons using a HSV-1 vector system enhances NMDA neurotoxicity. Brain Res Mol Brain Res 1996; 40:285–296.

59. Rainov NG, Sena-Esteves M, Fraefel C, Dobberstein KU, Chiocca EA, Breakefield XO. A chimeric fusion protein of cytochrome CYP4B1 and green fluorescent protein for detection of pro-drug activating gene delivery and for gene therapy in malignant glioma. Adv Exp Med Biol 1998; 451:393–403.

60. Herrlinger U, Jacobs A, Quinones A, et al. Helper virus-free helper simplex virus type 1 amplicon vectors for granulocyte-macrophage colony-stimulating factor-enhanced vaccination therapy for experimental glioma. Hum Gene Ther 2000; 11:1429–1438.

61. Shah K, Tang Y, Breakefield XO, Weissleder R. Real-time imaging of TRAIL-induced apoptosis of glioma tumors in vivo. Oncogene 2003; 22:6865–6872.

62. Johnston KM, Jacoby D, Pechan PA, et al. HSV-1/AAV hybrid amplicon vectors extend transgene expression in human glioma cells. Hum Gene Ther 1997; 10:359–370.

63. Lam P, Hui KM, Wang Y, et al. Dynamics of transgene expression in human glioblastoma cells mediated by herpes simplex virus/adeno-associated virus amplicon vectors. Hum Gene Ther 2002; 13:2147–2159.

64. Pechan PA, Herrlinger U, Aghi M, Jacobs A, Breakefield XO. Combined HSV-1 recombinant and amplicon piggyback vectors: replication-competent and defective forms, and therapeutic efficacy for experimental gliomas. J Gene Med 1999; 1:176–185.

65. Ho IA, Hui KM, Lam PY. Glioma-specific and cell cycle-regulated herpes simplex virus type 1 amplicon viral vector. Hum Gene Ther 2004; 15:495–508.

66. During MJ, Naegele JR, O'Malley KL, Geller AI. Long-term behavioural recovery in parkinsonian rats by an HSV vector expressing tyrosine hydroxylase. Science 1994; 266:1399–1403.

67. Geller AI, During MJ, Oh YJ, Fresse A, O'Malley K. An HSV-1 vector expressing tyrosine hydroxylase causes production and release of L-DOPA from cultured rat striatal cells. J Neurochem 1995; 64:487–496.
68. Song S, Wang Y, Bak SY, et al. Modulation of rat rotational behavior by direct gene transfer of constitutively active proteine kinase C into nigrostriatal neurons. J Neurosci 1998; 18:4119–4132.
69. Sun M, Zhang GR, Kong L, et al. Correction of a rat model of Parkinson's disease by coepression of tyrosine hydroxylase and aromatic amino acid decarboxylase from a helper virus-free herpes simplex virus type 1 vector. Human Gene Ther 2003; 14:415–424.
70. Costantini LC, Jacoby DR, Wang S, Fraefel C, Breakefield XO, Isakson O. Gene transfer to the nigrostriatal system by hybrid herpes simplex virus/adeno-associated virus amplicon vectors. Hum Gene Ther 1999; 10:2481–2494.
71. Brooks AI, Cory-Slechta DA, Bowers WJ, Murg SL, Federoff HJ. Enhanced learning in mice parallels vector-mediated nerve growth factor expression in hippocampus. Hum Gene Ther 2000; 11:2341–2352.
72. Neill JC, Sarkisian MR, Wang Y, et al. Enhanced auditory reversal learning by genetic activation of protein kinase C in small groups of rat hippocampal neurons. Brain Res Mol Brain Res 2001; 93:127–136.
73. Adrover M, Revol-Guyot V, Cheli V, et al. Hippocampal infection with HSV-1-derived vectors expressing a NMDAR1 antisense modifies behavior. Genes Brain Behav 2003; 2:103–113.
74. Cheli VT, Adrover MF, Blanco C, et al. Gene transfer of NMDAR1 subunit sequences to the rat CNS using herpes simplex virus vectors interfered with habituation. Cell Mol Neurobiol 2002; 3:303–314.
75. Clark MS, Sexton TJ, McClain M, Root D, Kohen R, Neumaier JF. Overexpression of 5-HT1B receptor in dorsal raphe nucleus using herpes simplex virus gene transfer increases anxiety behaviour after inescapable stress. J Neurosci 2002; 22:4550–4562.
76. Antunes-Bras J, Epstein AL, Bourgoin S, Hamon M, Cesselin F, Pohl M. Herpes simplex virus 1-mediated transfer of preproenkephalin A in rat dorsal root ganglia. J Neurochem 1998; 70:1299–1303.

3

Adeno Associated Viral Vectors for the Nervous System

Brian K. Kaspar
Department of Gene Therapy and Neuromuscular Research, Columbus Children's Research Institute and Department of Pediatrics, The Ohio State University, Columbus, Ohio, U.S.A.

Fred H. Gage
The Salk Institute for Biological Studies, La Jolla, California, U.S.A.

The realization of gene therapy for the central nervous system has advanced to the realms of clinical practice. The brain and spinal cord, once inaccessible to certain therapies, have been unlocked by gene therapy vectors allowing medical practitioners to target areas of the brain in a manner never before attainable. For example, certain vectors can target tumors, replicate in those cells, and deliver toxic substances to rid the brain of cancers. Also, we can now deliver genes to certain cell types of the brain and allow continuous gene delivery, delivering a therapeutic gene to the exact cells that are perishing in neurological disorders or injury. These discoveries have advanced the concept of gene therapy for the nervous system to a clinical reality.

This review will focus on one of the most promising vectors to date for nervous system gene therapy, the adeno-associated virus (AAV) and its development towards clinical practice.

ADENO ASSOCIATED VIRUS FOR NERVOUS SYSTEM GENE THERAPY

In recent years, a viral vector has been developed that satisfies many of the requirements of an "ideal" gene therapy vector. An ideal gene therapy vector will be safe, non-toxic, and replication incompetent. It will be capable of expressing a transgene long term, of infecting multiple cell types, and of expressing small and large transgenes. AAV has recently been shown to be an attractive, safe vector for gene therapy and has demonstrated long-term gene expression in the brain with no associated immune response (1,2).

AAV is a single-stranded DNA virus that is packaged as a plus and a minus strand. The parental wild-type virus is defective and requires helper functions from other viruses such as Adenovirus (AdV) or Herpes Simplex Virus (HSV) to complete the viral life cycle of rescuing, replicating, and packaging new progeny virions (3,4). Recombinant vectors based on AAV have all the viral sequences eliminated except the 145-bp inverted terminal repeats (ITRs). The removal of all viral sequences provides a significant safety advantage that prevents the generation of wild-type helper virus and also minimizes the possibility of immune reactions caused by viral gene expression that other recombinant viral vector systems experience. Therefore, the potential for vector replication and spread is minimized because a recombinant infected cell would require two separate hits from wild-type virus and AdV to initiate replication. More importantly, AAV is nonpathogenic and has no etiology association with any known diseases (5). Although wild-type AAV integrates specifically into human chromosome 19, recombinant vectors do not have this specific integration site (6,7). The integration capability of recombinant AAV vectors into the genome has been shown, although the quantification and role of genomic integration versus stable episomal concatamer forms on long-term expression have yet to be discerned (8).

In the early 1990s, brain studies utilizing AAV vectors were initiated to develop therapies for neurodegenerative diseases. An initial study showed neuron-selective gene expression from an AAV vector containing the cytomegalovirus promoter (9). Many studies have shown substantial promise using AAV in the nervous system to efficiently target neurons in multiple regions (1,10–13). The rapid uptake of virus exclusively in neurons was recently shown by labeling AAV virions with fluorescent molecules, indicating that AAV was suitable for transgene expression in neurons (14). Recent pre-clinical successes utilizing AAV have been shown for a number of neurodegenerative diseases, including Parkinson's disease, Alzheimer's disease, and spinal cord injury (9,15–19). Additionally, AAV has been successfully used to express therapeutic genes in the brains of primates (20,21).

Direct injection of a virus into various regions of the brain has shown great promise in a number of pre-clinical studies. Efficiently targeting projection neurons that are affected in many disease states has been difficult, however, because the broad anatomical distribution of these neurons and their relative inaccessibility have made local delivery difficult. Numerous strategies have been used in attempts to target specific cell types such as neurons. For example, certain types of viruses have been pseudotyped to allow them to infect a particular population of cells (18,22). Another approach to target specific cells utilizes promoters that are specific for expression in a particular cell type (23,24). For example, the neuron-specific enolase promoter has been used to direct transgene expression in the brain and spinal cord (11,25). However, these approaches have not been successful in efficiently targeting areas beyond the injection site. Since multiple injections are cumbersome and may not completely target entire neuronal projection pathways, the use of retrograde transport of the therapeutic agent warrants further investigation. To date, gene therapy studies have only used AdV, HSV, and pseudo-rabies virus for delivering transgenes in a targeted retrograde delivery strategy (26–29). In fact, a gene-delivery method using retrograde axonal transport of adenoviral vectors has been proposed to overexpress therapeutic proteins in motorneurons after intramuscular (i.m.) injections of these vectors (1,30). Despite the denervation and impairment of axonal transport discovered in mouse models of ALS, there is an improvement in axonal retrograde transport of AdV following the onset of the disease as well as the demonstration of increased uptake properties of MNs in response to botulinum neurotoxin treatment (31,32). While these studies have shown very encouraging results targeting large number of cells by utilizing the transport properties of the virus, AdV, HSV, and pseudo-rabies virus all cause immune responses resulting in transient transgene expression. Recently, our laboratory has discovered a unique property of AAV vectors: they are efficiently transported in the nervous system in a retrograde manner. There have been numerous reports that AAV vectors of any serotype are not retrogradely transported or are transported only in a limited fashion (10–12). Our laboratory has studied some potential mechanisms of viral transport within the nervous system and also utilized a retrograde delivery approach to efficiently deliver a therapeutic anti-apoptotic gene to prevent cell death in an Alzheimer's disease model. Further support for AAV retrograde transport is also gaining attention (33–36). Recently, the strategy of retrograde transport has been incorporated into lentiviral vectors by rabies virus glycoprotein that is showing great promise (37,38). The ability to target areas within the nervous system by a safe, long-term expressing vector such as AAV or pseudotyped lentiviral vectors may permit development of more efficient delivery strategies to target diseased areas within the brain.

ADENO ASSOCIATED VIRUS PRODUCTION AND PURIFICATION

AAV vectors can be produced in very high titers. Many laboratories are now able to generate substantial AAV titers between 10^{12}–10^{13} viral particles/ml with low particle to transduction ratios. Production of virus is usually performed by transient cotransfection of two plasmids. The vector plasmid contains the foreign transgene that is flanked by the AAV 145 bp ITRs, which are the only cis-elements necessary for AAV DNA replication, packaging, and integration. The second helper plasmid provides in trans the AAV genes; *rep* for viral DNA replication and *cap* for encapsidation. Subsequent infection with a helper virus such as AdV or HSV activates the helper plasmid that provides *rep* and *cap* to excise, replicate, and package the rAAV DNA from the vector plasmid, resulting in AAV virions containing the therapeutic gene. Vector production has been substantially improved by eliminating the requirements of helper AdV for virus production. An AdV-free production method was recently developed utilizing a plasmid construct that contains a mini-AdV genome capable of propagating AAV in the presence of the AAV *rep* and *cap* gene. The adenoviral construct was designed to be devoid of some of the early and most of the late AdV genes and is, therefore, incapable of producing infectious AdV. This development significantly simplified the production process and may provide a more defined reagent for clinical use (39). Another recent advance in the production process has been the development of column chromatography for purifying viral particles. Following gradient centrifugation by cesium chloride or iodixanol, viral preparations have been further purified on a heparin/agarose column utilizing the recent finding that AAV binds to a heparin sulfate proteoglycan cell surface molecule. The virus is then eluted in high salt, concentrated, and dialyzed. These recent advancements have allowed greater purity, consistency, and convenience of AAV vectors.

CLINICAL DEVELOPMENT OF AAV VECTORS

In pre-clinical studies, a disease target is identified and therapeutic factors tested usually in the context of an animal model of the disease for delaying disease onset or progression, correcting a genetic defect or delaying/curing the disease. Once a candidate therapy is identified, a plethora of activities are initiated to advance the gene therapy into the clinic.

To enter a clinical trial, an Investigational New Drug Application (IND) must be filed with the Food and Drug Administration. Within this application, detailed information is provided; including the preclinical data along with manufacturing/virus testing processes, pharmacology, toxicology, and biodistribution data with Phase I clinical trial plans outlined. The initial goals for entering the clinic in a Phase I clinical trial are to ensure that the product is safe. These safety studies will provide information that will ultimately be used for product labeling. Among the important studies to be performed are safety pharmacology and toxicology assessments.

Safety pharmacology tests the effects of the virus and gene on vital functions such as the cardiovascular, central nervous system, and respiratory system of animals. In tandem, a toxicology program is required to determine the safety of gene therapy agents and to provide information for the eventual product label used to communicate any possible risks to the prescribing physician. Toxicology programs for a gene therapy vector are somewhat different than the small molecule drugs developed by pharmaceutical companies. Gene therapy vectors are more complex in design such that the gene product itself, as well as the vector system used for gene delivery is tested in the context of the application for the clinical trial for potential toxicities. Biodistribution studies are performed to identify where the gene therapy product is distributed within the body after administration. Typically, a time course for evaluating target organs for vector persistence is performed. A major evaluation of the gene therapy product determines whether the vector has integrated into the germline.

The final goal is the preparation and submission of the IND to the Food and Drug Administration/Center for Biologics Evaluation and Research including the Division of Cell and Gene Therapies and Division of Clinical Trial Design and Analysis. A major portion of the IND submission includes sections related to Chemistry, Manufacturing and Control Information (CMC) describing the composition, manufacture and control of the product as well as labeling. Within the CMC, extensive details need to be documented. An example of the required sections are; (1) a detailed description of the cells used for production, (2) the cell culturing conditions, (3) cell storage and cell banking conditions, (4) cell stability issues, (5) safety and identity testing procedures (addressing genetic, phenotypic and viability measures), (6) thorough description of the vector including the sequence and vector map, (7) detailed history on the derivation of the construct, and (8) other reagents used during manufacturing process. Furthermore, product testing will include product characterization, specifically focusing on safety including sterility, mycoplasma clearance, pyrogenicity/endotoxin clearance, and freedom from adventitious agents, including in vitro and in vivo viral testing, species specific viral testing and replication competent virus (RCV) testing. The product will be characterized for identity, purity, potency, stability, and the development of specifications for ultimate licensure and labeling of the product. An IRB approved consent form is also included. The remainder of the IND includes the detailed clinical protocols, study design, patient monitoring and endpoint evaluations for the trial.

In summary, the information obtained above will provide the basis for IND filing and subsequent initiation of a Phase I clinical trial testing the safety, tolerability, and potential efficacy in human patients.

CONCLUSION

As we move forward with understanding the complexities of gene function within the nervous system and the role of genetics in human disease, the nervous system represents the opportunity for many therapeutic applications. Many diseases of the nervous system are localized to distinct regions of the brain, such as the spinal cord in ALS, the substantia nigra in Parkinson's, and the striatum in Huntington's. Not only will we have to focus on the disease pathways, but we will have to develop safer and more effective ways to target therapies to the defined cellular populations, sometimes requiring multiple populations of cells for therapeutic delivery. For example, in ALS, it appears that astrocytes are playing a role in disease pathogenesis in addition to motor neuron degeneration. New basic research will allow for new targets and cell types for optimal therapeutic development.

The costs for the development of gene therapy vectors are extremely high mainly due to the vast development and regulatory costs incurred for safety studies. The costs of today's research include the lessons learned that will allow for more efficient and less costly studies to be done in the future. Indeed we are at a pioneering time in gene therapy.

REFERENCES

1. Xiao X, Li J, McCown TJ, Samulski RJ. Gene transfer by adeno-associated virus vectors into the central nervous system. Exp Neurol 1997; 144:113–124.
2. Kaspar BK, Vissel B, Bengoechea T, et al. Adeno-associated virus effectively mediates conditional gene modification in the brain. Proc Natl Acad Sci USA 2002; 99:2320–2325.
3. Atchison RW, Casto BC, Hammon WM. Adenovirus-associated defective virus particles. Science 1965; 149:754–756.
4. Buller RM, Janik JE, Sebring ED, Rose JA. Herpes simplex virus types 1 and 2 completely help adenovirus-associated virus replication. J Virol 1981; 40:241–247.
5. Berns KI, Bohenzky RA. Adeno-associated viruses: an update. Adv Virus Res 1987; 32:243–306.
6. Kotin RM, Siniscalco M, Samulski RJ, et al. Site-specific integration by adeno-associated virus. Proc Natl Acad Sci USA 1990; 87:2211–2215.
7. Samulski RJ, Zhu X, Xiao X, et al. Targeted integration of adeno-associated virus (AAV) into human chromosome 19. EMBO J 1991; 10:3941–3950.
8. Weitzman MD, Young SM, Jr., Cathomen T, Samulski RJ. Targeted integration by adeno-associated virus. Methods Mol Med 2003; 76:201–219.
9. Kaplitt MG, Leone P, Samulski RJ, et al. Long-term gene expression and phenotypic correction using adeno-associated virus vectors in the mammalian brain. Nat Genet 1994; 8:148–154.
10. Chamberlin NL, Du B, de Lacalle S, Saper CB. Recombinant adeno-associated virus vector: use for transgene expression and anterograde tract tracing in the CNS. Brain Res 1998; 793:169–175.
11. Klein RL, Meyer EM, Peel AL, et al. Neuron-specific transduction in the rat septohippocampal or nigrostriatal pathway by recombinant adeno-associated virus vectors. Exp Neurol 1998; 150:183–194.
12. Davidson BL, Stein CS, Heth JA, et al. Recombinant adeno-associated virus type 2, 4, and 5 vectors: transduction of variant cell types and regions in the mammalian central nervous system. Proc Natl Acad Sci USA 2000; 97:3428–3432.
13. McCown TJ, Xiao X, Li J, Breese GR, Samulski RJ. Differential and persistent expression patterns of CNS gene transfer by an adeno-associated virus (AAV) vector. Brain Res 1996; 713:99–107.
14. Bartlett JS, Samulski RJ, McCown TJ. Selective and rapid uptake of adeno-associated virus type 2 in brain. Hum Gene Ther 1998; 9:1181–1186.
15. Bjorklund A, Kirik D, Rosenblad C, Georgievska B, Lundberg C, Mandel RJ. Towards a neuroprotective gene therapy for Parkinson's disease: use of adenovirus, AAV and lentivirus vectors for gene transfer of GDNF to the nigrostriatal system in the rat Parkinson model. Brain Res 2000; 886:82–98.
16. Mandel RJ, Spratt SK, Snyder RO, Leff SE. Midbrain injection of recombinant adeno-associated virus encoding rat glial cell line-derived neurotrophic factor protects nigral neurons in a progressive 6-hydroxydopamine-induced degeneration model of Parkinson's disease in rats. Proc Natl Acad Sci USA 1997; 94:14083–14088.
17. Klein RL, Hirko AC, Meyers CA, Grimes JR, Muzyczka N, Meyer EM. NGF gene transfer to intrinsic basal forebrain neurons increases cholinergic cell size and protects from age-related, spatial memory deficits in middle-aged rats. Brain Res 2000; 875:144–151.
18. Manning WC, Murphy JE, Jolly DJ, Mento SJ, Ralston RO. Use of a recombinant murine cytomegalovirus expressing vesicular stomatitis virus G protein to pseudotype retroviral vectors. J Virol Methods 1998; 73:31–39.

19. Peel AL, Klein RL. Adeno-associated virus vectors: activity and applications in the CNS. J Neurosci Methods 2000; 98:95–104.

20. During MJ, Samulski RJ, Elsworth JD, et al. In vivo expression of therapeutic human genes for dopamine production in the caudates of MPTP-treated monkeys using an AAV vector. Gene Ther 1998; 5:820–827.

21. Bankiewicz KS, Eberling JL, Kohutnicka M, et al. Convection-enhanced delivery of AAV vector in parkinsonian monkeys; in vivo detection of gene expression and restoration of dopaminergic function using pro-drug approach. Exp Neurol 2000; 164:2–14.

22. Kurre P, Morris J, Miller AD, Kiern HP. Envelope fusion protein binding studies in an inducible model of retrovirus receptor expression and in CD34(+) cells emphasize limited transduction at low receptor levels. Gene Ther 2001; 8:593–599.

23. Chen H, McCarty DM, Bruce AT, Suzuki K. Gene transfer and expression in oligodendrocytes under the control of myelin basic protein transcriptional control region mediated by adeno-associated virus. Gene Ther 1998; 5:50–58.

24. Millecamps S, Kiefer H, Navarro V, et al. Neuron-restrictive silencer elements mediate neuron specificity of adenoviral gene expression. Nat Biotechnol 1999; 17:865–869.

25. Peel AL, Zolotukhin S, Schrimsher GW, Muzyczka N, Reier PJ. Efficient transduction of green fluorescent protein in spinal cord neurons using adeno-associated virus vectors containing cell type-specific promoters. Gene Ther 1997; 4:16–24.

26. Choi-Lundberg DL, Lin Q, Schaller T, et al. Behavioral and cellular protection of rat dopaminergic neurons by an adenoviral vector encoding glial cell line-derived neurotrophic factor. Exp Neurol 1998; 154:261–275.

27. Hermens WT, Giger RJ, Holtmaat AJ, Dijkhuizen PA, Houweling DA, Verhaagen J. Transient gene transfer to neurons and glia: analysis of adenoviral vector performance in the CNS and PNS. J Neurosci Methods 1997; 71:85–98.

28. Soudais C, Laplace-Bulhc C, Kissa K, Kremer EJ. Preferential transduction of neurons by canine adenovirus vectors and their efficient retrograde transport in vivo. FASEB J 2001; 15:2283–2285.

29. Breakefield XO, DeLuca NA. Herpes simplex virus for gene delivery to neurons. New Biol 1991; 3:203–218.

30. Alisky JM, Hughes SM, Sauter SL, et al. Transduction of murine cerebellar neurons with recombinant FIV and AAV5 vectors. Neuroreport 2000; 11:2669–2673.

31. Summerford C, Samulski RJ. Membrane-associated heparan sulfate proteoglycan is a receptor for adeno-associated virus type 2 virions. J Virol 1998; 72:1438–1445.

32. Zolotukhin S, Byrne BJ, Mason E, et al. Recombinant adeno-associated virus purification using novel methods improves infectious titer and yield. Gene Ther 1999; 6:973–985.

33. Boulis NM, Willmarth NE, Song DK, Feldman EL, Imperiale MJ. Intraneural colchicine inhibition of adenoviral and adeno-associated viral vector remote spinal cord gene delivery. Neurosurgery 2003; 52:381–387 discussion 387.

34. Rubin AD, Hogikyan ND, Sullivan K, Boulis N, Feldman EL. Remote delivery of rAAV-GFP to the rat brainstem through the recurrent laryngeal nerve. Laryngoscope 2001; 111:2041–2045.

35. Paterna JC, Feldon J, Bueler H. Transduction profiles of recombinant adeno-associated virus vectors derived from serotypes 2 and 5 in the nigrostriatal system of rats. J Virol 2004; 78:6808–6817.

36. Burger C, Gorbatyuk OS, Velardo MJ, et al. Recombinant AAV viral vectors pseudotyped with viral capsids from serotypes 1, 2, and 5 display differential efficiency and cell tropism after delivery to different regions of the central nervous system. Mol Ther 2004; 10:302–317.

37. Mazarakis ND, Azzouz M, Rohll JB, et al. Rabies virus glycoprotein pseudotyping of lentiviral vectors enables retrograde axonal transport and access to the nervous system after peripheral delivery. Hum Mol Genet 2001; 10:2109–2121.

38. Azzouz M, Ralph GS, Storkebaum E, et al. VEGF delivery with retrogradely transported lentivector prolongs survival in a mouse ALS model. Nature 2004; 429:413–417.

39. Xiao X, Li J, Samulski RJ. Production of high-titer recombinant adeno-associated virus vectors in the absence of helper adenovirus. J Virol 1998; 72:2224–2232.

4

Heat Shock Proteins for Neurological Gene Therapy

Joanna Howarth, Stephen Kelly, and James B. Uney
Henry Wellcome Laboratories for Integrative Neuroscience and Endocrinology, University of Bristol, Bristol, U.K.

INTRODUCTION

Many human degenerative diseases are characterized by the progressive degeneration of neurons and accompanying production of abnormal intracellular inclusions. These inclusions are composed of once normal cellular proteins [e.g., neurofibrillary tangles in Alzheimer's disease (AD)] and are also generally found to contain the small heat shock protein (hsp's) ubiquitin and hsp70. These observations suggest that hsp's are associated with the etiology of these diseases, or that their up-regulation represents an unsuccessful attempt to remove the abnormal protein aggregates. A number of recent studies (and novel data presented in this review) have shown that the overexpression of hsp70 and/or hsp40 is neuroprotective for the polyglutamine disorders. Furthermore, genetic studies clearly show that abnormalities in the ubiquitin proteosome system (UPS) underlie some forms of Parkinson's disease (PD). These observations suggest that manipulating hsp expression to facilitate both the refolding and removal of abnormal proteins could be therapeutic for many human neurodegenerative conditions.

THE HEAT SHOCK RESPONSE

Background

The heat shock response (HSR), characterized by the increased expression of genes primarily involved with protein stabilization and metabolism, is a protection mechanism elicited by cells in reaction to noxious stimuli. The HSR was first defined in *Drosophila melanogoster* where it was reported that upon exposure to elevated temperatures the polytene chromosomes changed their pattern of chromosomal expansion due to the synthesis of mRNA's coding for "heat shock proteins" (hsp). It is now known that all cells respond to a sub-lethal heat shock by suppressing normal cellular transcription and translation and activating the transcription of hsp which buffer them from damage (1,2). Furthermore, cells not only induce the synthesis of hsps in response to a heat shock but also in response to exposure to a great variety of other metabolic challenges (e.g., ethanol, free radicals, excitotoxic challenge, viral infection, heavy metals and arsenic), (1,3,4) and hence the response is now sometimes referred to as a stress response and the proteins produced as stress proteins. The functions of hsp's have only recently been elucidated and hence remain named according to their molecular weight, the majority belonging to the 20, 30, 60, 70, 90, and 110 kDa hsp families. Furthermore, although referred to as hsp, many hsp's are actually constitutive and there is only a moderate increase in their expression following a stress. However, there is a rapid and much more dramatic increase in the synthesis of some inducible hsps and members of the hsp70 family are the most inducible and highly expressed. The induction of all hsp genes is due to the presence of specific DNA sequence elements located upstream of the $5'$-terminal of the gene. These heat shock elements (HSE) are consecutive arrays (of variable numbers) of the 5 base-pair sequence NGAAN arranged in altering orientation (N denotes less strongly conserved nucleotides). Induction of hsp gene transcription in response to stress is mediated by the binding of a transcriptional activator protein called the heat shock factor (HSF) to the HSE. The exact mechanism of HSR activation in neurons is still unclear. It is thought that pre-existing HSF exists in a non-active form when bound to hsp90 and/or highly inducible hsp70. However, damaged proteins produced by a cellular stress bind hsp70/90 with high affinity and thus mediate HSF release. Free HSF monomers then trimerise and translocate to the nucleus, whereupon they bind to the HSE and initiate the transcription of various hsp genes (Fig. 1). Misfolded proteins can then be eliminated by hsp's, either by refolding or degradation primarily via the UPS. The trimeric forms of HSF dissociate from the DNA and are converted back into nonactive monomers that bind to hsp70 family members, awaiting a subsequent heat shock (5).

Heat Shock Protein Function

The majority of hsp's function constitutively in the metabolically unstressed cell and are involved in multiple "housekeeping" roles to maintain cellular homeostasis. For example, hsp's ensure the correct folding of nascent polypeptide chains during protein translocation across organelle membranes. They also modulate protein activity by changing protein conformation and promoting multi-protein complex assembly or disassembly and also ensure the correct confirmation of inactive, unbound receptor proteins. Hsp's also play an active role in regulating protein degradation, directing misfolded or mutant proteins to proteolysis via the UPS (6). Generally the high molecular weight hsp chaperones (ranging from 50–100 kDa in size) assist in the folding of newly synthesized or damaged proteins in an active ATP-dependent process. The small hsp's (10–40 kDa) facilitate the actions of the hsp70 molecular chaperone family and/or can also sequester damaged proteins in an ATP-independent manner for refolding or digestion. A great deal of research to date has focused on the highly inducible hsp70 family of proteins that are thought to function to process nascent protein polypeptides or refold damaged or misfolded proteins (Fig. 2).

The hsp70 family constitutes the most conservative of the high molecular weight hsp's in both non-neuronal and neuronal systems. Human cells contain several hsp70 family members including the stress-inducible hsp70, constitutively expressed hsc70, mitochondrial hsp75 and GRP78, localized in the endoplasmic reticulum. These have been extensively studied in non-neuronal and neuronal systems and shown to catalyze the disassembly of clathrin cages that are involved in intracellular protein transport; mediate the transport of proteins across intracellular membranes, working in the cytosol to maintain proteins in a translocation-competent state, and working in the endoplasmic

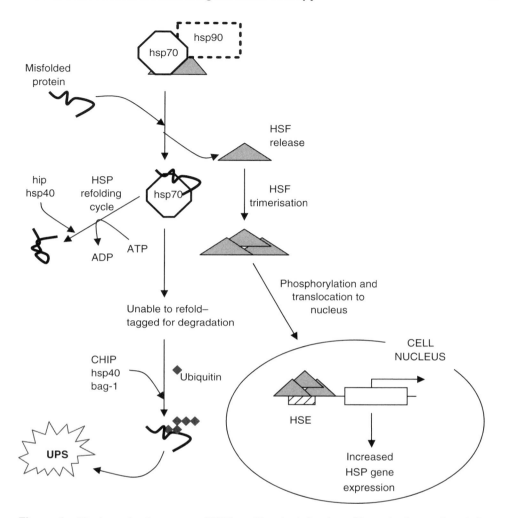

Figure 1 The heat shock response (HSR) enables the induction of heat shock proteins via heat shock factor (HSF) trimerisation and phosphorylation. Pre-existing HSF is believed to exist in a non-active form when bound to hsp90 and/or highly inducible hsp70. In the event of an environmental stress or during a disease process, levels of damaged proteins within the cell increase. These subsequently bind to hsp70/hsp90, mediating the release of HSF. Free HSF molecules form trimers that are phosphorylated and translocate to the nucleus. HSF trimers then bind to heat shock elements (HSE, found upstream of HSF-induced genes) leading to upregulation of these genes and increased production of HSP molecules to aid in refolding of abnormal proteins. In some instances HSP70 is unable to refold the abnormal proteins. These proteins are processed for degradation by the ubiquitin-proteasome system (UPS). Recent research has implicated some cochaperones, such as Carboxyl-terminus of hsp70-interacting protein (CHIP) and Bcl-2-associated athanogene (Bag-1), in this process. These molecules and others are now being investigated to understand the links between the HSP cycle and the UPS.

rectculum or mitochondrial matrix to accept the nascent polypeptide chain as it traverses the membrane (1). All of the hsp70's appear to be ATPases, and it has been hypothesised that hsc70 and hsp70 proteins have the general characteristic of binding hydrophobic surfaces, preventing adventitious associations and stabilizing target proteins in a fully or

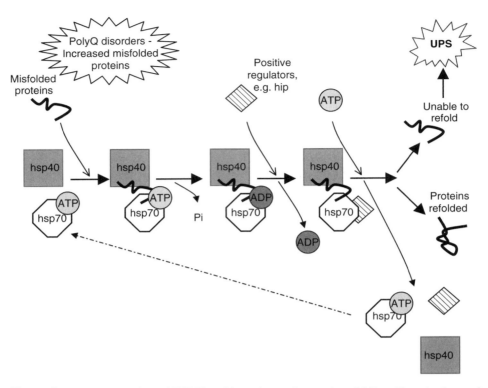

Figure 2 Basic mechanism of HSP70 and its cofactors in protein refolding. Heat shock proteins (HSP) bind to hydrophobic surfaces, such as those exposed on misfolded proteins. This interaction prevents adventitious associations with other proteins (or in the case of protein aggregation additional similar proteins) and stabilizes the target proteins in a fully or partially unfolded state. Following binding, hydrolysis of ATP promotes release of the HSP substrate protein, allowing additional folding, transport, or assembly into a normal conformation state. The presence of HSP40 family members (also known as DnaJ proteins) stabilize the ADP-bound state of HSP70 and aid refolding. Additional cofactors such as HSP70 interacting protein (HIP) are also involved. Often referred to as positive regulators, these cofactors play a major role in assisting HSP70 mediated refolding of target proteins. It is now known that the complement of cofactors present can determine the fate of the misfolded protein. The misfolded proteins are either successfully refolded or targeted to the UPS degradation pathway via ubiquitination. *Abbreviations*: ATP, adenosine triphosphate; UPS, ubiquitin proteosome system.

partially unfolded state. The hydrolysis of ATP then promotes the release of the hsp70 substrate protein, allowing folding, transport, or assembly (1,7). Other high molecular weight molecular chaperone families include hsp60 and hsp90. Hsp60, (acting with its co-chaperone partner, hsp10) is primarily localized to the matrix of the mitochondria, and it plays a major role in facilitating the translocation of proteins across the mitochondrial membrane (8,9). Hsp90 family members promote the conformational maturation of transcription factors, both ligand-dependent (steroid receptors) and ligand-independent (MyoD), and signalling transducing kinases (i.e., tyrosine kinases).

Recent work has shown that some of the high molecular weight chaperone proteins may be directed to different protein substrates by interacting with co-chaperone proteins. Studies on prokaryotic systems showed that dnaK (the bacterial homologue of hsc70) was directed to different protein substrates by interacting with proteins known collectively as

DnaJ's (10). Many eukaryotic DnaJ (termed hsp40's) homologues have now been isolated, suggesting that DnaJ proteins participate in the reactions catalyzed by eukaryotic hsp70 family members. In addition to a co-chaperone function, many DnaJ proteins have also been shown to act as chaperones. Cheetham et al. (1992) isolated a human alternatively spliced DnaJ/hsp40 homologue (hsj1a and hsj1b) and showed that the isoforms were stress inducible and preferentially expressed in the brain (10,11). Hsp40 was isolated from Hela cells, and was shown to be highly induced by stress in neurons and to accumulate in the nucleus and nucleolus during stress. Recently, a number of groups have shown that proteins of the hsp40 family increase hsp70 chaperone activity by enhancing the ATPase activity of hsp70 (12,13). This action is dependent on the interaction of the J-domain of hsp40 with the ATP binding domain of hsc70/hsp70 (14,15). A number of negative and additional positive regulators of hsc70 and hsp70 have been identified. Hsp70 interacting protein (hip) facilitates refolding by stabilizing the ADP-bound state of hsp70/hsc70. Hip directly binds to the ATPase domain of hsp70 when it is converted to the ADP-bound state by proteins of the hsp40 family (16). Hip alone can also bind to unfolded proteins and prevent their aggregation. Bcl-2-associated athanogene-1 (Bag-1) proteins and carboxyl-terminus of hsp70-interacting protein (CHIP) have been identified as negative regulators of hsp70. Bag-1 was originally identified as a Bcl-2 associated protein and has been shown to inhibit hsp70-refolding activity, exerting a dominant inhibitory effect when both hip and Bag-1 are present (17). Furthermore, co-chaperone molecules can also target proteins for degradation via the UPS rather than mediating refolding. Such co-chaperone molecules include the ubiquitin E3 ligase, CHIP (18). This co-chaperone forms an important link between the molecular chaperone and ubiquitin protein degradation systems (19,20) and is in turn assisted by Bag-1.

Ubiquitin Targeted Protein Degradation

Ubiquitin is a particularly important small hsp that tags proteins for degradation via distinct proteolytic pathways. The conjugation of ubiquitin to a substrate involves a complex cascade of enzymatic reactions, usually involving three separate types of enzymes. Initially the C-terminus of ubiquitin is activated in an ATP-dependent fashion by an ubiquitin-specific E1 enzyme or ubiquitin-activating enzyme. The activated ubiquitin is then transferred to an ubiquitin-conjugating enzyme (E2), which accepts the ubiquitin bound intermediate protein from the E1 enzyme and passes it on to a downstream protein. In some cases, E2 can directly transfer ubiquitin to the target proteins, but the reaction often requires the participation of a third factor, E3 or ubiquitin–protein ligase, which catalyzes the transfer of ubiquitin to a lysine residue in the protein substrate. This UPS can also be a target of substrate proteins via its interaction with the molecular chaperone system. The E3 ligase CHIP (mentioned above) provides the perfect example of this close collaboration. CHIP uses the molecular chaperones of the 70- and 90-kDa heat shock protein families to recognize misfolded protein substrates, which it then targets for degradation via the UPS. This mode of recognition enables CHIP to target diverse proteins that resemble one another only by virtue of their unfolded states, e.g., the cystic fibrosis transmembrane receptor, the glucocorticoid receptor, and tau (21–23).

The accumulation of ubiquitin conjugates and/or inclusion bodies associated with ubiquitin have been reported in a broad array of chronic neurodegenerative diseases. These include the neurofibrillary tangles of AD, brainstem Lewy bodies (LBs)—the neuropathological hallmark in PD, LBs in LB dementia, Bunina bodies in Amyotrophic Lateral Sclerosis (ALS), as well as the characteristic (often nuclear) inclusions in polyglutamine disorders (24). Importantly, mutations in the Parkin gene (identified as an ubiquitin protein ligase) and in the ubiquitin carboxy-terminal hydrolase L1 (UCH-L1) have been found to be associated with autosomal recessive juvenile parkinsonism (AR-JP) and autosomal dominant PD, respectively. Furthermore, the mutation in Parkin was found to result in an accumulation of one of its substrates, the Pael receptor. It was also found that when this receptor is overexpressed in cells it becomes misfolded and forms aggregates, which in turn elicits cell death. In the light of these findings abnormal UPS function has been hypothesized to underlie neurodegenerative disorders defined by the abnormal deposition of misfolded polypeptides (24,25).

ABNORMAL PROTEIN METABOLISM IN HUMAN NEURODEGENERATIVE DISEASE AND THE POTENTIAL PROTECTIVE ROLE OF HSP

Many human degenerative diseases are characterized by the progressive degeneration of neurons (with their eventual death) and accompanying production of abnormal intracellular inclusions containing hsps and once normal cellular proteins (e.g., neurofibrillary tangles in AD). These observations suggest that either stress proteins are associated with the aetiology of these diseases, or that their upregulation represents an unsuccessful attempt to remove the abnormal protein aggregates. A number of recent studies have also shown that the overexpression of hsp70 and hsp40 genes could be neuroprotective for stroke (26–28) and the polyglutamine (PolyQ) disorders (29,30). These observations together with other reports that implicate the UPS system in PD suggest that manipulating hsp expression could be prophylactic for many human neurodegenerative conditions. To expand on this hypothesis we have detailed the aetiology of the polyglutamine expansion diseases and discussed how abnormal protein aggregates are formed. Data is also presented and reviewed to detail how the overexpression of hsp genes can be used to reduce the accumulation of protein aggregates and increase the targeting of proteins to the UPS.

The Polyglutamine Disorders

The family of inherited polyglutamine (PolyQ) disorders form part of a larger family of at least 15 neurological disorders. Discovered in 1991, these disorders are characterized by the expansion of unstable triplet repeats in mutated genes (31,32) and are further classified into polyQ disorders and non-polyQ disorders, depending on the triplet repeat codon that is expanded and its localization within the affected gene. In the case of polyglutamine disorders this is always a CAG (glutamine) tract within the coding region of the gene. A brief overview of the most studied polyQ disorders and the gene mutated in each case is given in Table 1. Huntington's disease (HD), various forms of dominantly inherited spinocerebellar ataxia (SCAs) and Spinal and Bulbar Muscular Atrophy (SBMA, which was the first triplet repeat disease to be identified) are among these disorders (33–36). Several additional SCAs have been identified but are not as yet well characterized (i.e., SCA 8, 10, 12, 16, and 17). Some (i.e., SCA8 and SCA10) are not considered true polyQ disorders and are now classified as non-polyglutamine disorders. All polyQ disorders are characterized by selective neuronal loss, typically beginning in mid-life, involving a specific subset of neurons. It is now known that the CAG expansion confers a toxic gain-of-function and leads to the translation of a mutant protein (37). The mutant protein ultimately leads to the production of protein aggregates that are a characteristic

Table 1 Polyglutamine Disorders

Disorder	Alternative name	Protein involved	Gene map locus	Pattern of inheritance	Number of repeats		Protein localization	Clinical symptoms	Frequency	Brain regions most affected
					Normal	Disease				
Huntington disease (HD)	Huntington chorea	Huntingtin	4p16.3	Autosomal dominant	6–34	36–121	Cytoplasmic	Dementia, motor and psychiatric problems, seizures	4 to 7 per 100,000	Striatum, cerebral cortex
Spinal-bulbar muscular atrophy (SBMA)	Kennedy's disease	Androgen Receptor	Xq11-q12	X-linked recessive	9–36	>38	Nuclear and cytoplasmic	Progressive neuromuscular disease; proximal muscle weakness, atrophy	1/40 000 men	Anterior horn and bulbar neurons, dorsal root ganglia
Spinocerebellar ataxia-1 (SCA1)	Type I ADCA (autosomal dominant cerebellar ataxia), Olivopontocerebellar atrophy 1 (OPCA 1), menzel type OPCA	Ataxin-1 (ATX1)	6p21.3–p21.2	Autosomal dominant	6–44	39–82	Nuclear in neurons	Ataxia, dysarthria, cerebellar signs, upper motor neuron signs and extensor plantar responses. Involuntary choreiform movements may occur	6% of ADCA[a]	Cerebellar Purkinje cell, dentate nucleus, brainstem

(Continued)

Table 1 Polyglutamine Disorders (*Continued*)

Disorder	Alternative name	Protein involved	Gene map locus	Pattern of inheritance	Number of repeats		Protein localization	Clinical symptoms	Frequency	Brain regions most affected
					Normal	Disease				
SCA 2	Type I ADCA, OPCA II	Ataxin-2 (ATX2)	12q24	Autosomal dominant	15–31	36–63	Cytoplasmic	Ataxia, dysarthria, hypo- or areflexia, slow saccadic eye movements, peripheral neuropathy	15% of ADCA	Cerebellar Purkinje cell, brain stem, fronto-temporal lobes
SCA 3	MJD (Machado-Joseph disease), Type II ADCA	Ataxin-3 (MJD-1)	14q24.3–q31	Autosomal dominant	12–41	62–84	Cytoplasmic	Ataxia, dysarthria, bulging eyes, early faciolingual fasciculations, parkinsonism	21% of ADCA	Cerebellar dentate neurons, basal ganglia, brainstem, spinal cord.
SCA 6	None	Alpha-1A-voltage-dependent Ca^{2+} channel	19p13	Autosomal dominant	4–18	21–33	Cell membrane	Slow progressive or episodic ataxia, no extrapyramidal signs, spasticity, cognitive impairment and visual defeats	12–15% of ADCA	Cerebellar Purkinje cell, dentate nucleus, inferior olive

SCA 7	Type II ADCA	Ataxin-7	3p21.1–p12	Autosomal dominant	4–35	37–306	Nuclear	Ataxia, dysarthria, visual defects, pigmentary macular degeneration, auditory hallucinations and progressive psychoses in some	5% of ADCA	Cerebellum, brain stem, macula, visual cortex
Dentato-rubro-pallido-luysian atrophy (DRPLA)	Myoclonic epilepsy with choreathetosis, Naito-Oyanagi Disease (NOD)	Atrophin-1	12p13.31	Autosomal dominant	6–36	49–84	Cytoplasmic	Choreoathetosis, myoclonic epilepsy, ataxia and dementia	0.2–0.7 per 100,000	Cerebellum, cerebral cortex, basal ganglia, Luys body

Note: Since their discovery, triplet repeat disorders have been further classified into two distinct groups, polyglutamine repeat disorders and non-polyglutamine disorders. The eight best-studied polyglutamine disorders are detailed in this table. Many additional Spinocerebellar Ataxias have also been identified but are not well documented (i.e., SCA 8, 10, 12, 16 and 17). Some (i.e., SCA8 and SCA10) are not considered to be true CAG triplet repeat disorders, as their mode of inheritance is not that of "gain of function" at the protein level. Such disorders, along with the classic non-polyglutamine disorders have been omitted from this table.

[a] A japanese study estimated the prevalence of the various forms of spinocerebellar degeneration to be 4.53 per 100,000 (75).

hallmark of these disorders. The disease gene products are all distinct proteins, with only the polyglutamine repeat being common to all diseases. Importantly, although early studies demonstrated that the polyQ expansion is itself causative, the expression profile of the unique protein (that the repeat lies within) undoubtedly contributes to defining the specific pattern of neurodegeneration in each disorder (38). This was highlighted by the generation of a 146 CAG repeat construct inserted into the hypoxanthine phosphoribosyl-transferase gene (HPXT, a gene that does not contain a CAG repeat). The presence of the polyQ expansion led to a conformational change of the affected protein, leading to protein misfolding and the production of SDS resistant protein aggregates combined with an expression pattern that resulted from the natural expression pattern of HXPT gene (38). The protein aggregation itself is probably a critical molecular component of these diseases, and can be nuclear and/or cytoplasmic (39).

Huntington's Disease

The majority of polyQ research has focused on HD. Early studies using cell culture models clearly demonstrated that HD shows true dominance, with protein aggregate formation being used as an indicator of pathology (40). This study also confirmed that the rate of protein aggregation was dependent on the number of repeats and that the presence of wild type huntingtin neither enhanced nor interfered with protein aggregation. As with all polyQ disorders generally, several chaperone molecules are sequestered within the aggregates (Table 2). Ubiquitin was found associated with inclusion bodies within affected neurons, suggesting that abnormal huntingtin is targeted for proteolysis but is resistant to removal (41). While Chan et al. (2000) demonstrated that hsp70 and Hdj1 (the Drosophila homolog of human hsp40) showed substrate specificity for polyQ proteins as well as synergy in suppression of neurotoxicity. These chaperone molecules also suppressed aggregate formation and protected against cell death (Table 2) (42,43). Hsp27 has also been identified as a suppressor of polyQ-mediated cell death (30). However, in contrast to hsp40 and hsp70, hsp27 was found to suppress polyQ death without decreasing polyQ aggregation. Hsp27 decreased levels of reactive oxygen species (ROS) in cells expressing mutant huntingtin, suggesting that this chaperone may protect cells against oxidative stress.

The R6/2 Huntington's (containing 115–156 CAG repeats) disease mouse contains nuclear aggregates that contain expanded huntingtin protein colocalized with ubiquitin (44,45). In this model aggregates also induce hsp70 expression and redistribute it to the site of aggregation, along with HSJ-2/HSDJ and components of the proteosome. Various other transgenic models of HD have also been produced (46,47). The R6/2 mice are however the most established model and have now been used to produce double transgenic models that over-express several hsp's. Overexpression of hsp70 reversed the decrease in hsp70 at the protein level and moderately slowed HD progression, noticeably improving body weight (48,49). As the mice aged, however, increased hsp70 sequestration within nuclear aggregates was observed, suggesting that the expanded polyQ eventually negated the therapeutic actions of hsp70.

Spinocerebellar Ataxia

SCA1 and SCA3 have been the most extensively studied cerebellar ataxias. Cummings et al. (1998) found that there were large nuclear inclusions of ataxin-1 in the neurons of patients with SCA1 and that the 20S proteosome co-localized with HSJ2 (a member of the hsp40 family) (50). Similar results were shown in SCA1 transgenic mice containing 82 glutamine

Table 2 Recent Research on Chaperone Molecules in Polyglutamine Disease

Condition	Model/Species	HSPs	Findings	Refs
HD	Transgenic mouse model	Ubiquitin	Pronounced nuclear aggregates produced that contain expanded htt and ubiquitin	(44,45)
	In vitro yeast cell models	HSP70, HSP40	Chaperones inhibit self-assembly of polyQ proteins into amyloid-like fibrils	(72)
	Cell model	HSP27	HSP27 suppressed polyQ death without suppressing polyQ aggregation. Protection by HSP27 was regulated by its phosphorylation state and was independent of its ability to bind to cytochrome c.	(30)
	Ecdysone-inducible stable mouse neuro2A cell line	HSP40 and HSP70 families	Truncated huntingtin fragment interacts with HSP40 and HSP70 families. Expression of Hdj1 and HSC70 suppressed aggregate formation and protect against cell death	(42)
	Transgenic drosophila models	HSP70 and Hdj1HSP40	Chaperones altered the solubility properties of the mutant polyglutamine protein, demonstrating substrate specificity for polyglutamine proteins and synergy in suppression of neurotoxicity	(73)
	Double transgenic model	HSP70	R2/6 mice overexpressing huntingtin and HSP70. Improved body weight and modest effects on HD progression, together with the reversal of decrease in HSP70 at the protein level in R6/2 mice	(48,49)
SBMA	HeLa cell model	HDJ2/HSDJ	Coexpression causes significant reduction in aggregate formation	(56)
	Mouse neuroblastoma (N2A) cell model	HSP70, HSP40	Overexpression decreases aggregate formation and suppresses apoptosis	(55)
	Mouse motor neuron cell line	HSP70, HSP40	HSPs increase solubility of AR containing expanded repeat and enhance its degradation through the proteasome.	(54)
	Stable cell lines	HSP40	JNK activation caused by polyQ is reduced by HSPs	(58)
	Cos7 and SKNSH cells	HSP105	HSP05 colocalises with aggregates. The β-sheet and α-helix domains (but not ATPase domain) of HSP105 reduce aggregation and cell toxicity	(57)
	Double transgenic mouse model	HSP70	Motor function phenotype markedly reduced, decreased nuclear localized AR protein aggregates, enhanced mutant AR degradation	(59)

(Continued)

Table 2 Recent Research on Chaperone Molecules in Polyglutamine Disease (*Continued*)

Condition	Model/Species	HSPs	Findings	Refs
SCA1	Transgenic mouse model	HSP70, HSJ2/HSDJ, Proteasome chomponents	Pathological changes due to polyQ expression, later papers demonstrate Ataxin-1 induced HSP70 expression and redistributes it to the site of aggregation, along with HSJ2/HSDJ and proteasome components	(50,52)
	Double transgenic mouse model	HSP70	HSP70 overexpression protects against NDG, improved motor function and delayed phenotype development	(53)
SCA3	Transgenic Drosophila models	HSP70 and Hdj1 (HSP40)	Chaperones altered the solubility properties of the mutant polyglutamine protein, demonstrating substrate specificity for polyglutamine proteins and synergy in suppression of neurotoxicity	(73)
	Drosophila	HSP70	Demonstrated that HSP70 is a potent suppressor of both polyQ and PD pathogenicity	(74)
	Cell models	HSP70, HSP40	HSP and UPS involved in formation of intracellular aggregates in polyQ disorders	(18)

Note: This table highlights the main findings of recent research investigating the role of chaperone molecules in polyglutamine diseases. Early studies (not all are referenced) used immunohistochemistry techniques to establish the involvement of heat shock proteins in the disease process. Subsequent studies, utilizing stable cell lines, transgenic mice models, and viral vectors, enabled the effects of chaperone overexpression to be studied.

repeats with nuclear inclusions staining for hsc70. HeLa cells transfected with ataxin-1 also showed nuclear staining for hsc70 and the overexpression of HSJ2 reduced the aggregation of ataxin-1. Similar work was demonstrated in SCA3 cell models. Hsp40 and hsp70 co-localized with intranuclear ataxin-3 aggregates and aggregation was suppressed by the expression of HDJ-1 and HDJ-2 (51) as well as hsp70. The first transgenic mice model encoding full-length ataxin-1 (52) clearly demonstrated that the pathological changes were caused by the expression of ataxin-1 with an expanded tract. Cummings et al. (2001) crossbred SCA1 mice with mice over-expressing inducible hsp70 (53). Although the amount of nuclear inclusions in Purkinje cells persisted, they reported that chronic transgenic overexpression of hsp70 protected against neurodegeneration and led to improved motor function. The development of the neurological phenotype was delayed and hsp70 overexpression also inhibited the development of neuronal pathology without affecting formation of neuronal intranuclear aggregates of ataxin-1.

Spino-Bulbar Muscular Atrophy (SBMA)

As with HD, various cell culture models have been produced for SBMA and hsps were found sequestered within the polyQ aggregates (54). Furthermore, the overexpression of hsps in these models was found to decrease aggregation formation and suppress apoptosis (55,56). Hsp70 and hsp40, specifically, were shown to increase the solubility of androgen receptor (AR) containing expanded repeat and enhance its degradation through the proteosome (54). Hsp105 was also found to co-localize with aggregates, reducing aggregation and cell toxicity (57). Furthermore, hsp40 reduced polyQ related JNK activation that is associated with PolyQ mediated toxicity and disease (58). The overexpression of hsp70 in a mouse model of SBMA (59), was shown to markedly reduce the abnormal motor function phenotype of the SBMA transgenic mouse model. The nuclear localization of AR protein aggregates and the monomeric form of mutant AR were also decreased, suggesting that there is enhanced degradation of mutant AR in these double transgenics.

USING VIRAL VECTORS TO INVESTIGATE THE THERAPEUTIC POTENTIAL OF HSP40 PROTEINS IN POLYQ DISEASE

In recent years major steps have been taken to improve the safety, ease of production, and efficacy of adenoviral (Ad), lentiviral and adeno-associated virus (AAV) vectors. Furthermore, these vector systems have been developed in an attempt to optimize: (i) transduction efficiency (without altering normal cellular physiology); (ii) regulatable gene expression; (iii) targeting to specific cell types; (iv) long-term expression in the CNS. For example, we have recently shown that an Ad system incorporating the synapsin promoter and woodchuck hepatitis virus post-transcriptional regulatory element (WPRE) could mediate long-term transgene expression exclusively in neurons (60,61). In addition we have also developed a VSVG pseudotyped HIV lentiviral system incorporating the synapsin promoter to ensure entirely neuron specific expression. These advances in viral vectors technology mean they can be used to investigate, model, and potentially treat polyQ disorders (62). Deglon reviews how viral vectors can be used to both model and treat neurodegenerative disorders in Deglon & Hantraye 2005 (63).

We are currently investigating the neuroprotective effects of the human neuronal HSJ proteins using Ad and lentiviral vectors. HSJ1a and HSJ1b are spice variants

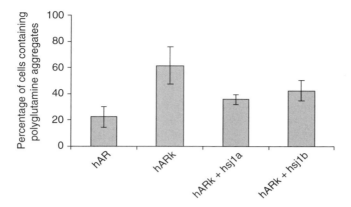

Figure 3 HSP40s decrease levels of polyQ aggregation. Neuro2A neuroblastoma cells were transfected with either a "wildtype" human Androgen Receptor (hAR) construct composed of a 20 glutamine repeat fragment upstream of the human Androgen Receptor DNA and ligand binding domains, or an expanded AR (human Androgen Receptor knock-in/hARk) composed of a 51 glutamine repeat fragment. The hAR construct caused localization of hAR within the nucleus whereas the expression of hARk caused the production of polyglutamine aggregates within the cytoplasm. Adenoviral vectors were then used to overexpress various chaperone molecules. Initial findings show that neuronal HSP40 family members, HSJ1a and HSJ1b, reduce the percentage of cells containing aggregates. Our most recent work (data not shown) implies that the HSJ proteins are relatively poor molecular chaperones and that the aggregates are being reduced due to increased ubiquitination.

generated from a single copy gene that differ in their C-termini. HSJ1a and HSJ1b are expressed in neuronal tissues but have distinct intracellular localizations. HSJ1a is cytoplasmic and nuclear, whereas the larger HSJ1b isoform is targeted to the cytoplasmic face of the ER. Importantly, both proteins can regulate the ATPase activity and substrate binding of hsp70. However, both HSJ1a and HSJ1b contain ubiquitin-interacting motifs (UIMs) that bind mono or polyubiquitinated. Proteins containing UIMs are generally involved in mediating ubiquitination (or known to interact with ubiquitin modifiers); or receptor mediated endocytosis. The functions the UIM-ubiquitin interaction of HSJ1 fulfill are currently being elucidated and it has been suggested that, like CHIP, they mediate ubiquitination and use hsp70 chaperones to target proteins for degradation.

In our studies rather than using relatively inefficient transfection methods we used highly efficient Ad mediated transfection to study chaperone function in a cell model of SBMA. N2a neuroblastoma cells were transfected with "wildtype" human Androgen Receptor (hAR) construct, composed of a 20 glutamine repeat fragment upstream of the hAR DNA and ligand binding domains, or expanded AR (human Androgen Receptor knock-in/hARk) containing an expanded Polyglutamine coding region with 51 repeats. The hAR construct caused localization of hAR within the nucleus whereas the expression of hARk caused the production of polyglutamine aggregates within the cytoplasm. Ad vectors were then used to express HSJ1a and HSJ1b and our results (Fig. 3) show that these previously uncharacterized hsp40 molecules can reduce the level of aggregation of expanded AR. Interestingly, our results (not shown) show the HSJ proteins are relatively poor molecular chaperones and it is, therefore, likely that the aggregates are being reduced due to increased ubiquitination.

DISCUSSION

The characteristic protein aggregation seen in polyQ diseases is a key pathological hallmark of many other neurodegenerative conditions (including AD, PD, and prion disease). The underlying cause and, therefore, the actual mechanism(s) leading to the deposition of protein inclusions are different for each disease. However, a general therapeutic strategy that tackles the build up of aggregates, irrespective of their protein content and method of deposition, could potentially be used to delay or prevent the development of one or more of these diseases. The evidence and data discussed in this chapter supports the hypothesis that manipulating hsp/chaperone protein expression could potentially delay or prevent the progress of such diseases. The data also shows that increasing chaperone activity and/or enhancing protein removal via the UPS are strategies that could be used to reduce the accumulation of protein aggregates. To achieve the former it would be logical to target the expression of hsp70 and/or its co-chaperones to the disease-affected areas of the brain using viral vectors that ideally mediated regulatable expression. It would similarly be possible to encourage the removal of protein aggregates via the UPS by overexpressing E3 ligases such as CHIP or other hsp's containing UIMs (e.g., HSJ1a). In addition to the molecular data already detailed, small molecule and pharmacological studies also support the use of hsp's for the treatment of neuro-degenerative disease. For example, Trehalose and other disaccharide molecules have been shown to stabilize the proteins containing the polyQ tract and show specific binding to the expanded repeats (25). Benzothiazoles have also been shown to suppress polyQ aggregation in a dose-dependent manner (64) by binding to the beta sheet structures. A mechanism of action similar to that of Congo red, which has been reported to decrease physical aggregates in cultured cells and reduce toxicity of polyglutamines in both cell culture and mouse models (65–67).

Several groups have shown that pharmacological agents can also be used to mediate an increase in chaperone molecule expression by targeting the HSF and have also shown these compounds could potentially be used to treat neurodegenerative diseases. Geldanamycin is a naturally occurring benzoquinone ansamycin that specifically binds to and interferes with the activity of HSP90 (68), a negative regulator of the HSF. Hence in animals, geldanamycin increases HSR activity and thereby increases the expression of HSP40, HSP70, and HSP90. Using geldanamycin, several groups have shown that aggregate formation can be inhibited in models of HD (49,69) and PD (70) in a dose-dependent manner (69). Another coinducer of HSPs, arimoclomol, produced similar results in delaying disease progression in ALS mice (71). These therapies highlight the potential for modulating the expression of HSPs to alleviate neurodegenerative disease, in this case via the HSR. However, hsps are not only involved in maintaining protein structure and function but are also involved in many other cellular processes, e.g., mediating endocytosis, nuclear transport and signalling, maintaining signalling pathways, and regulating apoptosis. The continued overexpression of one or more molecular chaperones could itself disturb cellular homeostasis. Future research should therefore also explore methods by which the potential adverse effects of prolonged hsp expression could be minimized.

In summary, a general strategy that tackles the build-up of aggregates, irrespective of their protein content and method of deposition, could potentially be used to delay or prevent the development of many human neurodegenerative diseases. Data to date suggests that hsps that facilitate protein disaggregation and/or increase protein degradation via the UPS would be potential therapeutic targets for the treatment of Huntington's and other human neurodegenerative diseases.

REFERENCES

1. Gething MJ, Sambrook J. Protein folding in the cell. Nature 1992; 355:33–45.
2. Parsell DA, Taulien J, Lindquist S. The role of heat-shock proteins in thermotolerance. Philos Trans R Soc Lond B Biol Sci 1993; 339:279–285.
3. Uney JB, Leigh PN, Marsden CD, Lees A, Anderton BH. Stereotaxic injection of kainic acid into the striatum of rats induces synthesis of mRNA for heat shock protein 70. FEBS Lett 1988; 235:215–218.
4. Uney JB, Anderton BH, Thomas SM. Changes in heat shock protein 70 and ubiquitin mRNA levels in C1300 N2A mouse neuroblastoma cells following treatment with iron. J Neurochem 1993; 60:659–665.
5. Morimoto RI. Cells in stress: transcriptional activation of heat shock genes. Science 1993; 259:1409–1410.
6. Bercovich B, Stancovski I, Mayer A, et al. Ubiquitin-dependent degradation of certain protein substrates in vitro requires the molecular chaperone Hsc70. J Biol Chem 1997; 272:9002–9010.
7. Jaattela M. Heat shock proteins as cellular lifeguards. Ann Med 1999; 31:261–271.
8. Samali A, Cai J, Zhivotovsky B, Jones DP, Orrenius S. Presence of a pre-apoptotic complex of pro-caspase-3, Hsp60 and Hsp10 in the mitochondrial fraction of jurkat cells. EMBO J 1999; 18:2040–2048.
9. Xanthoudakis S, Roy S, Rasper D, et al. Hsp60 accelerates the maturation of pro-caspase-3 by upstream activator proteases during apoptosis. EMBO J 1999; 18:2049–2056.
10. Silver PA, Way JC. Eukaryotic DnaJ homologs and the specificity of Hsp70 activity. Cell 1993; 74:5–6.
11. Cheetham ME, Brion JP, Anderton BH. Human homologues of the bacterial heat-shock protein DnaJ are preferentially expressed in neurons. Biochem J 1992; 284:469–476.
12. Freeman BC, Myers MP, Schumacher R, Morimoto RI. Identification of a regulatory motif in Hsp70 that affects ATPase activity, substrate binding and interaction with HDJ-1. EMBO J 1995; 14:2281–2292.
13. Minami Y, Hohfeld J, Ohtsuka K, Hartl FU. Regulation of the heat-shock protein 70 reaction cycle by the mammalian DnaJ homolog, Hsp40. J Biol Chem 1996; 271:19617–19624.
14. Michels AA, Kanon B, Konings AW, Ohtsuka K, Bensaude O, Kampinga HH. Hsp70 and Hsp40 chaperone activities in the cytoplasm and the nucleus of mammalian cells. J Biol Chem 1997; 272:33283–33289.
15. Michels AA, Kanon B, Bensaude O, Kampinga HH. Heat shock protein (Hsp) 40 mutants inhibit Hsp70 in mammalian cells. J Biol Chem 1999; 274:36757–36763.
16. Hohfeld J, Minami Y, Hartl FU. Hip, a novel cochaperone involved in the eukaryotic Hsc70/Hsp40 reaction cycle. Cell 1995; 83:589–598.
17. Nollen EA, Kabakov AE, Brunsting JF, Kanon B, Hohfeld J, Kampinga HH. Modulation of in vivo HSP70 chaperone activity by Hip and Bag-1. J Biol Chem 2001; 276:4677–4682.
18. Garrido C, Solary E. A role of HSPs in apoptosis through "protein triage"? Cell Death Differ 2003; 10:619–620.
19. Connell P, Ballinger CA, Jiang J, et al. The co-chaperone CHIP regulates protein triage decisions mediated by heat-shock proteins. Nat Cell Biol 2001; 3:93–96.
20. Jiang J, Ballinger CA, Wu Y, et al. CHIP is a U-box-dependent E3 ubiquitin ligase: identification of Hsc70 as a target for ubiquitylation. J Biol Chem 2001; 276:42938–42944.
21. Petrucelli L, Dawson TM. Mechanism of neurodegenerative disease: role of the ubiquitin proteasome system. Ann Med 2004; 36:315–320.
22. Petrucelli L, Dickson D, Kehoe K, et al. CHIP and Hsp70 regulate tau ubiquitination, degradation and aggregation. Hum Mol Genet 2004; 13:703–714.
23. Shimura H, Schwartz D, Gygi SP, Kosik KS. CHIP-Hsc70 complex ubiquitinates phosphorylated tau and enhances cell survival. J Biol Chem 2004; 279:4869–4876.
24. Ciechanover A, Schwartz AL. The ubiquitin system: pathogenesis of human diseases and drug targeting. Biochim Biophys Acta 2004; 1695:3–17.

25. Tanaka K, Suzuki T, Hattori N, Mizuno Y. Ubiquitin, proteasome and parkin. Biochim Biophys Acta 2004; 1695:235–247.

26. Giffard RG, Xu L, Zhao H, et al. Chaperones, protein aggregation, and brain protection from hypoxic/ischemic injury. J Exp Biol 2004; 207:3213–3220.

27. Kelly S, McCulloch J, Horsburgh K. Minimal ischaemic neuronal damage and HSP70 expression in MF1 strain mice following bilateral common carotid artery occlusion. Brain Res 2001; 914:185–195.

28. Klettner A. The induction of heat shock proteins as a potential strategy to treat neurodegenerative disorders. Drug News Perspect 2004; 17:299–306.

29. Ho LW, Carmichael J, Swartz J, Wyttenbach A, Rankin J, Rubinsztein DC. The molecular biology of Huntington's disease. Psychol Med 2001; 31:3–14.

30. Wyttenbach A, Carmichael J, Swartz J, et al. Effects of heat shock, heat shock protein 40 (HDJ-2), and proteasome inhibition on protein aggregation in cellular models of Huntington's disease. Proc Natl Acad Sci USA 2000; 97:2898–2903.

31. Fu YH, Kuhl DP, Pizzuti A, et al. Variation of the CGG repeat at the fragile X site results in genetic instability: resolution of the Sherman paradox. Cell 1991; 67:1047–1058.

32. La Spada AR, Taylor JP. Polyglutamines placed into context. Neuron 2003; 38:681–684.

33. Bossy-Wetzel E, Schwarzenbacher R, Lipton SA. Molecular pathways to neurodegeneration. Nat Med 2004; 10:S2–S9.

34. Merienne K, Helmlinger D, Perkin GR, Devys D, Trottier Y. Polyglutamine expansion induces a protein-damaging stress connecting heat shock protein 70 to the JNK pathway. J Biol Chem 2003; 278:16957–16967.

35. Michalik A, Van BC. Pathogenesis of polyglutamine disorders: aggregation revisited. Hum Mol Genet 2003; 12:R173–R186.

36. Tarlac V, Storey E. Role of proteolysis in polyglutamine disorders. J Neurosci Res 2003; 74:406–416.

37. Zoghbi HY, Orr HT. Glutamine repeats and neurodegeneration. Annu Rev Neurosci 2000; 23:217–247.

38. Ordway JM, Tallaksen-Greene S, Gutekunst CA, et al. Ectopically expressed CAG repeats cause intranuclear inclusions and a progressive late onset neurological phenotype in the mouse. Cell 1997; 91:753–763.

39. Ross CA. Intranuclear neuronal inclusions: a common pathogenic mechanism for glutamine-repeat neurodegenerative diseases? Neuron 1997; 19:1147–1150.

40. Narain Y, Wyttenbach A, Rankin J, Furlong RA, Rubinsztein DC. A molecular investigation of true dominance in Huntington's disease. J Med Genet 1999; 36:739–746.

41. DiFiglia M, Sapp E, Chase KO, et al. Aggregation of huntingtin in neuronal intranuclear inclusions and dystrophic neurites in brain. Science 1997; 277:1990–1993.

42. Jana NR, Tanaka M, Wang G, Nukina N. Polyglutamine length-dependent interaction of Hsp40 and Hsp70 family chaperones with truncated N-terminal huntingtin: their role in suppression of aggregation and cellular toxicity. Hum Mol Genet 2000; 9:2009–2018.

43. Muchowski PJ. Protein misfolding, amyloid formation, and neurodegeneration: a critical role for molecular chaperones? Neuron 2002; 35:9–12.

44. Davies SW, Turmaine M, Cozens BA, et al. Formation of neuronal intranuclear inclusions underlies the neurological dysfunction in mice transgenic for the HD mutation. Cell 1997; 90:537–548.

45. Mangiarini L, Sathasivam K, Seller M, et al. Exon 1 of the HD gene with an expanded CAG repeat is sufficient to cause a progressive neurological phenotype in transgenic mice. Cell 1996; 87:493–506.

46. Bates GP, Mangiarini L, Mahal A, Davies SW. Transgenic models of Huntington's disease. Hum Mol Genet 1997; 6:1633–1637.

47. Bates GP, Mangiarini L, Davies SW. Transgenic mice in the study of polyglutamine repeat expansion diseases. Brain Pathol 1998; 8:699–714.

48. Hansson O, Nylandsted J, Castilho RF, Leist M, Jaattela M, Brundin P. Overexpression of heat shock protein 70 in R6/2 Huntington's disease mice has only modest effects on disease progression. Brain Res 2003; 970:47–57.

49. Hay DG, Sathasivam K, Tobaben S, et al. Progressive decrease in chaperone protein levels in a mouse model of Huntington's disease and induction of stress proteins as a therapeutic approach. Hum Mol Genet 2004; 13:1389–1405.

50. Cummings CJ, Mancini MA, Antalffy B, DeFranco DB, Orr HT, Zoghbi HY. Chaperone suppression of aggregation and altered subcellular proteasome localization imply protein misfolding in SCA1. Nat Genet 1998; 19:148–154.

51. Chai Y, Koppenhafer SL, Bonini NM, Paulson HL. Analysis of the role of heat shock protein (Hsp) molecular chaperones in polyglutamine disease. J Neurosci 1999; 19:10338–10347.

52. Burright EN, Clark HB, Servadio A, et al. SCA1 transgenic mice: a model for neurodegeneration caused by an expanded CAG trinucleotide repeat. Cell 1995; 82:937–948.

53. Cummings CJ, Sun Y, Opal P, et al. Over-expression of inducible HSP70 chaperone suppresses neuropathology and improves motor function in SCA1 mice. Hum Mol Genet 2001; 10:1511–1518.

54. Bailey CK, Andriola IF, Kampinga HH, Merry DE. Molecular chaperones enhance the degradation of expanded polyglutamine repeat androgen receptor in a cellular model of spinal and bulbar muscular atrophy. Hum Mol Genet 2002; 11:515–523.

55. Kobayashi Y, Kume A, Li M, et al. Chaperones Hsp70 and Hsp40 suppress aggregate formation and apoptosis in cultured neuronal cells expressing truncated androgen receptor protein with expanded polyglutamine tract. J Biol Chem 2000; 275:8772–8778.

56. Stenoien DL, Cummings CJ, Adams HP, et al. Polyglutamine-expanded androgen receptors form aggregates that sequester heat shock proteins, proteasome components and SRC-1, and are suppressed by the HDJ-2 chaperone. Hum Mol Genet 1999; 8:731–741.

57. Ishihara K, Yamagishi N, Saito Y, et al. Hsp105alpha suppresses the aggregation of truncated androgen receptor with expanded CAG repeats and cell toxicity. J Biol Chem 2003; 278:25143–25150.

58. Cowan KJ, Diamond MI, Welch WJ. Polyglutamine protein aggregation and toxicity are linked to the cellular stress response. Hum Mol Genet 2003; 12:1377–1391.

59. Adachi H, Katsuno M, Minamiyama M, et al. Heat shock protein 70 chaperone overexpression ameliorates phenotypes of the spinal and bulbar muscular atrophy transgenic mouse model by reducing nuclear-localized mutant androgen receptor protein. J Neurosci 2003; 23:2203–2211.

60. Glover CP, Bienemann AS, Heywood DJ, Cosgrave AS, Uney JB. Adenoviral-mediated, high-level, cell-specific transgene expression: a SYN1-WPRE cassette mediates increased transgene expression with no loss of neuron specificity. Mol Ther 2002; 5:509–516.

61. Glover CP, Bienemann AS, Hopton M, Harding TC, Kew JN, Uney JB. Long-term transgene expression can be mediated in the brain by adenoviral vectors when powerful neuron-specific promoters are used. J Gene Med 2003; 5:554–559.

62. de Almeida LP, Ross CA, Zala D, Aebischer P, Deglon N. Lentiviral-mediated delivery of mutant huntingtin in the striatum of rats induces a selective neuropathology modulated by polyglutamine repeat size, huntingtin expression levels, and protein length. J Neurosci 2002; 22:3473–3483.

63. Deglon N, Hantraye P. Viral vectors as tools to model and treat neurodegenerative disorders. J Gene Med 2005.

64. Heiser V, Engemann S, Brocker W, et al. Identification of benzothiazoles as potential polyglutamine aggregation inhibitors of Huntington's disease by using an automated filter retardation assay. Proc Natl Acad Sci USA 2002; 99:16400–16406.

65. Bao YP, Sarkar S, Uyama E, Rubinsztein DC. Congo red, doxycycline, and HSP70 overexpression reduce aggregate formation and cell death in cell models of oculopharyngeal muscular dystrophy. J Med Genet 2004; 41:47–51.

66. Ross CA, Pickart CM. The ubiquitin-proteasome pathway in Parkinson's disease and other neurodegenerative diseases. Trends Cell Biol 2004; 14:703–711.

67. Sanchez I, Mahlke C, Yuan J. Pivotal role of oligomerization in expanded polyglutamine neurodegenerative disorders. Nature 2003; 421:373–379.
68. Stebbins CE, Russo AA, Schneider C, Rosen N, Hartl FU, Pavletich NP. Crystal structure of an Hsp90-geldanamycin complex: targeting of a protein chaperone by an antitumor agent. Cell 1997; 89:239–250.
69. Sittler A, Lurz R, Lueder G, et al. Geldanamycin activates a heat shock response and inhibits huntingtin aggregation in a cell culture model of Huntington's disease. Hum Mol Genet 2001; 10:1307–1315.
70. Auluck PK, Bonini NM. Pharmacological prevention of Parkinson disease in Drosophila. Nat Med 2002; 8:1185–1186.
71. Kieran D, Kalmar B, Dick JR, Riddoch-Contreras J, Burnstock G, Greensmith L. Treatment with arimoclomol, a coinducer of heat shock proteins, delays disease progression in ALS mice. Nat Med 2004; 10:402–405.
72. Muchowski PJ, Schaffar G, Sittler A, Wanker EE, Hayer-Hartl MK, Hartl FU. Hsp70 and hsp40 chaperones can inhibit self-assembly of polyglutamine proteins into amyloid-like fibrils. Proc Natl Acad Sci USA 2000; 97:7841–7846.
73. Chan HY, Warrick JM, Gray-Board GL, Paulson HL, Bonini NM. Mechanisms of chaperone suppression of polyglutamine disease: selectivity, synergy and modulation of protein solubility in Drosophila. Hum Mol Genet 2000; 9:2811–2820.
74. Bonini NM. Drosophila as a genetic approach to human neurodegenerative disease. Parkinsonism Relat Disord 2001; 7:171–175.
75. Hirayama K, Takayanagi T, Nakamura R, et al. Spinocerebellar degenerations in Japan: a nationwide epidemiological and clinical study. Acta Neurol Scand Suppl 1994; 153:1–22.

5

iBAC Technologies for Neurological Disease

Sean E. Lawler, Yoshinaga Saeki, and E. Antonio Chiocca
The Dardinger Laboratory for Neuro-oncology and Neurosciences, Department of Neurological Surgery, The Ohio State University Medical Center, Columbus, Ohio, U.S.A.

Richard Wade-Martins
The Wellcome Trust Centre for Human Genetics, University of Oxford, Oxford, U.K.

INTRODUCTION

The ability to efficiently deliver complete genomic DNA loci to mammalian cells will have important applications in functional genomics and gene therapy. Recent studies in our laboratories have led to the development of a novel gene delivery system named the infectious BAC, or iBAC system, in which human genetic loci cloned as bacterial artificial chromosomes (BACs), are packaged into herpes simplex virus type 1 (HSV-1) amplicons, allowing infectious delivery of genomic DNA to a broad range of cell types and tissues (1–3). Genomic transgenes delivered by iBACs behave in a similar fashion to genes in their native chromosomal state in terms of expression levels, RNA splicing and promoter regulation. Because of the natural tropism of HSV-1 for neuronal cells, the iBAC system may find uses in the treatment of certain neurological disorders. This chapter will discuss the development of the iBAC system, and its potential application in the treatment of diseases affecting the central nervous system (CNS).

THE TROUBLE WITH TRANSGENES

Sustained and regulated transgene expression at suitable therapeutic levels can be difficult to achieve using conventional gene therapy vectors in which cDNA expression is driven by a strong heterologous viral promoter, because expression is often compromised by vector loss and transcriptional silencing (4–6). In addition, the random chromosomal integration of vector DNA causes unpredictable transgene expression and can disrupt host gene expression by insertional mutagenesis (7) with potentially serious consequences, as in the cases of leukemia observed due to the insertional activation of the *LMO2* oncogene in the human severe X-linked combined immunodeficiency clinical trial (8). Alterations in DNA methylation patterns have been observed in transgenic DNA—causing

59

transcriptional silencing, and in chromosomal DNA at sites distant from transgene insertion leading to perturbations in cellular protein levels (9).

Novel approaches are being developed to overcome these problems, by site specific integration (10) or by extrachromosomal (episomal) maintenance of vector sequences. For example, the Epstein-Barr virus nuclear antigen-1 (*EBNA-1*) gene mediates nuclear retention of vector DNA carrying the EBV latent origin of replication, *oriP*. These vectors replicate and segregate autonomously in human and primate cells thereby allowing long-term episomal maintenance (11). EBV-based episomes carrying large (> 10–15 kb) mammalian genomic DNA fragments (up to 660 kb) are stably maintained in both human and murine cell lines (11–14) and in vivo in mice (15).

In addition to the difficulties associated with random insertion and loss of transgene expression, cDNA-based gene therapy vectors cannot reproduce normal physiological regulation of gene expression. In therapies that involve the replacement of a mutated gene, appropriately controlled, developmentally regulated, and tissue-specific gene expression may be critical for long-term optimal therapeutic benefit. For example, normal physiological negative feedback of LDL receptor gene expression by cholesterol could be vital for its effectiveness in clinical applications (see iBACs in Action: Promotor Regulation-LDLR).

The iBAC system has been designed to alleviate the drawbacks of cDNA-based vectors through efficient delivery of complete genomic loci to target cells. Transgene expression is, therefore, under the control of the native promoter and regulated by endogenous enhancer and silencer elements in the correct genomic context, including all introns, allowing physiological control and expression of all splice variants. In addition, our iBAC vectors incorporate the *EBNA-1* gene and *oriP*, allowing long-term episomal maintenance.

GENOMIC TRANSGENES

Genomic transgenes are known to function well in various systems. Long-term expression from genomic transgenes has now been demonstrated both in vitro (16) and in vivo (4,17–20). There are some unique technical challenges arising when working with genomic loci; these are outlined briefly below.

Genomic DNA Clone Identification

As a result of the human genome project, the identification of well characterized genomic DNA clones is quite straightforward. The strategy undertaken by the publicly funded International Human Genome Consortium involved sequencing a minimum tiling path of overlapping ~ 100–200 kb clones derived from human chromosomal DNA (21). These clones are all catalogued and maintained as single copy number plasmids in *E. coli* as either BACs or PACs (P1-based artificial chromosomes), which are able to stably carry large DNA inserts of up to 300 kb (22,23). The entire human genome sequence is, therefore, covered by series of fully sequenced BAC and PAC clones. These can be readily identified through database searches, and are freely available to the research community (24). The vast majority of genetic loci can be accommodated by a single BAC clone, and their usefulness has been demonstrated by increasing numbers of examples of gene expression from BAC and PAC clones, both in vitro (16,25) and in transgenic mice (26–28). Furthermore, every BAC and PAC plasmid includes a *loxP* site allowing manipulation by recombination with other *loxP* containing sequences (22,23).

Handling Large DNA Inserts

The use of BAC and PAC clones in gene expression studies has been hampered by their large size, which requires some specialized techniques. Fortunately, in recent years there have been advances in manipulation of large DNA by homologous recombination in bacteria, allowing easier vector construction and site-directed mutagenesis of large DNA clones (26,29–32).

Delivery of Genomic Clones to Mammalian Cells

The efficient delivery of therapeutic genes to specific cell types is a major challenge in gene therapy, and large genomic transgenes present a greater challenge still. Current transfection/electroporation methods are inefficient at introducing large genomic sequences into cells. Much more efficient gene delivery can be achieved using viral vectors. However, an average genetic locus, with all the regulatory regions included, can span over 100 kb of chromosomal DNA (33,34), far too large for most currently used viral vectors. The capacity of retroviral, lentiviral, and adeno-associated viral vectors is less than 10 kb (35). The "gutless" adenovirus has a theoretical capacity of around 36 kb, and has been used to express a 19 kb genomic transgene (19) but is too small to deliver larger loci. The viruses of the Herpes family have a particularly large capacity; these include HSV-1 (152 kb), EBV (172 kb), and cytomegalovirus (CMV) (230 kb). Of these, HSV-1 has been particularly well studied as a gene delivery vehicle. HSV-1 infects a broad range of cell types, both dividing and non-dividing, and has natural tropism for neurons, for which it has been proposed as a particularly suitable vector for therapeutic gene delivery (36).

The development of the amplicon system gives HSV-1 a major advantage in the delivery of large genes (37,38). The system is based on the observation that, in the presence of co-expressed helper functions, a vector containing DNA linked to two HSV-1 non-coding sequences, packaging/cleavage (*pac*) and origin of replication (*ori$_s$*), can be packaged into complete HSV-1 virions without any other viral DNA (39). HSV-1 amplicons have been widely used for in vivo and in vitro gene delivery of cDNA-based transgenes (40). Importantly, this system has been optimized so that contaminating helper virus is undetectable (41), thereby minimizing immune responses and cytotoxicity. HSV-1 amplicons can be produced at high titer, and have a theoretical capacity of ∼150 kb, high enough to accommodate 95% of predicted human gene loci (see http://www.ensembl.org/Homo_sapiens/martview). Low toxicity, neural tropism, ease of construction and high capacity, make HSV-1 amplicons ideal for the delivery of large DNA sequences to the nervous system and other cell types. Genomic transgene delivery using HSV-1 amplicons forms the basis of the iBAC system.

BUILDING AN iBAC

This section briefly outlines the steps involved in making an iBAC. Starting with the identification and characterization of a BAC clone to retrofitting with HSV-1 amplicon sequences via recombination, and packaging into amplicons (Fig. 1). Complete experimental details for iBAC construction and packaging can be found in Refs. 1 and 41.

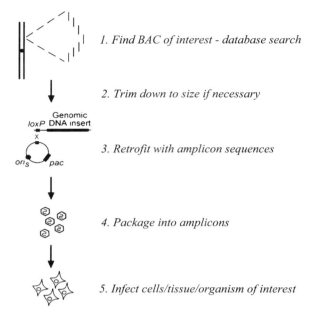

1. *Find BAC of interest - database search*

2. *Trim down to size if necessary*

3. *Retrofit with amplicon sequences*

4. *Package into amplicons*

5. *Infect cells/tissue/organism of interest*

Figure 1   Outline of the steps required to build an iBAC.

Step One: Identify and Characterize BAC of Interest

Because the human genome sequence is based on a series of overlapping BAC clones, it is highly likely that a suitable BAC or PAC clone can be identified for the large majority of genes. This can be done using public databases such as http://www.ensembl.org, or http://genome.ucsc.edu. Furthermore, clones have also been placed in databases in addition to the original sequenced minimal tiling path, therefore genomic BAC and PAC clones are now at a high depth of coverage on the human genome sequence. Often a number of clones will be available and can be ordered at http://www.ncbi.nlm.nih.gov/genome/clone/nomen.html, and at http://bacpac.chori.org. Clones should be checked on arrival for the presence of all exons by PCR, and by restriction digestion. The digested DNA can be resolved by pulsed-field gel electrophoresis (PFGE).

Step Two: Modify BAC Clone

The total packaging capacity of an HSV-1 amplicon is about 155–160 kb. If the BAC insert is less than the maximum recommended insert size of 140 kb it is possible to simply retrofit the library clone with a plasmid containing the HSV-1 amplicon elements (see step three below). For larger clones it may be necessary to trim the BAC insert to remove excess $5'$ or $3'$ sequence along with any sequences from neighboring genes, if present, prior to retrofitting. The simplest approach is to use suitable uncommon restriction sites to excise the intact genomic locus (14,16). However, with large DNA inserts this is not always possible, and strategies such as RecA-assisted restriction endonuclease (RARE) cleavage may be used (3,42). Homologous recombination in bacteria has also been used to simultaneously subclone and remove unwanted flanking sequences from entire loci (32). With further refinements in iBAC vector design, it is anticipated that genomic inserts of $\sim$150 kb will be deliverable.

Step Three: Retrofitting with HSV-1 Amplicon Sequences

The HSV-1 amplicon retrofitting plasmids, such as pHG, which are used to make iBAC vectors have a number of key features (Fig. 2). These include the HSV-1 *pac* and *ori$_s$* sequences necessary for packaging, a GFP expression cassette for tracking infected cells, and a *loxP* site allowing recombination with BAC clones in *Cre* expressing *E. coli* (1,41). Other elements, such as the EBV *EBNA-1* gene, can also be included. After transformation and selection of recombined clones in bacteria, the iBAC DNA should be checked by exon-specific PCR, and restriction digestion followed by PFGE.

Step Four: Package Retrofitted BACs as Infectious Amplicons

The final iBAC vector is packaged into amplicons using the improved helper virus free system (41). The iBAC vector is cotransfected into mammalian cells together with helper plasmids expressing the HSV-1 genes necessary for virus formation and packaging (Fig. 2). Three safety features present in the packaging construct fHSV $\triangle$ pac $\triangle$ 27 0^{++} ensure that no contaminating helper virus is detectable in the iBAC amplicon preparation (41). First, the fHSV $\triangle$ pac $\triangle$ 27 0^{++} plasmid containing the entire HSV-1 genome is deleted for the HSV-1 packaging signals; second, the plasmid is deleted for the essential ICP27 gene (which is supplied in trans by the second plasmid, pEBHICP27); third, the plasmid has been oversized to 178 kb by the addition of two extra copies of the HSV-1 ICP0 gene. This is well in excess of the maximum amplicon packaging capacity. At 60 hr post-transfection the amplicon is harvested and concentrated by ultracentrifugation. This method yields stocks of $\sim 2 \times 10^7$ transducing units/ml (t.u./ml) for iBAC amplicons.

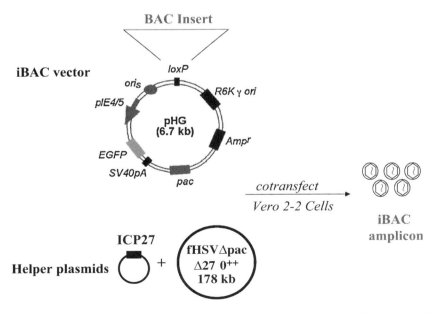

Figure 2 (*See color insert*) HSV-1 amplicon production scheme. Detail is shown of the amplicon plasmid pHG.

Step Five: Infect a Suitable Cell Type

Finally, the amplicon can be used to infect the cells or tissue of choice and infected live cells can be monitored by expression of GFP. iBAC locus gene expression can be measured by RT-PCR, antibody-based methods, and functional assays.

iBACs IN ACTION

The iBAC gene delivery system has been developed in the hope of efficiently transducing mammalian cells with complete genomic loci. At present, iBACs have been successfully used to express a number of human genomic transgenes in a variety of different cell types, which are discussed individually below.

Proof of Principle—HPRT

A *hypoxanthine phosphoribosyltransferase* (*HPRT*) locus containing iBAC was the first vector of this kind constructed, and successfully demonstrated that the system can deliver the native form of a large gene to complement a human genetic defect (1). The *HPRT* gene encodes a ubiquitously expressed enzyme involved in the purine salvage pathway. *HPRT* mutations cause Lesch-Nyhan syndrome and gouty arthritis (43). A previous study used non-viral transfection to deliver a 115 kb region encompassing the human *HPRT* locus to cultured cells (16). The locus corrected the deficiency in *HPRT* deficient cells as measured in hypoxanthine incorporation assays. Delivery of *HPRT* by iBAC led to functional HPRT expression as measured by hypoxanthine incorporation assays, with gene delivery efficiency greatly increased from 15% with non-viral transfection to 80% in *HPRT*⁻ human fibroblast cells. Also, the transduced iBAC-*HPRT* DNA was present at 1 copy/cell in clonal lines, close to the physiological situation. Importantly, the efficiency of *HPRT* locus delivery to primary mouse hepatocytes was orders of magnitude greater by iBAC-*HPRT* transduction than by transfection. The increased efficiency of gene transduction allowed the restoration of HPRT function in primary mouse hepatocytes defective for *HPRT* (1).

Promoter Regulation—LDLR

Low-density lipoprotein receptor (LDLR) deficiency is considered a strong candidate for gene therapy (44). Loss of *LDLR* function causes familial hypercholesterolemia (FH), a classic monogenic loss of function disorder that is amenable to the iBAC approach. The LDLR is responsible for importing cholesterol into the cell, and is under tight regulation by negative feedback to regulate cholesterol import (45,46). High intracellular cholesterol levels block LDLR expression through sterol response elements present within the *LDLR* promoter. Previous studies using cDNA based vectors with heterologous promoters typically showed short-lived (47,48) or very low gene expression levels (49). In addition, strong overexpression of LDLR is toxic, leading to intracellular accumulation of cholesterol, with subsequent cell death (50). The results of these studies suggest that alternative approaches such as the iBAC may have significant advantages.

Wade-Martins et al. (2) constructed an iBAC-*LDLR* vector using a 135 kb BAC insert encompassing the *LDLR* locus. The study showed close to physiological LDLR expression in *ldlr-/-* a7 CHO cells. In addition, co-expression of *EBNA-1* allowed episomal maintenance of the *LDLR* iBAC for at least 3 mo. The iBAC-*LDLR* was delivered to fibroblasts from FH patients—these are virtually untransfectable by lipofection (0.1%) but showed 50% transduction using the iBAC system. Importantly, the transduced *LDLR* locus was appropriately regulated by sterol levels. Expression was reduced strongly (75%) by cholesterol, compared with 80–90% in control MRC9 cells. This demonstrates that iBACs can retain their ability to respond to natural physiological signals in their extra-chromosomal state.

Complex Splicing—CDKN2

The *CDKN2* locus contains 6 exons, which by complex gene splicing, express five different proteins; $p16^{INK4A}$, $p14^{ARF}$, $p15^{INK4b}$, p12 (specifically expressed in the pancreas) and p10, an alternatively spliced form of $p15^{INK4b}$ (51,52). $p16^{INK4A}$ and $p14^{ARF}$ are expressed from overlapping genes in the *CDKN2* locus by alternative splicing and promoter usage. They share the same final two exons, which are translated in different reading frames, thus producing two proteins with no amino acid similarity, and different functions. $p16^{INK4a}$ and $p14^{ARF}$ are known to be major tumor suppressors and are the focus of intense research (51,52). The *CDKN2* locus is one of the most common deletions in human cancer, and is particularly common in glioblastomas (53–56). A *CDKN2* iBAC was constructed using a 132 kb BAC insert, which was used to efficiently infect both primary and immortalized human glioma cell lines carrying homozygous deletions of the *CDKN2* region. Expression of $p14^{ARF}$, $p15^{INK4B}$ and $p16^{INK4A}$ at approximately physiological levels was observed by RT-PCR, indicating that physiological splicing was taking place. Expression led to cell growth inhibition, demonstrating that functional gene products were being produced. This study shows that complex splicing events from a single locus are recapitulated in the iBAC system, and further demonstrates that genes delivered in this way can be controlled in an appropriate fashion.

Cell Differentiation—BMP2

Xing et al. (57) constructed an iBAC using a 128 kb sequence encompassing the *BMP2* locus in order to study the effect of BMP2 on development of preosteoblasts. BMP2 expression was clearly observed by Western blotting, and caused enhancement of osteoblast differentiation.

Taken together, these data clearly demonstrate that genomic loci can be delivered by iBAC vectors at high efficiency, express genes within a physiological range, and show physiological promoter regulation and gene splicing. The above examples suggest that iBACs may find broad applications in genomics research, which could ultimately lead to therapeutic applications. Some of these are discussed below.

APPLICATIONS IN NEUROLOGICAL DISORDERS

Recent years have seen great developments in CNS disease genetics, and experimental gene therapy approaches are being investigated for treatment of many disorders in which mutations have been identified. Gene therapy also has potential applications in nervous system repair, pain management, and cancer treatment. Some major challenges in CNS gene therapy include immune reactions, long-term gene expression, and the delivery of genes to non-dividing cells.

iBAC technology is most likely to find a use in gene replacement applications, such as in the many autosomal recessive and X-linked disorders that affect the nervous system. iBACs may also be useful in the delivery of neurotrophins, some of which exist in multiple splice forms, and finally could also be used to transduce stem cells.

HSV-1 has long been considered a strong candidate as a gene delivery vehicle for diseases of the CNS, due to its natural neuronal tropism (58). It has been shown that most neurons are efficiently infected by HSV-1 based vectors, as are astrocytes and oligodendrocytes (59). Injection of HSV-1 amplicons into the cerebellum efficiently transduces Purkinje cells (60,61). Moreover, injection into the inferior olive has been reported to allow efficient transduction of both cerebellar hemispheres by retrograde transport (60). Efficient transduction and GFP expression in rodents has been detected from HSV-1 amplicons injected into various areas of the CNS (40). Transgene expression can occur over an extended period of time with no apparent toxicity. With further regard to safety, HSV-1 amplicons generated using the helper virus free method were recently shown to have very low immunogenicity. This is in contrast with amplicons generated using helper viruses, which, in the same study, elicited a robust immune response (62). Importantly, iBACs can infect many cell types with no cytotoxic effects (1–3), including cultured cortical neurons (Fig. 3).

Autosomal-Recessive and X-linked Disorders

One route by which iBACs could be used to explore novel therapies is in the treatment of diseases caused by homozygous mutations in a single gene, where appropriate re-establishment of normal gene function would be the ideal approach. In these disorders heterozygotes are normally healthy, therefore if a functional gene can be delivered to the affected cells of a homozygous individual, a long-term therapeutic effect would likely be achieved (63). There are many such diseases that affect the nervous system, including some metabolic diseases, lysosomal storage disorders, spinal muscular atrophies, ataxias, retinal degenerations, muscular dystrophies, and familial amyotrophic lateral sclerosis (ALS). These involve a wide range of mutations in single genes, many of which have now

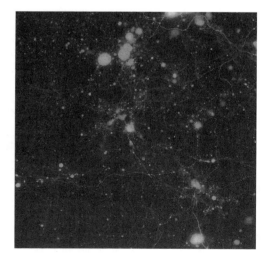

Figure 3   (*See color insert*) Cultured mouse cortical neurons infected with an empty iBAC vector. The image was taken 48 hours post-infection and shows strong GFP staining in the majority of neurons.

Table 1   A Selection of Autosomal Recessive and X-Linked Disorders, Including Minimum Locus Size and the Number of Splice Variants

Disease	Gene	Locus size (kb)	Transcripts
Ataxia telangiectasia	ATM	138.4	2
Friedreich's ataxia	Frataxin	38.5	1
X-linked retinitis pigmentosa 2	RP2	45.4	1
X-linked retinitis pigmentosa 3	RPGPR	58.4	7
Spinal muscular atrophies	SMN1/SMN2	26.9	2
Familial ALS	Cu, Zn SOD	6.4	1
Kennedy's disease	Androgen receptor	178.8	1
Charcot-Marie tooth type X1 (X-linked)	Connexin-32	10.3	3
Becker and Duchenne muscular Dystrophy (X-linked)	Dystrophin	1040.4	3
Familial dysautonomia	IKBKAP	86.6	1
Generalized myotonia	CLC1	35.9	1
Phenylketonurea	PAH	79.3	1
Lesch-Nyhan	HPRT	40.5	1
GM1 gangliosidoses	Beta-galactosidase	100.6	2
Tay-Sachs	HexosaminidaseA	32.6	1
Sandhoffs	HexosaminidaseB (and A)	36.1	1
Gauchers	Glucocerebrosidase	10.2	1
Niemann-Pick A,B	Acid sphingomyeli-nase	4.5	3
Neuronal Ceroid lipofuscinosis	CLN1	24.6	1
	CLN2	6.7	1
	CLN3	17.3	9
	CLN5	11.9	1
MPS1 (hurlers disease)	Alpha-l-iduronidase	17.5	1
MPSII (hunters syndrome)	Iduronate sulfatase	28.4	7
MPSIIIB(sanfilippo syndromes)	N-acetylglucosamini-dase	8.5	1
Krabbe disease	Galactosylceramidase	60.5	3
Metachromatic leukodystrophy	Arylsulfatase A	3.1	2
Adrenoleukodystrophy	ALD protein	19.9	1
Canavan disease	Aspartoacylase	23.4	1
Fragile X, A (X-linked)	FMR1	39.1	10
Fragile X, E (X-linked)	FMR2	520.1	3

Source: Data from http://www.ensembl.org.

been characterized and been used to test potential gene therapies in animal models. A selection of these diseases and associated genes is presented in Table 1, which also shows the number of known transcripts for each gene, and the minimum size of the genetic locus as described at http://www.ensembl.org. These sizes represent the length of DNA between the first and last exons, and for expression purposes extra flanking DNA should be included to ensure the presence of all regulatory regions. For example, from first exon to last, the *HPRT* gene is 40 kb, and in iBAC-*HPRT* a 115 kb region encompassing the locus was used (1). The exact length of DNA used depends on the size of the coding region, the presence of neighboring genes and their regulatory regions, and also to some extent experimental convenience. It has been estimated that 10 kb of $5'$ sequence will likely encompass the endogenous promoter sequence in most genes (64,65). Table 1 shows that genetic loci differ widely in their sizes, from 4.49 kb for the acid sphingomyelinase gene to 1040 kb for the dystrophin gene, which is too large for the iBAC system. The androgen receptor in Kennedy's disease and FMR2 are also too large for packaging into iBACs, but the rest are a suitable size. In fact, many genes, particularly those involved in lysosomal storage diseases, are small enough for packaging in "gutless" adenovirus, should be a useful delivery vector for the disease in question. Table 1 shows that 12 of the 31 genes have multiple transcripts, and up to nine (CLN3) and ten transcripts (FMR1) have been observed. The function of these splice variants is often not well understood, is probably biologically relevant, and may be important in therapeutic applications. In these cases delivery of a complete genetic locus may be of great benefit.

Lysosomal storage diseases have been well studied as potential targets for gene therapy. Many of the proteins involved are secreted and can spread throughout the body, and only 10% of normal levels may be required for a therapeutic effect. Some studies have described problems in the maintenance of gene expression (66,67), which could potentially be solved by the use of genomic transgenes. Also, transplantation of allogeneic hematopoietic stem cells has provided a good therapy for many of these diseases, removing the necessity for gene therapeutic approaches (68).

A large number of ataxias are autosomal recessive, and their genes are known (69). Some of these, such as ataxia telangiectasia, are linked directly to the cerebellum and are thus extremely attractive targets for therapy using HSV-1 based vectors, due to the high infectability of this area by HSV amplicons (60). Thus ataxia telangiectasia, caused by mutations in the *ATM* gene (70), may be an excellent candidate for iBAC gene therapy. The ATM genetic locus is large (138 kb), close to the upper limit of the iBAC system, but an iBAC-*ATM* construct may be a promising therapeutic vector. HSV-1 amplicon delivery for ataxias is promising because it combines unique vector capacity and route of delivery by retrograde transport for efficient delivery to the cerebellum.

Repair and Regeneration

iBACs may also find broader applications, for example in neurotrophin delivery, where authentic splicing may be beneficial. Many neurotrophins have been explored as therapeutic agents (71,72) in a wide range of neurodegenerative conditions, including Alzheimer's disease, Parkinson's disease, ALS, and brain or spinal cord injury. Several neurotrophic factors have multiple splice variants that may be crucial for maximum biological activity. For example, GDNF has three, and BDNF has six splice variants. It has been proposed that alternative splicing plays an especially important role in cells of the nervous system, and is necessary for the complexity observed in the CNS (73). It will be interesting to explore whether the simultaneous expression of multiple splice variants would improve the efficacy of gene therapy with these factors. In these cases, it may be of benefit to use iBACs engineered for higher expression levels in order to ensure sufficient transgene expression.

Stem Cell Transplantation

The transplantation of cells carrying specific genetic modifications has much potential for the treatment of diseases of the CNS (74–76). In this way therapeutic genes can be delivered to stem cells ex vivo—which could be preferable to injecting a virus directly.

Stem cells have the valuable property of being able to migrate to damaged areas of the brain (77), where they could deliver trophic support, or immunomodulatory molecules in cancer treatment. Studies in our laboratory show that neural stem cells derived from new-born mice are transducible with HSV-1 amplicons (S. Lawler and D. Gianni unpublished observations). Further study is required to examine the maintenance of genetic material in stem cells, but they could be a useful vehicle for the delivery of genes expressed by iBACs, and expand the range in which HSV-1 amplicons are of use in gene delivery.

DISCUSSION

The repair or replacement of pathogenic genes in their properly functioning form remains a difficult goal. As illustrated in this chapter, expression of genomic transgenes delivered by HSV-1 amplicons could provide some benefits through tissue-specific, appropriately regulated gene expression. iBACs overcome several obstacles in genomic locus delivery, and the system has several important advantages:

1. Capacity—iBACs allow delivery of genomic DNA sequences up to ~150 kb in size, large enough to express 95% of known genes.
2. Delivery—HSV-1 can infect a broad range of cells, both dividing and non-dividing, and is an excellent candidate for neuronal gene delivery. Genes delivered by iBACs and maintained as episomes remain largely intact—unlike those delivered by chemical methods. The helper free amplicon system also delivers genes with minimal toxicity and immune reactions in vivo. The high in vitro efficiency of transduction allows straightforward initial testing of iBAC vectors in cell culture models.
3. Regulation—Genes delivered by iBACs show appropriate regulation, in their extrachromosomal state. They are maintained at a low copy number allowing physiologic expression levels (1).
4. Long-term expression—Episomal BAC vectors carrying the EBV*oriP* sequence are retained at 96–98% efficiency in the absence of selection when EBNA-1 is co-expressed (13). Gene expression from iBACs retained using the *EBNA-1/oriP* system has been detected after more than 3 mo of continuous cell culture (1,3).
5. Ease of production—Making an iBAC is a straightforward process, using well-described methodologies. There is also flexibility in the system as iBACs can be shuttled between mammalian cells and bacteria, potentially allowing fine manipulation of genomic sequences (32). The transgene capacity of HSV-1 allows flexibility in the plasmid backbone, so that marker genes, and other modifications such as the addition of *EBNA-1*, can be incorporated. The ease of making iBACs could be useful in functional genomics studies to examine the functions of multiple SNPs.

iBACs form part of a second generation of transgene vectors—delivering genes based on genomic DNA sequences. Short of directly correcting genetic defects, approaches such as the iBAC system could ultimately find a major role in moving towards the treatment of human disease. Indeed, the iBAC system was recently recognized as an important breakthrough in gene therapy research (78,79).

The number of examples of iBAC-based expression is limited at present and awaits in vivo testing. One of the main challenges to overcome, as with many potential gene therapies of the nervous system is widespread delivery, and the number of cells which must be transduced in order to gain therapeutic benefit will likely vary from disease to disease. Even though the capacity of HSV-1 amplicons is impressive, some genes are too large for packaging, and larger capacity vectors with different cell specificity—such as EBV (80) or CMV may yet be needed. Amplicon systems are in development based on various large viruses including CMV, which was shown to package 210 kb with titers of 2×10^4 tfu/ml (81). An EBV amplicon was recently used to deliver a 120 kb insert carrying the complete Nijmegen breakage syndrome (NBS1) genomic locus (80). Amplicons based on Human herpes viruses 6 and 7 have been used to infect T lymphocytes (82,83). These systems represent exciting alternatives, but do not possess the same neuronal infectivity as HSV-1 based amplicons. In recent years, there have also been advances in the development of human artificial chromosomes for stable delivery of genomic DNA (84), although delivery remains a difficult problem.

Gene expression is a complex process involving alternative splicing mechanisms, alternative promoter-enhancer usage, intronic gene expression, expression of inhibiting RNAs, and effects of DNA polymorphisms. Conventional gene therapy vectors employing a cDNA transgene and a strong viral promoter are not able to replicate the complexity and subtlety of normal gene regulation. This is particularly relevant in therapies involving gene replacement. iBAC technology could be a major step in overcoming these difficulties. At the present time, iBACs may be the best method available for functional study of genetic loci, and their possible utility in gene therapy applications.

REFERENCES

1. Wade-Martins R, Smith ER, Tyminski E, et al. An infectious transfer and expression system for genomic DNA loci in human and mouse cells. Nat Biotechnol 2001; 19:1067–1070.
2. Wade-Martins R, Saeki Y, Chiocca EA. Infectious delivery of a 135 kb LDLR genomic locus leads to regulated complementation of low-density lipoprotein receptor deficiency in human cells. Mol Ther 2003; 7:604–612.
3. Inoue R, Moghaddam KA, Ranasinghe M, et al. Infectious delivery of the 132 kb CDKN2A/CDKN2B genomic DNA region results in correctly spliced gene expression and growth suppression in glioma cells. Gene Ther 2004; 11:1195–1204.
4. Kaplan JM, Armentano D, Sparer TE, et al. Characterization of factors involved in modulating persistence of transgene expression from recombinant adenovirus in the mouse lung. Hum Gene Ther 1997; 8:45–56.
5. Rozmahel R, Gyomorey K, Plyte S, et al. Incomplete rescue of cystic fibrosis transmembrane conductance regulator deficient mice by the human CFTR cDNA. Hum Mol Genet 1997; 6:1153–1162.
6. Robertson G, Garrick D, Wilson M, et al. Age-dependent silencing of globin transgenes in the mouse. Nucleic Acids Res 1996; 24:1465–1471.
7. Pravtcheva DD, Wise TL. A postimplantation lethal mutation induced by transgene insertion on mouse chromosome 8. Genomics 1995; 30:529–544.
8. Cavazzana-Calvo M, Thrasher A, Mavilio F. The future of gene therapy. Nature 2004; 427:779–781.
9. Doerfler W, Schubert R, Heller H, et al. Integration of foreign DNA and its consequences in mammalian systems. TIBTECH 1997; 15:297–301.
10. Heister T, Heid I, Ackermann M, et al. Herpes simplex virus type 1/adeno-associated virus hybrid vectors mediate site specific integration at the adeno-associated virus preintegration site, AAVS1, on chromosome 19. J Virol 2002; 76:7163–7173.
11. Yates J, Warren N, Sugden B. Stable replication of plasmids derived from Epstein-Barr virus in mammalian cells. Nature 1985; 313:812–815.
12. Simpson K, McGuigan A, Huxley C. Stable episomal maintenance of yeast artificial chromosomes in human cells. Mol Cell Biol 1996; 16:5117–5126.

13. Westphal EM, Sierakowska H, Livanos E, et al. A system for shuttling 200 kb BAC/PAC clones into human cells: stable extrachromosomal persistence and long-term ectopic gene expression. Hum Gene Ther 1998; 9:1863–1873.

14. Wade-Martins R, Frampton J, James MR. Long-term stability of large insert genomic DNA episomal shuttle vectors in human cells. Nucleic Acids Res 1999; 27:1674–1682.

15. Stoll SM, Sclimenti CR, Baba EJ, et al. Epstein-Barr virus/human vector provides high-level long-term expression of alpha-1 antitrypsin in mice. Mol Ther 2001; 4:122–129.

16. Wade-Martins R, White RE, Kimura H. Stable correction of a genetic deficiency in human cells by an episome carrying a 115 kb genomic transgene. Nat Biotechnol 2000; 18:1311–1314.

17. Schedl A, Ross A, Lee M, et al. Influence of PAX6 gene dosage on development: overexpression causes severe eye abnormalities. Cell 1996; 86:71–82.

18. Manson AL, Trezise AE, MacVinish LJ, et al. Complementation of null CF mice with a human CFTR YAC transgene. EMBO J 1997; 16:4238–4249.

19. Schiedner G, Morral N, Parks SJ, et al. Genomic gene transfer with a high capacity adenovirus vector results in improved in vivo gene expression and reduced toxicity. Nat Genet 1998; 18:180–183.

20. Rowntree RK, Vassaux G, McDowell TL, et al. An element in intron 1 of the CFTR gene augments intestinal expression in vivo. Hum Mol Genet 2001; 10:1455–1464.

21. Lander ES, Linton LM, Birren B, et al. Initial sequencing and analysis of the human genome. Nature 2001; 409:860–921.

22. Shizuya H, Birren B, Kim UJ, et al. Cloning and stable maintenance of 300-kilobase-pair fragments of human DNA in Escherichia coli using an F-factor based vector. Proc Natl Acad Sci USA 1992; 89:8794–8797.

23. Ioannou PA, Amemiya CT, Garnes J, et al. A new bacteriophage P1 vector for the propagation of large human DNA fragments. Nat Genet 1994; 6:84–89.

24. Karolchik D, Hinrichs AS, Furey TS. The UCSC table browser data retrieval tool. Nucleic Acids Res 2004; 32:D493–D496.

25. Compton SH, Mecklenbeck S, Mejia JE, et al. Stable integration of large (>100 kb) PAC constructs in HaCaT keratinocytes using an integrin-targeting peptide delivery system. Gene Ther 2000; 7:1600–1605.

26. Yang XW, Model P, Heintz N. Homologous recombination based modification in Escherichia coli, and germline transmission in transgenic mice of a bacterial artificial chromosome. Nat Biotechnol 1997; 15:859–865.

27. Yang XW, Wynder C, Doughty ML, et al. BAC-mediated gene-dosage analysis reveals a role for Zipro1 (Ru49/Zfp38) in progenitor cell proliferation in cerebellum and skin. Nat Genet 1999; 22:327–335.

28. Gong S, Zheng C, Doughty ML, et al. A gene expression atlas of the central nervous system based on bacterial artificial chromosomes. Nature 2003; 425:917–925.

29. Narayanan K, Williamson R, Zhang Y, et al. Efficient and precise engineering of a 200 kb beta globin human/bacterial artificial chromosome in E.coli DH10B using an inducible homologous recombination system. Gene Ther 1999; 6:442–447.

30. Zhang Y, Muyrers JPP, Testa G, et al. DNA cloning by homologous recombination in Escherichia coli. Nat Biotechnol 2000; 18:1314–1317.

31. Muyrers JPP, Zhang Y, Benes V, et al. Point mutation of bacterial artificial chromosomes by ET recombination. EMBO Rep 2000; 1:239–243.

32. Muyrers JPP, Zhang Y, Stewart AF. Techniques: recombinogenic engineering—new options for cloning and manipulating DNA. Trends Biochem Sci 2001; 26:325.

33. Blackwood EM, Kadonaga JT. Going the distance: a current view of enhancer action. Science 1998; 281:60–63.

34. Li Q, Harju S, Peterson KR. Locus control regions—coming of age at a decade plus. Trends Genet 1999; 15:403–408.

35. Thomas CE, Ehrhardt A, Kay MA. Progress and problems with the use of viral vectors for gene therapy. Nat Rev Genet 2003; 4:346–358.

36. Chiocca EA, Choi BB, Cai W. Transfer and expression of the LacZ gene in rat brain mediated by herpes simplex virus mutants. New Biol 1990; 2:739–746.

37. Spaete RR, Frenkel N. The herpes simplex virus amplicon: a new eukaryotic defective-virus cloning-amplifying vector. Cell 1982; 30:295–304.

38. Geller AI. A new method to propagate defective HSV-1 vectors. Nucleic Acids Res 1998; 16:5690.

39. Sena-Estevez M, Saeki Y, Fraefel C, et al. HSV-1 amplicon vectors—simplicity and versatility. Mol Ther 2002; 2:9–15.

40. Oehmig A, Fraefel C, Breakefield X. Update on herpes virus amplicon vectors. Mol Ther 2004; 10:630–643.

41. Saeki Y, Fraefel C, Ichikawa T, et al. Improved helper virus-free packaging system for HSV amplicon vectors using an ICP27-deleted, oversized HSV-1 DNA in a bacterial artificial chromosome. Mol Ther 2001; 3:591–601.

42. Boren J, Lee I, Callow MJ, et al. A simple and efficient method for making site-directed mutants, deletions, and fusions of large DNA such as P1 and BAC clones. Genome Res 1996; 6:1123–1130.

43. Caskey CT, Kruh GD. The HPRT locus. Cell 1979; 16:1–9.

44. Rader DJ. Gene therapy for familial hypercholesterolemia. Nutr Metab Cardiovasc Dis 2001; 11:40–44.

45. Brown MS, Goldstein L. Regulation of the activity of the low density lipoprotein receptor in human fibroblasts. Cell 1975; 6:307–316.

46. Russell DW, Yamamoto T, Schneider WJ, et al. cDNA cloning of the bovine lipoprotein receptor: feedback regulation of a receptor mRNA. Proc Natl Acad Sci USA 1983; 80:7501–7505.

47. Kozarsky KF, Jooss K, Donahee M, et al. Effective treatment of familial hypercholesterolemia in the mouse model using adenovirus mediate transfer of the VLDL receptor gene. Nat Genet 1996; 13:54–62.

48. Chen SJ, Rader DJ, Tazelaar J, et al. Prolonged correction of hyperlipidemia in mice with familial hypercholesterolemia using an adenovirus vector expressing very-low-density lipoprotein receptor. Mol Ther 2000; 2:256–261.

49. Chowdhury JR, Grossman M, Gupta S, et al. Long-term improvement of hypercholesterolemia after ex vivo gene therapy. Science 1991; 254:1802–1805.

50. Heeren J, Steinwaerder DS, Schneiders F, et al. Nonphysiological overexpression of low density lipoprotein receptors cause pathological intracellular lipid accumulation and the formation of cholesterol and cholesteryl ester crystals in vitro. J Mol Med 1999; 77:735–743.

51. Sharpless NE, DePinho RA. The *INK4A/ARF* locus and its two gene products. Curr Opin Genet Dev 1999; 9:22–30.

52. Sherr CJ. The INK4A/ARF network in tumor suppression. Nat Rev Mol Cell Biol 2001; 2:731–737.

53. Caldas C, Hahn SA, da Costa LT, et al. Frequent somatic mutations and homozygous deletions of the p16 (MTS1) gene in pancreatic adenocarcinoma. Nat Genet 1994; 8:27–32.

54. Schmidt EE, Ichimura K, Reifenberger G, et al. CDKN2 (p16/MTS1) gene deletion or CDK4 amplification occurs in the majority of glioblastomas. Cancer Res 1994; 54:6321–6324.

55. Moulton T, Samara G, Chung WY, et al. MTS1/p16/CDKN2 lesions in primary glioblastoma multiforme. Am J Pathol 1995; 146:613–619.

56. Simon M, Koster G, Menon AG, et al. Functional evidence for a role of combined CDKN2A (p16-14(ARF)/CDKN2B(p15) gene inactivation in malignant gliomas. Acta Neuropathol (Berl) 1999; 98:444–452.

57. Xing W, Baylink D, Kesaven C, et al. HSV-1 amplicon-mediated transfer of 128-kb BMP-2 genomic locus stimulates osteoblast differentiation in vitro. Biochem Biophys Res Commun 2004; 319:781–786.

58. Lilley CE, Branston RH, Coffin RS. Herpes simplex virus vectors for the nervous system. Curr Gene Ther 2001; 1:339–358.

59. Marsh DR, Dekaban GA, Tan W, et al. Herpes simplex viral and amplicon vector-mediated gene transfer into glia and neurons in organotypic spinal cord and dorsal root ganglion cultures. Mol Ther 2000; 1:464–478.

60. Agudo M, Trejo JL, Lim F, et al. Highly efficient and specific gene transfer to Purkinje cells in vivo using a herpes simplex virus amplicon. Hum Gene Ther 2002; 13:665–674.

61. Cortes ML, Bakkenist CJ, Di Maria MV, et al. Gene Ther 2003; 10:1321–1327.

62. Olschowka JA, Bowers WJ, Hurley SD, et al. Helper-free HSV-1 amplicons elicit a markedly less robust innate immune response in the CNS. Mol Ther 2003; 7:218–227.

63. MacMillan JC, Lowenstein PR. Gene therapy approaches to the treatment of human neurological disease: the future of neurological therapies. In: Lowenstein PR, Enquist LW, eds. Protocols for Gene Transfer in Neuroscience. U.K.: John Wiley and Sons, 1995:379–407.

64. Praz V, Perier R, Bonnard C. The Eukaryotic Promoter Database, EPD: new entry types and links to gene expression data. Nucleic Acids Res 2002; 30:322–324.

65. Ureta-Vidal A, Ettwiller L, Birney E. Comparative genomics: genome-wide analysis in metazoan eukaryotes. Nat Rev Genet 2003; 4:251–262.

66. Ding EY, Hodges BL, Hu H, et al. Long-term efficacy after [E1-polymerase] adenovirus-mediated transfer of human acid-alpha-glucosidase gene into glycogen storage disease type II knockout mice. Hum Gene Ther 2001; 12:955–965.

67. Hodges BL, Taylor KM, Joseph MF, et al. Long-term transgene expression from plasmid DNA gene therapy vectors is negatively affected by CpG dinucleotides. Mol Ther 2004; 10:269–278.

68. Krivit W. Allogeneic stem cell transplantation for the treatment of lysosomal and peroxisomal metabolic diseases. Springer Semin Immunopathol 2004; 26:119–132.

69. Taroni F, DiDonato S. Pathways to motor incoordination: the inherited ataxias. Nat Rev Neurosci 2004; 5:641–655.

70. Savitsky K, Bar-Shira A, Gilad S, et al. A single ataxia telangiectasia gene with a product similar to PI-3 kinase. Science 1995; 268:1749–1753.

71. Hendriks WT, Ruitenberg MJ, Blits B, et al. Viral vector-mediated gene transfer of neurotrophins to promote regeneration of the injured spinal cord. Prog Brain Res 2004; 146:451–476.

72. Tuszynski MH. Gene therapy for neurological disease. Expert Opin Biol Ther 2003; 3:815–828.

73. Grabowski PJ. Splicing regulation in neurons: tinkering with cell specific control. Cell 1998; 92:709–712.

74. Burton EA, Glorioso JC, Fink DJ. Gene therapy progress and prospects: Parkinson's disease. Gene Ther 2003; 10:1721–1727.

75. Flax JD, Aurora S, Yang C, et al. Engraftable human neural stem cells respond to developmental cues, replace neurons, and express foreign genes. Nat Biotechnol 1998; 16:1033–1039.

76. Park KI, Ourednik J, Ourednik V, et al. Global gene and cell replacement strategies via stem cells. Gene Ther 2002; 9:613–624.

77. Aboody KS, Brown A, Rainov NG, et al. Neural stem cells display extensive tropism for pathology in adult brain: evidence from intracranial gliomas. Proc Natl Acad Sci 2000; 97:12846–12851.

78. Steele FR. Gene therapy tools for functional genomics. Genomics 2002; 80:1.

79. Ackerman M, Fraefel C. One giant leap for gene transfer technology. Mol Ther 2003; 7:571.

80. White RE, Wade-Martins R, James MR. Infectious delivery of 120 kb genomic DNA by an Epstein-Barr virus amplicon vector. Mol Ther 2002; 5:427–435.

81. Borst EM, Messerle M. Construction of a cytomegalovirus-based amplicon: a vector with a unique transfer capacity. Hum Gene Ther 2003; 14:959–970.

82. Romi H, Singer O, Rapaport D, et al. Tamplicon-7, a novel T-lymphotropic vector derived from human herpes virus 7. J Virol 1999; 73:7001–7007.

83. Borenstein R, Singer O, Moseri A, et al. Use of amplicon-6 vectors derived from human herpes virus 6 for efficient expression of membrane-associated and -secreted proteins in T cells. J Virol 2004; 78:4730–4743.

84. Larin Z, Mejia T. Advances in human artificial chromosome technology. Trends Genet 2002; 18:313–319.

6

Targeted Gene Modification of the Nervous System

Maria L. Cortes and Xandra O. Breakefield

Departments of Neurology and Radiology, Massachusetts General Hospital,
Charlestown and Program in Neuroscience, Harvard Medical School, Boston,
Massachusetts, U.S.A.

INTRODUCTION

This review will cover direct modification of the neuronal cell genome to achieve therapeutic intervention, as well as elucidation of neuronal functions. Targeted engineering of the mammalian genome can be accomplished using viral vectors, oligonucleotides, and DNA fragments, as well as proteins, such as recombinases and rare restriction enzymes, which recognize specific nucleotide sequences. Topics covered include: adeno-associated virus (AAV) mediated integration of transgenes into the AAVS1 site; oligonucleotide site-directed gene mutagenesis and correction; homologous recombination (HR) using small and larger DNA sequences, and use of recombinases, such as Cre, Flp and the ϕC31 integrase to insert or delete genes or alter gene structure, so as to turn off or on informative genes. Therapeutic interventions are discussed, such as replacement and correction of defective genes, as well as introduction of modulating genes. Elucidation of neuronal functions covers marking of specific neuronal subtypes, tracing neuronal circuitry and monitoring of neuronal activity. The review is intended to inform gene therapists as to the multipotential approaches currently available to expand the ability to understand and treat human disease.

METHODS TO TARGET SPECIFIC SITES IN THE GENOME AND THERAPEUTIC APPLICATIONS

AAV and Integration into AAVS1 Site

The challenge of gene therapy to the nervous system is to develop non-toxic vectors that can achieve stable, regulated transgene expression in post-mitotic cells (1). AAV has the potential for insertion of genes into a specific site (AAVS1) in the mammalian genome, which is a unique property among mammalian viruses. Retrovirus and derivative lentivirus vectors can integrate transgenes into a variety of dividing and non-dividing cell types (2,3), but they are limited by their relatively small transgene capacity ($\sim$8 kb), random integration into the genome and deposition of viral sequences within the host genome. Random integration has the potential to disrupt the expression of endogenous genes, and activate proto-oncogenes (4). Adenovirus and herpes simplex type 1 (HSV) vectors have a larger transgene capacity (30 kb and 150 kb, respectively) in their "gutless," "helper dependent" (HD) or amplicon versions (5–10), and also infect a wide range of dividing and non-dividing cells, but do not have an intrinsic integrative mechanism into the host cell genome.

Methods

AAV is a nonpathogenic parvovirus with a single-stranded (ss) DNA genome that can enter either a lytic or latent state after infecting cells (11). Efficient replication of the AAV genome occurs in the presence of coinfection with a helper virus, either adenovirus or HSV (12). In the absence of a helper virus, the AAV genome can integrate into a specific AAVS1 site in the human host cell genome located on chromosome 19q13.3 and establish a latent infection (13,14). Site-specific integration can occur in non-dividing cells, although at a lower frequency than in dividing cells (15,16). AAV has a 4.7 kb DNA genome containing two open reading frames (ORFs): Rep, encoding four regulatory proteins (Rep 40, 52, 68, 78); and Cap, encoding three structural capsid proteins, which are flanked by 145 bp inverted terminal repeats (ITRs) (17). Both the ITRs and Rep68 or Rep78 proteins are essential for AAV replication and site-specific integration into the host genome (18–21). In the absence of Rep proteins, long-term expression of ITR-flanked cassettes results from random integration(s) into the host genome (22–24) and/or persistence as an extrachromosomal element (25,26).

The mechanism of site-specific integration of AAV into the human genome is not completely understood; however, in vitro models support the involvement of Rep proteins and specific elements present within the ITRs and AAVS1 site (27,28). Linden et al. (27) showed that the first 125 bp of the ITR constitute an overall palindrome interrupted by two smaller internal palindromes of 21 bp. The ITRs fold into hairpin structures, and the long stem of the hairpin contains a Rep binding site (RBS). The two large viral proteins (Rep68 and Rep78) bind both to the RBS in the ITR and to a homologous RBS in the AAVS1 site (Fig. 1). This alignment initiates a nonhomologous recombination event between AAV and AAVS1 sequences. Rep then introduces a nick into the AAVS1 terminal resolution site (TRS) and DNA synthesis initiates, displacing a ss of AAVS1 (27–29). The AAVS1 sequence itself, and not the secondary structure of human chromosome 19, is sufficient for AAV site-specific integration, as AAVS1 sequences introduced into either plasmid vectors (27) or animal genomes (30–32) can serve as platforms for site-specific integration of AAV ITR-flanked cassettes in the presence of Rep proteins. Transgenic mouse models bearing the human AAVS1 site have been established, containing varying length fragments of this site—1.6 kb (31), 3.5 kb (30), and the full-length, 8.2 kb (32) in the mouse genome. In addition, Dutheil et al. (33) has identified a mouse ortholog of the AAVS1 sequence in the mouse genome, which should be capable of mediating ITR integration.

Applications and Therapeutic Potential

Most of the work being carried out with AAV for gene therapy uses the virus in a recombinant form (rAAV) deleted of all viral genes thus having lost the Rep-mediated, site-specific integration property of the wild-type virus (34,35). rAAV vectors maintain a residual capacity for ITR-mediated integration in some target cells (e.g., liver), although at low efficiency and with virtually no site-specificity (36–38). Like retroviruses, AAV vectors appear to have a preference for integration into transcriptionally active regions (39).

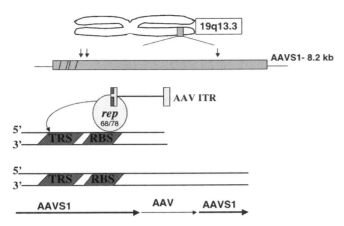

Figure 1 Model for AAV site-specific integration. AAV genome can integrate into the specific AAVS1 site in the human host cell genome located on chromosome 19q13.3. The two larger viral proteins (Rep68 and Rep78) both bind to the RBS in the ITR and to a homologous RBS at the AAVS1 site. Rep introduces a strand-specific nick at the TRS in AAVS1 and DNA synthesis initiates by single-strand displacement at the TRS. This alignment initiates a nonhomologous recombination event between AAV and AAVS1 sequences that result in integrated copies of AAV DNA within the AAVS1 site. *Abbreviations*: AAV, adeno-associated virus; ITR, inverted terminal repeat; RBS, rep binding site; TRS, terminal resolution site. *Source*: Dr. Bakowska, Harvard Medical School, Boston, Massachusetts and Ref. 27.

The major limitation of rAAV vectors is their size capacity, as vectors can package only about 4.7 kb of exogenous DNA. This size constraint can be overcome by using dual vector strategies that exploit intermolecular concatemerization of rAAV genomes (40,41) and combining viral elements from different viruses. AAV ITRs and Rep functions have been incorporated into hybrid, large-capacity viral vectors, such as baculovirus (42), HSV-1 amplicon (32,43,44), and adenovirus (45,46) vectors. However, the inhibitory effect of Rep on viral replication (47–49) significantly reduces the production of adenovirus and HSV-1 vectors that incorporate elements of the AAV integration machinery (43–45).

In addition, large Rep proteins affect viral and cellular gene expression at transcriptional and post-transcriptional levels and continued expression can be toxic to cells (47,50–53). This toxicity can be curtailed in several ways: (1) by limiting the presence of Rep activity by using a temperature sensitive mutant (54) or conditionally functional form of Rep (55); (2) by using a Cre/loxP-expression-switching system to regulate the expression of the *rep* gene (56,57); (3) by delivery of chimeric proteins based on Rep fused to different oligomerization motifs and transcriptional activation domains (58) or to virion proteins (59); (4) or by introducing the *rep* gene in plasmids separately from the viral vectors (35).

The HSV/AAV hybrid amplicon contains the AAV ITRs flanking the transgene(s) of choice with Rep-coding sequences placed outside the ITR cassette (Fig. 2) to reduce the chance of integration of the *rep* gene that could result in continued expression of this cytotoxic protein and promote excision of the integrated transgene (60,61). Several versions of the HSV/AAV hybrid amplicon vector have been designed for targeted integration of transgenes into the human genome. One version that prolongs transgene expression in dividing and nondividing cells contains, through inadvertent construction, partial ITRs and interrupted *rep* sequences resulting in no expression of Rep proteins

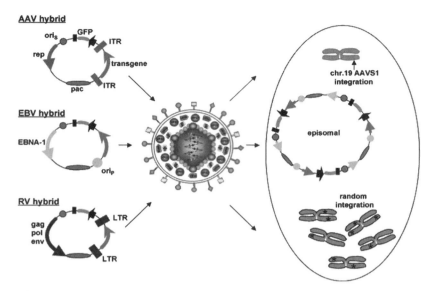

Figure 2 (*See color insert*) Structures and properties of HSV-1 amplicon-based hybrid vectors. HSV/AAV, HSV/EBV and HSV/RV hybrid amplicon DNA with HSV-1-specific elements (oriS and pac) and AAV (ITR and rep), EBV (EBNA-1 and oriP) and RV (gag-pol-env and LTR)-specific elements, respectively. The DNA is packaged as concatenates into HSV-1 virions. In the host cell nucleus, the DNA either integrates site-specifically into chromosome 19 (HSV/AAV), persists episomally (HSV/EBV) or integrates randomly into chromosomes (HSV/RV). *Source*: From Ref. 240.

(62,63). Other versions contain full-length ITRs and *rep* gene sequences that express either all four Rep proteins (60,44) or the two largest Rep proteins (43).

HSV/AAV hybrid amplicon vectors have been shown to integrate the ITR-flanked transgene cassette into the AAVS1 locus in human glioma and fibroblast cells in culture with frequencies up to 30% of infected cells (43,44), although there has been no assessment of site-specific integration in the nervous system. Immortalized fibroblasts from homozygous transgenic mice containing multiple copies of the human AAVS1 site at a single locus showed an overall 10-fold higher integration frequency with HSV/AAV vectors containing *rep* compared to control HSV amplicon vectors, and most of these integration events were into the AAVS1 locus (32). The creation of transgenic mouse models bearing the human AAVS1 site provides new opportunities in the study of gene therapy for neurologic disorders. Mice homozygous for the AAVS1 site can be crossed to mouse models of neurologic disorders to assess whether transduction with AAV or hybrid vectors carrying the *rep* gene in *cis* or *trans* to the transgene will be incorporated into the AAVS1 site, as a model of gene replacement in the human genome.

AAV ITRs and Rep functions have also been incorporated into a split adenovirus/AAV vector system, in which an AAV ITR-flanked integration cassette and a Rep78/68 expression cassette are carried by two different HD adenovirus vectors (45). This system has been improved by incorporating an ITR flanked integration cassette and a tightly regulated, drug-inducible Rep expression cassette into a single HD adenovirus vector. Using this vector, site-specific integration was obtained in vivo in liver cells following a single tail vein administration in an AAVS1 transgenic mouse model.

In addition to integration at AASV1 sites in the presence of Rep, Miller et al. (64) found randomly integrated AAV vector provirus at increased frequency in sites of spontaneous double-strand breaks (DSB) in the absence of Rep. Exposure of cells to DNA-damaging agents increases DSB and stable transduction by AAV in parallel (65). DSB are also increased in ataxia–telangiectasia (A–T), an autosomal recessive disease with a complex phenotype involving cerebellar degeneration, immunodeficiency, chromosomal instability, radiosensitivity, and cancer predisposition (66). Cells defective in the A–T gene product (ATM) have an increase in genomic DSB, as ATM is involved in DNA damage sensing and checkpoint signaling, and this is associated with an increased number of integrated proviral genomes after rAAV gene transfer (67). In addition to providing a means of gene replacement this vector integration could be used to capture DSB events, thus providing insight into the extent and location of DNA damage. This rAAV integration system could potentially be used in a number of other neurological disorders, such as xeroderma pigmentosum with DNA instability to assess the levels of DNA damage in the brain and to promote integration of corrective genes.

Site-Specific Recombinases

Site-specific recombinases (SSRs) are enzymes derived from prokaryotic and eukaryotic microorganisms that mediate efficient "cut-and-paste" type recombination between recognition sites in the range of 30–40 bp or longer (68). These allow integration and rearrangement of genes modified to incorporate recognition elements.

Methods

SSR are divided into two large families based on amino acid sequence homology and catalytic residues, either tyrosine or serine (69–71). The tyrosine SSR family, also known as the integrase family for its prototypical member λ integrase, uses a tyrosine to attack the DNA backbone during cleavage. This family includes more than 300 recombinases, with the two currently available for genomic manipulation being Cre recombinase and Flp invertase (68). Cre normally mediates recombination of the bacteriophage P1 genome (72), and Flp inverts, or "flips," a DNA segment in the yeast *S. cerevisae* (73). The serine recombinase family possess a catalytic serine residue, and also comprises a large family that includes invertases, resolvases, transposases, and phage integrases, like φC31, which has been used for genetic modifications in mammalian cells (71,74,75).

Cre and Flp are able to recombine specific sequences of DNA without the need for cofactors (74,76) and have been used effectively in flies (77,78), mammalian cell culture (79,80), and mice (81,82). Cre and Flp recombine DNA at defined target sites, termed loxP (locus of crossover in P1) and FRT (Flp recombinase recognition target), respectively, in both actively dividing and postmitotic cells in most tissue types (83). These sites share an overall structure that includes two 13 bp inverted repeats, separated by an 8 bp asymmetric spacer. In the presence of two target sites, recombinase monomers bound to the inverted repeats promote DNA complex formation and recombination between the two sites (84,85). Flp invertase functions at only 10–25% efficiency compared to Cre in generating genomic deletions (86). The DNA segment between two sites is either excised or inverted depending on the orientation of the paired sites. For example, when two loxP sites are in the same orientation, Cre excises the intervening DNA segment, resulting in a single remaining loxP site. If the repeats are in opposite orientations, the DNA segment undergoes inversion and the two loxP sites remain (87). This integration reaction is reversible, because the recombination product harbors two identical target sites that are themselves substrates for recombination (34). By contrast, the excision reaction is effectively irreversible and has been exploited extensively in generating mouse mutants.

The Cre/loxP system is the most widely used approach for generating tissue-specific gene knockout mice. In most cases, Cre- and loxP-containing strains of mice are developed independently then crossed to generate offspring with tissue-specific gene knockouts (87).

Cre and Flp each tolerate certain variations in their target sequences that fall in two classes: spacer variants and inverted repeat variants (88). The first class contains nucleotide substitution within the spacer sequence, as it is spacer length not sequence per se that is critical for efficient recombination (89–91). This is the basis for the insertion strategy called "recombinase-mediated cassette exchange" (92,93) and the inversion strategy called "FLEx" switch, where the fragment is inverted once and to prevent further inversions the DNA fragment is flanked by heterotypic target sites (94). The second class contains nucleotide substitutions within the inverted repeats that compromise binding of the recombinase to DNA thus allowing stable DNA insertions (91,95,96). In order to maximize recombination efficiency, Cre activity has been increased by modifying the Cre gene to be more eukaryotic-like, including a reduced CpG content and improved Kozak translation initiation consensus sequence (97). Ligand-regulated forms of Cre and Flp have also been developed to control temporal SSR activity thus enabling the induction of genetic changes late in embryogenesis and/or in adult tissues. Successful strategies include fusing a mutant estrogen receptor (ER) ligand binding domain (LBD) to the C-terminus of Flp (98) or Cre (99–103) such that they enter the nucleus upon binding to estrogen, or regulating SSR transcription by placing Cre and Flp under the tetracycline (tet) regulatory system (104).

Members of the serine SSR family, including the *Streptomyces* phage-derived φC31 have also proven effective for genomic modification in mammalian cells (105). φC31 mediates recombination between two different sites, *att*B (34 bp) and *att*P (39 bp) (106,107). The names of the sites derive from the attachment sites for the phage integrase on the bacterial (*att*B) and phage genomes (*att*P). The sites contain a core TTG cross-over region flanked by different ITRs in *att*B and *att*P (108) that are bound by φC31 homodimers (106). The product, two hybrid sites, *att*L and *att*R, are no longer substrates for recombination by the integrase, so the reactions are unidirectional and irreversible (109,110). In contrast to the tyrosine family, these SSRs make a 2 bp staggered cut in each *att* site breaking all four strands at once followed by a 180° rotation and DNA ligation (111). When considering designing experiments using φC31, an important consideration is the presence of multiple pseudo *att*P sites in the genomes of both human and mouse cell lines (107).

Applications and Therapeutic Potential

SSRs are transforming mouse genetics by providing a means to manipulate chromosomal DNA with high fidelity, thus advancing the understanding of gene function in development and disease. The generation of conditional knockout mouse models using SSR technology overcomes problems of embryonic lethality associated with loss of some genes. Combined with conditional turn-on of reporter genes it allows the study of gene function selectively within the mammalian nervous system, as well as the development of novel therapeutic strategies. Among SSRs, the Cre-loxP system has been employed the most for investigating neurologic diseases and neural functions. Cre has been placed under the control of different brain specific promoters like Thy-1, CamKIIα, synapsin, GluRδ2 (112–115) and mice have been engineered to allow Cre to be regulated spatially and temporally using inducible promoters specific for neuronal populations in different brain regions (88,116–119). Numerous transgenic lines expressing Cre SSR in the central nervous system have been published to date (120).

The Nagy Laboratory (http://www.mshri.on.ca/nagy/default.htm) and Jackson Laboratories (http://jaxmice.jax.org/models/cre_flp_loxp.html) web sites provide an up-to-date list of existing lines bearing Cre and floxed genes. Activation, as well as deletion of, genes can be achieved in the nervous system by the Cre-loxP method. Inserting a floxed transcriptional stop cassette $5'$ to the gene of interest silences the locus, with Cre mediated removal of the floxed stop allowing the gene to be transcribed (121).

However, some reports had indicated that Cre can cause a reduction in cell proliferation or even induce chromosomal aberrations (122,123). These effects strongly depend on the level and the length of time of expression of Cre, and they have not been observed to date in transgenic mice (124). A possible explanation for these toxic effects is the presence of pseudo-loxP sequences throughout the genome, such that expression of Cre can lead to genomic rearrangement (125–127).

Several neurologic disorders caused by a known genetic mutation have been modeled in mice using SSR technology. For example, to determine whether onset of the disease relates to the developmental or adult function of a gene, it is possible to induce reversible mutations. Yamamoto et al. (128) demonstrated in a conditional mouse model of Huntington's disease that symptoms and cellular inclusions which increased in early life could be diminished when the mutated gene was switched off in the adult animal. This reversal of neuropathology has also been achieved in early stages of another disease model, spinocerebellar ataxia type 1; however, in this case halting expression of the mutated gene at later stages yielded only partial recovery of neurologic function (129).

The ϕC31 SSR can potentially be used like Cre, with *att* sites placed into the genome of an organism and used as a target for recombination, as it has been shown in cultured mammalian cells (107). Belteki et al. (110) demonstrated the ability of ϕC31 to integrate an *att*B-flanked transgene cassette into an *att*P-flanked cassette in the genome of mouse embryonic stem (ES) cells. Several studies have also demonstrated the use of ϕC31 for gene therapy, including transduction of cells containing genomic *att*P sites with a combination of *att*B/transgene and integrase plasmids to achieve correction of gene defects and long-term expression of secreted proteins (130,131).

Oligonucleotide Site-Directed Gene Targeting

A number of oligonucleotide site-directed gene targeting strategies have been developed with the primary aim of correcting human genetic disorders caused by simple base alterations in a single gene. The advantage of gene repair is that the corrected gene can be maintained, expressed, and regulated as a normal endogenous gene. Several approaches, including chimeric RNA–DNA oligonucleotides (RDO), short ss oligodeoxynucleotides (ODN), and triple-helix-forming oligonucleotides (TFO), have been used for targeted modification of the genome.

Methods

RDOs are ss molecules, usually 70–80 bases in length, with RNA and DNA nucleotides in a self-complementary sequence that folds into a double-hairpin configuration, termed a chimera, which is resistant to nuclease digestion and concatenation (132,133). The upper strand of the chimera consists of $2'$-0-methylRNA residues, and the lower strand contains the DNA targeting region (134,135). The feasibility of gene correction by RDOs was first demonstrated in 1996 by correction of a point mutation in an alkaline phosphatase cDNA integrated in the genome of cultured CHO cells (136). Since then, it has been shown to repair genes at the episomal and chromosomal levels in mammalian, yeast, and plant cells

(136,137), including in vivo correction of mutations in cells in a variety of tissues, including liver, lung, muscle, and skin (138–141). However, variability and lack of reproducibility in the conversion frequencies (<1–50%) in culture and in vivo are a major criticism of this strategy (142–144).

Studies on the structure–activity of the RDOs suggested that the lower band of the chimera was responsible for DNA repair, so ss ODN were tested for their ability to effect genomic alterations in diverse culture systems, including mammalian, yeast and plant cells (145–148). The mechanism of action is unclear, but appears to involve endogenous mismatch repair proteins, polymerases, ligases, and recombinases (149). The conversion frequencies in this strategy are reproducible, but still low (<1%) for effective gene repair. Further studies are required to evaluate the feasibility and application of this approach in vivo.

TFOs bind in the major groove of a duplex DNA target that consist of homopurine or homopyridine stretches (15–30 bp) (150). These regions occur about every kilobase or so in the mammalian genome, so it is likely that the majority of genes (average size 10 kb) contain multiple TFO targets (151). TFOs have been used in a number of ways to mediate transcriptional regulation, mutagenesis, and recombination (152,153). By coupling crosslinking agents to the TFOs (e.g., the mutagen, psoralen), the DNA sequence can be disrupted through a chemical or physical reaction (154). The resultant DNA damage stimulates the genomic repair system and thereby can increase the frequency of HR in the presence of the correct gene sequence (155) or by gene conversion.

Applications and Therapeutic Potential

The use of oligonucleotides for site-directed gene targeting in the nervous system is currently limited by a low frequency of correction, although this remains a promising strategy. Global delivery to the brain in vivo would probably require direct injection of oligonucleotides incorporated in liposomes with expanded distribution facilitated by inclusion of mannitol and convection-enhanced delivery (156). Pegylated immunoliposomes coupled to antibodies to the transferrin receptor have also been used to transfer DNA from the blood stream across the blood-brain-barrier (157). To improve the efficiency of delivery, nucleotides can be modified, such as by linking with peptides or configuring them in a locked nucleic acid state, to increase their resistance to nuclease degradation (158). Translocating peptides, such as the HIV TAT peptide, herpes simplex VP22, and antenopedia peptides, may improve entry of coupled molecules into cells and on to the nucleus bypassing endosomal compartments (159). Parekh-Olmedo et al. (146) have suggested the possibility that Huntington's disease, characterized by an expansion of the polyglutamine tract in the huntingtin protein (160), could be treated by mutating a CAG in the repeat to a CTG using a gene repair vector and thereby disrupting the repeat or by creating a stop codon (CAG→TAG) in the coding sequence, therefore, producing a protein less likely to aggregate.

Ex vivo approaches could include the electroporation or transduction of cells cultured from affected individuals, including neural stem cells (146). Stem cells can provide a propagating source of corrected neural cells, which could be reintroduced into the patient and would have the ability to differentiate into different cell types. Growth advantage and migrational capacity of corrected stem cells could translate into symptomatic improvement by "relocalization" and neural cell replacement in diseased brain (161–163). The application of ODNs to target gene repair in stem cells supports the goal of long-term correction through clonal expansion (142). Richardson et al. (149)

proposed the use of this strategy in utero with vascular delivery of stem cells to take advantage of the increased permeability of the blood-brain-barrier in embryos, so that it might be possible to "correct" certain neurologic disorders even before birth. Early intervention could prevent the damage to the nervous system that occurs during the embryonic period in developmental disorders like Tay-Sachs and Gaucher's disease.

Homologous Recombination

There are a number of intrinsic properties of chromatin DNA that can be used to deliver or replace genes in the genome, including the DNA sequence itself, DSB sites, secondary structure, and transcriptionally active regions. Specific DNA sequences can be targeted by HR. This is the primary means used to modify the genome of ES cells to introduce targeting sequences into specific gene loci (164). It also provides a means for repair of mutations in endogenous genes.

Methods

HR is believed to proceed by DSB in endogenous and exogenous DNA, gap enlargement by 5' and 3' endonucleases, as annealing of DNA strands from endogenous and exogenous elements, DNA replication to fill gaps, and ligation of free DNA ends (165). This process is fairly inefficient in most transient DNA delivery paradigms, with frequencies of "classical" HR in one out of $1/10^5$ cells using 10 kb sequences with complete homology (166–168). There is a rough logarithmic relationship between the length of the homologous sequence, between 3–15 kb, and the frequency of HR, with a less marked increase in HR for fragments > 15 kb (169).

The frequency of HR also increases with DSB and an open DNA configuration in the transgene fragments and the genome (170). Other factors important for HR in mammalian cells include Rad51, which is involved in a critical step in strand exchange when the 3' end invades the donor duplex (171,172); in addition, overexpression of Rad51 alone or together with DNA polymerase β can increase the frequency of HR (173–175). Delivery of ds DNA by viral vectors, such as adenovirus (176) and AAV (177) also increases the frequency of HR beyond that of DNA transfection, possibly due to the configuration of the virally delivered DNA. Although most targeted gene-repair efforts have focused on non-viral methods, rAAV has been used to correct a single bp substitution in an enhanced green fluorescent protein (eGFP) expression cassette in cultured cells by HR with an efficiency of 0.1% (178).

Small fragment homologous replacement (SFHR) was developed to address fundamental problems associated with classical HR, such as difficult construction and delivery of targeting vectors, high rates of non-HR events, and low levels of HR (149). SFHR involves ssDNA or dsDNA fragments hundreds of bases in length that are homologous to the target sequence with specific mismatches designed to alter the genomic sequence by one or even several nucleotides (179–181).

Applications and Therapeutic Potential

HR is increased in certain mutant cell types, such as those expressing the dominant negative form of p53 (182), those from patients with Fanconi's anemia who have a defect in the removal of interstrand crosslinks (183), and those from patients with A–T (see above). The increased levels of genetic instability observed in A–T patients may be the result of an increased frequency of HR stimulated by oxidative damage to DNA causing DSBs (184,185). HR is decreased in other mutant cells, for example from patients with xeroderma pigmentosum F which lack an endonuclease required for excision repair (186). An increase in DSB, and hence of HR, can be achieved by treatment of cells with gamma irradiation or drugs, like etoposide that causes random breaks in DNA, but with the risk of an increased mutation rate and DNA rearrangements (187). HR can also be increased by cleaving exogenous DNA introduced into cells, for example by flanking homologous sequences with rare "meganucleases," such as 18 bp restriction sites for yeast I-SceI combined with expression of I-SceI endonuclease (188). In an attempt to increase the site specific integration of AAV vector sequences into mammalian cells, Miller et al. (64) introduced the I-SceI site into the genome of human cells and expressed this endonuclease via infection with a MLV vector, yielding a low frequency of site specific integrations. Potentially, breaks in specific regions of the genome could also be achieved by introducing proteins, such as transcription factors and DNA binding proteins that

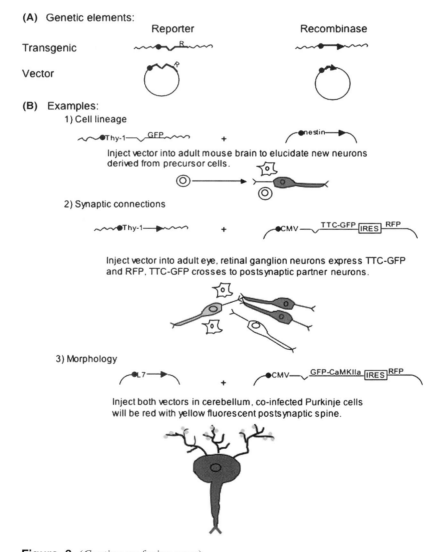

(A) Genetic elements:

Reporter   Recombinase

Transgenic

Vector

(B) Examples:

1) Cell lineage

Inject vector into adult mouse brain to elucidate new neurons derived from precursor cells.

2) Synaptic connections

Inject vector into adult eye, retinal ganglion neurons express TTC-GFP and RFP, TTC-GFP crosses to postsynaptic partner neurons.

3) Morphology

Inject both vectors in cerebellum, co-infected Purkinje cells will be red with yellow fluorescent postsynaptic spine.

Figure 3 (*Caption on facing page*)

recognize specific sequences in the genome (189) and coupling them to endonucleases or other agents, such as psoralen or chromophores (coupled with laser inactivation) (190), that could potentiate DSB. In general, DNA that has an open configuration, either through replication or transcriptional activity, has a higher chance of undergoing recombination events. For example, several studies have shown that integration of retrovirus vectors occurs most commonly in transcriptionally active regions of the genome (191).

SFHR have been successfully used to correct deletions, insertions, and point mutations in mammalian cells in culture with a frequency of < 1–20% (148,192–194) and $< 2\%$ in vivo (195,196). It is probable that SFHR functions by HR, but the precise mechanism is still unknown. The low correction efficiencies achieved using this technique is unlikely to prove useful for gene therapy without further improvements (34).

ELUCIDATION OF NEURONAL FUNCTIONS

Targeting the Genome to Elucidate Neuronal Properties

Many fundamental questions in neurobiology and neurologic disease require marking specific neuronal subtypes and following their fate in development and degeneration, as well as elucidating neuronal morphology, tracing neuronal pathways, and monitoring neuronal functions. The ability to answer these questions has been dramatically improved by new methods designed to modify the genome of neuronal cells combined with the use of vectors and "informative" reporter proteins. The basic elements in these combinatorial methods include: (1) cell specific and regulatable promoters; (2) SSRs and target sites, such as Cre/loxP and Flp/FRT, which can be incorporated either into the host cell genome or virus vectors; and (3) fluorescent or bioluminescent proteins that report, for example, on specific neuronal responses and synaptic dynamics (Fig. 3). There are numerous examples of combinatorial investigations using these elements, and a few examples are given here to show the versatile potential of this technology. Typically, enrichment of transgenic mouse

Figure 3 (*Figure on facing page*) Genetic modifications to elucidate neuronal structure and function. (**A**) Genetic elements that can be used in combination to control the timing and cell type of reporter gene expression can be encoded within the genome (*wavy lines*) of transgenic mice or within virus vectors (*circular line*). The reporter cassette (R) is constructed such that a recombination event mediated by a recombinase (*dark arrow*) is needed to either turn-on or turn-off expression. Specificity is conferred by the promoter elements (*solid black circle*) controlling the reporter and the recombinases. (**B**) Three examples are given to show how various combinations can be used to generate information. (1) *Cell lineage.* The Thy-1 promoter (active in neurons) is placed upstream of a GFP expression cassette and integrated into the genome of a transgenic mouse line. A vector expressing a recombinase under the nestin promoter (active in neuroprecursor cells) in injected into the brains of adult transgenic animals. Neuroprecursor cells infected with the vector that later differentiate into neurons will be marked by GFP expression. (2) *Synaptic connections.* In this case the transgenic mouse bears the recombinase under the Thy-1 promoter and the vector contains a conditional expression cassette for TTC-GFP-IRES-RFP under a strong constitutive promoter. Injection of the vector into the eye leads to expression of both reporter proteins selectively in retinal ganglion cells. The TTC-GFP protein can cross synapses to label the postsynaptic partner neurons of these retinal ganglion cells. (3) *Morphology.* Co-injection of two vectors into the cerebellum is used to define the morphology of individual neurons. In this case only Purkinje cells infected with both vectors will allow L7-driven (Purkinje cell specific) expression of the recombinase. This will activate expression of both RFP, which will label the whole cell, and GFP-CamKIIα, which will highlight postsynaptic dendritic spines.

genomes with informational reporters has been achieved through creating and breeding transgenic mouse lines, now complemented by the use of virus vectors.

Cell-Specific and Regulatable Promoters

Given the complexity of the nervous system, with a vast number of different neuronal subtypes and with morphologically similar neurons performing different functions, it is important to target expression of reporters or recombinases to specific neuronal subtypes. Typical examples of neuronal specific promoters include L7 (or pcp) that has been used in transgenic mice to specifically label Purkinje cells and retinal bipolar neurons, as well as to kill essentially all Purkinje cells starting in the first two postnatal weeks when this promoter is active (121). The Thy-1 promoter is active in many regions throughout the brain, but within the eye it is specific to retinal ganglion cells. Placing reporter genes under this promoter in transgenic animals has allowed elucidation of developmental events in these cells (197). However, even with a defined neuronal specific promoter, the site of genomic integration results in a different pattern of labeled neurons in different transgenic mouse strains (198). This latter study demonstrates, on one hand, that even cell specific promoter elements can vary in phenotypic expression depending on surrounding DNA sequences and, on the other hand, that additional, albeit randomly generated, information on cell specificity can be obtained via influences of surrounding chromatin. One reason for direct transgene integration to specific genomic sites is to try to achieve reproducibility in expression pattern for the same promoter across transgenic lines, unfortunately the influence of surrounding sequences, although consistent, is still an issue. Integration of transgenes into the hypoxanthine phosphoribosyl transferase locus has proven especially permissive to promoter integrity (199). Cell specific expression can also be combined with drug regulated expression in transgenic mice. This is typically achieved with a tet-regulatable promoter system allowing drug induction or inhibition of transgene expression.

Recombinases and Hit Sites

Another means to control expression of transgenes is by the use of recombinases and their target sites associated with specific genes or promoter elements. These control elements can be combined with other regulatory proteins to achieve developmental or refined cell specific and regulated expression. For example, a fusion of Cre recombinase and the progesterone receptor was created such that its entry into the nucleus is controlled by addition of a synthetic steroid, with resultant loxP recombination yielding expression of a reporter (*lacZ*) under the control of a neuronal specific promoter (113). A dual level of steroid regulation was achieved by placing this fusion protein under a steroid responsive promoter (200). In another example, transgenic mice expressing Cre under a tet-on responsive promoter were crossed to transgenic mice that both encoded the tet-transactivator protein under the CamKIIα neuronal promoter and a floxed *lacZ* reporter (201). This paradigm was used to demonstrate the ability of drug responsive control to allow activation of expression at different points in development, hence targeting different neuronal cell populations at various points of differentiation. Lineage fate-mapping in the developing nervous system has been carried out using the Cre-loxP system to activate a reporter protein under the engrailed-2 promoter (202) and, in a similar paradigm, with Flp-FRT to activate a reporter under the Wnt-1 promoter (203). The advantages of combinatorial interaction among promoters includes: high cell specificity, with two (or potentially more) promoter elements plus the site of integration restricting expression to defined cell types; the ability to temporarily regulate levels of gene expression and to permanently turn on or off genes; and the capacity for developmental timing of expression.

Virus Vectors

Virus vectors have been used to introduce reporter genes into ES cells to create transgenic mice, as in the introduction of a Cre-progesterone receptor expression cassette into ES cells with a retrovirus vector derived from murine embryonal stem cell virus (MESV) (204) or lentivirus (205), both of which allow stable, albeit random, integration into the host cell genome and efficient creation of transgenic mice. Viral vectors have also been used to deliver Cre to the adult rodent nervous system with on-site targeted recombination events in neurons. In pioneering studies, Brooks et al. (206–208) injected an HSV amplicon vector encoding Cre into the brains of transgenic mice bearing a loxP-activatable cassette for nerve growth factor and demonstrated an association of transgene activation with an increased locomotor activity and changes in cholinergic learning paradigms. A number of other groups have documented Cre mediated activation of floxed reporter genes in discrete neurons using AAV (209–211), lentivirus (123,211,212), and adenovirus (213–215). In order to eliminate any toxicity due to Cre expression, Pfeiffer et al. (123) designed a lentivirus vector in which Cre is active only for a limited time and then deleted by mediating a loxP excision on itself. Delivery of Cre by virus vectors has a number of advantages: it allows targeting of recombination events to focal regions within the brain (Fig. 4), thus providing an additional degree of specificity; it creates a mosaic of gene expression in the targeted region such that a one-on-one comparison can be made of the same type of neuron with and without expression of a transgene; and it eliminates the time consuming mouse breeding needed in transgenic crosses. In addition, it is possible and possibly even more efficient to put the floxed gene in the vector and infect transgenic mice expressing Cre in specific, well characterized cell types.

Reporter Proteins

Reporter proteins can allow both detection of cells expressing transgenes (either in transgenic mice or vector-infected cells) and assessment of morphology and functional

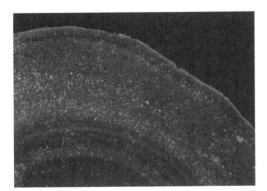

Figure 4 (*See color insert*) GFP expression after in utero AAV1-mediated delivery of Cre recombinase in Z/EG mice. One µl of AAV1 vector stock expressing Cre recombinase was injected into the lateral ventricle of E15 Z/EG mouse embryos. Brains were harvested at P27 and tissue sections stained with anti-EGFP (*green*) and anti-NeuN (*red*). The picture shows the cortex and the CA1 region of the hippocampus. Magnification 10×. *Source*: Drs. Broekman and Sena-Esteves, Harvard Medical School, Boston, Massachusetts and from Ref. 241.

activity of neurons. Such molecular imaging agents, including fluorescent proteins (FPs) and luciferases, can report from living cells to allow monitoring of dynamic events in dissociated cell and explant cultures, and even in vivo. FPs have been most useful for culture experiments and two photon fluorescent microscopy, as on the one hand, they allow fine cellular resolution and, on the other, the emission spectrum does not penetrate well through tissues. The range of available fluorescent reporters is expanding dramatically (162) with a host of new hues (216) and a form of red fluorescent protein, mPlum, with emission at 660 nm that increases in vivo applications (217). A wide range of fusion proteins have also been generated which combine FPs with proteins that can elucidate spatial organization and activity in neurons to monitor intracellular dynamics. For example, GFP-tubulin and GFP-NgCAM (218) can be used to monitor neurite outgrowth and the axonal surface, respectively. These can be combined to visualize protein–protein interactions as, for example, the first step in synapse formation, with presynaptic β-neurexin-RFP and postsynaptic neuroligin-1-GFP interacting on the cell surface to give yellow punctuate signals of synaptic contact (219). "Smarter" versions of these FPs have been engineered such that they are sensitive to their environment, like synapto-pHlourin which consists of a pH-sensitive variant of GFP fused to the intralumenal terminus of the synaptic vesicle protein, VAMP (220), such that fluorescence is quenched within synaptic vesicles and activated upon transmitter release with exposure to the extracellular space. Other FPs have been designed to report biochemical events in cells, such as calcium levels (221,222), redox potential (223), kinase specific phosphorylation (224) and chloride levels (225). Fusion of FPs to other peptides/proteins, such as the heavy chain fragment of tetanus toxin (226,227), lectins (228) and BDNF (229) may allow transfer of reporters across synapses to label synaptically connected neurons. Proteins can also be engineered to allow tagging with fluorescent ligands, for example, by incorporating a tetracysteine peptide motif that binds to a membrane permeant fluorescent dye and fluoresces only after it binds to these cysteine thiols (230).

High tissue penetrating signals can be achieved with bioluminescence (231,232). There are several luciferases currently in use that serve as robust reporters in vivo and which, through different substrates, e.g., D-luciferin for firefly luciferase and coelenterazine for *Renilla* luciferase and the extracellularly active *Gaussia* luciferase, can allow dual imaging of two dynamic events in parallel (233–235). To date bioluminescence imaging in vivo has been used primarily to monitor growth and regression of tumor cells stably expressing luciferases (233,236), migration of neuroprecursor cells to tumors in the brain (237), gene delivery via viral vectors (233,238) and promoter activity (239). In this exploding field it is hard to predict the next generation of in vivo molecular reporters, but these, in combination with viral vectors, transgenic mice and site specific recombinases will provide a new level of genetic instrumentation to allow finer dissection of neurobiologic events and facilitate evaluation of therapeutic initiatives.

CONCLUSION

The combination of molecular genetic and imaging technologies now allows direct modification of the mammalian genome to elucidate the function of normal neurobiological processes in living cells and to determine the effects of disease genes on these processes. Further, it allows for the exciting possibility of correcting disease genes in the brains of patients, which even a few years ago seemed like a very remote possibility.

REFERENCES

1. Hsich G, Sena-Esteves M, Breakefield XO. Critical issues in gene therapy for neurologic disease. Hum Gene Ther 2002; 13:579–604.
2. Kay MA, Glorioso J, Naldini L. Viral vectors for gene therapy: the art of turning infectious agents into vehicles of therapeutics. Nature 2001; 7:33–40.
3. Naldini L, Blomer U, Gallay P, et al. In vivo gene delivery and stable transduction of nondividing cells by a lentiviral vector. Science 1996; 272:263–267.
4. Verma IM. Success and setback: another adverse event. Mol Ther 2002; 6:565–566.
5. Kumar-Singh R, Chamberlain JS. Encapsidated adenovirus minichromosomes allow delivery and expression of a 14 kb dystrophin cDNA to muscle cells. Hum Mol Genet 1996; 5:913–921.
6. Kochanek S, Clemens PR, Mitani K, Chen HH, Chan S, Caskey CT. A new adenoviral vector: replacement of all viral coding sequences with 28 kb of DNA independently expressing both full length dystrophin and beta-galactosidase. Proc Natl Acad Sci USA 1996; 93:5731–5736.
7. Schneider DB, Fly CA, Dichek DA, Geary RI. Adenoviral gene transfer in arteries of hypercholesterolemic nonhuman primates. Hum Gene Ther 1998; 9:815–821.
8. Fraefel C, Song S, Lim F, et al. Helper virus-free transfer of herpes simplex virus type 1 plasmid vectors into neural cells. J Virol 1996; 70:7190–7197.
9. Fraefel C, Breakefield XO, Jacoby D. The HSV-1 amplicon. In: Breakefield XO, Chiocca EA, eds. Gene Therapy for Neurological Disorders and Brain Tumors. Totowa, NJ: Humana Press Inc., 1998:63–82.
10. Sena-Esteves M, Saeki Y, Fraefel C, Breakefield XO. HSV-1 amplicon vectors—simplicity and versatility. Mol Ther 2000; 2:9–15.
11. Berns KI, Linden RM. The cryptic life style of adeno-associated virus. Bioessays 1995; 17:237–245.
12. Berns KI. Parvoviridae: the viruses and their replication. In: Fields BN, Knipe DM, Howley PM, eds. Virology. Philadelphia: Lippincott-Raven, 1996:2173–2197.
13. Kotin RM, Sinscalco M, Samulski RJ, et al. Site-specific integration of adeno-associated virus. Proc Natl Acad Sci USA 1990; 87:2211–2215.
14. Samulski RJ, Zhu X, Xiao X, et al. Targeted integration of adeno-associated virus (AAV) into human chromosome 19. EMBO J 1991; 10:3941–3950.
15. Podsakoff G, Wong KKJ, Chatterjee S. Efficient gene transfer into nondividing cells by adeno-associated virus-based vectors. J Virol 1994; 68:5656–5666.
16. Russell DW, Miller AD, Alexander IE. Adeno-associated virus vectors preferentially transduce cells in S phase. Proc Natl Acad Sci USA 1994; 91:8915–8919.
17. Srivastava A, Lusby EW, Berns KI. Nucleotide sequence and organization of the adeno-associated virus 2 genome. J Virol 1983; 45:555–564.
18. Im DS, Muzyczka N. Factors that bind to adeno-associated virus terminal repeats. J Virol 1989; 63:3095–3104.
19. Surosky RT, Urabe M, Godwin SG, et al. Adeno-associated virus Rep proteins target DNA sequences to a unique locus in the human genome. J Virol 1997; 71:7951–7959.
20. Weitzman MD, Kyostio SRM, Kotin RM, Owens RA. Adeno-associated virus (AAV) Rep proteins mediate complex formation between AAV DNA and its integration site in human DNA. Proc Natl Acad Sci USA 1994; 91:5808–5812.
21. Philpott NJ, Gomos H, Berns KI, Flack-Pedersen E. A p5 integration efficiency element mediates Rep-dependent integration into AAVS1 at chromosome 19. Proc Natl Acad Sci USA 2002; 99:12381–12385.
22. Kearns WG, Afione SA, Fulmer SB, et al. Recombinant adeno-associated virus (AAV-CFTR) vectors do not integrate in a site-specific fashion in an immortalized epithelial cell line. Gene Ther 1996; 3:748–755.
23. Xiao X, Xiao W, Li J, Samulski RJ. A novel 165-base-pair terminal repeat sequence is the sole cis requirement for the adeno-associated virus life cycle. J Virol 1997; 71:941–948.

24. Yang CC, Xiao X, Zhu X, et al. Cellular recombination pathways and viral terminal repeat hairpin structures are sufficient for adeno-associated virus integration in vivo and in vitro. J Virol 1997; 71:9231–9247.

25. Duan D, Sharma P, Yang J, et al. Circular intermediates of recombinant adeno-associated virus have defined structural characteristics responsible for long-term episomal persistence in muscle tissue. J Virol 1998; 72:8568–8577.

26. Nakai H, Yant SR, Strom TA, Fuess S, Meuse L, Kay MA. Extrachromosomal recombinant adeno-associated virus vector genomes are primarily responsible for stable liver transduction in vivo. J Virol 2001; 75:6969–6976.

27. Linden RM, Winocour E, Berns KI. The recombination signals for adeno-associated virus site-specific integration. Proc Natl Acad Sci USA 1996; 93:7966–7972.

28. Young SMJ, Samulski RJ. Adeno-associated virus (AAV) site-specific recombination does not require a Rep-dependent origin of replication within the AAV terminal repeat. Proc Natl Acad Sci USA 2001; 98:13525–13530.

29. Weitzman MD, Young SMJ, Cathomen T, Samulski RJ. Targeted integration by adeno-associated virus. In: Machida CA, ed. Methods in Molecular Medicine, Vol. 76. Totowa, NJ: Humana Press Inc., 2003:201.

30. Rizzuto G, Gorgoni B, Cappelletti M, et al. Development of animal models for adeno-associated virus site-specific integration. J Virol 1999; 73:2517–2526.

31. Young SMJ, McCarty DM, Degtyareva N, Samulski RJ. Roles of adeno-associated virus Rep protein and human chromosome 19 in site-specific recombination. J Virol 2000; 74:3953–3966.

32. Bakowska JC, DiMaria MV, Camp SM, Wang Y, Allen PD, Breakefield XO. Targeted transgene integration into transgenic mouse fibroblasts carrying the full-length human AAVS1 locus mediated by HSV/AAV rep(+) hybrid amplicon vector. Gene Ther 2003; 10:1691–1702.

33. Dutheil N, Yoon-Robarts M, Ward P, et al. Characterization of the mouse adeno-associated virus AAVS1 ortholog. J Virol 2004; 78:8917–8921.

34. Portlock JL, Calos MP. Site-specific genomic strategies for gene therapy. Curr Opin Mol Ther 2003; 5:376–382.

35. Huttner NA, Girod A, Schnittger S, Schoch C, Hallek M, Buning H. Analysis of site-specific transgene integration following cotransduction with recombinant adeno-associated virus and a rep encoding plasmid. J Gene Med 2003; 5:120–129.

36. Miao CH, Snyder RO, Schowalter DB, et al. The kinetics of rAAV integration in the liver. Nat Genet 1998; 19:13–15.

37. Ponnazhagan S, Erikson D, Kearns WG, et al. Lack of site-specific integration of the recombinant adeno-associated virus 2 genomes in human cells. Hum Gene Ther 1997; 8:275–284.

38. Miller DG, Rutledge EA, Russell DW. Chromosomal effects of adeno-associated virus vector integration. Nat Genet 2002; 30:147–148.

39. Nakai H, Montini E, Fuess S, Storm TA, Grompe M, Kay MA. AAV serotype 2 vectors preferentially integrate into active genes in mice. Nat Genet 2003; 34:297–302.

40. Duan D, Yue Y, Yan Z, Yang J, Engelhardt JF. Endosomal processing limits gene transfer to polarized airway epithelia by adeno-associated virus. J Clin Investig 2000; 105:1573–1587.

41. Sun L, Li J, Xiao X. Overcoming adeno-associated virus vector size limitation through viral DNA heterodimerization. Nat Med 2000; 6:599–602.

42. Palombo F, Monciotti A, Recchia A, Cortese R, Ciliberto G, LaMonica N. Site-specific integration in mammalian cells mediated by a new hybrid baculovirus-adeno-associated virus vector. J Virol 1998; 72:5025–5034.

43. Wang Y, Camp SM, Niwano M, et al. Herpes simplex virus type 1/adeno-associated virus rep(+) hybrid amplicon vector improves the stability of transgene expression in human cells by site-specific integration. J Virol 2002; 76:7150–7162.

44. Heister T, Heid I, Ackermann M, Fraefel C. Herpes simplex virus type 1/adeno-associated virus hybrid vectors mediate site-specific integration at the adeno-associated virus preintegration site, AAVS1, on human chromosome 19. J Virol 2002; 76:7163–7173.

45. Recchia A, Parks RJ, Lamartina S, et al. Site-specific integration mediated by a hybrid adenovirus-adeno/associated virus. Proc Natl Acad Sci USA 1999; 96:2615–2620.

46. Recchia A, Perani L, Sartori D, Olgiati C, Mavilio F. Site-specific integration of functional transgenes into the human genome by adeno/AAV hybrid vectors. Mol Ther 2004; 10:660–670.

47. Antoni BA, Rabson AB, Miller IL, Trempe JP, Chejanovsky N, Carter BJ. Adeno-associated virus Rep protein inhibits human immunodeficiency virus type 1 production in human cells. J Virol 1991; 65:396–404.

48. Hermonat PL. Inhibition of bovine papillomarvirus plasmid DNA replication by adeno-associated virus. Virology 1992; 189:329–333.

49. Weitzman MD, Fisher KJ, Wilson JM. Recruitment of wild-type and recombinant adeno-associated virus into adenovirus replication centers. J Virol 1996; 70:1845–1854.

50. Khleif SN, Myers T, Carter BJ, Trempe JP. Inhibition of cellular transformation by the adeno-associated virus rep gene. Virology 1991; 181:738–741.

51. Tratschin JD, Tal J, Carter BJ. Negative and positive regulation in trans of gene expression from adeno-associated virus vectors in mammalian cells by a viral rep gene product. Mol Cell Biol 1986; 6:2884–2894.

52. Yang Q, Chen F, Ross J, Trempe JP. Inhibition of cellular and SV40 DNA replication by the adeno-associated virus Rep proteins. Virology 1995; 207:246–250.

53. Saudan P, Vlach J, Beard P. Inhibition of S-phase progression by adeno-associated virus Rep78 protein is mediated by hypophosphorylated pRb. EMBO J 2000; 19:4351–4361.

54. Gavin DK, Young SMJ, Xiao W, et al. Charge-to-alanine mutagenesis of the adeno-associated virus type 2 Rep 78/68 proteins yields temperature-sensitive and magnesium-dependent variants. J Virol 1999; 73:9433–9445.

55. Rinaudo D, Lamartina S, Roscilli G, Ciliberto G, Toniatti C. Conditional site-specific integration into human chromosome 19 by using a ligand-dependent chimeric adeno-associated virus/Rep protein. J Virol 2000; 74:281–294.

56. Ueno T, Matsumura H, Tanaka K, et al. Site-specific integration of a transgene mediated by a hybrid adenovirus/adeno-associated virus vector using the Cre/loxP-expression-switching system. Biochem Biophys Res Commun 2000; 273:473–478.

57. Satoh W, Hirai Y, Tamayose K, Shimada T. Site-specific integration of an adeno-associated virus vector plasmid mediated by regulated expression of rep based on Cre-loxP recombination. J Virol 2000; 74:10631–10638.

58. Cathomen T, Collete D, Weitzman MD. A chimeric protein containing the N terminus of the adeno-associated virus Rep protein recognizes its target site in an in vivo assay. J Virol 2000; 74:2372–2382.

59. Oehmig A, Schuback DE, Grandi P, Fraefel C, Breakefield XO. Delivery of AAV rep protein as VP16-REP fusion proteins in HSV-1 virions. In: 29th Int'l Herpesvirus Workshop 2004. Abst. 1.69.

60. Johnston KM, Jacoby D, Pechan P, et al. HSV/AAV hybrid amplicon vectors extend transgene expression in human glioma cells. Hum Gene Ther 1997; 8:359–370.

61. Lam P, Hui KM, Wang Y, et al. Dynamics of transgene expression in human glioblastoma cells mediated by herpes simplex virus/adeno-associated virus amplicon vectors. Hum Gene Ther 2002; 13:2147–2159.

62. Fraefel C, Jacoby DR, Lage C, et al. Gene transfer into hepatocytes mediated by helper virus-free HSV/AAV hybrid vectors. Mol Med 1997; 3:813–825.

63. Costantini LC, Jacoby DR, Wang S, Fraefel C, Breakefield XO, Isacson O. Gene transfer to the nigrostriatal system by hybrid herpes simplex virus/adeno-associated virus amplicon vectors. Hum Gene Ther 1999; 10:2481–2494.

64. Miller DG, Petek LM, Russell DW. Adeno-associated virus vectors integrate at chromosome breakage sites. Nat Genet 2004; 36:767–773.

65. Kuzminov A. Single-strand interruptions in replicating chromosomes cause double-strand breaks. Proc Natl Acad Sci USA 2001; 98:8241–8246.

66. Lavin MF, Shiloh Y. The genetic defect in ataxia-telangiectasia. Annu Rev Immunol 1997; 15:177–202.

67. Sanlioglu S, Benson P, Engelhardt JF. Loss of ATM function enhanced recombinant adeno-associated virus transduction and integration through pathways similar to UV irradiation. Virology 2000; 268:68–78.

68. Groth AC, Calos MP. Phage integrases: biology and applications. J Mol Biol 2004; 335:667–678.

69. Esposito D, Scocca JJ. Purification and characterization of HP1 Cox and definition of its role in controlling the direction of site-specific recombination. J Biol Chem 1997; 272:8660–8670.

70. Nunes-Dudy SE, Kwon HJ, Tirumalai RS, Ellenberger T, Landy A. Similarities and differences among 105 members of the Int family of site-specific recombinases. Nucleic Acids Res 1998; 26:391–406.

71. Smith MC, Thorpe HM. Diversity in the serine recombinases. Mol Microbiol 2002; 44:299–307.

72. Austin S, Ziese M, Sternberg N. A novel role for site-specific recombination in maintenance of bacterial replicons. Cell 1981; 25:729–736.

73. Broach JR, Guarascio VR, Jayaram M. Recombination within the yeast plasmid 2 mu circle is site-specific. Cell 1982; 29:227–234.

74. Stark WM, Boocock MR, Sherratt DJ. Catalysis by site-specific recombinases. Trends Genet 1992; 8:432–439.

75. Hallet B, Sherratt DJ. Transposition and site-specific recombination: adapting DNA cut-and-paste mechanisms to a variety of genetic rearrangements. FEMS Microbiol Rev 1997; 21:157–178.

76. Dymecki SM. Site-specific recombination in cells and mice. In: Joyner AL, ed. Gene Targeting, a Practical Approach. Oxford: Oxford University Press, 2000:37–99.

77. Golic KG, Lindquist S. The FLP recombinase of yeast catalyzes site-specific recombination in the Drosophila genome. Cell 1989; 59:499–509.

78. Xu T, Rubin GM. Analysis of genetic mosaics in developing and adult Drosophila tissues. Development 1993; 117:1223–1237.

79. Sauer B, Henderson N. Site-specific DNA recombination in mammalian cells by the Cre recombinase of bacteriophage P1. Proc Natl Acad Sci USA 1988; 85:5166–5170.

80. O'Gorman S, Fox DT, Wahl GM. Recombinase-mediated gene activation and site-specific integration in mammalian cells. Science 1991; 251:1351–1355.

81. Orban PC, Chui D, Marth JD. Tissue- and site-specific DNA recombination in transgenic mice. Proc Natl Acad Sci USA 1992; 89:6861–6865.

82. Dymecki SM. Flp recombinase promotes site-specific DNA recombination in embryonic stem cells and transgenic mice. Proc Natl Acad Sci USA 1996; 93:6191–6196.

83. McLeod M, Craft S, Broach JR. Identification of the crossover site during Flp-mediated recombination in the Saccharomyces cerevisiae plasmid 2 microns circle. Mol Cell Biol 1986; 6:3357–3367.

84. Hoess RH, Ziese M, Sternberg N. P1 site-specific recombination: nucleotide sequence of the recombining sites. Proc Natl Acad Sci USA 1982; 79:3398–3402.

85. Hoess RH, Wierzbicki A, Abremski K. Formation of small circular DNA molecules via an in vitro site-specific recombination system. Gene 1985; 40:325–329.

86. Andreas S, Schwenk F, Kuter-Luks B, Faust N, Kuhn R. Enhanced efficiency through nuclear localization signal fusion of phage PhiC31-integrase: activity comparison with Cre and FLPe recombinase in mammalian cells. Nucleic Acids Res 2002; 30:2299–2306.

87. Kos CH. Cre/loxP system for generating tissue-specific knockout mouse models. Nutr Rev 2004; 62:243–246.

88. Branda CS, Dymecki SM. Talking about a revolution: the impact of site-specific recombinases on genetic analyses in mice. Dev Cell 2004; 6:7–28.

89. Hoess RH, Wierzbicki A, Abremski K. The role of the loxP spacer region in P1 site-specific recombination. Nucleic Acids Res 1986; 14:2287–2300.

90. Senecoff JF, Cox MM. Directionality in FLP protein-promoted site-specific recombination is mediated by DNA–DNA pairing. J Biol Chem 1986; 261:7380–7386.

91. Senecoff JF, Rossmeissl PJ, Cox MM. DNA recognition by the FLP recombinase of the yeast 2 mu plasmid. A mutational analysis of the FLP binding site. J Mol Biol 1988; 201:405–421.

92. Bode J, Schlake T, Iber M, et al. The transgeneticist's toolbox: novel methods for the targeted modification of eukaryotic genomes. Biol Chem 2000; 381:801–813.

93. Baer A, Bode J. Coping with kinetic and thermodynamic barriers: RMCE, an efficient strategy for the targeted integration of transgenes. Curr Opin Biotechnol 2001; 12:473–480.

94. Schnutgen F, Doerflinger N, Calleja C, Wendling O, Chambon P, Ghyselinck NB. A directional strategy for monitoring Cre-mediated recombination at the cellular level in the mouse. Nat Biotechnol 2003; 21:562–565.

95. Albert H, Dale EC, Lee E, Ow DW. Site-specific integration of DNA into wild-type and mutant lox sites placed in the plant genome. Plant J 1995; 7:649–659.

96. Araki K, Araki M, Yamamura K. Targeted integration of DNA using mutant lox sites in embryonic stem cells. Nucleic Acids Res 1997; 25:868–872.

97. Shimshek DR, Kim J, Hubner MR, et al. Codon-improving Cre recombinase (iCre) expression in the mouse. Genesis 2002; 32:19–26.

98. Logie C, Stewart AF. Ligand-regulated site-specific recombination. Proc Natl Acad Sci USA 1995; 92:5940–5944.

99. Metzger D, Clifford J, Chiba H, Chambon P. Conditional site-specific recombination in mammalian cells using a ligand-dependent chimeric Cre recombinase. Proc Natl Acad Sci USA 1995; 92:6991–6995.

100. Feil R, Brocard J, Mascrez B, LeMeur M, Metzger D, Chambon P. Ligand-activated site-specific recombination in mice. Proc Natl Acad Sci USA 1996; 93:10887–10890.

101. Kellendonk C, Tronche F, Monaghan AP, Angrand PO, Stewart F, Schutz G. Regulation of Cre recombinase activity by the synthetic steroid RU 486. Nucleic Acids Res 1996; 24:1404–1411.

102. Brocard J, Warot X, Wendling O, et al. Spatio-temporally controlled site-specific somatic mutagenesis in the mouse. Proc Natl Acad Sci USA 1997; 94:14559–14563.

103. Schwenk F, Kuhm R, Angrand PO, Rajewski K, Stewart AF. Temporally and spatially regulated somatic mutagenesis in mice. Nucleic Acids Res 1998; 26:1427–1432.

104. Gossen M, Bujard H. Tight control of gene expression in mammalian cells by tetracycline-responsive promoters. Proc Natl Acad Sci USA 1992; 89:5547–5551.

105. Hollis RP, Stoll SM, Sclimenti CR, Lin J, Chen-Tsai Y, Calos MP. Phage integrases for the construction and manipulation of transgenic mammals. Reprod Biol Endocrinol 2003; 1:79.

106. Groth AC, Olivares EC, Thyagarajan B, Calos MP. A phage integrase directs efficient site-specific integration in human cells. Proc Natl Acad Sci USA 2000; 97:5995–6000.

107. Thyagarajan B, Olivares EC, Hollis RP, Ginsburg DS, Calos MP. Site-specific genomic integration in mammalian cells mediated by phage phiC31 integrase. Mol Cell Biol 2001; 21:3926–3934.

108. Kuhstoss S, Rao RN. Analysis of the integration function of the streptomycete bacteriophage phi C31. J Mol Biol 1991; 222:897–908.

109. Thorpe HM, Smith MC. In vitro site-specific integration of bacteriophage DNA catalyzed by a recombinase of the resolvase/invertase family. Proc Natl Acad Sci USA 1998; 95:5505–5510.

110. Belteki G, Gertsenstein M, Ow DW, Nagy A. Site-specific cassette exchange and germline transmission with mouse ES cells expressing phiC31 integrase. Nat Biotechnol 2003; 21:321–324.

111. Sadowski P. Site-specific recombinases: changing partners and doing the twist. J Bacteriol 1986; 165:341–347.

112. Tsien JZ, Chen DF, Gerber D, et al. Subregion- and cell type-restricted gene knockout in mouse brain. Cell 1996; 87:1317–1326.

113. Kellendonk C, Tronche F, Casanova E, Anlag K, Opherk C, Schutz G. Inducible site-specific recombination in the brain. J Mol Biol 1999; 285:175–182.

114. Zhu Y, Romero MI, Ghosh P, et al. Ablation of NF1 function in neurons induces abnormal development of cerebral cortex and reactive gliosis in the brain. Genes Dev 2001; 15:859–876.

115. Kitayama K, Abe M, Kakizaki T, et al. Purkinje cell-specific and inducible gene recombination system generated from C57BL/6 mouse ES cells. Biochem Biophys Res Commun 2001; 281:1134–1140.

116. Kuhn R, Schwenk F, Aguet M, Rajewski K. Inducible gene targeting in mice. Science 1995; 269:1427–1429.

117. Sauer B. Inducible gene targeting in mice using the Cre/lox system. Methods 1998; 14:381–392.

118. Weber P, Metzger D, Chambon P. Temporally controlled targeted somatic mutagenesis in the mouse brain. Eur J Neurosci 2001; 14:1777–1783.

119. Vooijs M, Jonkers J, Berns A. A highly efficient ligand-regulated Cre recombinase mouse line shows that LoxP recombination is position dependent. EMBO Rep 2001; 2:292–297.

120. Morozov A, Kellendonk C, Simpson E, Tronche F. Using conditional mutagenesis to study the brain. Biol Psychiatry 2003; 54:1125–1133.

121. Barski JJ, Morl K, Meyer M. Conditional inactivation of the calbindin D-28k (Calb1) gene by Cre/loxP-mediated recombination. Genesis 2002; 32:165–168.

122. Schmidt EE, Taylor DS, Prigge JR, Barnett S, Capecchi MR. Illegitimate Cre-dependent chromosome rearrangements in transgenic mouse spermatids. Proc Natl Acad Sci USA 2000; 97:13702–13707.

123. Pfeifer A, Brandon EP, Kootstra DN, Gage FH, Verma IM. Delivery of the Cre recombinase by a self-deleting lentiviral vector: efficient gene targeting in vivo. Proc Natl Acad Sci USA 2001; 98:11450–11455.

124. Loonstra A, Vooijs M, Beverloo HB, et al. Growth inhibition and DNA damage induced by Cre recombinase in mammalian cells. Proc Natl Acad Sci USA 2001; 98:9209–9214.

125. Sternberg N, Hamilton D, Hoess R. Bacteriophage P1 site-specific recombination. II. Recombination between loxP and the bacterial chromosome. J Mol Biol 1981; 150:487–507.

126. Sauer B. Identification of cryptic lox sites in the yeast genome by selection for Cre-mediated chromosome translocations that confer multiple drug resistance. J Mol Biol 1992; 223:911–928.

127. Thyagarajan B, Guimaraes MJ, Groth AC, Calos MP. Mammalian genomes contain active recombinase recognition sites. Gene 2000; 244:47–54.

128. Yamamoto A, Lucas JJ, Hen R. Reversal of neuropathology and motor dysfunction in a conditional model of Huntington's disease. Cell 2000; 101:57–66.

129. Zu T, Duvick LA, Kaytor MD, et al. Recovery from polyglutamine-induced neurodegeneration in conditional SCA1 transgenic mice. J Neurosci 2004; 24:8853–8861.

130. Olivares EC, Hollis RP, Chalberg TW, Meuse L, Kay MA, Calos MP. Site-specific genomic integration produces therapeutic Factor IX levels in mice. Nat Biotechnol 2002; 20:1124–1128.

131. Ortiz-Urda S, Thyagarajan B, Keene DR, et al. Stable nonviral genetic correction of inherited human skin disease. Nat Med 2002; 8:1166–1170.

132. Igoucheva O, Yoon K. Targeted single-base correction by RNA–DNA oligonucleotides. Hum Gene Ther 2000; 11:2307–2312.

133. Wu XS, Liu DP, Liang CC. Prospects of chimeric RNA–DNA oligonucleotides in gene therapy. J Biomed Sci 2001; 8:439–445.

134. Gamper HBJ, Cole-Strauss A, Metz R, Parekh H, Kumar R, Kmiec EB. A plausible mechanism for gene correction by chimeric oligonucleotides. Biochemistry 2000; 39:5808–5816.

135. Gamper HB, Parekh H, Rice MC, Bruner M, Youkey H, Kmiec EB. The DNA strand of chimeric RNA/DNA oligonucleotides can direct gene repair/conversion activity in mammalian and plant cell-free extracts. Nucleic Acids Res 2000; 28:4332–4339.

136. Yoon K, Cole-Strauss A, Kmiec EB. Targeted gene correction of episomal DNA in mammalian cells mediated by a chimeric RNA. DNA oligonucleotide. Proc Natl Acad Sci USA 1996; 93:2071–2076.

137. Cole-Strauss A, Yoon K, Xiang Y, et al. Correction of the mutation responsible for sickle cell anemia by an RNA–DNA oligonucleotide. Science 1996; 273:1386–1389.

138. Bankyopadhyay P, Ma X, Linehan-Stieers C, Kren BT, Steer CJ. Nucleotide exchange in genomic DNA of rat hepatocytes using RNA/DNA oligonucleotides. Targeted delivery of liposomes and polyethyleneimine to the asialoglycoprotein receptor. J Biol Chem 1999; 274:10163–10172.

139. Alexeev V, Igoucheva O, Domashenko A, Cotsarelis G, Yoon K. Localized in vivo genotypic and phenotypic correction of the albino mutation in skin by RNA–DNA oligonucleotide. Nat Biotechnol 2000; 18:43–47.

140. Rando TA, Disatnik MH, Zhou LZ. Rescue of dystrophin expression in mdx mouse muscle by RNA/DNA oligonucleotides. Proc Natl Acad Sci USA 2000; 97:5363–5368.

141. Lai LW, Lien YH. Chimeric RNA/DNA oligonucleotide-based gene therapy. Kidney Int 2002; 61:47–51.

142. Zhang Z, Eriksson M, Falk G, et al. Failure to achieve gene conversion with chimeric circular oligonucleotides: potentially misleading PCR artifacts observed. Antisense Nucleic Acid Drug Rev 1998; 8:531–536.

143. Albuquerque-Silva J, Vassart G, Lavinha J, Abramowicz MJ. Chimeraplasty validation. Nat Biotechnol 2001; 19:1011.

144. Kmiec EB. Targeted gene repair—in the arena. J Clin Investig 2003; 112:632–636.

145. Igoucheva O, Alexeev V, Yoon K. Targeted gene correction by small single-stranded oligonucleotides in mammalian cells. Gene Ther 2001; 8:391–399.

146. Parekh-Olmedo H, Drury M, Kmiec EB. Targeted nucleotide exchange in Saccharomyces cerevisiae directed by short oligonucleotides containing locked nucleic acids. Chem Biol 2002; 9:1073–1084.

147. Pierce EA, Liu Q, Igoucheva O, et al. Oligonucleotide-directed single-base DNA alterations in mouse embryonic stem cells. Gene Ther 2003; 10:24–33.

148. Nickerson HD, Colledge WH. A comparison of gene repair strategies in cell culture using a lacZ reporter system. Gene Ther 2003; 10:1584–1591.

149. Richardson PD, Augustin LB, Kren BT, Steer CJ. Gene repair and transposon-mediated gene therapy. Stem Cells 2002; 20:105–118.

150. Chan PP, Glazer PM. Triplex DNA: fundamentals, advances, and potential applications for gene therapy. J Mol Med 1997; 75:267–282.

151. Vasquez KM, Dagle JM, Weeks DL, Glazer PM. Chromosome targeting at short polypurine sites by cationic triplex-forming oligonucleotides. J Biol Chem 2001; 276:38536–38541.

152. Knauert MP, Glazer PM. Triplex forming oligonucleotides: sequence-specific tools for gene targeting. Hum Mol Genet 2001; 10:2243–2251.

153. Vasquez KM, Glazer PM. Triplex-forming oligonucleotides: principles and applications. Q Rev Biophys 2002; 35:89–107.

154. Cimino GD, Gamper HBJ, Isaacs ST, Hearst JE. Psoralens as photoactive probes of nucleic acid structure and function: organic chemistry, photochemistry, and biochemistry. Annu Rev Biochem 1985; 54:1151–1193.

155. Raha M, Lacroix L, Glazer PM. Mutagenesis mediated by triple helix-forming oligonucleotides conjugated to psoralen: effects of linker arm length and sequence context. Photochem Photobiol 1998; 67:289–294.

156. Mamot C, Nguyen JB, Pourdehnad M, et al. Extensive distribution of liposomes in rodent brains and brain tumors following convection-enhanced delivery. J Neurooncol 2004; 68:1–9.

157. Pardridge WM. Gene targeting in vivo with pegylated immunoliposomes. Methods Enzymol 2003; 373:507–528.

158. Sangiuolo F, Novelli G. Sequence-specific modification of mouse genomic DNA mediated by gene targeting techniques. Cytogenet Genome Res 2004; 105:435–441.

159. Derossi D, Chassaing G, Prochiantz A. Trojan peptides: the penetratin system for intracellular delivery. Trends Cell Biol 1998; 8:84–87.

160. Wexler NS, Young AB, Tanzi RE, et al. Homozygotes for Huntington's disease. Nature 1987; 326:194–197.

161. Halene S, Kohn DB. Gene therapy using hematopoietic stem cells: sisyphus approaches the crest. Hum Gene Ther 2000; 11:1259–1267.

162. Zhang J, Campbell RE, Ting AY, Tsien RY. Creating new fluorescent probes for cell biology. Nat Rev Mol Cell Biol 2002; 3:906–918.

163. Zwaka TP, Thomson JA. Homologous recombination in human embryonic stem cells. Nat Biotechnol 2003; 21:319–321.

164. Misra RP, Duncan SA. Gene targeting in the mouse: advances in introduction of transgenes into the genome by homologous recombination. Endocrine 2002; 19:229–238.

165. Valancius V, Smithies O. Double-strand gap repair in a mammalian gene targeting reaction. Mol Cell Biol 1991; 11:4389–4397.

166. Capecchi MR. Altering the genome by homologous recombination. Science 1989; 244:1288–1292.

167. Deng C, Capecchi MR. Reexamination of gene targeting frequency as a function of the extent of homology between the targeting vector and the target locus. Mol Cell Biol 1992; 12:3365–3371.

168. Hatada S, Nikkuni K, Bentley SA, Kirby S, Smithies O. Gene correction in hematopoietic progenitor cells by homologous recombination. Proc Natl Acad Sci USA 2000; 97:13807–13811.

169. Fujitani Y, Yamamoto K, Kobayashi I. Dependence of frequency of homologous recombination on the homology length. Genetics 1995; 140:797–809.

170. Ganguly A, Smelt S, Mewar R, et al. Targeted insertions of two exogenous collagen genes into both alleles of their endogenous loci in cultured human cells: the insertions are directed by relatively short fragments containing the promoters and the 5′ ends of the genes. Proc Natl Acad Sci USA 1994; 91:7365–7369.

171. Haber JE. DNA repair. Gatekeepers of recombination. Nature 1999; 398:665–667.

172. Nishinaka T, Shinohara A, Ito Y, Yokoyama S, Shibata T. Base pair switching by interconversion of sugar puckers in DNA extended by proteins of RecA-family: a model for homology search in homologous genetic recombination. Proc Natl Acad Sci USA 1998; 95:11071–11076.

173. Vispe S, Cazaux C, Lesca O, Defais M. Overexpression of Rad51 protein stimulates homologous recombination and increases resistance of mammalian cells to ionizing radiation. Nucleic Acids Res 1998; 26:2859–2864.

174. Lanzov VA. Gene targeting for gene therapy: prospects. Mol Genet Met 1999; 68:276–282.

175. Canitrot Y, Capp JP, Puget N, et al. DNA polymerase beta overexpression stimulates the Rad51-dependent homologous recombination in mammalian cells. Nucleic Acids Res 2004; 32:5104–5112.

176. Mitani K, Wakamiya M, Hasty P, Graham FL, Bradley A, Caskey CT. Gene targeting in mouse embryonic stem cells with an adenoviral vector. Somat Cell Mol Genet 1995; 21:221–231.

177. Russell DW, Hirata RK. Human gene targeting by viral vectors. Nat Genet 1998; 18:325–330.

178. Liu X, Yan Z, Lou M, et al. Targeted correction of single-base-pair mutations with adeno-associated virus vectors under nonselective conditions. J Virol 2004; 78:4165–4175.

179. Goncz KK, Gruenert DC. Site-directed alteration of genomic DNA by small-fragment homologous replacement. Methods Mol Biol 2000; 133:85–99.

180. Goncz KK, Colosimo A, Dallapiccola B, et al. Expression of DeltaF508 CFTR in normal mouse lung after site-specific modification of CFTR sequences by SFHR. Gene Ther 2001; 8:961–965.

181. Gruenert DC, Bruscia E, Novelli G, et al. Sequence-specific modification of genomic DNA by small DNA fragments. J Clin Investig 2003; 112:637–641.

182. Bertrand P, Rouillard D, Boulet A, Levalois C, Soussi T, Lopex BS. Increase of spontaneous intrachromosomal homologous recombination in mammalian cells expressing a mutant p53 protein. Oncogene 1997; 14:1117–1122.

183. Thyagarajan B, Campbell C. Elevated homologous recombination activity in Fanconi anemia fibroblasts. J Biol Chem 1997; 272:23328–23333.

184. Bishop AJ, Barlow C, Wynshaw-Boris AJ, Schiestl RH. Atm deficiency causes an increased frequency of intrachromosomal homologous recombination in mice. Cancer Res 2000; 60:395–399.

185. Bishop AJ, Schiestl RH. Homologous recombination as a mechanism for genome rearrangements: environmental and genetic effects. Hum Mol Genet 2000; 9:2427–2334.

186. Yao XD, Matecic M, Elias P. Direct repeats of the herpes simplex virus a sequence promote nonconservative homologous recombination that is not dependent on XPF/ERCC4. J Virol 1997; 71:6842–6849.

187. Carroll D. Using nucleases to stimulate homologous recombination. Methods Mol Biol 2004; 262:195–207.

188. Rouet P, Smih F, Jasin M. Expression of a site-specific endonuclease stimlates homologous recombination in mammalian cells. Proc Natl Acad Sci USA 1994; 91:6064–6068.

189. Barski A, Frenkel B. ChIP Display: novel method for identification of genomic targets of transcription factors. Nucleic Acids Res 2004; 32:e104.

190. Grate D, Wilson C. Laser-mediated, site-specific inactivation of RNA transcripts. Proc Natl Acad Sci USA 1999; 96:6131–6136.

191. Wu XS, Li Y, Burgess SM. Transcription start regions in the human genome are favored targets for MLV integration. Science 2003; 300:1670–1671.

192. Colosimo A, Goncz KK, Novelli G, Dallapiccola B, Gruenert DC. Targeted correction of a defective selectable marker gene in human epithelial cells by small DNA fragments. Mol Ther 2001; 3:178–185.

193. Bruscia E, Sangiuolo F, Sinibaldi P, Goncz KK, Novelli G, Gruenert DC. Isolation of CF cell lines corrected at DeltaF508-CFTR by SFHR-mediated targeting. Gene Ther 2002; 9:683–685.

194. Thorpe PH, Stevenson BJ, Porteous DJ. Functional correction of episomal mutations with short DNA fragments and RNA–DNA oligonucleotides. J Gene Med 2002; 4:195–204.

195. Kapsa R, Quigley A, Lynch GS, et al. In vivo and in vitro correction of the mdx dystrophin gene nonsense mutation by short-fragment homologous replacement. Hum Gene Ther 2001; 12:629–642.

196. Kapsa RM, Quigley AF, Vadolas J, et al. Targeted gene correction in the mdx mouse using short DNA fragments: towards application with bone marrow-derived cells for autologous remodeling of dystrophic muscle. Gene Ther 2002; 9:695–699.

197. Kollias G, Spanopoulou E, Grosveld F, Ritter M, Beech J, Morris R. Differential regulation of a Thy-1 gene in transgenic mice. Proc Natl Acad Sci USA 1987; 84:1492–1496.

198. Feng G, Mellor RH, Bernstein M, et al. Imaging neuronal subsets in transgenic mice expressing multiple spectral variants of GFP. Neuron 2000; 28:41–51.

199. Farhadi HF, Lepage P, Forghani R, et al. A combinatorial network of evolutionarily conserved myelin basic protein regulatory sequences confers distinct glial-specific phenotypes. J Neurosci 2003; 23:10214–10223.

200. Kyrkanides S, Miller JH, Bowers WJ, Federoff HJ. Transcriptional and posttranslational regulation of Cre recombinase by RU486 as the basis for an enhanced inducible expression system. Mol Ther 2003; 8:790–795.

201. Lindeberg J, Mattsson R, Ebendal T. Timing the doxycycline yields different patterns of genomic recombination in brain neurons with a new inducible Cre transgene. J Neurosci Res 2002; 68:248–253.

202. Zinyk DL, Mercer EH, Harris E, Anderson DJ, Joyner AL. Fate mapping of the mouse midbrain–hindbrain constriction using a site-specific recombination system. Curr Biol 1998; 8:665–668.

203. Dymecki SM, Tomasiewicz H. Using Flp-recombinase to characterize expansion of Wnt1-expressing neural progenitors in the mouse. Dev Biol 1998; 201:57–65.

204. Psarras S, Karagianni N, Kellendonk C, et al. Gene transfer and genetic modification of embryonic stem cells by Cre- and Cre-PR-expressing MESV-based retroviral vectors. J Gene Med 2004; 6:32–42.

205. Pfeifer A, Ikawa M, Dayn Y, Verma IM. Transgenesis by lentiviral vectors: lack of gene silencing in mammalian embryonic stem cells and preimplantation embryos. Proc Natl Acad Sci USA 2002; 99:2140–2145.

206. Brooks AI, Muhkerjee B, Panahian N, Cory-Slechta D, Federoff HJ. Nerve growth factor somatic mosaicism produced by herpes virus-directed expression of cre recombinase. Nat Biotechnol 1997; 15:57–62.

207. Brooks AI, Cory-Slechta DA, Bowers WJ, Murg SL, Federoff HJ. Enhanced learning in mice parallels vector-mediated nerve growth factor expression in hippocampus. Hum Gene Ther 2000; 11:2341–2352.

208. Brooks AI, Cory-Slechta DA, Federoff HJ. Gene-experience interaction alters the cholinergic septohippocampal pathway of mice. Proc Natl Acad Sci USA 2000; 97:13378–13383.

209. Kaplitt MG, Leone P, Samulski RJ, et al. Long-term gene expression and phenotypic correction using adeno-associated virus vectors in the mammalian brain. Nat Genet 1994; 8:148–154.

210. Kaspar BK, Vissel B, Bengoechea T, et al. Adeno-associated virus effectively mediates conditional gene modification in the brain. Proc Natl Acad Sci USA 2002; 99:2320–2325.

211. Ahmed BY, Chakravarty S, Eggers R, et al. Efficient delivery of Cre-recombinase to neurons in vivo and stable transduction of neurons using adeno-associated and lentiviral vectors. BMC Neurosci 2004; 5:4.

212. Blömer U, Naldini L, Kafri T, Trono D, Verma IM, Gage FH. Highly efficient and sustained gene transfer in adult neurons with lentivirus vector. J Virol 1997; 71:6641–6649.

213. Wang Y, Krushel LA, Edelman GM. Targeted DNA recombination in vivo using an adenovirus carrying the cre recombinase gene. Proc Natl Acad Sci USA 1996; 93:3932–3936.

214. Thevenot E, Cote F, Colin P, et al. Targeting conditional gene modification into the serotonin neurons of the dorsal raphe nucleus by viral delivery of the Cre recombinase. Mol Cell Neurosci 2003; 24:139–147.

215. Sinnayah P, Lindley TE, Staber PD, Davidson BL, Cassell MD, Davisson RL. Targeted viral delivery of Cre recombinase induces conditional gene deletion in cardiovascular circuits of the mouse brain. Physiol Genomics 2004; 18:25–32.

216. Shaner NC, Campbell RE, Steinbach PA, Giepmans BN, Palmer AE, Tsien RY. Improved monomeric red, orange and yellow fluorescent proteins derived from Discosoma sp. red fluorescent protein. Nat Biotechnol 2004; 22:1567–1572.

217. Wang L, Jackson WC, Steinbach PA, Tsien RY. Evolution of new nonantibody proteins via iterative somatic hypermutation. Proc Natl Acad Sci USA 2004;101.

218. Sampo B, Kaech S, Kunz S, Banker G. Two distinct mechanisms target membrane proteins to the axonal surface. Neuron 2003; 37:611–624.

219. Dean C, Scholl FG, Choih J, et al. Neurexin mediates the assembly of presynaptic terminals. Nat Neurosci 2003; 6:708–716.

220. Miesenbock G, de Angelis DA, Rothman JE. Visualizing secretion and synaptic transmission with pH-sensitive green fluorescent proteins. Nature 1998; 394:192–195.

221. Palmer AE, Jin C, Reed JC, Tsien RY. Bcl-2-mediated alterations in endoplasmic reticulum Ca2+ analyzed with an improved genetically encoded fluorescent sensor. Proc Natl Acad Sci USA 2004; 101:17404–17409.

222. Miyawaki A, Griesbeck O, Heim R, Tsien RY. Dynamic and quantitative Ca2+ measurements using improved cameleons. Proc Natl Acad Sci USA 1999; 96:2135–2140.

223. Hanson GT, Aggeler R, Oglesbee D, et al. Investigating mitochondrial redox potential with redox-sensitive green fluorescent protein indicators. J Biol Chem 2004; 279:13044–13053.

224. Kunkel MT, Ni Q, Tsien RY, Zhang J, Newton AC. Spatio-temporal dynamics of protein kinase B/Akt signaling revealed by a genetically-encoded fluorescent reporter. J Biol Chem 2004.

225. Kuner T, Augustine GJ. A genetically encoded ratiometric indicator for chloride: capturing chloride transients in cultured hippocampal neurons. Neuron 2000; 27:447–459.

226. Kissa K, Mordelet E, Soudais C, et al. In vivo neuronal tracing with GFP-TTC gene delivery. Mol Cell Neurosci 2002; 20:627–637.

227. Coen L, Osta R, Maury M, Brulet P. Construction of hybrid proteins that migrate retrogradely and transynaptically into the central nervous system. Proc Natl Acad Sci USA 1997; 94:9400–9405.

228. Zou Z, Horowitz LF, Montmayeur JP, Snapper S, Buck LB. Genetic tracing reveals a stereotyped sensory map in the olfactory cortex. Nature 2001; 414:173–179.

229. Kohara K, Kitamura A, Morishima M, Tsumoto T. Activity-dependent transfer of brain derived neurotrophic factor to postsynaptic neurons. Science 2001; 291:2419–2423.

230. Adams SR, Campbell RE, Gross LA, et al. New biarsenical ligands and tetracysteine motifs for protein labeling in vitro and in vivo: synthesis and biological applications. J Am Chem Soc 2002; 124:6063–6076.

231. Contag CH, Bachmann MH. Advances in in vivo bioluminescence imaging of gene expression. Annu Rev Biomed Eng 2002; 4:235–260.

232. Shah K, Jacobs A, Breakefield XO, Weissleder R. Molecular imaging of gene therapy for cancer. Gene Ther 2004; 11:1175–1187.

233. Shah K, Tang Y, Breakefield X, Weissleder R. Real-time imaging of TRAIL-induced apoptosis of glioma tumors in vivo. Oncogene 2003; 22:6865–6872.

234. Tannous BA, Kim DE, Fermandez JL, Weissleder R, Breakefield XO. Codon optimized *Gaussia* luciferase cDNA for mammalian gene expression in culture and in vivo. Mol Ther 2005; 11:435–443.

235. Bhaumik S, Gambhir SS. Optical imaging of Renilla luciferase reporter gene expression in living mice. Proc Natl Acad Sci USA 2002; 99:377–382.

236. Rehemtulla A, Stegman LD, Cardozo SJ, Gupta S, Hall DE, Contag CH, Ross BD. Rapid and quantitative assessment of cancer treatment response using in vivo bioluminescence imaging. Neoplasia 2000; 2:491–495.

237. Tang Y, Shah K, Messerli SM, Snyder E, Breakefield XO, Weissleder R. In vivo tracking of neuronal progenitor cell migration to glioblastomas. Hum Gene Ther 2003; 14:1247–1254.

238. Rehemtulla A, Hall DE, Stegman LD, et al. Molecular imaging of gene expression and efficacy following adenoviral-mediated brain tumor gene therapy. Mol Imag 2002; 1:43–55.

239. Collaco AM, Geusz ME. Monitoring immediate-early gene expression through firefly luciferase imaging of HRS/J hairless mice. BMC Physiol 2003; 3:8.

240. Oehmig A, Fraefel C, Breakefield XO, Ackermann M. Herpes simplex virus type 1 amplicons and their hybrid virus partners, EBV, AAV, and retrovirus. Curr Gene Ther 2004; 4:385–408.

241. Novak A, Guo C, Yang W, Nagy A, Lobe CG. Z/EG, a double reporter mouse line that expresses enhanced green fluorescent protein upon Cre-mediated excision. Genesis 2000; 28:147–155.

7

Astrocytes as Targets for Neurological Gene Therapy

Tetsuya Imura
*Department of Neurobiology and Brain Research Institute, UCLA School of Medicine,
University of California, Los Angeles, California, U.S.A. and Department of Pathology
and Applied Neurobiology, Graduate School of Medical Science, Kyoto Prefectural
University of Medicine, Kawaramachi-Hirokoji, Kamigyo-ku, Kyoto, Japan*

Michael V. Sofroniew
*Department of Neurobiology and Brain Research Institute, UCLA School of Medicine,
University of California Los Angeles, Los Angeles, California, U.S.A.*

INTRODUCTION

Despite the great advances in our knowledge about basic neuroscience, many neurological diseases still remain refractory to existing treatments and as a consequence, functional preservation and recovery after insults is unsatisfactory. Most research attempting to develop an effective therapy has been focused on neurons and oligodendrocytes trying to prevent their death and restore functions. On the other hand, astrocytes, the most abundant cell type in the central nervous system (CNS), have been largely ignored. This is presumably because astrocytes are widely believed to be more resistant to neurological insults, and also because the roles of astrocytes have been considered less critical for brain function compared to their more specialized partners. Nevertheless, progress in understanding astrocyte biology, especially during the last decade, has revealed their importance in both physiological and pathological states of brain function. The development of glia is closely correlated with brain evolution. Only 10% of cells in the fly nervous system are glia whereas glial cells vastly outnumber neurons in human brains (1). Astrocytes are more expanded and differentiated as brain size gets bigger and neural circuits become more complicated. From a phylogenic point of view, the primitive role of glia in intervertebrates is likely to be the insulation of each neural circuit to prevent crosstalk. But elaborate coordination and plasticity of neural circuits are required for complex behavior of higher vertebrates and the development of astrocytes may be the result of evolutionary pressure to establish these functions. Indeed recent findings have supported this notion (2,3).

    This chapter focuses on the potential of astrocytes in neurological gene therapy. We first review recent advances about the roles of astrocytes under physiological and pathological conditions. We then summarize the usefulness and limitation of animal models to study the functions of astrocytes. Finally, strategies to target astrocytes for gene therapy are discussed.

PHYSIOLOGICAL ROLES OF ASTROCYTES IN THE MATURE CNS

Astrocytes are morphologically and spatially classified into two populations; protoplasmic astrocytes in the gray matter and fibrous astrocytes in the white matter. There are also more specialized astrocyte-related cells in anatomically distinct regions, such as Bergmann glia in cerebellum, Muller cells in retina, tanycytes along the ventricles, and possibly adult neural progenitor cells that are discussed later. Lineage relationship and functional divergence among those populations remain largely unknown but are important issues for future studies.

At a cellular level, astrocytes extend their end-feet to make contact with blood vessels, and their processes also envelop synaptic elements. This anatomical composition led to the suggestion that astrocytes are involved in the formation of the blood brain barrier (BBB), the maintenance of ion homeostasis, and the clearance of neurotransmitters. These ideas are still basically true, but recent studies have revealed that astrocytes regulate neural activity by controlling these functions more actively than previously considered. For instance, the major excitatory neurotransmitter glutamate is taken up via specific transporters on astrocytes and recycled back to neurons as glutamine. This function is crucial for limiting glutamate's actions and preventing excitotoxicity, but in addition to a scavenging role this uptake and recycling is also directly involved in regulating neural activity (4). Astrocytes retract and extend their processes at synaptic cleft to modulate the clearance rate of glutamate, which in turn alters synaptic strength and determines glutamate spillover to neighboring synapses (5–8). Furthermore, glutamate transport into astrocytes stimulates glucose uptake from their end-feet and enhances the production of lactate by aerobic glycolysis. Then astrocytes release lactate as an energy substrate for neighboring neurons to meet their activity-dependent energy demand (9–11). Astrocytes also express a wide variety of neurotransmitter receptors including glutamate and voltage-gated ion channels, which enable them to monitor synaptic activity. In particular, cytosolic Ca^{2+} elevation and its propagation to neighboring astrocytes through gap junctions (known as Ca^{2+} wave) are a major machinery to provoke various feedback reactions in astrocytes (12). In response to these signals, astrocytes release neuroactive substances such as glutamate and ATP and promote arteriole dilation, resulting in a change in synaptic efficacy and an increase in local blood flow (13,14). Astrocytes further modulate synaptic function by influencing on the morphology of dendritic spines, controlling the number of synapses, and secreting growth factors and extracellular matrix molecules (15–17).

The participation of astrocytes in the Blood-brain barrier (BBB) has been of great interest but still remains controversial. The induction of tight junction in endothelial cells is the essential component of the BBB, but this property is not intrinsic to brain endothelial cells, and the contact with astrocytes appears to be necessary. Several grafting and tissue culture studies have indicated that astrocytes are critical for the BBB formation (18,19). Although the contrary claim has been made that the BBB remains intact after astrocytes are injured by immunotoxin (20), genetically targeted ablation of astrocytes leads to failure of BBB repair after injury, and grafts of astrocytes can restore BBB after such astrocyte ablation (21). Mechanisms in the BBB induction by astrocytes are unknown, but the contribution of astrocyte-produced factors such as transforming growth factor-beta (TGF-β) (22), gial cell line-derived neurotrophic factor (GDNF) (23), and basic fibroblast growth factor (bFGF) (24) has been postulated. Even though there is a disagreement on the direct role of astrocytes for the induction and maintenance of the BBB (25), it seems generally accepted that extensive communications between astrocytes and endothelium are involved in a number of important brain functions such as regulation of immune cells, water transport, blood flow control, energy supply, and antioxidant defense (19).

Thus, all of these findings strongly support the dynamic roles of astrocytes for regulating ongoing neural activity and plasticity. This implies that the dysfunction of astrocytes is an important potential cause of various pathological states of the CNS.

ASTROCYTES IN NEUROLOGICAL DISEASES

It is generally believed that astrocytes are more resistant to neurological insults than neurons and oligodendrocytes, and that therefore they are not the primary target of diseases except for only a few cases such as hepatic encephalopathy and Alexander disease. Nevertheless, the death of neurons and oligodendrocytes, a hallmark of many neurological diseases, is not likely to be exclusively cell-autonomous and complex cell to cell interactions including astrocytes can play a critical role. Because of the importance of astrocytes in maintaining brain homeostasis, even the subtle change of astrocyte functions may disrupt it followed by pathological changes of the CNS. One of the best examples is Alexander disease in which a missense mutation in the glial fibrillary acidic protein (GFAP) gene has been recently identified (26). Even though this is a primary disorder of astrocytes, extensive demyelination is the prominent neuropathological characteristic (27). In this section, we review recent progress regarding the involvement of astrocytes in neurological diseases and their potential as a therapeutic target.

The effects of astrocytes on acute insults such as ischemia and trauma may be due to the loss of their normal functions. Ultrastructral changes of astrocytes including swelling of processes and mitochondria are one of the earliest findings after the onset of insults, suggesting that the dysfunction of astrocytes may precede the death of neurons and olidodendrocytes (28,29). Membrane depolarization and energy crisis in astrocytes results in dysregulation of ionic homeostasis, reversal of glutamate transporter, and loss of antioxidant glutathione, all of which are likely to accelerate neuronal cell death (30). Astrocyte-to-astrocyte gap junctional communication may facilitate the propagation of cell injury and increase neuronal vulnerability to insults (4,31–33) although other studies have proposed the protective roles of astrocytic gap junctions for neuronal survival (34,35). Moreover, astrocyte dysfunction may play a crucial role for the formation of vasogenic brain edema, a common cause of mortality in many neurological diseases. Pathological conditions either physically disrupt astrocyte-endothelial junctions at the BBB or induce astrocytic expression of some factors such as metalloproteases and vascular endothelial growth factor (VEGF) to increase the permeability of the BBB (36,37). Recent studies suggest that water channels aquaporins (AQPs) concentrated in the end-feet of astrocytes regulate influx and efflux of water between brain and vessels in coupling with K^+ buffering (38). AQPs are upregulated in astrocytes under pathological conditions, and the genetic disruption of AQP4, a major AQP isoform in the CNS, suppresses brain edema and improves outcome after ischemia (39). Thus, the genetic or pharmacological manipulation of AQPs is a promising target for preventing brain edema.

The effects of astrocytes on subacute and chronic neurological disease conditions appear to be more complicated and sometimes paradoxical, but have important implications in gene therapy because of a wide time window. Rather than the loss of their normal functions, the aberrant regulation of astrocyte functions can be involved in the pathogenesis of these conditions. The responses of astrocytes are commonly called as "reactive astrocytes" or "astrogliosis," which is characterized by cellular hypertrophy, proliferation, and an increased expression of GFAP. Although reactive astrocytes are often referred as a stereotyped reaction to insults, a growing body of evidence indicates that considerable heterogeneity exists in regard to both function and phenotype (40,41). One of the well-known properties of reactive astrocytes is the formation of the structural barrier for axonal regeneration by producing inhibitory molecules such as proteoglycans (42), leading to the notion that reactive astrocytes are detrimental to neurological outcome. Exaggeration of inflammatiory brain injury may be another harmful effect of reactive astrocytes. They produce potentially neurotoxic molecules such as nitric oxide (NO) and tumor necrosis factors (43,44), and also up-regulate adhesion molecules and chemokines that are known to recruit lymphocytes and monocytes into the CNS (45,46). In addition, they could act as antigen-presenting cells by expressing major histocompatibility (MHC) class II molecules like microglia (47). Thus, these results suggest the role of reactive astrocytes as an inflammatory mediator. Conversely, a number of studies have shown that reactive astrocytes posses beneficial properties. They produce a wide variety of neurotrophic molecules such as NGF, CNTF, GDNF, etc. (48). Paradoxical findings exist regarding "detrimental" aspects of reactive astrocytes. Antigen presentation and production of potentially toxic molecules such as NO may control the replication of some parasites such as Toxoplasma gondii (49,50). NO production in astrocytes also could promote the release of neuroprotective glutathione (51). Targeted ablation of dividing reactive astrocytes using the transgenic strategy has further demonstrated their beneficial roles. Removal of reactive astrocytes results in increased infiltration of leukocytes, delayed BBB repair, and neuronal degeneration after injury, although it also increases axonal sprouting (21,52).

How can we interpret those complicated and ambivalent observations? The most plausible explanation is that the roles of astrocytes are multiple and different depending on the pathogenesis of diseases even though their cellular phenotype ("reactive astrocytes") looks similar. In addition, there could be spatial and temporal differences even in a single disease. Therefore, it is necessary to dissociate the roles of astrocytes in each disease condition at different time points. Consistent with this notion, a number of different studies indicate that astrocytes exhibit disease-specific properties in some neurological diseases (Table 1). Those are of a considerable interest as therapeutic targets for gene therapy. However, it remains to be clarified how much is their contribution to the entire pathogenesis of each disease. Furthermore, astrocytes are not the only cell type to express specific molecules in most cases. For instance, proinflammatory cytokines are postulated to play an important role in several neurological diseases, but multiple cell types express those cytokines in the CNS. The importance of specific molecules needs to be assessed in a cell-type specific manner. To address these questions, it is required to develop animal models in which functions of astrocytes can be dissociated and manipulated.

ANIMAL MODELS TO STUDY THE ROLES OF ASTROCYTES

There are at present two major strategies to analyze the functions of astrocytes in models of neurological disease conditions in vivo. First is the cellular ablation strategy in which astrocytes are either pharmacologically or genetically eliminated, which allows us to analyze the entire roles of astrocytes as a cell population. Second is the cellular targeting in

Table 1 Specific Roles of Astrocytes for the Pathogenesis of Neurological Diseases

Disease	Potential roles for pathogenesis	References
Alexander disease	Gene mutation in the GFAP gene, Rosenthal fiber formation	(26)
Alzheimer disease	Degradation of extracellular amyloid-beta deposits	(80,81)
ALS (Motor neuron disease)	Loss of glutamate transporters	(Howland et al. 2002; Rothstein et al. 1995)
Multiple sclerosis	Syncytin expression and the release of redox reactants Loss of β2-adrenergic receptor	(Antony et al. 2004; De Keyser et al. 1999)
Hepatic encephalopathy	Accumulation of glutamine and water	(Norenberg et al. 1992)
HIV dementia	Production of stromal cell-derived factor 1	(Zhang et al. 2003)

which specific molecules are either expressed or deleted only in astrocytes, with a goal that roles of specific molecules in astrocytes can be identified. Gliotoxins such as fluorocitrate have been used as a pharmacological tool for the ablation of astrocytes over 30 years, but the selectivity of toxicity is always relative in this method, such that at high doses effects on other cell types can not be excluded, and at low doses negative results may be due to insufficient ablation of astrocytes themselves. With advancements in genetic technologies, astrocyte-specific gene manipulation has been developed. In most studies, the GFAP promoter is applied to target astrocytes (53), advantages and potential problems using this promoter are discussed below.

To ablate astrocytes using transgenic strategies, two different models have been reported to date. In the first of these, herepes simplex virus thymidine kinase (HSV–TK) is expressed under the control of the GFAP promoter (21,54). In this model, the application of the antiviral agent gancyclovir (GCV) kills dividing HSV–TK expressing astrocytes. This is a well-characterized system, and it has been shown that GCV effectively eliminates dividing reactive astrocytes after injury. The other model expresses *E. coli* nitroreductase from the GFAP promoter. In this model, even non-dividing astrocytes can be ablated by the administration of the prodrug, and cerebellar Bergmann glia are especially sensitive to the treatment of adult mice, presumably because of their high GFAP expression (55).

To study the function of specific molecules in astrocytes, the GFAP promoter-driven expression of these molecules has been most commonly used. Some of these models are listed in Table 2. This gain-of-function experiment may have two limitations. First, it is possible that the effects mediated by such over-expression is artificial and does not reflect the significance of their endogenous expression in astrocytes. Second, transgene expression is always dependent on the GFAP promoter activity. Sufficient transgene expression may not be achieved in low-GFAP expressing astrocytes like gray matter protoplasmic astrocytes, whereas higher expression is expected in hippocampal astrocytes or Bergmann glia. The cell-type specific conditional gene manipulation using the Cre-loxP system is one of the promising strategies to solve these problems (56). In these models, Cre recombinase, whose expression is controlled in a cell-type specific (e.g., the GFAP promoter) and/or an inducible manner (e.g., TetO), recognizes a short DNA sequence called loxP and excises the genomic region flanked by two loxP sites. This system enables the generation of astrocyte-specific deletion of a gene of interest to determine the significance of its expression in astrocytes. Moreover, this system can be also applied to generate transgenic

Table 2 Animal Models to Study Astrocyte Functions

	Promoter[a]	Gene	Phenotype	References
Cell ablation	HGFAP	HSV–TK	Ganciclovir treatment in newborn caused cerebellar abnormality (Bergmann glia disorganization, ectopic Purkinje cells, and granule cell loss)	(54)
	MGFAP	HSV–TK	Ganciclovir treatment caused death of enteric glia, reduction of adult CNS neurogenesis, and ablation of reactive astrocytes after injury	(62,67)
	MGFAP	nitroreductase	Prodrug CB1954 treatment in adult caused loss of cerebellar Bergmann glia and granule cell degeneration	(55)
Cytokines	MGFAP	IL–6	Neuronal dendric atrophy, GFAP elevation, neovascularization, and abnormal BBB development	(87)
	MGFAP	TGF-β1	Hydrocephalus, premature death	(88)
	HGFAP	TGF-β1	Hydrocephalus, extracellular matrix protein deposition	(89)
	MGFAP	IL–3	Primary demyelination and accumulation of macrophage/microglia	(90)
Infection	MGFAP	HIV gp120	Loss of pyramidal neurons in cortex, reactive changes of astrocytes, and microglial activation	(91)
	TetO-mGFAP	HIV Tat	Doxycycline-dependent Tat expression in astrocytes, abnormal behavior and premature death	(92)
	HGFAP	BDV phosphoprotein	Abnormal behavior and decreased synaptic density	(93)
	MGFAP	hamster PrP	Spongiform encephalopathy induced by hamster scrapie	(94)
Neurodegenerative disease	HGFAP	human APOE (ε3 and 4)	Poor neurite outgrowth in vitro co-culture withε4 transgenic astrocytes	(95)
	HGFAP	ALS-mutant SOD1	Reactive changes of astrocytes but no motor neuron death	(59)
Gene transfer	HGFAP	TVA	Avian leukosis virus A receptor expression for astrocyte specific gene delivery	(96)
Conditional	HGFAP	Cre	Cre excision occurred in the majority of neural cells in cortex	(64,65)
	MGFAP	Cre	Cre excision occurred in late-born neurons and astrocytes	(67)

[a] hGFAP, human glial fibrillary acidic protein; mGFAP, mouse glial fibrillary acidic protein.

models. The STOP signal flanked by loxP is inserted to prevent transgene expression (e.g., reporter), but Cre excision activates its expression only in astrocytes. Since transgene expression, once activated, is controlled by the ubiquitous promoter, a constant level of the expression is expected in astrocytes independently of their GFAP promoter activity. As shown in Figure 1, the reporter expressing astrocytes are more broadly distributed than GFAP-immunoreactive astrocytes in GFAP-Cre-Reporter mouse cortex. This is especially useful when continuous and ubiquitous transgene expression in astrocytes is required. For example, forced expression of human amyotrophic lateral sclerosis (ALS) -related mutant superoxide dismutase 1 (mSOD1) in mice causes motor neuron death. Non cell-autonomous mechanisms including the contribution of astrocytes are postulated (57,58), but the GFAP-promoter driven mSOD1 fails to induce motor neuron death (59). It remains possible that the GFAP promoter activity is not enough to produce a sufficient amount of mSOD1 and the application of the Cre-loxP system has a considerable advantage to further address this question.

Even though the GFAP promoter is the most effective and practical way of targeting astrocytes to date, it should be noted that potential problems also exist in its application. GFAP is an intermediate filament predominantly localized in astrocytes in the CNS, but it is also expressed by other cell types inside and outside the CNS such as retinal Muller cells, Schwann cells, enteric glia, hepatic stellate cells, pancreatic peri-islet cells, and chondrocytes (53,60,61). These cells can be affected as well. For example,

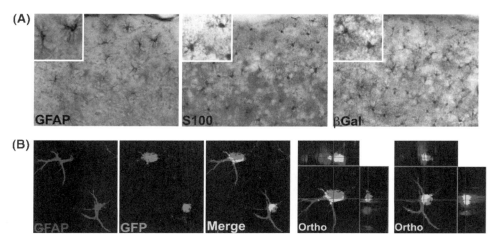

Figure 1 (*See color insert*) Astrocytes are effectively targeted in GFAP-Cre mice. GFAP-Cre mice that express Cre recombinase from the mouse GFAP promoter were crossed with two strains of reporter mice in which the expression of the reporter protein, either β-galactosidase (β-gal) or green fluorescent protein (GFP), is controlled by a ubiquitous promoter, either ROSA or pCAGGS respectively, under regulation of a STOP signal. In offspring of these mice, the Cre recombinase excises the STOP signal to activate the reporter protein, either βgalalactosidase (βgal) or green fluorescent protein (GFP), whose expression is then controlled by the ubiquitous promoter, either ROSA or pCAGGS, respectively. (**A**) Bright-field immunohistochemistry shows βgal expression in somatosensory cortex of GFAP-Cre reporter mice. βgal-positive cells exhibit a multipolar morphology typical for astrocytes (*inset*). There are more βgal-positive cells in cortex than GFAP-positive astrocytes, but comparable numbers to S100-positive astrocytes. In these cells, reporter expression continues even though GFAP has been down regulated. (**B**) Confocal orthogonal three-dimensional analysis of GFAP-positive (*red*) astrocytes expressing the reporter protein GFP (*green*), shows clear expression of reporter by GFAP positive cells.

the cellular ablation using the mouse GFAP promoter resulted in the elimination of not only reactive astrocytes in the CNS but also enteric glia in gut to cause fulminant jejuno-ileitis resemble to human inflammatory bowel disease (62). In addition, there exist different GFAP promoter fragments and each has different expression profiles. The human 2kb GFAP promoter targets neural progenitor cells in embryonic mouse cortex (63), and as a result gene excision occurs in the vast majority of neurons as well as astrocytes in the human GFAP-Cre mouse cortex (64,65). The use of the mouse 15 kb promoter may be more relevant to mouse endogenous GFAP expression, but still targets postnatal neural progenitor cells (66–68). Even though this unexpected feature of the GFAP promoter can be useful in targeting specific population of neural progenitor cells, one should take into consideration this issue when analyzing the functions of astrocytes. S100β is another astrocyte marker and the S100β promoter-driven transgenic mice have been recently generated. Reporter expression, however, can be found not only in astrocytes but also in subsets of neurons and oligodendrocytes, indicating that the same potential problem exists as the GFAP promoter (69).

STRATEGY FOR TARGETING ASTROCYTES IN NEUROLOGICAL GENE THERAPY

In considering astrocytes as a target for gene therapy, two distinct approaches can be proposed. First is to target astrocytes simply as a vehicle for the gene delivery. They may have higher chance to get genes introduced into the CNS since they are the most numerous cells and can be efficiently transduced by various viral and non-viral vectors (70–72). It seems that astrocytes are more tolerant to insults and their functions are less specialized compared to neurons and oligodendrocytes, therefore higher efficiency and less adverse effects under various conditions can be expected. In the case of ex vivo gene therapy, astrocytes are expandable ex vivo and survive better after grafting in vivo. Cultured neural progenitor cells, another promising vehicle for ex vivo gene therapy (73,74), favor to differentiate into astrocytes after transplanted into adult brains (75,76). Thus, astrocytes are good candidates as a "factory" to produce exogenous molecules. In this context, these molecules do not need to be related to the functions of astrocytes, but should produce secreted molecules. Most attempts targeting astrocytes for gene therapy to date have been conducted along this line such as GDNF and tyrosine hydroxylase for Parkinson's disease, and beta-glucuronidase for a lysosomal storage dsease (77–79).

A second approach is to regulate the functions of astrocytes by gene therapy. As already reviewed in this chapter, astrocytes exert various important functions under both physiological and pathological conditions. To potentiate their beneficial roles and suppress their detrimental roles would be a promising approach for future gene therapy. To bring this strategy into realistic clinical application, it is necessary to elucidate what are the specific roles of astrocytes and how important are these roles in the pathogenesis of each disease. For example, it has been recently reported that astrocytes contribute to the degradation of Alzheimer disease (AD)-related amyloid-beta (Aβ) deposits and apoE expression in astrocytes is involved in this process (80,81). Even though the impact of Aβ degradation by astrocytes on the pathogenesis of AD awaits further studies, the reinforcement of this ability would be one potential therapeutic target in the future.

To manipulate astrocytes effectively but avoid undesirable effects on other cells, it is important to construct a vector selectively targeting astrocytes. Each viral and non-viral vector may have some degree of cell-type specificity (72,82–84), but it is controversial and incomplete. As is the case with animal models, the expression regulation by the GFAP promoter is a most commonly applied and presumably most effective way at this time. However the use of the GFAP promoter for gene therapy potentially has the same problems as indicated in animal models discussed above. That is, inefficient gene expression in some astrocytes with low levels of GFAP, ectopic expression in other types of cells, and unexpected targeting neural progenitor cells. It has been recently reported that neural progenitor cells in adult human brains also express GFAP (85). Inappropriate manipulation of these cells may disrupt physiological neurogenesis or induce tumorgenesis (86). The advance of basic knowledge about the behavior of neural cells and the technical development to improve cell-type specificity would provide reasonable solution to these concerns.

CONCLUDING REMARKS

Astrocytes have long been obscured by their more glamorous partners, neurons and oligodendrocytes, but recent and ongoing research is revealing important roles of these cells. While the final goal of any therapeutic attempt against neurological diseases is to normalize brain functions, and there can be no doubt that neurons and their circuitry are the primary functional units of brain, it may however not always be true that direct manipulation of neurons is the most effective way to normalize brain functions after insults. Instead, regulating or modifying astrocyte functions may in some cases represent an alternative and effective therapeutic strategy. Clarifying specific roles of astrocytes in different disease conditions may help to develop novel approaches for neurological gene therapy. In addition, astrocytes may be useful targets for gene therapy as vehicles for gene delivery.

ACKNOWLEDGMENTS

This work was supported by National Institutes of Health (NIH) grants NS42039 and NS042693, and fellowships from Uehara Memorial Foundation and Japan Heart Foundation (T.I.). We thank N.B. Doan, M.E. Sislak, T. Chiem and R.A. Korsak for technical assistance.

REFERENCES

1. Rowitch DH. Glial specification in the vertebrate neural tube. Nat Rev Neurosci 2004; 5:409–419.
2. Laming PR, Kimelberg H, Robinson S, et al. Neuronal-glial interactions and behaviour. Neurosci Biobehav Rev 2000; 24:295–340.
3. Iino M, Goto K, Kakegawa W, et al. Glia-synapse interaction through Ca2+-permeable AMPA receptors in Bergmann glia. Science 2001; 292:926–929.
4. Mitchell SJ, Silver RA. Glutamate spillover suppresses inhibition by activating presynaptic mGluRs. Nature 2000; 404:498–502.
5. Oliet SH, Piet R, Poulain DA. Control of glutamate clearance and synaptic efficacy by glial coverage of neurons. Science 2001; 292:923–926.
6. Semyanov A, Kullmann DM, Mitchell SJ, Silver RA. Modulation of GABAergic signaling among interneurons by metabotropic glutamate receptors. Neuron 2000; 25:663–672.
7. Bergles DE, Jahr CE. Synaptic activation of glutamate transporters in hippocampal astrocytes. Neuron 19 1997; 19:1297–1308.

8. Kasischke KA, Vishwasrao HD, Fisher PJ, Zipfel WR, Webb WW. Neural activity triggers neuronal oxidative metabolism followed by astrocytic glycolysis. Science 2004; 305:99–103.

9. Pellerin L, Magistretti PJ. Glutamate uptake into astrocytes stimulates aerobic glycolysis: a mechanism coupling neuronal activity to glucose utilization. Proc Natl Acad Sci USA 1994; 91:10625–10629.

10. Auld DS, Robitaille R. Glial cells and neurotransmission: an inclusive view of synaptic function. Neuron 2003; 40:389–400.

11. Mulligan SJ, MacVicar BA. Calcium transients in astrocyte endfeet cause cerebrovascular constrictions. Nature 2004; 431:195–199.

12. Zonta M, Angulo MC, Gobbo S, Rosengarten B, Hossmann KA, Pozzan T, Carmignoto G. Neuron-to-astrocyte signaling is central to the dynamic control of brain microcirculation. Nat Neurosci 2003; 6:43–50.

13. Dityatev A, Schachner M. Extracellular matrix molecules and synaptic plasticity. Nat Rev Neurosci 2003; 4:456–468.

14. Murai KK, Nguyen LN, Irie F, Yamaguchi Y, Pasquale EB. Control of hippocampal dendritic spine morphology through ephrin-A3/EphA4 signaling. Nat Neurosci 2003; 6:153–160.

15. Ullian EM, Sapperstein SK, Christopherson KS, Barres BA. Control of synapse number by glia. Science 2001; 291:657–661.

16. Abbott NJ. Astrocyte-endothelial interactions and blood-brain barrier permeability. J Anat 2002;629–638.

17. Ballabh P, Braun A, Nedergaard M. The blood–brain barrier: an overview: structure, regulation, and clinical implications. Neurobiol Dis 2004; 16:1–13.

18. Bush TG, Puvanachandra N, Horner CH, et al. Leukocyte infiltration, neuronal degeneration, and neurite outgrowth after ablation of scar-forming, reactive astrocytes in adult transgenic mice. Neuron 1999; 23:297–308.

19. Tran ND, Correale J, Schreiber SS, Fisher M. Transforming growth factor-beta mediates astrocyte-specific regulation of brain endothelial anticoagulant factors. Stroke 1999; 30:1671–1678.

20. Igarashi Y, Utsumi H, Chiba H, et al. Glial cell line-derived neurotrophic factor induces barrier function of endothelial cells forming the blood-brain barrier. Biochem Biophys Res Commun 1999; 261:108–112.

21. Sobue K, Yamamoto N, Yoneda K, et al. Induction of blood-brain barrier properties in immortalized bovine brain endothelial cells by astrocytic factors. Neurosci Res 1999; 35:155–164.

22. Holash JA, Noden DM, Stewart PA. Re-evaluating the role of astrocytes in blood-brain barrier induction. Dev Dyn 1993; 197:14–25.

23. Brenner M, Johnson AB, Boespflug-Tanguy O, Rodriguez D, Goldman JE, Messing A. Mutations in GFAP, encoding glial fibrillary acidic protein, are associated with Alexander disease. Nat Genet 2001; 27:117–120.

24. Delaney CL, Brenner M, Messing A. Conditional ablation of cerebellar astrocytes in postnatal transgenic mice. J Neurosci 1996; 16:6908–6918.

25. Schiffmann R, Boespflug-Tanguy O. An update on the leukodsytrophies. Curr Opin Neurol 2001; 14:789–794.

26. Garcia JH, Yoshida Y, Chen H, et al. Progression from ischemic injury to infarct following middle cerebral artery occlusion in the rat. Am J Pathol 1993; 142:623–635.

27. Liu D, Smith CL, Barone FC, et al. Astrocytic demise precedes delayed neuronal death in focal ischemic rat brain. Brain Res Mol Brain Res 1999; 68:29–41.

28. Chen Y, Swanson RA. Astrocytes and brain injury. J Cereb Blood Flow Metab 2003; 23:137–149.

29. Cotrina ML, Kang J, Lin JH, et al. Astrocytic gap junctions remain open during ischemic conditions. J Neurosci 1998; 18:2520–2537.

30. Frantseva MV, Kokarovtseva L, Naus CG, Carlen PL, MacFabe D, Perez Velazquez JL. Specific gap junctions enhance the neuronal vulnerability to brain traumatic injury. J Neurosci 2002; 22:644–653.

31. Lin JH, Weigel H, Cotrina ML, et al. Gap-junction-mediated propagation and amplification of cell injury; Astrocytic gap junctions remain open during ischemic conditions. Nat Neurosci 1998; 1:494–500.

32. Blanc EM, Bruce-Keller AJ, Mattson MP. Astrocytic gap junctional communication decreases neuronal vulnerability to oxidative stress-induced disruption of Ca2+ homeostasis and cell death. J Neurochem 1998; 70:958–970.

33. Siushansian R, Bechberger JF, Cechetto DF, Hachinski VC, Naus CC. Connexin43 null mutation increases infarct size after stroke. J Comp Neurol 2001; 440:387–394.

34. Papavassiliou E, Gogate N, Proescholdt M, et al. Vascular endothelial growth factor (vascular permeability factor) expression in injured rat brain. J Neurosci Res 1997; 49:451–460.

35. Rosenberg GA, Estrada EY, Dencoff JE. Matrix metalloproteinases and TIMPs are associated with blood-brain barrier opening after reperfusion in rat brain. Stroke 1998; 29:2189–2195.

36. Amiry-Moghaddam M, Ottersen OP. The molecular basis of water transport in the brain. Nat Rev Neurosci 2003; 4:991–1001.

37. Hoke A, Silver J. Heterogeneity among astrocytes in reactive gliosis. Perspect Dev Neurobiol 1994; 2:269–274.

38. Ridet JL, Malhotra SK, Privat A, Gage FH. Reactive astrocytes: cellular and molecular cues to biological function. Trends Neurosci 1997; 20:570–577.

39. Silver J, Miller JH. Regeneration beyond the glial scar. Nat Rev Neurosci 2004; 5:146–156.

40. Hewett SJ, Csernansky CA, Choi DW. Selective potentiation of NMDA-induced neuronal injury following induction of astrocytic iNOS. Neuron 1994; 13:487–494.

41. Lieberman AP, Pitha PM, Shin HS, Shin ML. Production of tumor necrosis factor and other cytokines by astrocytes stimulated with lipopolysaccharide or a neurotropic virus. Proc Natl Acad Sci USA 1989; 86:6348–6352.

42. Babcock AA, Kuziel WA, Rivest S, Owens T. Chemokine expression by glial cells directs leukocytes to sites of axonal injury in the CNS. J Neurosci 2003;7922–7930.

43. Ransohoff RM, Hamilton TA, Tani M, et al. Astrocyte expression of mRNA encoding cytokines IP-10 and JE/MCP-1 in experimental autoimmune encephalomyelitis. Faseb J 1993; 7:592–600.

44. Dong Y, Benveniste EN. Immune function of astrocytes. Glia 2001; 36:180–190.

45. Schwartz JP, Sheng JG, Mitsuo K, Shirabe S, Nishiyama N. Trophic factor production by reactive astrocytes in injured brain. Ann NY Acad Sci 1993; 679:226–234.

46. Peterson PK, Gekker G, Hu S, Chao CC. Human astrocytes inhibit intracellular multiplication of Toxoplasma gondii by a nitric oxide-mediated mechanism. J Infect Dis 1995; 171:516–518.

47. Wilson EH, Hunter CA. The role of astrocytes in the immunopathogenesis of toxoplasmic encephalitis. Int J Parasitol 2004; 34:543–548.

48. Gegg ME, Beltran B, Salas-Pino S, et al. Differential effect of nitric oxide on glutathione metabolism and mitochondrial function in astrocytes and neurones: implications for neuroprotection/neurodegeneration? J Neurochem 2003; 86:228–237.

49. Faulkner JR, Herrmann JE, Woo MJ, Tansey KE, Doan NB, Sofroniew MV. Reactive astrocytes protect tissue and preserve function after spinal cord injury. J Neurosci 2004; 24:2143–2155.

50. Brenner M, Messing A. GFAP Transgenic Mice. Methods 1996; 10:351–364.

51. Delaney CL, Brenner M, Messing A. Conditional ablation of cerebellar astrocytes in postnatal transgenic mice. J Neurosci 1996; 16:6908–6918.

52. Cui W, Allen ND, Skynner M, Gusterson B, Clark AJ. Inducible ablation of astrocytes shows that these cells are required for neuronal survival in the adult brain. Glia 2001; 34:272–282.

53. Krum JM, Kenyon KL, Rosenstein JM. Expression of blood-brain barrier characteristics following neuronal loss and astroglial damage after administration of anti-Thy-1 immunotoxin. Exp Neurol 1997; 146:33–45.

54. Morozov A, Kellendonk C, Simpson E, Tronche F. Using conditional mutagenesis to study the brain. Biol Psychiatry 2003; 54:1125–1133.

55. Bruijn LI, Becher MW, Lee MK, et al. ALS-linked SOD1 mutant G85R mediates damage to astrocytes and promotes rapidly progressive disease with SOD1-containing inclusions. Neuron 1997; 18:327–338.

56. Clement AM, Nguyen MD, Roberts EA, et al. Wild-type nonneuronal cells extend survival of SOD1 mutant motor neurons in ALS mice. Science 2003; 302:113–117.

57. Gong YH, Parsadanian AS, Andreeva A, Snider WD, Elliott JL. Restricted expression of G86R Cu/Zn superoxide dismutase in astrocytes results in astrocytosis but does not cause motoneuron degeneration. J Neurosci 2000; 20:660–665.

58. Viale G, Doglioni C, Dell'Orto P, et al. Glial fibrillary acidic protein immunoreactivity in human respiratory tract cartilages and pulmonary chondromatous hamartomas. Am J Pathol 1988; 133:363–373.

59. Winer S, Tsui H, Lau A, et al. Autoimmune islet destruction in spontaneous type 1 diabetes is not beta-cell exclusive. Nat Med 2003; 9:198–205.

60. Bush TG, Savidge TC, Freeman TC, et al. Fulminant jejuno-ileitis following ablation of enteric glia in adult transgenic mice. Cell 1998; 93:189–201.

61. Malatesta P, Hartfuss E, Gotz M. Isolation of radial glial cells by fluorescent-activated cell sorting reveals a neuronal lineage. Development 2000; 127:5253–5263.

62. Malatesta P, Hack MA, Hartfuss E, et al. Neuronal or glial progeny: regional differences in radial glia fate. Neuron 2003; 37:751–764.

63. Manley GT, Fujimura M, Ma T, et al. Aquaporin-4 deletion in mice reduces brain edema after acute water intoxication and ischemic stroke. Nat Med 2000; 6:159–163.

64. Zhuo L, Theis M, Alvarez-Maya I, Brenner M, Willecke K, Messing A. hGFAP-cre transgenic mice for manipulation of glial and neuronal function in vivo. Genesis 2001; 31:85–94.

65. Doetsch F, Caille I, Lim DA, Garcia-Verdugo JM, Alvarez-Buylla A. Subventricular zone astrocytes are neural stem cells in the adult mammalian brain. Cell 1999; 97:703–716.

66. Garcia AD, Doan NB, Imura T, Bush TG, Sofroniew MV. GFAP-expressing progenitors are the principal source of constitutive neurogenesis in adult mouse forebrain. Nat Neurosci 2004; 7:1233–1241.

67. Imura T, Kornblum HI, Sofroniew MV. The predominant neural stem cell isolated from postnatal and adult forebrain but not early embryonic forebrain expresses GFAP. J Neurosci 2003; 23:2824–2832.

68. Vives V, Alonso G, Solal AC, Joubert D, Legraverend C. Visualization of S100B-positive neurons and glia in the central nervous system of EGFP transgenic mice. J Comp Neurol 2003; 457:404–419.

69. Jakobsson J, Ericson C, Jansson M, Bjork E, Lundberg C. Targeted transgene expression in rat brain using lentiviral vectors. J Neurosci Res 2003; 73:876–885.

70. Nedergaard M, Ransom B, Goldman SA, et al. New roles for astrocytes: redefining the functional architecture of the brain. Trends Neurosci 2003; 26:523–530.

71. Le Gal La Salle G, Robert JJ, Berrard S, et al. An adenovirus vector for gene transfer into neurons and glia in the brain. Science 1993; 259:988–990.

72. Shi N, Zhang Y, Zhu C, Boado RJ, Pardridge WM. Brain-specific expression of an exogenous gene after i.v. administration. Proc Natl Acad Sci U.S.A. 2001; 98:12754–12759.

73. Park KI, Ourednik J, Ourednik V, et al. Global gene and cell replacement strategies via stem cells. Gene Ther 2002; 9:613–624.

74. Tai YT, Svendsen CN. Stem cells as a potential treatment of neurological disorders. Curr Opin Pharmacol 2004; 4:98–104.

75. Fricker RA, Carpenter MK, Winkler C, Greco C, Gates MA, Bjorklund A. Site-specific migration and neuronal differentiation of human neural progenitor cells after transplantation in the adult rat brain. J Neurosci 1999; 19:5990–6005.

76. Suhonen JO, Peterson DA, Ray J, Gage FH. Differentiation of adult hippocampus-derived progenitors into olfactory neurons in vivo. Nature 1996; 383:624–627.

77. Segovia J, Vergara P, Brenner M. Astrocyte-specific expression of tyrosine hydroxylase after intracerebral gene transfer induces behavioral recovery in experimental parkinsonism. Gene Ther 1998; 5:1650–1655.

78. Serguera C, Sarkis C, Ridet JL, Colin P, Moullier P, Mallet J. Primary adult human astrocytes as an ex vivo vehicle for beta-glucuronidase delivery in the brain. Mol Ther 2001; 3:875–881.
79. Rami A, Volkmann T, Winckler J. Effective reduction of neuronal death by inhibiting gap junctional intercellular communication in a rodent model of global transient cerebral ischemia. Exp Neurol 2001; 170:297–304.
80. Wang ZH, Ji Y, Shan W, et al. Therapeutic effects of astrocytes expressing both tyrosine hydroxylase and brain-derived neurotrophic factor on a rat model of Parkinson's disease. Neuroscience 2002; 113:629–640.
81. Koistinaho M, Lin S, Wu X, et al. Apolipoprotein E promotes astrocyte colocalization and degradation of deposited amyloid-beta peptides. Nat Med 2004; 10:719–726.
82. Wyss-Coray T, Loike JD, Brionne TC, et al. Adult mouse astrocytes degrade amyloid-beta in vitro and in situ. Nat Med 2003; 9:453–457.
83. Davidson BL, Stein CS, Heth JA, et al. Recombinant adeno-associated virus type 2 4, and 5 vectors: transduction of variant cell types and regions in the mammalian central nervous system. Proc Natl Acad Sci U.S.A. 2000; 97:3428–3432.
84. Naldini L, Blomer U, Gage FH, Trono D, Verma IM. Efficient transfer, integration, and sustained long-term expression of the transgene in adult rat brains injected with a lentiviral vector. Proc Natl Acad Sci U.S.A. 1996; 93:11382–11388.
85. Peltekian E, Parrish E, Bouchard C, Peschanski M, Lisovoski F. Adenovirus-mediated gene transfer to the brain: methodological assessment. J Neurosci Methods 1997; 71:77–84.
86. Sanai N, Tramontin AD, Quinones-Hinojosa A, et al. Manuel-Garcia Verdugo, J. Unique astrocyte ribbon in adult human brain contains neural stem cells but lacks chain migration. Nature 2004; 427:740–744.
87. Galbreath E, Kim SJ, Park K, Brenner M, Messing A. Overexpression of TGF-beta 1 in the central nervous system of transgenic mice results in hydrocephalus. J Neuropathol Exp Neurol 1995; 54:339–349.
88. Wyss-Coray T, Feng L, Masliah E, et al. Increased central nervous system production of extracellular matrix components and development of hydrocephalus in transgenic mice overexpressing transforming growth factor-beta 1. Am J Pathol 1995; 147:53–67.
89. Chiang CS, Powell HC, Gold LH, Samimi A, Campbell IL. Macrophage/microglial-mediated primary demyelination and motor disease induced by the central nervous system production of interleukin-3 in transgenic mice. J Clin Invest 1996; 97:1512–1524.
90. Toggas SM, Masliah E, Rockenstein EM, Rall GF, Abraham CR, Mucke L. Central nervous system damage produced by expression of the HIV-1 coat protein gp120 in transgenic mice. Nature 1994; 367:188–193.
91. Kim BO, Liu Y, Ruan Y, Xu ZC, Schantz L, He JJ. Neuropathologies in transgenic mice expressing human immunodeficiency virus type 1 Tat protein under the regulation of the astrocyte-specific glial fibrillary acidic protein promoter and doxycycline. Am J Pathol 2003; 162:1693–1707.
92. Kamitani W, Ono E, Yoshino S, et al. Glial expression of Borna disease virus phosphoprotein induces behavioral and neurological abnormalities in transgenic mice. Proc Natl Acad Sci U.S.A. 2003; 100:8969–8974.
93. Jeffrey M, Goodsir CM, Race RE, Chesebro B. Scrapie-specific neuronal lesions are independent of neuronal PrP expression. Ann Neurol 2004; 55:781–792.
94. Sun Y, Wu S, Bu G, et al. Glial fibrillary acidic protein-apolipoprotein E (apoE) transgenic mice: astrocyte-specific expression and differing biological effects of astrocyte-secreted apoE3 and apoE4 lipoproteins. J Neurosci 1998; 18:3261–3272.
95. Gong YH, Parsadanian AS, Andreeva A, Snider WD, Elliott JL. Restricted expression of G86R Cu/Zn superoxide dismutase in astrocytes results in astrocytosis but does not cause motoneuron degeneration. J Neurosci 2000; 20:660–665.
96. Malatesta P, Hack MA, Hartfuss E, et al. Neuronal or glial progeny: regional differences in radial glia fate. Neuron 2003; 37:751–764.

8

Non-viral Mediated Gene Delivery for Therapeutic Applications

Lali K. Medina-Kauwe
The Gene Therapeutics Research Institute, Cedars-Sinai Medical Center, Los Angeles, California, U.S.A.

INTRODUCTION

Non-viral vector development has expanded into a broad area of research incorporating diverse fields and technologies to essentially mimic what the virus does well: deliver nucleic acids into cells. Viruses have evolved into highly efficient gene transfer agents that exploit the cellular machinery to deliver the viral genome to the nucleus and ensure viral propagation. As such, they have become useful recombinant agents for delivery of therapeutic genes. One might wonder, then, why it is desirable to attempt an alternative non-viral approach to gene delivery given the evolutionary advantage of the virus. One major reason is simply that non-viral vectors are not viruses: they are not pathogenic agents prone to mutation or recombination that could potentially produce emergent species. Additionally, non-viral vectors are often less cytotoxic and immunogenic than viruses. Moreover, for practical reasons, it is more facile to produce and test non-viral vectors in pharmacologic amounts than attempt to manipulate the viral genome without disrupting the ability to propagate the virus. A major drawback to non-viral vectors in vivo, however, is the typically low yield of gene transfer compared to viruses. In some cases, the stability of non-viral vectors in vivo is also questionable. Thus, to appreciate the exploration of non-viral delivery to such specialized tissue as neuronal cells, it is worthwhile examining the molecular and cellular requirements that one must consider for non-viral vector development.

In this chapter, we will review the concepts and advancements in non-viral vector design, with an emphasis on the requirements for optimized non-viral gene transfer. Importantly, we will highlight the elements that have been cleverly borrowed from naturally evolved systems, such as viruses and other pathogens, to effect non-viral vector delivery. Among the considerations for gene delivery that will be discussed here are physico-chemical requirements, such as vector size, charge, and stability; and vector-cell interactions, such as cell binding, entry, intracellular trafficking, and nuclear delivery. We will then present the therapeutic applications of non-viral gene transfer vectors, highlighting studies performed in neurological tissues.

A Brief History of Non-viral Vector Development

Initial chemical methods of in vitro DNA transfer began in the 1950s and 1960s, and included the use of basic proteins (1), DEAE dextran (2), and calcium phosphate precipitation (3) for the delivery of infectious viral nucleic acid into cells (Fig. 1). The first report of the cloning of a human gene (encoding β-globin) in 1976 (4) advanced the concept of "gene therapy" toward an actual possibility, and fueled the accelerating development of both viral and non-viral vectors for the delivery of recombinant genes. The first liposome-mediated transfection, reported in 1980 (5), followed by the development of cationic lipid formulations (6), opened up possibilities in the production of synthetic gene delivery systems. While these methods had proven efficient for gene transfer in many cell types in vitro, a therapeutic potential in vivo required additional features of improved delivery. Foremost, even if the plasmid contained cell-specific gene promoters, the non-specificity of vector uptake by these methods would dilute out the chances of sufficient amounts of vector reaching the target tissue, thus requiring high, and potentially toxic, doses of vector (7). Physical targeting of non-viral (and viral) vectors could potentially alleviate this problem by allowing lower, thus safer, doses of vector to circulate systemically and hone in on its target tissue. In the first demonstrations of receptor targeting, polylysine-condensed DNA plasmids were directed to asialoglycoprotein and transferrin (Tf) receptors, respectively, by specific ligands (8,9). It became clear, however, that while receptor-targeting proved effective for cell binding and internalization, once inside the cell, transport to the degradative lysosomal compartment prevented high levels of nuclear delivery and gene expression. Knowing that certain viruses could prevent this fate by penetrating the endosomal vesicle after receptor-mediated endocytosis, Curiel et al. (1991) demonstrated that whole adenovirus (Ad) could enhance Tf-targeted non-viral gene transfer (10). In follow-up studies using transcriptionally-inactive Ad, it was confirmed that the adenovirus capsid shell actually possessed the capacity for endosomal penetration (11), and underscored the importance of an endosomal-escape (or "endosomolysis") mechanism as part of non-viral vector design. It also became clear, however, that

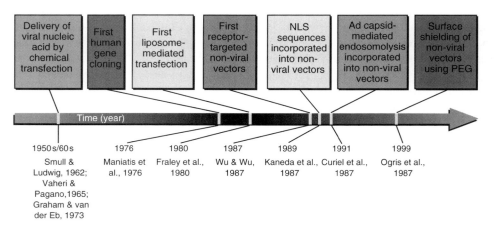

Figure 1 A brief history of non-viral vector development. Arrow indicates the chronology of vector development, with important milestones highlighted above (*boxes*). The year or years of each milestone is/are indicated below the arrow, corresponding to each box, and references for these milestones are indicated.

penetration into the cytosol was not enough, and that the DNA had to be directed to the nucleus for efficient gene expression. The incorporation of proteins containing nuclear localization signal (NLS) sequences to enhance nuclear delivery was demonstrated by Kaneda et al. (1989) (12), and since then, numerous proteins and peptides have been tested for nuclear targeting of non-viral vectors after cell entry (13–15). In the 1990s, more sophisticated advances in the design of synthetic systems, such as polyethylenimine (16) and dendrimers (17), as well as recombinant multicomponent systems containing DNA transport, receptor binding, and endosomolytic activities in a single molecule (18), produced a wide variety of vectors utilizing diverse strategies for gene transfer. Subsequent studies on vector-host interactions have more recently aided the development of surface shielding using polyethylene glycol (PEG) to reduce interactions with serum components (19), thus further advancing non-viral gene delivery as a realistic option for in vivo gene therapy.

Types of Non-viral Vectors

While the repertoire of non-viral vectors has grown in diversity, they share the property of binding plasmid DNA for transport into cells. The term "molecular conjugate" has become a catch-all definition for a wide variety of non-viral vectors that combine a cell entry agent with DNA. These vectors may incorporate recombinant proteins, peptides, or synthetic polymers attached in a variety of ways, either covalently or non-covalently, to DNA. Importantly, many such conjugates incorporate cell targeting ligands, such as transferrin, to mediate cell binding and cell entry of DNA. In many of the examples provided here, the payload of choice is plasmid DNA, though it is altogether possible for many of the vectors in this discussion to combine with oligonucleotides or linear DNA as well. Alternative to protein-based conjugates are liposomal formulations that can form DNA/liposome complexes called "lipoplexes" (Fig. 2) (20). A mixture of a polymer, such as polylysine, with DNA has been called a "polyplex" (21,22). The combination of liposomes with polymers and DNA has been given the term "lipopolyplex" (23,24).

Overview of Vector Hurdles

Non-viral gene transfer systems face common hurdles (Fig. 3). Such systems require DNA condensation to evade serum and cytosolic degradation, thus requiring the incorporation

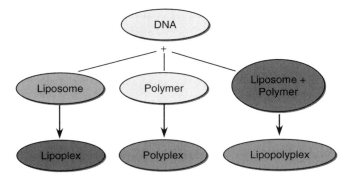

Figure 2 Types of synthetic non-viral vectors.

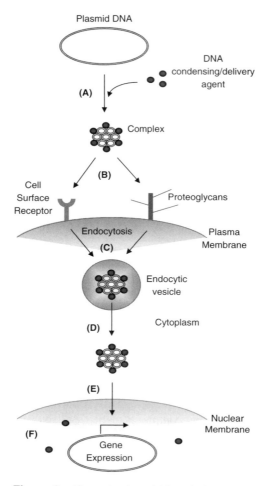

Figure 3   (*See color insert*) Non-viral gene transfer vector hurdles. Each sequential step of gene transfer is indicated by a letter. (**A**) Assembly of DNA with delivery agents to form non-viral complex. (**B**) Binding of complex to cell surface molecules or receptors. (**C**) Cell entry via endocytosis. (**D**) Endosomal escape. (**E**) Nuclear targeting. (**F**) Gene expression.

of reagents into the vector complex that bind, condense, and protect the DNA from extracellular and intracellular hazards. These vectors must bind to cells either through charge interaction with anionic cell surface molecules, such as proteoglycans, or through the incorporation of receptor-specific ligands. After cell binding, it is well accepted that cell entry occurs via endocytosis, resulting in entrapment of the vector in endocytic vesicles. To escape from these vesicles, agents must be incorporated into the vector to induce endosomolysis and enable penetration into the cytosol. Once in the cytosol, the vector must traffic to the nucleus either as a condensed or uncondensed particle. If the vector enters the nucleus as a condensed particle, it must undergo decondensation to release the DNA molecule and enable gene expression. Thus, for effective gene transfer, DNA must successfully proceed through six steps: (1) Assembly (with delivery agents); (2) Cell binding; (3) Cell entry; (4) Cytosolic entry; (5) Nuclear delivery; and (6) DNA decondensation for gene expression.

PHYSICO-CHEMICAL PARAMETERS: PACKAGING THE PAYLOAD

Important to the efficiency of viral infection is the capacity of the virus capsid to package the viral genome into a discrete particle that can navigate through, and remain stable in, the circulatory system. To achieve this end by non-viral means, factors taken into consideration are: vector size, charge, and stability.

Size

One of the many features of viruses that promote efficient delivery is size. Viruses range in size from 300 Å to 200 nm in diameter (25), which is key to enabling passage through capillaries, fenetrations, into tissues, and between cells. Yet, the sizes of some viral genomes are as large as 100–200 kb. Efficient compaction of the genome requires the neutralization of the negatively charged DNA phosphate backbone to counteract charge repellance both from within the DNA itself (26,27), and from the cell surface (28). Thus, appropriate condensation by charge neutralization can collapse the DNA into a particle that promotes cell entry. A variety of methods employing electrostatic interaction with DNA phosphates have been used to achieve this end in non-viral vectors (Fig. 4). Polyplexes incorporate hydrophilic polymers that are either linear, such as polylysine or spermine, or branched, such as polyethyleneimine (PEI) (16). The cationic liposomes incorporated into lipoplexes bind DNA by the same principle of electrostatic interaction and also have the benefit of hydrophobic moieties that can interact with the plasma membrane and enable cell entry. Still other approaches take advantage of naturally occurring basic proteins, such as protamine (29) and histones (30), which tightly compact DNA and may enable nuclear delivery by virtue of their endogenous NLSs (31).

While the concept of mixing polycations with DNA is straightforward enough for producing DNA complexes, in practice, particle size during formation is greatly affected by environmental factors such as salt concentration. The DNA binding and compaction efficiency of some polycations, such as protamine, is so great that it is difficult to control the reaction in order to produce small particles of homogeneous size or solubility (32). For some types of polylysine/DNA conjugates, low (below physiological) or no salt concentration promotes the formation of aggregates whereas raising the salt concentration

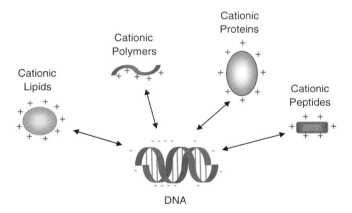

Figure 4 Complex assembly showing the types of cationic molecules that can be added non-covalently to DNA for phosphate backbone neutralization and condensation.

(at or above physiological levels) prevents the formation of aggregates in favor of homogeneous particles (8,33). Likewise, dilute concentrations of DNA (i.e., ≥ 50 µg/ml) favor the formation of kinetically controlled complexes of uniform size (34). These conditions have been tested with specific types of vectors, and the rules do not always hold true across the board. For example, transferrin-PEI conjugates form large aggregates of several hundred nanometers at physiological salt concentration whereas small particles of 40 nm are formed in water (33).

Charge

In the formation of non-viral complexes, the ratio of positive to negative charges, known as the charge ratio, is taken into consideration. This ratio reflects the number of cations to the number of DNA phosphates. A polycation to DNA ratio resulting in a net positive charge of the overall complex can promote cell binding by counteracting the net negative charge of the cell surface. While this may enhance gene transfer, it also promotes non-specific uptake of the vector by endocytic engulfment, which may not be the best in vivo approach to target specific tissues. Strategies to avoid non-specific uptake include forming complexes with a neutral or slightly negative charge in addition to adding a cell targeting ligand. An advantage to forming complexes with a net positive charge, however, is that it enables the incorporation of additional molecules, such as cell entry peptides, by electrostatic binding. In complexes receiving an excess of polylysine, for example, the net positive charge enabled further binding of a negatively charged endosomolytic peptide, to enhance gene transfer (35). Of course, the addition of negatively charged peptides helps to further neutralize the excess cations on such complexes. In a similar approach, anionic liposomes could be added to polylysine/DNA complexes containing a net positive charge (36). These additional negatively charged liposomes reduced non-specific cell binding and entry. The conjugation of receptor-specific ligands further honed these vectors toward cell-targeted delivery.

Stability

It has been shown that naked DNA can activate complement (37) as well as become degraded by serum nucleases if not sufficiently protected or condensed (38). On the other hand, while a net positive charge may enhance cell binding, in vivo, this may also encourage interaction with certain blood components (39), induce complement (40), and destabilize or aggregate the vector. Certain lipopolyplexes can induce cytokines, such as TNFα and IFNγ, regardless of transgene expression (41), and form aggregates with mouse serum proteins, which has correlated with poor gene transfer in vivo (42). It has been shown that Tf-targeted lipoplexes are bound by plasma proteins, such as IgM, fibrinogen, fibronectin, and complement, in vivo (19). The opsonization of vectors by serum proteins induces rapid clearance from the circulation by the reticuloendothelial system (43). An approach to prevent this has been to coat non-viral vectors with PEG (44,45). Not only does this strategy prolong circulation time in the blood (46), but it also has proven to reduce vector cytotoxicity and interaction with blood components (19).

Once inside the cytoplasm, the DNA faces further threats from cytoplasmic nucleases, as demonstrated by the degradation of naked plasmids microinjected into the cytoplasm of HeLa and COS cells (47). Thus, it may be important for the DNA condensing agent to remain bound to the plasmid en route to the nucleus, not just for nuclear delivery but also to protect against these nucleases. Finally, while efficient DNA condensation protects the plasmid from serum and cytosolic nucleases and promotes cell entry, it is possible that a condensing agent may be unable to release the DNA once it reaches the nucleus, thus reducing gene expression. This possibility was suggested when it was shown that, after microinjection into the nucleus, gene expression from liposome/DNA complexes was inhibited compared to DNA alone (48). It is unclear whether polycations release DNA in the cytoplasm or remain bound to the DNA during transit to the nucleus. In the case where complexes enter cells by endocytosis, it is thought that the anionic lipids found in endosomal vesicle membranes displace the DNA by electrostatic interaction with the polycations, thus enabling release into the cytoplasm (49). On the other hand, it has also been suggested that, if the complex reaches the nucleus intact, genomic DNA can displace the plasmid and interact with the polycations, thus enabling release in the nucleus (50) and gene expression.

VECTOR-CELL INTERACTIONS: THE PATHWAY TO GENE EXPRESSION

Among the most important advances in non-viral vector development is the incorporation of elements that enhance gene transfer *after* cell binding. Highly evolved mechanisms of avoiding cellular defenses such as cytosolic and lysosomal degradation can be found in the capsid and associated proteins of the virus, as well as in specialized proteins of pathogenic bacteria. These proteins can lend themselves toward overcoming the remaining hurdles for a non-viral vector after it has reached its target cell. These hurdles are: receptor binding, endocytosis, endosomolysis, and nuclear delivery.

Cell Binding

By incorporating a ligand to non-viral vectors, specific physical targeting of non-viral gene delivery to certain tissues could theoretically be obtained in vivo. Polycations have in some cases provided a necessary point of linkage to additional molecules, such as receptor ligands, for targeting gene transfer. Such linkages may occur covalently, utilizing sulfhydryl groups (8,9). In other cases, ligands have been linked directly to DNA (51). Alternatively, peptide nucleic acids have been designed to take advantage of the ability of short synthetic sequences to hybridize to a transcriptionally active plasmid, thus providing an additional possibility for attaching external molecules directly to DNA (52). Still other approaches have taken advantage of sequence-specific DNA binding domains, such as that of the GAL4 protein, to link fusion proteins to plasmids bearing the GAL4 binding site (18). The incorporation of exogenous moieties to non-viral vectors to facilitate receptor-targeted cell binding and enhanced cell entry has increasingly become an important area of non-viral vector development.

The earliest targeted vector incorporated asialoorosomucoid (ASOR) as a chemically coupled conjugate to polylysine, thus linking the targeting ligand to the plasmid DNA through the non-covalent interaction of the polycation with the plasmid (8,53). The proof-of-principle that the vector bound to asialoglycoprotein receptors specifically expressed on hepatocytes was demonstrated by the competitive inhibition of gene expression by free asialoglycoprotein. Similarly, it was shown that transferrin could be conjugated, through disulfide linkage, to polycations of varying length, as well as protamine (9). In each case, the vector facilitated DNA entry into the target cells by receptor-mediated endocytosis.

Other such ligands have since been tested for receptor-targeted delivery of genes. The choice of ligand has been largely dictated by whether or not the target receptor undergoes endocytosis, as not all cell surface proteins are triggered to internalize after ligand binding. Among the additional ligands that have been tested are TGFα (54), insulin (55,56), folate (36,57,58), basic FGF (59), integrin-binding motifs (60–62), and heregulin (63). Antibodies generated against certain cell-specific ligands also have been used to direct gene transfer. Among the targets against which antibody-directed molecular conjugates have been produced are: CD3 (64–67), CD5 (68), EGF-R (69,70), and ErbB2 (71). Key to the efficacy of an antibody-directed molecular conjugate, however, is the ability of the antibody to trigger or enable receptor internalization.

Alternative to receptor-ligand interaction is the electrophilic attraction between vector cations and highly anionic cell surface proteoglycans, which are among the most negatively charged components of the cell. Sulfated proteoglycans are composed of a core protein covalently linked to one or more sulfated glycosaminoglycans (72), and thus are likely targets of non-viral assemblies carrying a net positive charge. It has been shown that certain polyplexes and lipoplexes transfect cells through proteoglycan binding through the demonstration that: (1) proteoglycan inhibitors prevent gene transfer, and (2) proteoglycan-deficient cells could not be transfected (73,74).

Cell Entry

Receptor endocytosis into clathrin-coated vesicles enables the cell entry of many ligands, including viruses (75). However, non-clathrin-mediated pathways, such as endocytosis through caveolae or macropinosomes, can also facilitate vector uptake. More recently, it has been evident that non-viral vectors may enter cells through multiple, clathrin- and non-clathrin -mediated endocytic pathways (Fig. 5).

Clathrin-Mediated Endocytosis

Clathrin-mediated endocytosis facilitates the internalization of a majority of receptor-ligand complexes (75), and involves the localized accumulation of clathrin on the cytoplasmic surface of the plasma membrane at the sites of receptor binding (Fig. 5). By rendering clathrin unavailable for localized accumulation, through the use of hypertonic

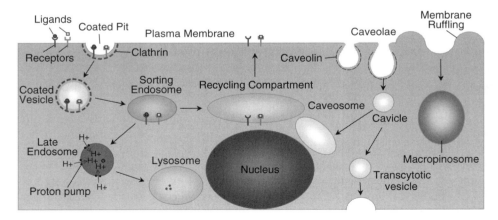

Figure 5 (*See color insert*) Endocytic pathways. Clathrin-mediated, caveolae-mediated, and macropinocytic pathways are shown. The clathrin-mediated pathway shows fates of receptor-ligand pairs as they transit through either a degradative pathway (leading to lysosomes) or recycling pathway (leading to the recycling compartment and back to the cell surface). Protons are indicated by H+.

medium (76), it was shown that certain targeted lipopolyplexes transfected cells via clathrin-dependent endocytosis (77).

As these localized sites begin to invaginate, forming clathrin-coated pits, the GTPase, dynamin (78,79) pinches off the pits into vesicles with the assistance of a number of different effector proteins (80). The internalization of certain lipoplexes and molecular conjugates through this pathway has been verified by showing that inhibitors of coated pit formation prevented gene transfer and expression (81,82).

These pinched-off vesicles then become uncoated by an enzymatic process (83), and the vesicle cargo is delivered to early (or sorting) endosomes that become acidified by ATP-dependent proton pumps (84). These endosomes then traffic to either recycling endosomes, where the cargo may recycle back to the cell surface, or to the lysosome, where the cargo gets degraded by lysosomal enzymes. Vectors internalizing through the latter pathway must avoid degradation by incorporating mechanisms of endosomal escape (85). To accomplish this, acid-triggered membrane penetration moieties have been incorporated into many types of non-viral vectors (86). Alternative internalization pathways, however, can also avoid delivery to the lysosome. Such pathways include non-clathrin-mediated endocytosis through caveolae and macropinosomes.

Caveolae-Mediated Endocytosis

Caveolae, which are flask-shaped invaginations in the plasma membrane marked by the integral membrane protein, caveolin, internalize large molecular complexes, toxins, bacteria, and some viruses (Fig. 5) (87). Mundy et al. (2002) showed that caveolae can be retained on the cell surface by cortical actin filaments (88), whose disruption facilitated the pinching off and internalization of caveolar vesicles, or "cavicles." These cavicles apparently require intact microtubules to migrate to pericentrisomal caveosomes (89), which cluster near the microtubule organizing center (MTOC), in close proximity to recycling endosomes. Studies on the caveolar-mediated uptake of Simian Virus 40 (SV40) suggest that this virus transits through caveosomes to arrive at the endoplasmic reticulum (ER) (89), from which viral DNA and associated viral proteins somehow escape into the cytoplasm to gain nuclear access. It is worthwhile investigating whether such a pathway could greatly benefit non-viral vector transfection, as little work has been done thus far on this area of research, though some studies have shown that inhibitors of caveolae formation, such as nystatin (90,91), could prevent transfection by polyplexes (92) and molecular conjugates (93).

The caveolar-endocytic pathway may not only provide an alternative means of vector uptake, but may also potentially enable delivery through the endothelium to tissues in vivo. A monoclonal antibody specific for lung caveolae could target lung endothelium in vivo after pulmonary artery perfusion (94), and mediate the delivery of a conjugated drug into lung tissue by transendothelial trafficking. As the endothelium presents a major barrier to systemically targeted in vivo gene transfer, the transcytosis ability of this antibody suggests that targeting the caveolar pathway may enhance vector delivery to desired tissue (95,96).

Macropinocytosis

Relatively large macromolecules may enter cells through macropinosomes, which are formed by actin-driven ruffling of the plasma membrane, followed by folding and pinching off of irregularly sized vesicles (Fig. 5) (97). Membrane ruffling is non-clathrin-mediated and inhibited by cytochalasin D, which disrupts actin filaments, or amiloride, which blocks the Na^+/H^+ exchanger (98,99). While macropinosomes can acidify, they do not intersect with lysosomes (100), thus presenting a possible alternative cell entry route for non-viral vectors. It has been shown that histidinylated polyplexes avoided late endosomes and lysosomes after cell entry, which could be substantially inhibited by amiloride (101), thus supporting a macropinocytic internalization pathway.

The protein transduction domain, or PTD, peptides may also enter cells through macropinocytosis. These peptides, which contain highly charged basic domains, were once thought to possess the capacity to translocate across cell membranes (102), but more recently, it has been shown that the actual mode of cell entry is endocytic (103). Transcriptional activators, such as the human immunodeficiency virus (HIV) transactivator of transcription (TAT) and antennapedia (Antp), are among the proteins from which these PTD peptides have been derived. A study on the trafficking of a TAT fusion protein demonstrated that cell entry was prevented by amiloride and cytochalasin D (104). Internalization was mediated by heparan sulfate proteoglycans endocytosis, as reported by others (105,106). Similarly, other studies have also shown that Antp and polyarginine peptides bind proteoglycans to gain cell entry (107,108). Taken together with studies showing that certain viral proteins undergo heparin-sensitive cell binding and actin-dependent cell entry into large vesicles (109), it is likely that proteoglycans mediate the majority of macropinocytic internalization events.

Endosomolysis

A major barrier to efficient gene transfer is the cellular endosome. For non-viral vectors internalizing through clathrin-mediated endocytosis, the inability to escape the endosome results in transport to the lysosome and proteolytic degradation. In the early stages of development, vectors targeted by asialoglycoprotein and Tf suffered this fate. However, the co-administration of Ad, even when transcriptionally inactive, enhanced Tf-targeted gene transfer and expression (10,11,110–112). Subsequent studies showing that the Ad capsid facilitated endosome escape highlighted the need for endosomolytic agents to enhance non-viral gene transfer.

It is now understood that a vesicle escape function is largely a necessary aspect of non-viral vector design. Several different mechanisms of vesicle escape have been developed and characterized.

Pore Formation

The human rhinovirus serotype 2 (HRV2) VP1 capsid protein contains an amino (N)-terminal segment that apparently forms pores within the endosomal membrane at low pH (i.e., pH 5.5), thus enabling the release of the RNA genome into the cytosol (113). A peptide derived from this N-terminal segment and incorporated into transferrin-targeted conjugates enhanced gene transfer (114). The hemagglutinin (HA) protein of influenza virus (INF) similarly mediates fusion with the endosomal membrane through its N-terminal portion, which also forms fusion pores in response to an acid environment (115,116). Likewise, peptides derived from this segment of HA have been used to enhance transferrin-targeted gene transfer (117).

The toxic domains of bacterial proteins represent a similar but alternative strategy of inducing endosomal membrane lysis for cytosolic entry of non-viral vectors. The toxic domain of diphtheria toxin (DT) has been produced as a recombinant protein coupled to polylysine and tested for gene transfer (118). Full-length DT contains an N-terminal toxic domain followed by an α-helical region and a carboxy (C) -terminal receptor binding domain (119,120). After receptor-mediated endocytosis, the DT toxic domain undergoes a conformational change in response to endosome acidification (121), forming channels in the endosomal membrane that allow the escape of entrapped contents (122,123). Gene transfer by an ASOR-targeted polylysine conjugate could be enhanced when incorporated with a diptheria toxin (DT) translocation domain (118). The DT toxic domain has also been produced as a targeted modular fusion protein containing a Gal4 DNA binding domain and a single-chain antibody targeted to the ErbB2 receptor (124). Gene transfer by this fusion protein was substantially reduced by inhibitors of vesicular proton import, indicating that endosome acidification was required for efficient transfection.

In similar fashion, the translocation domain of *Pseudomonas* exotoxin A (ETA) was produced as a fusion protein flanked by DNA binding and receptor targeting domains (18,54). The ETA translocation domain enables endosomal escape to the cytosol via pore formation (125). Importantly, the removal of the translocation domain significantly reduced gene transfer, thus emphasizing the requirement for endosome disruption during gene delivery (54).

Another pore forming peptide, melittin, which is a major component of bee venom, could enhance PEI-mediated gene transfer, up to 700-fold, over PEI alone (126). The toroidal pores thought to be induced by melittin (127,128) produce perturbations in the membrane that bend it so that the top and bottom layers of the bilayer join contiguously at the pore wall (Fig. 6). The pore-forming GALA peptide, which is comprised of a Glu-Ala-Leu-Ala repeat (129), also undergoes a conformational change from a random coil at neutral pH to an amphipathic alpha helix at acidic pH (130), promoting high membrane binding. At a certain threshold of membrane accumulation, GALA peptides aggregate and form pores (131), and can release a fluid phase marker co-internalized with Tf-targeted liposomes (132). The incorporation of this peptide into a polycation-condensed plasmid has enhanced gene transfer (35). Pore formation by both GALA and melittin peptides can accelerate an additional mechanism of membrane penetration by phospholipid "flip-flop," as described next (133).

Flip-Flop

Normally, anionic lipids are maintained on the cytoplasmic face of the membrane by cellular flippase enzymes (134), whereas channel forming antibiotics, such as amphotericin B (135) can induce the flipping of phospholipids to the apposing leaflet of the membrane

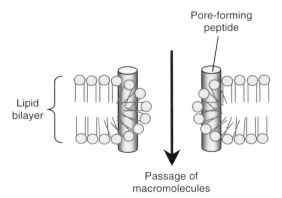

Figure 6 (*See color insert*) Endosomal escape via pore formation. Pore forming peptides induce the membrane to bend, causing the bilayer leaflets to become contiguous, and forming an opening in the endosomal membrane through which vesicular contents can escape into the cytosol.

bilayer. Pore-forming peptides, such as GALA and melittin, may stimulate flip-flop of phospholipids within the vicinity of the pore (133). Cationic lipoplexes may also induce phospholipid flipping to facilitate cytosolic release of the DNA (49). In the proposed mechanism for this reaction, the endosomal membrane encompassing a cationic lipoplex becomes destabilized by the complex, allowing anionic lipids facing the cytoplasmic side of the membrane (136) to flip and face the endosomal lumen (Fig. 7). As these anionic lipids diffuse into the complex, they form charge neutral ion pairs with the complex lipids, thus displacing the DNA from the complex, and releasing it into the cytoplasm.

Proton Sponge

An effect known as the "proton-sponge" is thought to enable endosomal disruption by polyplexes formed using the branched polymers, polyamidoamine (PAM) (137), or PEI (Fig. 8) (16). Every third atom of PEI, for example, is an amino nitrogen that can become protonated thus imparting a high buffering capacity over nearly the entire pH range. After endocytosis, PEI induces massive proton accumulation in the acidifying endosome. This in turn invokes a high influx of chloride ions into the endosome, causing osmotic swelling and eventual bursting of the endosomal vesicle. Inhibitors such as bafilomycin A_1, that block vacuolar proton pumps, can prevent PEI transfection in a cell type-specific manner (138). Proof of this endosomolytic mechanism was demonstrated in CHO-K1 cells, in which Cl^- and pH indicators were used to detect Cl^- accumulation and pH decrease during PEI or PAM uptake (139). An increase in size of polyplex-containing vesicles followed by dissipation of fluorescently-tagged polyplexes strongly suggested that the internalized polyplexes induced vesicle swelling and disruption.

Histidinylated polymers, such as polylysine partially substituted with histidyl residues, are thought to escape endosomes through a combination of membrane disruption and proton-sponge effects (140,141). Bafilomycin A_1 dramatically inhibited transfection by histidinylated polylysine, suggesting that these polymers may undergo imidazole protonation in endosomes (142). However, structural investigations indicated that these peptides undergo α-helical conformations and membrane insertion (143,144). It has also been shown that histidinylated peptides enable the transfer of fluorophores between liposomes (145).

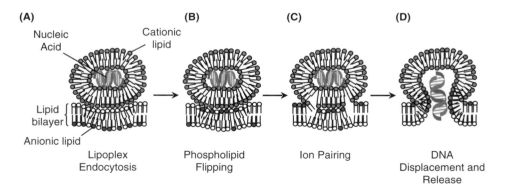

Figure 7 (*See color insert*) Endosomolysis via flip-flop. After lipoplex endocytosis (**A**) the endosomal membrane becomes destabilized, enabling anionic lipids facing the cytoplasm to flip and face the endosomal lumen. (**B**) The cationic lipids of the complex form charge neutral ion pairs with these anionic lipids (**C**) resulting in DNA displacement and (**D**) release into the cytoplasm.

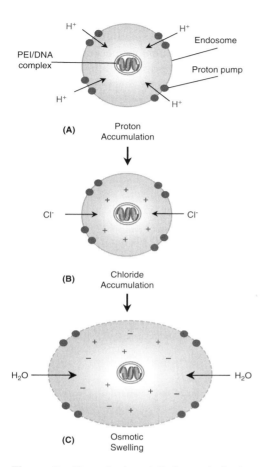

Figure 8 (*See color insert*) Endosomolysis via proton sponge. (**A**) Protons accumulate massively into the endosome due to the high buffering capacity of the polyplex (**B**) inducing passive influx of chloride ions (**C**) that cause osmotic swelling and vesicle rupture.

Membrane Fusion and General Disruption

The HA2 fusogenic protein of influenza virus has been incorporated into molecular conjugates, such as ASOR-targeted complexes, to enhance endosome escape and gene transfer (86,146). The HA2 protein contains an amino-terminal fusion peptide that is normally buried within the HA trimer on the virus coat (147). Endosome acidification provokes conformational rearrangements that expose the fusion peptide (115) and enable it to interact with the target membrane to induce fusion with the virus membrane. Fusion activity can be measured by lysis of erythrocyte membranes or by the production of heterokaryons in HA2-expressing cells. These assays have been used to test membrane fusion by mutant HA2 peptides and synthetic analogs (148).

Other types of viral coat proteins may enable endosome penetration through different mechanisms. The Ad penton base capsid protein is thought to be responsible for the endosomal penetration by the virus, thus, based on this designation, non-viral vectors have been developed from the penton base proteins of Ad3 (149), Ad5 (63,150), and Ad7 (151) capsids. A function in membrane disruption is supported by the observed conformational change of the penton base at low pH, exposing hydrophobic regions that bind non-ionic detergents (152). The penton base binds selectively to $\alpha_v\beta_5$ integrins under acidic conditions (153,154), and membrane penetration apparently requires a TVD motif in the cytoplasmic domain of the β_5 subunit (153). The exact mechanism of membrane penetration remains unclear. A comparison of rhinovirus (HRV2) and adenovirus membrane penetration suggested that the penton base may induce broad disruption of the membrane whereas the HRV2 VP1 protein induces pores of a distinct size (113). In both cases, however, endosome disruption was dependent on vesicle acidification.

Nuclear Targeting

Whereas small fragments of DNA ($<$250 base pairs, or bp) readily diffuse through the cytosol, naked plasmid DNA or DNA fragments $>$250 bp are immobile in the cytoplasm, likely due to molecular crowding (Fig. 9) (155). Thus, transit to the nucleus often requires an active transport mechanism. Naked plasmids incorporating the Simian Virus 40 (SV40) promoter and origin of replication (OriP) are reported to be transported to the nucleus, presumably by NLS-containing proteins that bind to these cis-acting sequences (156). This approach has been tested using plasmids that harbor an Epstein–Barr Virus (EBV) OriP binding site as well (157). Whereas some studies report nuclear uptake and expression of SV40 ori-containing plasmids in cells lacking SV40 T antigen (158), the expression of EBV nuclear antigen 1 (EBNA-1) was required for transgene expression from EBV

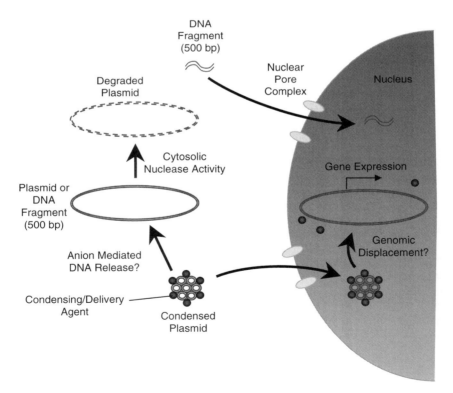

Figure 9   (*See color insert*) Intracellular fates of DNA after endosome escape. Pathways leading to DNA release in the cytoplasm or nucleus are shown.

ori-containing plasmids. In either case, the presence of cytosolic nucleases (47), makes the approach of using naked DNA impractical, and underscores the need to protect the DNA by condensing agents during cytosolic transport (Fig. 9).

Many types of DNA condensing proteins have the benefit of not only reducing the size of the non-viral particle, which likely enhances cytosolic motility, but also containing a NLS sequence to enable nuclear targeting (14). Such proteins are either naturally occurring nuclear proteins, such as histones (159), high mobility group (HMG) -1 proteins (160), or protamine; or derived from viruses, such as SV40 large T antigen (161), or Ad core proteins (162). In the case of using virally derived proteins, peptides containing the relevant protein segments for binding DNA and nuclear targeting were synthesized and harbor an NLS. A commonly used NLS is derived from the SV40 large T antigen and contains the sequence PKKKRKV (163).

Several soluble cytoplasmic proteins, known as karyopherins or importins, have been identified that contribute to nuclear import by binding to the NLS and docking to the nuclear pore complex (NPC) (164–166). The NPC is ~ 55 Å, or 25–30 nm (167), in diameter and permits the passage of molecules with a molecular weight (mw) of ≤ 40 kDa (168). Studies on the nuclear entry of Ad showed that the partially uncoated viral capsid interacts with fibrils extending from the cytoplasmic face of the NPC (169), where the capsid docks before extruding the viral DNA through the pore into the nucleus. It is thought that the NPC may undergo conformational changes in response to calcium levels that would enable passage through the pore (170). The lectin, wheat germ agglutinin (WGA), which binds to N-acetylglucosamine residues on NPC proteins, or antibodies that block the NPC, inhibit nuclear import of Ad DNA and karyophilic proteins (171–174).

A major paradox of non-viral vector development is designing a mechanism of plasmid decondensation that enables DNA release at an effective time point after cell entry. DNA release in the cytosol is likely to occur from lipoplexes if endosomal or cytosolic anions displace the DNA from the lipid (Fig. 9) (49). However, naked plasmid DNA is nearly immobile in the cytoplasm compared to small (≤ 500 bp) double-stranded fragments, likely due to cytosolic macromolecular crowding (155). Moreover, release in the cytoplasm can have a detrimental effect on gene transfer, as Ca^{2+}-dependent nucleases present in the cytoplasm, but not the nucleus, can degrade cytoplasmic DNA (Fig. 9) (47). On the other hand, condensing agents that would protect the DNA from cytosolic nucleases and enable transit to the nucleus may actually impede gene expression, as demonstrated when lipoplexes directly microinjected into nuclei displayed impaired gene expression compared to naked DNA (48). Studies showing that PEI promoted nuclear delivery and DNA release in the nucleus, whereas cationic lipids did not suggest that vector type may actually dictate whether DNA is released in the cytoplasm or nucleus (175).

NEURONAL APPLICATIONS

Cationic liposomes have been used to introduce genes into neuroblastoma and primary neuronal cells in vitro, resulting in a higher transfection efficiency in the former compared to the latter (176), likely due to the differing mitotic rates of these cell types. While methodologies to improve lipoplex-mediated gene expression within these cells have been explored, which include chemical modifications to enhance DNA release from the liposomes (177), targeting neuronal cells has been a major focus to address feasibility in vivo. In addition to concentrating the vector to the tissue site of interest, physical targeting may reduce the complications associated with exposing lipoplexes to serum, which include aggregation by serum components and selective expression in the lung (178–180).

To target lipoplexes to neuronal cells, Zhang et al. (2003) attached receptor-specific monoclonal antibodies recognizing specific cell surface proteins. These targeted immunoliposomes were formed by first coating lipoplexes with PEG, thus providing a point of linkage for chemical attachment of the antibodies. The PEG serves an additional purpose of protecting the lipoplexes in vivo from opsonization by serum proteins. Antibodies generated separately against the human insulin receptor (HIR) and TfR were tested with these complexes. Both of these receptor targets were desirable due to their apparent capacity to transcytose across the endothelium. As each neuron is fed by its own blood vessel, transport across the endothelium could potentially deliver vectors to every neuron, thus enabling systemic delivery to the brain. Additionally, these receptors are expressed on the cell surface of certain neuronal cells, thus antibody-directed targeting could enable the complex to penetrate both the blood vessel wall and plasma membrane of the target cell. The limited availability of antibodies across species prevented any comparisons between different targeted complexes. However, within the same species, certain patterns of tissue distribution were observed after intravenous delivery: HIR-targeted complexes preferentially transduced the liver and brain of the adult rhesus monkey, whereas TfR-targeted complexes preferentially transduced the liver, spleen, lung, and brain of the rat. A comparison to non-targeted complexes may have better distinguished whether the mechanism of delivery was through receptor targeting or whether the liposomes themselves substantially contributed to cell entry.

To assess the efficacy of immunoliposomes in disease models, Tf-targeted immunoliposomes delivering plasmids encoding tyrosine hydroxylase (TH) were intravenously injected into an experimental animal model of Parkinson's disease and produced enhanced levels of striatal TH activity compared to saline injected animals (181,182). Importantly in these studies, TH expression driven by the SV40 promoter, which produces ubiquitous gene expression, was detected in both brain and peripheral tissues, whereas the brain-specific glial fibrillary acidic protein (GFAP) promoter produced brain-preferential expression levels of TH. In other studies, the noncovalent assembly of Tf to lipoplexes apparently was sufficient to enhance delivery in vivo and has been applied in a brain injury model in which the complexes were stereotactically injected into the brain (183). Expression of nerve growth factor (NGF) from these vectors attenuated kainic acid-induced damage. While a benefit to noncovalent assembly of the targeting ligand with the lipoplex is the avoidance of chemical modifications that can impair activity, it was unclear from these studies whether these assemblies were highly stable in vivo.

Ligands that preferentially target the nervous system have been considered for directing non-viral gene transfer complexes to neuronal cells. Tetanus toxin (TeNT), for example, has a high specificity for neuronal tissue, and functions by binding cell surface gangliosides on presynaptic motor neuron terminals, followed by endocytic internalization, and trafficking to the cell body by axonal retrograde transport (184). As the non-toxic H_C fragment of the TeNT holotoxin is responsible for cell binding and internalization, this fragment has been used to target polylysine-complexed DNA to neuronal cell lines (185). While the H_C-targeted complexes exhibited preferential transfection of neuronal cell lines compared to non-neuronal cell lines, transfection efficiency could be enhanced by chloroquine, indicating that the complexes were largely trapped in endosomes after cell entry. The inclusion of the fusogenic H_N chain of the holotoxin, in hindsight, may have improved gene transfer by facilitating endosomal escape of the complexes.

In similar fashion, the cell entry domain of cholera toxin (CT) has been incorporated into polyplexes to target gene transfer to neuronal cells (186). Like many bacterial toxins, CT is composed of linked A and B subunits. While the A subunit imparts enzymatic (toxin) activity, the pentameric B subunit (or CTb) binds the ganglioside GM1 (187), inducing endocytic uptake and retrograde trafficking from sorting endosomes to the Golgi. This property has enabled the use of CTb as a neuronal tracer. Specific transfection of undifferentiated and NGF-differentiated PC12 cells was demonstrated by competitive inhibition by free CTb. In agreement with other studies, transfection of the undifferentiated cells was higher than of differentiated cells, likely because of differing mitotic states.

Whether receptor-targeted or not, an important consideration with any vector is whether the complex undergoes appropriate trafficking within the cell. To enhance nuclear delivery, basic peptides containing classical or putative NLS sequences have been incorporated into lipoplexes. Polylysine and protamine are among such peptides used in non-neuronal systems to enhance gene transfer. For testing in a neuronal system, Murray et al. (2001) (188) examined the utility of two viral proteins, the Ad Mu and polyoma virus VP1 proteins, for enhanced gene transfer, based on the rationale that these viral proteins assist viral infection by mediating the transit of the viral DNA to the nucleus. As with many multicomponent systems, testing titrated concentrations of the carrier molecules (i.e., mu or VP1, and liposome) against the DNA enabled the investigators to assess the ratios of DNA:protein:liposome required for optimal gene transfer. At the optimal ratios of complex components, mu increased lipoplex gene transfer and expression, whereas VP1 did not. In comparison to each identical complex in which mu was replaced with either protamine or polylysine, the level of gene transfer was similar between all three, and significantly enhanced over complexes lacking the proteins.

CONCLUSIONS AND FUTURE DIRECTIONS

It is clear that targeted non-viral gene transfer vectors must overcome a number of hurdles to produce a level of gene expression that approaches that of viruses, especially in neuronal cells. As our knowledge of viral cell entry mechanisms increases, it may increasingly become easier to apply key viral components to non-viral gene transfer to penetrate critical cellular barriers. Alternatively, the cell entry or intracellular translocation activities of certain viral proteins may lend themselves just as well to the targeted delivery of alternative therapeutics, in addition to genes, such as drugs, toxins, or small nucleic acids. Indeed, targeted toxins and "stealth liposomes" have already been explored and developed for in vivo delivery (189–191). While there are certainly fewer barriers to overcome in the delivery of such molecules, as many of these need only be delivered to the cytoplasm to be effective, the regulatory elements encoded in DNA add an additional layer of specificity, providing a fail-safe for gene expression in the target tissue. In light of recent gene therapy related adverse events, such measures to enhance the safety of gene delivery vectors is foremost in future developments.

ACKNOWLEDGMENTS

Support for this work has been provided by grants from the National Institutes of Health (CA102126), the Susan G. Komen Breast Cancer Foundation (BCTR02-1194), and the

Donna and Jesse Garber Award. I am grateful to Pedro Lowenstein and Maria Castro for their leadership, and to Dr. Shlomo Melmed, Mr. Richard Katzman, Dr. David Meyer, and the Cedars-Sinai Board of Governors for their support.

REFERENCES

1. Smull CE, Ludwig EH. Enhancement of the plaque-forming capacity of poliovirus ribonucleic acid with basic proteins. J Bacteriol 1962; 84:1035–1040.
2. Vaheri A, Pagano JS. Infectious poliovirus RNA: a sensitive method of assay. Virology 1965; 27:434–436.
3. Graham FL, van der Eb AJ. A new technique for the assay of infectivity of human adenovirus 5 DNA. Virology 1973; 52:456–467.
4. Maniatis T, Kee SG, Efstratiadis A, Kafatos FC. Amplification and characterization of a beta-globin gene synthesized in vitro. Cell 1976; 8:163–182.
5. Fraley R, Subramani S, Berg P, Papahadjopoulos D. Introduction of liposome-encapsulated SV40 DNA into cells. J Biol Chem 1980; 255:10431–10435.
6. Felgner PL, Gadek TR, Holm M, et al. Lipofection: a highly efficient, lipid-mediated DNA-transfection procedure. Proc Natl Acad Sci USA 1987; 84:7413–7417.
7. Felgner PL. Progress in Gene Delivery Research and Development. In: Huang L, Hung MC, Wagner E, eds. Nonviral Vectors for Gene Therapy. San Diego: Academic Press, 1999:25–38.
8. Wu GY, Wu CH. Receptor-mediated in vitro gene transformation by a soluble DNA carrier system. J Biol Chem 1987; 262:4429–4432 [erratum appears in J Biol Chem 1988 Jan 5; 263(1):588].
9. Wagner E, Zenke M, Cotten M, Beug H, Birnstiel ML. Transferrin-polycation conjugates as carriers for DNA uptake into cells. Proc Natl Acad Sci USA 1990; 87:3410–3414.
10. Curiel DT, Agarwal S, Wagner E, Cotten M. Adenovirus enhancement of transferring-polylysine-mediated gene delivery. Proc Natl Acad Sci USA 1991; 88:8850–8854.
11. Cotten M, Wagner E, Zatloukal K, Phillips S, Curiel DT, Birnstiel ML. High-efficiency receptor-mediated delivery of small and large (48 kilobase) gene constructs using the endosome-disruption activity of defective or chemically inactivated adenovirus particles. Proc Natl Acad Sci USA 1992; 89:6094–6098.
12. Kaneda Y, Iwai K, Uchida T. Increased expression of DNA cointroduced with nuclear protein in adult rat liver. Science 1989; 243:375–378.
13. Escriou V, Carriere M, Scherman D, et al. NLS bioconjugates for targeting therapeutic genes to the nucleus. Adv Drug Deliv Rev 2003; 55:295–306.
14. Chan CK, Jans DA. Using nuclear targeting signals to enhance non-viral gene transfer. Immunol Cell Biol 2002; 80:119–130.
15. Johnson-Saliba M, Jans DA. Gene therapy: optimising DNA delivery to the nucleus. Curr Drug Targets 2001; 2:371–399.
16. Boussif O, Lezoualc'h F, Zanta MA, et al. A versatile vector for gene and oligonucleotide transfer into cells in culture and in vivo: polyethylenimine. Proc Natl Acad Sci USA 1995; 92:7297–7301.
17. Tang MX, Redemann CT, Szoka FC, Jr. In vitro gene delivery by degraded polyamidoamine dendrimers. Bioconjug Chem 1996; 7:703–714.
18. Fominaya J, Wels W. Target cell-specific DNA transfer mediated by a chimeric multidomain protein. Novel non-viral gene delivery system. J Biol Chem 1996; 271:10560–10568.
19. Ogris M, Brunner S, Schuller S, Kircheis R, Wagner E. PEGylated DNA/transferrin-PEI complexes: reduced interaction with blood components, extended circulation in blood and potential for systemic gene delivery. Gene Ther 1999; 6:595–605.
20. Duzgunes N, De Ilarduya CT, Simoes S, Zhdanov RI, Konopka K, Pedroso de Lima MC. Cationic liposomes for gene delivery: novel cationic lipids and enhancement by proteins and peptides. Curr Med Chem 2003; 10:1213–1220.

21. Howard KA, Alpar HO. The development of polyplex-based DNA vaccines. J Drug Target 2002; 10:143–151.

22. Oupicky D, Ogris M, Seymour LW. Development of long-circulating polyelectrolyte complexes for systemic delivery of genes. J Drug Target 2002; 10:93–98.

23. Tsai JT, Furstoss KJ, Michnick T, Sloane DL, Paul RW. Quantitative physical characterization of lipid-polycation-DNA lipopolyplexes. Biotechnol Appl Biochem 2002; 36:13–20.

24. Yang J-P, Huang L. Novel Supramolecular Assemblies for Gene Delivery. In: Kabanov AV, Felgner PL, Seymour LW, eds. Self-Assembling Complexes for Gene Delivery. Chichester: John Wiley & Sons, 1998.

25. Flint SJ, Enquist LW, Krug RM, Racaniello VR, Skalka AM. In: Flint SJ, Enquist LW, Krug RM, Racaniello VR, Skalka AM, eds. Virus Structure. In: Principles of Virology. Washington, D.C.: ASM Press, 2000:59–98.

26. Manning GS. The molecular theory of polyelectrolyte solutions with applications to the electrostatic properties of polynucleotides. Q Rev Biophys 1978; 11:179–246.

27. Tang MX, Szoka FC, Jr. Characterization of Polycation Complexes with DNA. In: Kabanov AV, Felgner PL, Seymour LW, eds. Self-Assembling Complexes for Gene Delivery. Chichester: John Wiley & Sons, 1998.

28. Vigneron JP, Oudrhiri N, Fauquet M, et al. Guanidinium-cholesterol cationic lipids: efficient vectors for the transfection of eukaryotic cells. Proc Natl Acad Sci USA 1996; 93:9682–9686.

29. Warrant RW, Kim SH. alpha-Helix-double helix interaction shown in the structure of a protamine-transfer RNA complex and a nucleoprotamine model. Nature 1978; 271:130–135.

30. Stavridis JC, Psallidopoulos M. Use of transferrin as a gene-carrier to the erythroid cells of the marrow. Cell Mol Biol 1982; 28:15–18.

31. Thatcher DR, Haines A, Phillips R. Peptide-mediated gene delivery. In: Kabanov AV, Felgner PL, Seymour LW, eds. Self-Assemblying Complexes for Gene Delivery. Chichester: John Wiley & Sons, 1998:331–350.

32. Prieto MC, Maki AH, Balhorn R. Analysis of DNA-protamine interactions by optical detection of magnetic resonance. Biochemistry 1997; 36:11944–11951.

33. Ogris M, Steinlein P, Kursa M, Mechtler K, Kircheis R, Wagner E. The size of DNA/transferrin-PEI complexes is an important factor for gene expression in cultured cells. Gene Ther 1998; 5:1425–1433.

34. Wagner E, Cotten M, Foisner R, Birnstiel ML. Transferrin-polycation-DNA complexes: the effect of polycations on the structure of the complex and DNA delivery to cells. Proc Natl Acad Sci USA 1991; 88:4255–4259.

35. Gottschalk S, Sparrow JT, Hauer J, et al. A novel DNA-peptide complex for efficient gene transfer and expression in mammalian cells. Gene Ther 1996; 3:48–57.

36. Lee RJ, Huang L. Folate-targeted, anionic liposome-entrapped polylysine-condensed DNA for tumor cell-specific gene transfer. J Biol Chem 1996; 271:8481–8487.

37. Jiang H, Cooper B, Robey FA, Gewurz H. DNA binds and activates complement via residues 14–26 of the human C1q A chain. J Biol Chem 1992; 267:25597–25601.

38. Gao X, Huang L. Potentiation of cationic liposome-mediated gene delivery by polycations. Biochemistry 1996; 35:1027–1036.

39. Schwartz B, Benoist C, Abdallah B, Scherman D, Behr JP, Demeneix BA. Lipospermine-based gene transfer into the newborn mouse brain is optimized by a low lipospermine/DNA charge ratio. Hum Gene Ther 1995; 6:1515–1524.

40. Plank C, Mechtler K, Szoka FC, Jr., Wagner E. Activation of the complement system by synthetic DNA complexes: a potential barrier for intravenous gene delivery. Hum Gene Ther 1996; 7:1437–1446.

41. Whitmore M, Li S, Huang L. LPD lipopolyplex initiates a potent cytokine response and inhibits tumor growth. Gene Ther 1999; 6:1867–1875.

42. Li S, Rizzo MA, Bhattacharya S, Huang L. Characterization of cationic lipid-protamine-DNA (LPD) complexes for intravenous gene delivery. Gene Ther 1998; 5:930–937.

43. Oja CD, Semple SC, Chonn A, Cullis PR. Influence of dose on liposome clearance: critical role of blood proteins. Biochim Biophys Acta 1996; 1281:31–37.

44. Kim JK, Choi SH, Kim CO, Park JS, Ahn WS, Kim CK. Enhancement of polyethylene glycol (PEG)-modified cationic liposome-mediated gene deliveries: effects on serum stability and transfection efficiency. J Pharm Pharmacol 2003; 55:453–460.

45. Hong K, Zheng W, Baker A, Papahadjopoulos D. Stabilization of cationic liposome-plasmid DNA complexes by polyamines and poly(ethylene glycol)-phospholipid conjugates for efficient in vivo gene delivery. FEBS Lett 1997; 400:233–237.

46. Chonn A, Semple SC, Cullis PR. Association of blood proteins with large unilamellar liposomes in vivo. Relation to circulation lifetimes. J Biol Chem 1992; 267:18759–18765.

47. Lechardeur D, Sohn KJ, Haardt M, et al. Metabolic instability of plasmid DNA in the cytosol: a potential barrier to gene transfer. Gene Ther 1999; 6:482–497.

48. Zabner J, Fasbender AJ, Moninger T, Poellinger KA, Welsh MJ. Cellular and molecular barriers to gene transfer by a cationic lipid. J Biol Chem 1995; 270:18997–19007.

49. Xu Y, Szoka FC, Jr. Mechanism of DNA release from cationic liposome/DNA complexes used in cell transfection. Biochemistry 1996; 35:5616–5623.

50. Remy JS, Kichler A, Mordvinov V, Schuber F, Behr JP. Targeted gene transfer into hepatoma cells with lipopolyamine-condensed DNA particles presenting galactose ligands: a stage toward artificial viruses. Proc Natl Acad Sci USA 1995; 92:1744–1748.

51. Cheng S, Merlino GT, Pastan IH. A versatile method for the coupling of protein to DNA: synthesis of alpha 2-macroglobulin-DNA conjugates. Nucleic Acids Res 1983; 11:659–669.

52. Ray A, Norden B. Peptide nucleic acid (PNA): its medical and biotechnical applications and promise for the future. FASEB J 2000; 14:1041–1060.

53. Wu GY, Wu CH. Receptor-mediated gene delivery and expression in vivo. J Biol Chem 1988; 263:14621–14624.

54. Fominaya J, Uherek C, Wels W. A chimeric fusion protein containing transforming growth factor-a mediates gene transfer via binding to the EGF receptor. Gene Ther 1998; 5:521–530.

55. Huckett B, Ariatti M, Hawtrey AO. Evidence for targeted gene transfer by receptor-mediated endocytosis. Stable expression following insulin-directed entry of NEO into HepG2 cells. Biochem Pharmacol 1990; 40:253–263.

56. Rosenkranz AA, Yachmenev SV, Jans DA, et al. Receptor-mediated endocytosis and nuclear transport of a transfecting DNA construct. Exp Cell Res 1992; 199:323–329.

57. Mislick KA, Baldeschwieler JD, Kayyem JF, Meade TJ. Transfection of folate-polylysine DNA complexes: evidence for lysosomal delivery. Bioconjug Chem 1995; 6:512–515.

58. Gottschalk S, Cristiano RJ, Smith LC, Woo SL. Folate receptor mediated DNA delivery into tumor cells: potosomal disruption results in enhanced gene expression. Gene Ther 1994; 1:185–191.

59. Sosnowski BA, Gonzalez AM, Chandler LA, Buechler YJ, Pierce GF, Baird A. Targeting DNA to cells with basic fibroblast growth factor (FGF2). J Biol Chem 1996; 271:33647–33653.

60. Harbottle RP, Cooper RG, Hart SL, et al. An RGD-oligolysine peptide: a prototype construct for integrin-mediated gene delivery. [see comment]. Hum Gene Ther 1998; 9:1037–1047.

61. Hart SL, Harbottle RP, Cooper R, Miller A, Williamson R, Coutelle C. Gene delivery and expression mediated by an integrin-binding peptide. Gene Ther 1995; 2:552–554 [erratum appears in Gene Ther 1996 Nov;3(11):1032–3].

62. Harvie P, Dutzar B, Galbraith T, et al. Targeting of lipid-protamine-DNA (LPD) lipopolyplexes using RGD motifs. J Liposome Res 2003; 13:231–247.

63. Medina-Kauwe LK, Maguire M, Kasahara N, Kedes L. Non-viral gene delivery to human breast cancer cells by targeted Ad5 penton proteins. Gene Ther 2001; 8:1753–1761.

64. Buschle M, Cotten M, Kirlappos H, et al. Receptor-mediated gene transfer into human T lymphocytes via binding of DNA/CD3 antibody particles to the CD3 T cell receptor complex. Hum Gene Ther 1995; 6:753–761.

65. Finke S, Trojaneck B, Lefterova P, et al. Increase of proliferation rate and enhancement of antitumor cytotoxicity of expanded human CD3+ CD56+ immunologic effector cells by receptor-mediated transfection with the interleukin-7 gene. Gene Ther 1998; 5:31–39.

66. Ebert O, Finke S, Salahi A, et al. Lymphocyte apoptosis: induction by gene transfer techniques. Gene Ther 1997; 4:296–302.

67. Kircheis R, Kichler A, Wallner G, et al. Coupling of cell-binding ligands to polyethylenimine for targeted gene delivery. Gene Ther 1997; 4:409–418.

68. Merwin JR, Carmichael EP, Noell GS, et al. CD5-mediated specific delivery of DNA to T lymphocytes: compartmentalization augmented by adenovirus. J Immunol Methods 1995; 186:257–266.

69. Chen J, Stickles RJ, Daichendt KA. Galactosylated histone-mediated gene transfer and expression. Hum Gene Ther 1994; 5:429–435.

70. Cristiano RJ, Roth JA. Epidermal growth factor mediated DNA delivery into lung cancer cells via the epidermal growth factor receptor. Cancer Gene Ther 1996; 3:4–10.

71. Foster BJ, Kern JA. HER2-targeted gene transfer. Hum Gene Ther 1997; 8:719–727.

72. Hardingham TE, Fosang AJ. Proteoglycans: many forms and many functions. Faseb J 1992; 6:861–870.

73. Mislick KA, Baldeschwieler JD. Evidence for the role of proteoglycans in cation-mediated gene transfer. Proc Natl Acad Sci USA 1996; 93:12349–12354.

74. Mounkes LC, Zhong W, Cipres-Palacin G, Heath TD, Debs RJ. Proteoglycans mediate cationic liposome-DNA complex-based gene delivery in vitro and in vivo. J Biol Chem 1998; 273:26164–26170.

75. Mukherjee S, Ghosh RN, Maxfield FR. Endocytosis. Physiol Rev 1997; 77:759–803.

76. Heuser JE, Anderson RG. Hypertonic media inhibit receptor-mediated endocytosis by blocking clathrin-coated pit formation. J Cell Biol 1989; 108:389–400.

77. Colin M, Maurice M, Trugnan G, et al. Cell delivery, intracellular trafficking and expression of an integrin-mediated gene transfer vector in tracheal epithelial cells. Gene Ther 2000; 7:139–152.

78. Hinshaw JE, Schmid SL. Dynamin self-assembles into rings suggesting a mechanism for coated vesicle budding. [comment]. Nature 1995; 374:190–192.

79. Schmid SL, McNiven MA, De Camilli P. Dynamin and its partners: a progress report. Curr Opin Cell Biol 1998; 10:504–512.

80. Mousavi SA, Malerod L, Berg T, Kjeken R. Clathrin-dependent endocytosis. Biochem J 2004; 377:1–16.

81. Zuhorn IS, Kalicharan R, Hoekstra D. Lipoplex-mediated transfection of mammalian cells occurs through the cholesterol-dependent clathrin-mediated pathway of endocytosis. J Biol Chem 2002; 277:18021–18028. Epub 2002 Mar 01.

82. Coeytaux E, Coulaud D, Le Cam E, Danos O, Kichler A. The cationic amphipathic alpha-helix of HIV-1 viral protein R (Vpr) binds to nucleic acids, permeabilizes membranes, and efficiently transfects cells. J Biol Chem 2003; 278:18110–18116. Epub 2003 Mar 14.

83. Rothman JE, Schmid SL. Enzymatic recycling of clathrin from coated vesicles. Cell 1986; 46:5–9.

84. Van Dyke RW. Acidification of lysosomes and endosomes. Subcell Biochem 1996; 27:331–360.

85. Wattiaux R, Laurent N, Wattiaux-De Coninck S, Jadot M. Endosomes, lysosomes: their implication in gene transfer. Adv Drug Deliv Rev 2000; 41:201–208.

86. Wagner E. Application of membrane-active peptides for nonviral gene delivery. Adv Drug Deliv Rev 1999; 38:279–289.

87. Parton RG, Richards AA. Lipid rafts and caveolae as portals for endocytosis: new insights and common mechanisms. Traffic 2003; 4:724–738.

88. Mundy DI, Machleidt T, Ying YS, Anderson RG, Bloom GS. Dual control of caveolar membrane traffic by microtubules and the actin cytoskeleton. J Cell Sci 2002; 115:4327–4339.

89. Pelkmans L, Kartenbeck J, Helenius A. Caveolar endocytosis of simian virus 40 reveals a new two-step vesicular-transport pathway to the ER. Nat Cell Biol 2001; 3:473–483.

90. Tammi R, Rilla K, Pienimaki JP, et al. Hyaluronan enters keratinocytes by a novel endocytic route for catabolism. J Biol Chem 2001; 276:35111–35122. Epub 2001 Jul 12.

91. Schnitzer JE, Oh P, Pinney E, Allard J. Filipin-sensitive caveolae-mediated transport in endothelium: reduced transcytosis, scavenger endocytosis, and capillary permeability of select macromolecules. J Cell Biol 1994; 127:1217–1232.

92. Huth S, Lausier J, Gersting SW, et al. Insights into the mechanism of magnetofection using PEI-based magnetofectins for gene transfer. J Gene Med 2004; 6:923–936.

93. Eguchi A, Akuta T, Okuyama H, et al. Protein transduction domain of HIV-1 Tat protein promotes efficient delivery of DNA into mammalian cells. J Biol Chem 2001; 276:26204–26210. Epub 2001 May 09.

94. McIntosh DP, Tan XY, Oh P, Schnitzer JE. Targeting endothelium and its dynamic caveolae for tissue-specific transcytosis in vivo: a pathway to overcome cell barriers to drug and gene delivery. Proc Natl Acad Sci USA 2002; 99:1996–2001.

95. Carver LA, Schnitzer JE. Caveolae: mining little caves for new cancer targets. Nat Rev Cancer 2003; 3:571–581.

96. Schnitzer JE. Caveolae: from basic trafficking mechanisms to targeting transcytosis for tissue-specific drug and gene delivery in vivo. Adv Drug Deliv Rev 2001; 49:265–280.

97. Grimmer S, van Deurs B, Sandvig K. Membrane ruffling and macropinocytosis in A431 cells require cholesterol. J Cell Sci 2002; 115:2953–2962.

98. Dangoria NS, Breau WC, Anderson HA, Cishek DM, Norkin LC. Extracellular simian virus 40 induces an ERK/MAP kinase-independent signalling pathway that activates primary response genes and promotes virus entry. J Gen Virol 1996; 77:2173–2182.

99. Dowrick P, Kenworthy P, McCann B, Warn R. Circular ruffle formation and closure lead to macropinocytosis in hepatocyte growth factor/scatter factor-treated cells. Eur J Cell Biol 1993; 61:44–53.

100. Conner SD, Schmid SL. Regulated portals of entry into the cell. Nature 2003; 422:37–44.

101. Goncalves C, Mennesson E, Fuchs R, Gorvel JP, Midoux P, Pichon C. Macropinocytosis of polyplexes and recycling of plasmid via the clathrin-dependent pathway impair the transfection efficiency of human hepatocarcinoma cells. Mol Ther 2004; 10:373–385.

102. Schwarze SR, Hruska KA, Dowdy SF. Protein transduction: unrestricted delivery into all cells. Trends Cell Biol 2000; 10:290–295.

103. Lundberg M, Wikstrom S, Johansson M. Cell surface adherence and endocytosis of protein transduction domains. Mol Ther 2003; 8:143–150.

104. Wadia JS, Stan RV, Dowdy SF. Transducible TAT-HA fusogenic peptide enhances escape of TAT-fusion proteins after lipid raft macropinocytosis. Nat Med 2004; 10:310–315. Epub 2004 Feb 08.

105. Silhol M, Tyagi M, Giacca M, Lebleu B, Vives E. Different mechanisms for cellular internalization of the HIV-1 Tat-derived cell penetrating peptide and recombinant proteins fused to Tat. Eur J Biochem 2002; 269:494–501.

106. Tyagi M, Rusnati M, Presta M, Giacca M. Internalization of HIV-1 tat requires cell surface heparan sulfate proteoglycans. J Biol Chem 2001; 276:3254–3261. Epub 2000 Oct 06.

107. Console S, Marty C, Garcia-Echeverria C, Schwendener R, Ballmer-Hofer K. Antennapedia and HIV transactivator of transcription (TAT) "protein transduction domains" promote endocytosis of high molecular weight cargo upon binding to cell surface glycosaminoglycans. J Biol Chem 2003; 278:35109–35114.

108. Fuchs SM, Raines RT. Pathway for polyarginine entry into mammalian cells. Biochemistry 2004; 43:2438–2444.

109. Rentsendorj A, Agadjanian H, Chen X, et al. The Ad5 fiber mediates nonviral gene transfer in the absence of the whole virus, utilizing a novel cell entry pathway. Gene Ther 2005; 12:225–237.

110. Curiel DT. High-efficiency gene transfer mediated by adenovirus-polylysine-DNA complexes. Ann NY Acad Sci 1994; 716:36–56 discussion -8.

111. Fasbender A, Zabner J, Chillon M, et al. Complexes of adenovirus with polycationic polymers and cationic lipids increase the efficiency of gene transfer in vitro and in vivo. J Biol Chem 1997; 272:6479–6489.

112. Wagner E, Zatloukal K, Cotten M, et al. Coupling of adenovirus to transferrin-polylysine/DNA complexes greatly enhances receptor-mediated gene delivery and expression of transfected genes. Proc Natl Acad Sci USA 1992; 89:6099–6103.

113. Prchla E, Plank C, Wagner E, Blaas D, Fuchs R. Virus-mediated release of endosomal content in vitro: different behavior of adenovirus and rhinovirus serotype 2. J Cell Biol 1995; 131:111–123.

114. Zauner W, Blaas D, Kuechler E, Wagner E. Rhinovirus-mediated endosomal release of transfection complexes. J Virol 1995; 69:1085–1092.

115. Bullough PA, Hughson FM, Skehel JJ, Wiley DC. Structure of influenza haemagglutinin at the pH of membrane fusion. [see comment]. Nature 1994; 371:37–43.

116. White JM, Wilson IA. Anti-peptide antibodies detect steps in a protein conformational change: low-pH activation of the influenza virus hemagglutinin. J Cell Biol 1987; 105:2887–2896.

117. Wagner E, Plank C, Zatloukal K, Cotten M, Birnstiel ML. Influenza virus hemagglutinin HA-2 N-terminal fusogenic peptides augment gene transfer by transferrin-polylysine-DNA complexes: toward a synthetic virus-like gene-transfer vehicle. Proc Natl Acad Sci USA 1992; 89:7934–7938.

118. Fisher KJ, Wilson JM. The transmembrane domain of diphtheria toxin improves molecular conjugate gene transfer. Biochem J 1997; 321:49–58.

119. Choe S, Bennett MJ, Fujii G, et al. The crystal structure of diphtheria toxin. Nature 1992; 357:216–222.

120. Bennett MJ, Eisenberg D. Refined structure of monomeric diphtheria toxin at 2.3 A resolution. Protein Sci 1994; 3:1464–1475.

121. Blewitt MG, Chung LA, London E. Effect of pH on the conformation of diphtheria toxin and its implications for membrane penetration. Biochemistry 1985; 24:5458–5464.

122. Olsnes S, van Deurs B, Sandvig K. Protein toxins acting on intracellular targets: cellular uptake and translocation to the cytosol. Med Microbiol Immunol 1993; 182:51–61.

123. Zhan H, Oh KJ, Shin YK, Hubbell WL, Collier RJ. Interaction of the isolated transmembrane domain of diphtheria toxin with membranes. Biochemistry 1995; 34:4856–4863.

124. Uherek C, Fominaya J, Wels W. A modular DNA carrier protein based on the structure of diphtheria toxin mediates target cell-specific gene delivery. J Biol Chem 1998; 273:8835–8841.

125. Zalman LS, Wisnieski BJ. Characterization of the insertion of Pseudomonas exotoxin A into membranes. Infect Immun 1985; 50:630–635.

126. Ogris M, Carlisle RC, Bettinger T, Seymour LW. Melittin enables efficient vesicular escape and enhanced nuclear access of nonviral gene delivery vectors. J Biol Chem 2001; 276:47550–47555. Epub 2001 Oct 12.

127. Allende D, Simon SA, McIntosh TJ. Melittin-Induced Bilayer Leakage Depends on Lipid Material Properties: Evidence for Toroidal Pores. Biophys J 2004; 13:13.

128. Yang L, Harroun TA, Weiss TM, Ding L, Huang HW. Barrel-stave model or toroidal model? A case study on melittin pores Biophys J 2001; 81:1475–1485.

129. Li W, Nicol F, Szoka FC, Jr. GALA: a designed synthetic pH-responsive amphipathic peptide with applications in drug and gene delivery. Adv Drug Deliv Rev 2004; 56:967–985.

130. Parente RA, Nir S, Szoka FC, Jr. Mechanism of leakage of phospholipid vesicle contents induced by the peptide GALA. Biochemistry 1990; 29:8720–8728.

131. Nir S, Nicol F, Szoka FC, Jr. Surface aggregation and membrane penetration by peptides: relation to pore formation and fusion. Mol Membr Biol 1999; 16:95–101.

132. Kakudo T, Chaki S, Futaki S, et al. Transferrin-modified liposomes equipped with a pH-sensitive fusogenic peptide: an artificial viral-like delivery system. Biochemistry 2004; 43:5618–5628.

133. Fattal E, Nir S, Parente RA, Szoka FC, Jr. Pore-forming peptides induce rapid phospholipid flip-flop in membranes. Biochemistry 1994; 33:6721–6731.

134. Daleke DL. Regulation of transbilayer plasma membrane phospholipid asymmetry. J Lipid Res 2003; 44:233–242. Epub 2002 Dec 16.

135. Schneider E, Haest CW, Plasa G, Deuticke B. Bacterial cytotoxins, amphotericin B and local anesthetics enhance transbilayer mobility of phospholipids in erythrocyte membranes. Consequences for phospholipid asymmetry. Biochim Biophys Acta 1986; 855:325–336.

136. Devaux PF. Protein involvement in transmembrane lipid asymmetry. Annu Rev Biophys Biomol Struct 1992; 21:417–439.

137. Haensler J, Szoka FC, Jr. Polyamidoamine cascade polymers mediate efficient transfection of cells in culture. Bioconjug Chem 1993; 4:372–379.

138. Kichler A, Leborgne C, Coeytaux E, Danos O. Polyethylenimine-mediated gene delivery: a mechanistic study. J Gene Med 2001; 3:135–144.

139. Sonawane ND, Szoka FC, Jr., Verkman AS. Chloride accumulation and swelling in endosomes enhances DNA transfer by polyamine-DNA polyplexes. J Biol Chem 2003; 278:44826–44831. Epub 2003 Aug 27.

140. Midoux P, LeCam E, Coulaud D, Delain E, Pichon C. Histidine containing peptides and polypeptides as nucleic acid vectors. Somat Cell Mol Genet 2002; 27:27–47.

141. Kichler A, Leborgne C, Marz J, Danos O, Bechinger B. Histidine-rich amphipathic peptide antibiotics promote efficient delivery of DNA into mammalian cells. Proc Natl Acad Sci USA 2003; 100:1564–1568. Epub 2003 Jan 31.

142. Midoux P, Monsigny M. Efficient gene transfer by histidylated polylysine/pDNA complexes. Bioconjug Chem 1999; 10:406–411.

143. Vogt TC, Bechinger B. The interactions of histidine-containing amphipathic helical peptide antibiotics with lipid bilayers. The effects of charges and pH. J Biol Chem 1999; 274:29115–29121.

144. Bechinger B. Towards membrane protein design: pH-sensitive topology of histidine-containing polypeptides. J Mol Biol 1996; 263:768–775.

145. Kumar VV, Pichon C, Refregiers M, Guerin B, Midoux P, Chaudhuri A. Single histidine residue in head-group region is sufficient to impart remarkable gene transfection properties to cationic lipids: evidence for histidine-mediated membrane fusion at acidic pH. Gene Ther 2003; 10:1206–1215.

146. Nishikawa M, Yamauchi M, Morimoto K, Ishida E, Takakura Y, Hashida M. Hepatocyte-targeted in vivo gene expression by intravenous injection of plasmid DNA complexed with synthetic multi-functional gene delivery system. Gene Ther 2000; 7:548–555.

147. Wilson IA, Skehel JJ, Wiley DC. Structure of the haemagglutinin membrane glycoprotein of influenza virus at 3 A resolution. Nature 1981; 289:366–373.

148. Steinhauer DA, Wharton SA, Skehel JJ, Wiley DC. Studies of the membrane fusion activities of fusion peptide mutants of influenza virus hemagglutinin. J Virol 1995; 69:6643–6651.

149. Fender P, Ruigrok RW, Gout E, Buffet S, Chroboczek J. Adenovirus dodecahedron, a new vector for human gene transfer [see comments]. Nat Biotechnol 1997; 15:52–56.

150. Medina-Kauwe LK, Kasahara N, Kedes L. 3PO, a novel non-viral gene delivery system using engineered Ad5 penton proteins. Gene Ther 2001; 8:795–803.

151. Bal HP, Chroboczek J, Schoehn G, Ruigrok RW, Dewhurst S. Adenovirus type 7 penton purification of soluble pentamers from Escherichia coli and development of an integrin-dependent gene delivery system. Eur J Biochem 2000; 267:6074–6081.

152. Seth P, Willingham MC, Pastan I. Binding of adenovirus and its external proteins to Triton X-114. Dependence on pH. J Biol Chem 1985; 260:14431–14434.

153. Wang K, Guan T, Cheresh DA, Nemerow GR. Regulation of adenovirus membrane penetration by the cytoplasmic tail of integrin beta5. J Virol 2000; 74:2731–2739.

154. Wickham TJ, Filardo EJ, Cheresh DA, Nemerow GR. Integrin alpha v beta 5 selectively promotes adenovirus mediated cell membrane permeabilization. J Cell Biol 1994; 127:257–264.

155. Lukacs GL, Haggie P, Seksek O, Lechardeur D, Freedman N, Verkman AS. Size-dependent DNA mobility in cytoplasm and nucleus. J Biol Chem 2000; 275:1625–1629.

156. Dean DA. Import of plasmid DNA into the nucleus is sequence specific. Exp Cell Res 1997; 230:293–302.

157. Langle-Rouault F, Patzel V, Benavente A, et al. Up to 100-fold increase of apparent gene expression in the presence of Epstein-Barr virus oriP sequences and EBNA1: implications of the nuclear import of plasmids. J Virol 1998; 72:6181–6185.

158. Graessmann M, Menne J, Liebler M, Graeber I, Graessmann A. Helper activity for gene expression, a novel function of the SV40 enhancer. Nucleic Acids Res 1989; 17:6603–6612.

159. Chen J, Gamou S, Takayanagi A, Shimizu N. A novel gene delivery system using EGF receptor-mediated endocytosis. FEBS Lett 1994; 338:167–169.

160. Isaka Y, Akagi Y, Kaneda Y, Imai E. The HVJ liposome method. Exp Nephrol 1998; 6:144–147.

161. Sebestyen MG, Ludtke JJ, Bassik MC, et al. DNA vector chemistry: the covalent attachment of signal peptides to plasmid DNA. Nat Biotechnol 1998; 16:80–85.

162. Preuss M, Tecle M, Shah I, Matthews DA, Miller AD. Comparison between the interactions of adenovirus-derived peptides with plasmid DNA and their role in gene delivery mediated by liposome-peptide-DNA virus-like nanoparticles. Org Biomol Chem 2003; 1:2430–2438.

163. Kalderon D, Roberts BL, Richardson WD, Smith AE. A short amino acid sequence able to specify nuclear location. Cell 1984; 39:499–509.

164. Adam SA, Sterne-Marr R, Gerace L. Nuclear protein import using digitonin-permeabilized cells. Methods Enzymol 1992; 219:97–110.

165. Imamoto N. Diversity in nucleocytoplasmic transport pathways. Cell Struct Funct 2000; 25:207–216.

166. Conti E, Izaurralde E. Nucleocytoplasmic transport enters the atomic age. Curr Opin Cell Biol 2001; 13:310–319.

167. Pante N, Aebi U. Molecular dissection of the nuclear pore complex. Crit Rev Biochem Mol Biol 1996; 31:153–199.

168. Stoffler D, Fahrenkrog B, Aebi U. The nuclear pore complex: from molecular architecture to functional dynamics. Curr Opin Cell Biol 1999; 11:391–401.

169. Pante N, Aebi U. Sequential binding of import ligands to distinct nucleopore regions during their nuclear import. Science 1996; 273:1729–1732.

170. Greber UF, Suomalainen M, Stidwill RP, Boucke K, Ebersold MW, Helenius A. The role of the nuclear pore complex in adenovirus DNA entry. EMBO J 1997; 16:5998–6007.

171. Finlay DR, Newmeyer DD, Price TM, Forbes DJ. Inhibition of in vitro nuclear transport by a lectin that binds to nuclear pores. J Cell Biol 1987; 104:189–200.

172. Martin K, Helenius A. Transport of incoming influenza virus nucleocapsids into the nucleus. J Virol 1991; 65:232–244.

173. Pollard VW, Michael WM, Nakielny S, Siomi MC, Wang F, Dreyfuss G. A novel receptor-mediated nuclear protein import pathway. Cell 1996; 86:985–994.

174. Dabauvalle MC, Schulz B, Scheer U, Peters R. Inhibition of nuclear accumulation of karyophilic proteins in living cells by microinjection of the lectin wheat germ agglutinin. Exp Cell Res 1988; 174:291–296.

175. Pollard H, Remy JS, Loussouarn G, Demolombe S, Behr JP, Escande D. Polyethylenimine but not cationic lipids promotes transgene delivery to the nucleus in mammalian cells. J Biol Chem 1998; 273:7507–7511.

176. Ajmani PS, Hughes JA. 3Beta [N-(N′,N′-dimethylaminoethane)-carbamoyl] cholesterol (DC-Chol)-mediated gene delivery to primary rat neurons: characterization and mechanism. Neurochem Res 1999; 24:699–703.

177. Ajmani PS, Tang F, Krishnaswami S, Meyer EM, Sumners C, Hughes JA. Enhanced transgene expression in rat brain cell cultures with a disulfide-containing cationic lipid [3Beta N-(N′,N′-dimethylaminoethane)-carbamoyl]. cholesterol (DC-Chol)-mediated gene delivery to primary rat neurons: characterization and mechanism. Neurosci Lett 1999; 277:141–144.

178. Li S, Tseng WC, Stolz DB, Wu SP, Watkins SC, Huang L. Dynamic changes in the characteristics of cationic lipidic vectors after exposure to mouse serum: implications for intravenous lipofection. Gene Ther 1999; 6:585–594.

179. Sakurai F, Nishioka T, Saito H, et al. Interaction between DNA-cationic liposome complexes and erythrocytes is an important factor in systemic gene transfer via the intravenous route in mice: the role of the neutral helper lipid. Gene Ther 2001; 8:677–686.

180. Liu Y, Mounkes LC, Liggitt HD, et al. Factors influencing the efficiency of cationic liposome-mediated intravenous gene delivery. Nat Biotechnol 1997; 15:167–173.

181. Zhang Y, Calon F, Zhu C, Boado RJ, Pardridge WM. Intravenous nonviral gene therapy causes normalization of striatal tyrosine hydroxylase and reversal of motor impairment in experimental parkinsonism. Hum Gene Ther 2003; 14:1–12.

182. Zhang Y, Schlachetzki F, Zhang YF, Boado RJ, Pardridge WM. Normalization of striatal tyrosine hydroxylase and reversal of motor impairment in experimental parkinsonism with intravenous nonviral gene therapy and a brain-specific promoter. Hum Gene Ther 2004; 15:339–350.

183. Teresa Girao da Cruz M, Cardoso AL, de Almeida LP, Simoes S, Pedroso de Lima MC. Tf-lipoplex-mediated NGF gene transfer to the CNS: neuronal protection and recovery in an excitotoxic model of brain injury. Gene Ther 2005; 12:1242–1252.

184. Lalli G, Bohnert S, Deinhardt K, Verastegui C, Schiavo G. The journey of tetanus and botulinum neurotoxins in neurons. Trends Microbiol 2003; 11:431–437.

185. Knight A, Carvajal J, Schneider H, Coutelle C, Chamberlain S, Fairweather N. Non-viral neuronal gene delivery mediated by the HC fragment of tetanus toxin. Eur J Biochem 1999; 259:762–769.

186. Barrett LB, Berry M, Ying WB, et al. CTb targeted non-viral cDNA delivery enhances transgene expression in neurons. J Gene Med 2004; 6:429–438.

187. Lencer WI, Hirst TR, Holmes RK. Membrane traffic and the cellular uptake of cholera toxin. Biochim Biophys Acta 1999; 1450:177–190.

188. Murray KD, Etheridge CJ, Shah SI, et al. Enhanced cationic liposome-mediated transfection using the DNA-binding peptide mu (mu) from the adenovirus core. Gene Ther 2001; 8:453–460.

189. Cattel L, Ceruti M, Dosio F. From conventional to stealth liposomes: a new frontier in cancer chemotherapy. Tumori 2003; 89:237–249.

190. Frankel AE, Kreitman RJ, Sausville EA. Targeted toxins. Clin Cancer Res 2000; 6:326–334.

191. Moghimi SM, Szebeni J. Stealth liposomes and long circulating nanoparticles: critical issues in pharmacokinetics, opsonization and protein-binding properties. Prog Lipid Res 2003; 42:463–478.

9

Gene Therapy Applications for Parkinson's Disease

E. M. Torres, C. Monville, and S. B. Dunnett
The Brain Repair Group, School of Biosciences, Cardiff University, Cardiff, U.K.

INTRODUCTION

The degeneration of nigrostriatal dopamine neurons in the human brain is known to be the primary pathology of Parkinson's disease (PD) and underlies the profound motor syndrome associated with the disease, involving bradykinesia, rigidity and tremor. The discovery in the 1950s that administration of the dopamine precursor L-3, 4-dihydroxyphenylanaline (L-DOPA) could reverse a similar dopamine-denervation syndrome in experimental animals (1) rapidly led to the clinical application of L-DOPA. When administered orally, together with the peripheral decarboxylase inhibitor carbidopa, L-DOPA proved an effective therapy for this previously untreatable condition. Subsequent innovations have increased the potency and efficacy of L-DOPA therapy, such as the development of slow releasing forms of the drug, as well as the use of other dopamine agonists such as bromocriptine. Since the mid 1970s, countless thousands of Parkinson's sufferers have benefited from the treatment and to this day, L-DOPA remains the mainstay of treatment for PD.

However, despite the obvious benefits, pharmacological treatment of Parkinson's patients has serious limitations. It is not curative and the underlying disease progresses inexorably with time. In the early stages of the disease, a proportion of the degenerating dopamine neurons still survive and these contain the enzymes necessary to synthesize dopamine from L-DOPA once it arrives at the target area. In addition, there are intrinsic mechanisms that compensate for the progressive decrease in dopamine levels (2). There is up-regulation of the numbers of striatal dopamine receptors and an increase in dopamine receptor sensitivity. There is also down-regulation of dopamine degradation in nerve terminals. Together, these compensatory mechanisms have the overall effect of increasing the efficacy of smaller and smaller amounts of endogenous dopamine as the levels decrease with time. However, as the disease progresses, patients need increasing and more frequent doses of L-DOPA to obtain therapeutic benefit and the ameliorative properties of the drug become complicated by the development of debilitating side effects, mainly in the form of drug-induced dyskinesias and on-off fluctuations in drug response (3). These typically develop after 5–10 yr of drug therapy and arise from the interaction of the increasing drug load, in particular the peak and trough nature of drug levels in the blood, with the increased dopamine-sensitivity of the brain. Continuous intravenous delivery of low dose L-DOPA has been shown to dramatically reduce drug induced dyskinesias, but is in itself not a practical therapy for a predominantly elderly out–patient population (4). Inevitably, patients reach an end-stage of the disease when the side effects of therapy come to outweigh the benefits and drug treatment becomes increasingly problematic. Consequently, there has for a long time been the need for an alternative to L-DOPA for these end stage PD sufferers.

PD presents a tantalizing target for gene therapy mainly because the principal pathology arises from the degeneration of a single group of cells the consequences of which are manifested in a circumscribed and well characterized neural circuitry. Although the etiology of the disease is unknown, the root cause of the clinical pathology is known to be the death of dopamine containing cells in the substantia nigra pars compacta (SNc) and the subsequent loss of dopamine innervation to the principal target area, the striatum. The failure of the dopaminergic input to the striatum results in an up-regulation of the gamma-amino-butyric acid (GABA) output from this nucleus to the globus pallidus pars externa (GPe). As a consequence, there is down-regulation of the GABA output of the GPe to both subthalamic nucleus (STN) and the substantia nigra pars reticulata (SNr), resulting in disinhibition of both these nuclei. The resulting up-regulation in the glutamatergic output of the STN causes over excitation of efferent areas including the SNr and globus pallidus pars interna (GPi). It is the up-regulation of these two nuclei in particular that is thought to account for the characteristic symptoms of PD, in particular tremor, rigidity, and bradykinesia (See PD affected areas in Fig. 1) (5).

PD can be modeled in animals by lesioning of the dopamine cells of the SNc. This is done principally using dopamine cell-specific toxins such as 6-hydroxydopamine (6-OHDA), or 1-methyl-4-phenyl-1, 2, 3, 6-tetrahydropyridine (MPTP). Total bilateral destruction of the dopamine system in rats is seriously debilitating on the recipient animal and the animals need intensive care simply to remain alive (6). A more common approach therefore, is a hemi-Parkinsonian model in which 6-OHDA in injected unilaterally, either into the ascending nigrostriatal nerve bundle or into the striatal terminal field. The resulting dopamine asymmetry in the brain produces a corresponding motor asymmetry and a measurable rotational behavior in response to amphetamines or the dopamine agonist apomorphine (7,8). The magnitude of the rotational response is sensitive to therapeutic strategies and is widely used as the main index of functional recovery in this model. The unilateral 6-OHDA model has also been used in primates as has the peripheral injection of MPTP to produce a bilateral, partial dopamine lesion. Chronic peripheral administration of MPTP at low doses over extended periods of time can also produce an animal model in monkeys that is progressive and has many of the hallmarks of the idiopathic disease (9). Conversely, intracarotid administration can be used to produce a unilateral lesion similar to the 6-OHDA lesion in rats, without the need for surgical intervention in the brain (10).

While L-DOPA therapy in patients is targeted at dopamine replacement in the striatum, treatments aimed at correcting some of the downstream consequences of dopamine depletion have also enjoyed some success. Based on the direct and indirect pathways of the basal ganglia circuitry described above, lesions have been used to ablate downstream targets in order to "correct" the up-regulated outputs of the striatum in GPi and STN (11). Such experiments led to the introduction of pallidotomy and subthalamotomy as experimental surgical treatments for PD (12). This approach has not been without its problems, however, and in some patients there have been severe side effects. Except in a small number of patients who have a drug-resistant tremor, this treatment has now fallen out of favour (13). More promising has been a technique known as deep brain stimulation in which high-frequency timulating electrodes implanted to the

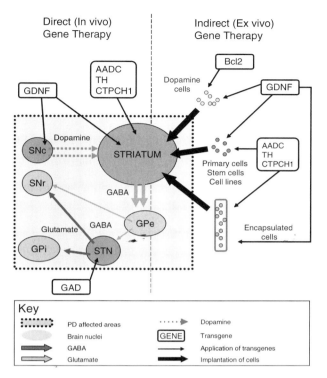

Figure 1 (*See color insert*) Parkinson's Disease affected brain areas and targets for gene therapeutic approaches. Parkinson's Disease affected areas are shown in the yellow shaded box. There is a degeneration of the nigrostriatal dopamine pathway (*dashed blue arrows*) and upregulation of GABAergic output from the striatum to the external segment of the globus pallidus (*double orange arrows*). This causes downregulation of GABAergic output from from this nucleus (*thin orange arrows*) and, in turn, upregulated glutamatergic output from the Subthalamic Nucleus to the SNr and Gpi (*pink arrows*). Strategies for CNS gene therapy may be 'direct' (*left*), where transgenes are injected directly into the host brain, or 'indirect' (*right*), where transgenes are introduced into accessory cells before implantation into the host brain. The diagram shows how these therapies might be applied to Parkinson's Disease. Genes of interest might be targeted at a number of affected areas. Direct application of neurotrophic genes such as GDNF to either the striatum or SNc might be used to rescue the degenerating dopamine system. Alternatively, dopamine synthesis might be established in the striatum by the introduction of genes for TH, AADC and GTPCH1. Another direct approach might be to downregulate the overactive STN by the introduction of a gene for GAD to enable synthesis of GABA in this nucleus. Indirect approaches fall into two main categories: Modification of primary cells and modification of cell lines. The survival of primary dopamine grafts might be enhanced by the introduction of GDNF or of anti-apoptotic genes such as Bcl2. GDNF and the dopamine synthetic enzymes TH, AADC and GTPCH1 might be introduced into primary cells such as host astrocytes, stem cell lines or cells contained within polymer capsules prior to implantation into the host striatum. *Abbreviations*: PD, parkinson's disease; STN, subthalamic nucleus; GABA, gamma-amino-butyric acid; SNr, substantia nigra pars reticulata; GPi, globus pallidus pars interna; GDNF, glial cell line derived neurotrophic factor; SNc, substantia nigra pars compacta; TH, tyrosine hydroxylase; AADC, L-aromatic aminoacid decarboxylase; GTPCH1, GTP cyclohydrolase 1; Bcl2, B cell lymphoma 2 proto-oncogene; GAD, glutamic acid decarboxylase.

sensorimotor region of either the GPi or STN of Parkinson's patients are able to inhibit the up-regulated output of these nuclei and to modulate most of the motor symptoms of the disease (14). Patients also gain better control of "on" time and are typically able to reduce their dopaminergic medication (15–17).

One of the most studied alternative therapies and one which still holds considerable promise has been neural transplantation. Dopaminergic cells, extracted from developing embryos, are implanted ectopically into the dopamine-depleted striatum. The implants are able to form dopamine cells in the host brain that send out axons into the surrounding tissue. They make appropriate synaptic connections, and most importantly, deliver dopamine to the target tissue. Originally developed in animal models in the 1980s and 1990s, such transplants have since been carried out in humans in a number of centers around the world (18,19). There have been successes as well as failures and the technique has had as many detractors as supporters. However, there is little doubt that, in a definable subset of patients, transplants derived from donor embryos of the correct age and implanted using a robust surgical protocol, are able to provide considerable therapeutic benefits. In successful cases the implanted dopamine cells provide a continuous low dose of dopamine to the denervated striatum in a manner that eliminates the peak-trough regime of orally administered L-DOPA. Patients are able to reduce their L-DOPA intake dramatically to a fraction of the previous dosage and in some cases L-DOPA treatment can be stopped altogether. The associated side effects are much reduced or eliminated altogether. Long- term studies of these patients have shown that transplantation therapy is long lasting, and that it has the potential to extend treatment of PD patients well beyond the therapeutic window provided by L-DOPA (20,21). However, despite its success, transplantation therapy is not widely or routinely used as a therapy for PD. The reasons for this are less to do with efficacy of the treatment itself and more to do with the complexity of the ethical, logistical, and quality control problems that surround the use of fetal donor tissues (22,23).

Targets for Parkinson's Disease Gene Therapy

The disrupted circuitry described above, defines the regions of the brain at which novel treatments for PD, including gene therapies might be targeted. Broadly speaking, gene therapies can be applied in one of two ways: either by direct in vivo injection of transgenes into the brain or blood stream using a suitable gene vector or indirectly ex vivo, by packaging transgenes into accessory cells for subsequent implantation into the affected areas. In the case of PD, there are a number of potential direct approaches (Fig. 1). Dopamine replacement in the striatum, a direct correlate of L-DOPA therapy, is an obvious one. A number of research groups have succeeded in transducing striatal cells with one or more of the genes involved in dopamine synthesis and have reported beneficial effects in animal models. The three principal genes thought to be required are tyrosine hydroxylase (TH), L-aromatic amino acid decarboxylase (AADC) (the first two enzymes involved in the conversion of tyrosine to dopamine) and GTP cyclohydrolase 1 (GTPCH1) the enzyme that synthesizes an important TH cofactor, tetrahydrobiopterin (BH_4). A further factor involved in the packaging and transport of dopamine, vesicular monoamine transporter (VMAT), may also be required (24). Transduction of TH alone will probably be insufficient for de-novo dopamine synthesis in vivo, although gene therapy using an adeno-associated virus (AAV) vector containing only the AADC gene, in conjunction with peripherally administered L-DOPA has been shown to partially reverse 6-OHDA induced deficits in rats (25,26).

However, novel synthesis of L-DOPA in vivo will almost certainly require transduction of two or more of the TH, AADC and GTPCH1 transgenes. Some promising work has already been carried out in this regard. In a rat model of PD, Mandel and colleagues (1999) showed that injection into rat striatum of AAV vectors containing genes for both TH and GTPCH1 led to demonstrable L-DOPA production in vivo over long periods of time and was able to ameliorate the deficits produced by the 6-OHDA lesions (27). Kirik et al. used a TH-containing AAV vector in combination with BH$_4$ in a partial lesion model to show good recovery on a range of behavioural tests (28). Transduction of TH and AADC using a *Herpes simplex* (HSV)-based vector was carried out by Sun et al. who succeeded in partially reversing apomorphine induced rotation and showed up to 10,000 TH/AADC positive cells in the striatum seven months after treatment (29).

Transduction of TH, AADC, and GTPCH1 in combination will likely be the optimal approach for dopamine replacement therapy, and several methods of gene delivery have already been investigated. AAV vectors have been used to introduce genes for TH AADC and GTPCH1 into rat (30) and monkey (31) striatum resulting in amelioration of lesion induced deficits. Azzouz and colleagues used a tricistronic lentivirus (LV) vector in a rat model with comparable results (32,33).

An alternative to the dopamine replacement strategy is the provision of neurotrophic factors to the Parkinsonian brain in an attempt to halt or reverse dopamine cell degeneration. Glial cell line derived neurotrophic factor (GDNF) is a prime candidate for a PD gene therapy. Direct administration of GDNF protein has been shown to have potent ameliorative and reparative effects in both rodent and primate models of PD (34–38) and a report of efficacy in a pilot clinical study has attracted particular interest (39). In animal models using gene therapy, GDNF has been reported to protect dopamine cells against the effects of a dopamine lesion when delivered using AAV (40,41) adenovirus (AV) vectors (42,43) and LV vectors (44–47). GDNF has also been used in combination with the anti-apoptotic Bcl-2 delivered using an HSV vector and found to be effective in protecting against the effects of 6-OHDA (48). Given the progressive nature of PD, it is likely that any growth factor therapy will need to be administered continuously over a long period of time in order to sustain dopamine neuron survival and function in the long term. Moreover, since GDNF does not cross the blood–brain barrier, and GDNF receptors are widely distributed throughout the body, delivery will need to be directly into the brain. Because the primary cellular pathology of PD is confined mainly to the dopaminergic neurons of the substantia nigra, supplying therapeutic genes to these neurons by injection of viral vectors into localized sites in the forebrain is the most obvious strategy.

An innovative strategy by Luo and colleagues targeted the deep brain areas at which electrical stimulation has been directed (49). They used AAV vectors to introduce the GABA-synthetic enzyme glutamic acid decarboxylase (GAD) into the STN in an attempt to inhibit the output of this region. Following success in animal models, the go-ahead has now been given for a clinical trial using this approach in patients (49).

In the ex vivo gene therapy approach, accessory cells are used as vehicles for the introduction of transgenes into the brain. Vectors similar to those used in direct therapies can be used to engineer primary cells, cell lines or stem cells, which can then be implanted into the target areas. There are several advantages to this approach. Firstly, the host tissues are not directly exposed to potentially harmful viral vectors and so safety and toxicity issues are of less concern. Secondly, with few exceptions, implanted cells stay at the site at which they are injected and, unlike some viral vectors, are not transported to other sites in the brain nor via the blood stream to peripheral tissues. Thirdly, in the event of problems arising, some cell-based therapies are reversible. Encapsulated cells can be withdrawn from the brain or drug-induced suicide genes can be introduced into the implanted cells (50–53). In the case of xenografts (implantation of cells from other species) implanted tissues survive only by continuous administration of immunosuppressant drugs and if necessary, death of the implant might be effected by removal of immunosuppression.

The targets for ex vivo therapies in PD remain the same, namely the replacement of dopamine in the striatum or the delivery of neurotrophic factors to the degenerating dopamine neurons (Fig. 1). Which might be the best cell to use, is a question which has yet to be answered. Several cell types have been investigated already. Primary rat fibroblasts or immortalized astrocyte cell lines transduced with genes for TH and GTPCH1 have been implanted successfully into the striatum of hemi-Parkinsonian rats (54,55). The same genes have also been shown to have functional effects when delivered using rat bone marrow stromal cells (56). Ex vivo GDNF protection against 6-OHDA lesions has also been demonstrated using adrenal chromaffin cells, (57) astrocytes, (58) and neural stem cells (59).

A final PD gene therapy strategy could be the enhancement of dopamine cell transplantation. One of the major and long-standing problems in the use of foetal transplants has been the relatively poor survival of implanted dopamine neurons. In animal models, although survival rates of 20% and even 40% have been reported, typically only 5–10% of implanted embryonic dopamine neurons survive in the host brain. Put another way, more than 90% of the implanted dopamine cells (or cells that have the potential to become dopamine cells) die, or never develop a dopaminergic phonotype following implantation into the host brain (60). Poor survival has also been confirmed in human patients (61–63) and is considered a major factor in the incomplete recovery seen in many clinical trials. In experimental models, the problem of poor survival can be simply overcome by increasing the amount of donor tissue used, since the degree of functional recovery has been shown to correlate with the number of dopaminergic cells surviving implantation in these models (64). However, in the clinic, the necessity for donor tissue from multiple embryos is problematic. Up to six embryos per patient, per side of the brain are now considered to be necessary for optimal therapy (65,66). The logistical difficulty of obtaining a sufficient quantity of fresh tissue has proved extremely problematic, such that over the fifteen years that this therapy has been actively explored, transplantation therapy for PD has been carried out in only a few centres around the world and to date only a few hundred patients have received implants.

A great deal of effort has been put into finding alternative sources of dopamine cells for implantation. Embryonic dopamine cells from pigs have been investigated (67,68). However cross species transplant studies still have problems of immune rejection and the theoretical possibility that contaminating strains of virus might be able to cross the species barrier have led to significant regulatory and safety concerns. Expansion of precursor cells derived from embryonic primary tissue to increase the number of dopamine cells has also received much attention. Fetal progenitor cells can be expanded indefinitely in the form of neurospheres that can then be differentiated into neurons and glia. However such cells have resisted attempts to encourage their differentiation down the dopaminergic lineage, despite more than a decade of research (69). More recently, embryonic stem (ES) cells have been considered. These are derived from the blastula stage of the developing embryo and in theory have the potential to form all cell types of the body. In spite of some promising preliminary reports in mouse models, using mouse ES cells (70,71), we are still a long way from achieving reliable control of the steps required to generate dopamine neurons from ES cells and for the cells to retain differentiation following transplantation in vivo. Nevertheless there remains widespread optimism that these problems are solvable, and the ES cell remains an exciting prospect for the future (72,73).

In theory, if the survival of implanted dopamine cells could be routinely boosted from 10% up to 50% or more, then an optimal therapy might still be achieved using a single embryo per patient, and the practical problems surrounding the limited availability of primary fetal tissue for PD therapy would be much reduced. To this end, several centres are exploring a variety of different approaches to reduce the processes involved in cell death and promote neuronal survival in tissues destined for transplantation (60).

Viral Vectors for Parkinson's Disease Gene Therapy

While it might be argued that the potential targets for PD gene therapy have largely been established, the optimal means of delivery of therapeutic genes into the brain is still far from decided and is the subject of vigorous research effort. The issue is complex, as evidenced by the wide range of vector systems that are currently being investigated. In the race to find the best vector for gene delivery for the central nervous system, the front-runners have already been mentioned; AAV, AV, LV, and HSV-based vectors appear to be the main contenders. Each vector system has benefits and drawbacks and we shall not go into a detailed comparison here (74). Ultimately, in the race for the perfect CNS gene therapy vector, there may be more than one winner. It is likely for example, that the optimal vector for in vivo delivery of one growth factor to the striatum may not be the one best suited for in ex vivo delivery of the same or another factor to embryonic dopamine cells. Efficient delivery of the genes for dopamine synthesis may well be best achieved using a third vector.

There are a number of issues to be considered when choosing the best vector for delivery of a particular transgene. Common to all is the issue of toxicity. The vector must not be cytotoxic itself, nor cause cell death by initiating a cycle of virus replication in host cells. As a consequence, all virus-based vector systems have genes deleted to reduce cytotoxicity and render them replication-deficient. In addition the vector, and the process used to produce it, must be non-immunogenic such that no potentially damaging immune response is induced in the host. The use of ex vivo gene therapy is one way of avoiding this.

The tropism of viral vectors is also an issue. For direct application, the vector must be able to infect non-dividing cells and transduce them successfully. Transduction relies both on successful delivery of the transgene to the cells of interest and on successful activation of the gene promoter, which may be cell specific. For example, genes driven by the glial-fibrillary-acidic-protein (GFAP) will express only in glial cells, while a neuron-specific-enolase promoter will only be switched on in neuronal cells. Control of promoter expression is more problematic. Viral gene promoters are prone to switching off after a short period of time. On the other hand promoters that drive gene expression indefinitely may have unforeseen consequences and many think that for gene therapy in humans, some form of controllable expression may well be required. The use of the gene promoters linked to tetracycline responsive elements has already shown some promise (75–77).

Hands-On Experience with Viral Vectors

In our laboratory, we are investigating alternative approaches to PD gene therapy using a variety of viral vector systems. Firstly, a GDNF delivery, dopamine cell protection approach using HSV-based vectors, in collaboration with Cantab Pharmaceuticals (Cambridge U.K) and with the group of Dr. Stacey Efstathiou at the University of Cambridge. Secondly a dopamine replacement strategy using a tricistronic LV vector containing gene inserts for TH, AADC, and GTPCH1, produced by Oxford Biomedica (Oxford, U.K). Thirdly, a strategy for increasing the survival of dopamine cell transplants using AV vectors containing genes for GDNF and Sonic hedgehog (Shh), in collaboration with P.R. Lowenstein and M.G. Castro of the Gene Therapeutics Research Institute, Cedars–Sinai Medical Center (University of California, Los Angeles, U.S.A).

All of our studies are carried out using a unilateral 6-OHDA lesion model of PD in the rat. Dopamine lesions are carried out using 6-OHDA (Hydrobromide) at a free base concentration of 3.5 mg/ml. All surgery is conducted under isoflurane anaesthesia in a Kopf stereotaxic frame, with the nose bar set 2.3 mm below the interaural line, The toxin is administered either as a single injection into the median forebrain bundle (MFB) (A = −4.4, L = −0.1, V = −7.8) or using the 4-site striatal injection paradigm based on that described by Kirik et al. (A = +1.3, L = −2.6; A = +0.4, L = −3.0; A = −0.4, L = −4.2; A = −1.3, L = −4.6; all injections at V = −5.0) (78). MFB injection of the toxin results in an acute lesion in which nigrostriatal dopamine function is disrupted immediately and dopamine cell death occurs within 1–2 days following injection, to produce a near-complete (>95%) unilateral lesion. The striatal injection paradigm induces dopamine cell death over 1–3 wk and is better suited to treatment strategies aimed at cell protection.

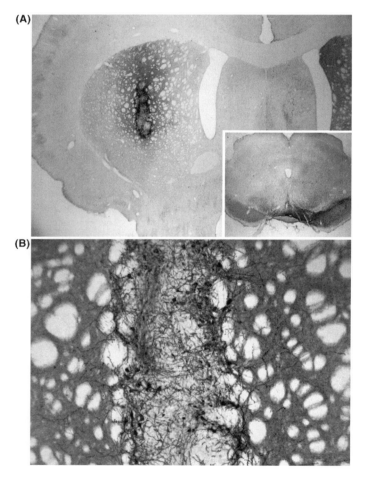

Figure 2 Typical appearance of dopamine grafts in rat model of Parkinson's disease. (**A**) Appearance of an E14 derived graft implanted into the dopamine depleted striatum, as visualized by TH immunohistochemistry. The graft contains many TH positive cells which re-innervate the surrounding striatum (dark halo around the graft). (**B**) Higher power photograph of the graft showing TH cell morphology and TH processes within and radiating from the graft. TH staining of the substantia nigra showing loss of dopamine cells unilaterally on the side of the lesion injection (*inset*).

Dopamine grafts are prepared from the dissected ventral mesencephalic (VM) of embryos aged E14 (14 days after formation of the post-copulatroy vaginal plug). Dissociation of the tissue is carried out using trypsin and mechanical triturating to produce a single cell suspension (79). When grafting, each rat receives an amount of tissue equivalent to one VM injected into the dopamine depleted striatum either as a single injection (A = +0.6, L = −3.0, V = −4.5) or as four injections at the same coordinates used for the striatal 6-OHDA administration.

Behavioural assessment of the lesions and grafts is undertaken by screening all animals for drug-induced rotation in a bank of rotometer bowls (8) over 90 min following intraperitoneal (i.p.) injection of 2.5 mg/kg methamphetamine i.p. and over 60 min after a subcutaneous (s.c.) injection of 0.05 mg/kg apomorphine. Anatomically, the lesions, grafts and vector injections are assessed by TH immunohistochemistry (Fig. 2).

GDNF GENE THERAPY FOR PARKINSON'S DISEASE USING HSV VECTORS

The progressive nature of Parkinson disease offers an opportunity for gene therapy aimed at slowing or blocking the degenerative process. As a candidate vector for gene delivery, vectors derrived from disabled *Herpes simplex* viruses (HSV) are potentially very attractive. HSV has a natural tropism for mammalian neurons. It has a large genome into which large or multiple transgenes can be inserted (80). More than 84 viral genes are encoded, approximately half of which are essential for viral replication in a permissive tissue culture environment (81). In the generation of gene therapy vectors, nonessential genes may be deleted, to allow the insertion of exogenous genetic material and vector toxicity can be reduced, and safety improved, by the simultaneous deletion of several immediate-early (IE) genes (82–85). Transgene sequences can be introduced into the defective vector genomes by homologous recombination, and it is possible using appropriate complementing cell lines to prepare high titre vector stocks that are free from contaminating replication-competent viruses and that have normal targeting character-istics without the ability to replicate or reactivate in vivo (86).

Safety is clearly a critical consideration in the development of any gene therapy designed to treat human disease. While many other vectors have yet to reach clinical trials, the safety of HSV vectors in humans has already been examined. In two separate trials, replication-competent HSV vectors were injected into the brain as a potential treatment for glioblastoma (87,88) and no significant vector-related adverse effects were reported.

Another factor in favor of the use of HSV is that its genome does not integrate into the mammalian genome but remains as an episomal element within the nucleus of the infected cell. The use of other viral vectors that insert into the host genome has potential problems. Two studies have shown insertional mutagenesis could lead to leukemia (89,90). Further, viral vectors that integrate into chromosomes have been shown to be more likely to insert into active genes than into non-coding regions (91). Thus, the non-integrating nature of HSV may well add to its suitability as a gene therapy candidate vector.

We have undertaken an investigation of the potential of different HSV vectors to deliver GDNF in a rat model of PD. The vectors involved in the work are summarized in Table 1. Viral vectors were obtained from two different collaborators and the construction of the vectors reflects the different approaches of each collaborating group. The vectors prefaced DH were obtained from Cantab Pharmaceuticals of Cambridge. The vectors prefaced gH and CS were obtained from the group led by Stacey Efstathiou, based in the Department of Virology of Cambridge University. Deletion of the essential

Table 1 Summary of HSV-Based Vectors Used in the Current Work

Vector[a]	Backbone	Transgene	Source
DH1J4	-gH/Multiple IE deletions GDNF	Cantab	
DH1J1	-gH/Multiple IE deletions LacZ	Cantab	
gHLAPGDNF	-gH/-Tk/-LAP	GDNF	U.C.
gHLAPLacZ	-gH/-Tk/-LAP	LacZ	U.C.
CS1	-gH/-Tk/-LAP	LacZ	U.C.

[a] All HSV transgenes are driven by the LAT promoter.
Abbreviations: Tk, thymidine kinase; LAP, latency associated promoter; U.C., University of Cambridge.

glycoprotein gH, which is important in viral entry and cell-to-cell spreading (92), restricts replication to a single cycle in both vectors. The endogenous latency-associated transcript (LAT) regions are also deleted to reduce the possibility of intra-genomic recombinations with wild type viruses. Transgene expression is driven by a 3.3 kb fragment of the LAT promoter (LAP) important in long-term transgene expression in the PNS (93,94). The LAP/transgene cassette is inserted into either the gH/Tk locus (DH vectors) or between the IRL sites separating the unique-long and unique-short regions of the genome (g/CS vectors). The main difference between the two vectors is the extent of viral gene deletion undertaken. As well as the gH and LAT deletions the gH/tk are deleted in the thymidine kinase (tk) locus, a non essential gene which is a known neuro-virulence determinant (95). Tk negative viruses are attenuated and reactivate poorly in animal models. The DH1J-based vectors have multiple deletions of the ICP4, ICP22, ICP47, and ICP27 immediate early genes and as a consequence have very limited IE gene expression which in theory should greatly decrease their cytotoxicity.

Previous studies have suggested that, when injected into the striatum, HSV is taken up by terminals and retrogradely transported to the cell bodies of afferent neurons (96) including the critical DA neuronal populations in the SN. In an initial study, (97) we compared the ability of GDNF to protect nigrostriatal neurons against the effects of a 6-OHDA lesion when delivered using either the DH1J4 or gHLAPGDNF constructs. DH1J1 and gHLAPLacZ were used as the respective controls. Striatal injection of both of the HSV-GDNF constructs was effective in protecting against a subsequent 6-OHDA lesion as measured by the number of surviving DA neurons in the substantia nigra (Fig. 3). However, only ghLAPGDNF constructs (the least deleted) were able to alleviate the behavioral deficits caused by the lesion, and then only partially.

An unexpected and as yet unexplained result was that injection of the DH1J1 and DH1J4 vectors was associated with severe cytotoxicity and tissue loss at the site of injection. While the data showed that the modest recovery of function on amphetamine rotation was specific to the GDNF vector, the inhibition of apomorphine-induced rotation was comparable with both GDNF and control viruses. This was probably due to either death or dysfunction of the striatal neurons wherein the receptor super-sensitivity responsible for this form of rotation lies (98). Although the anatomical observation of partial neuroprotection is in line with the hypothesis that GDNF could be neuroprotective, the cytotoxicity associated with the virus needed further investigation.

The second HSV-GDNF vector from the University of Cambridge (Table 1) was less deleted than the Cantab vector lacking only the gH, tk, and LAP genes. Previous studies using similar vectors containing the LacZ gene under the control of the LAP, have shown that following delivery in the striatum, β-galactosidase expression was detected within anatomically related CNS regions distal to the site of injection (99). In a second

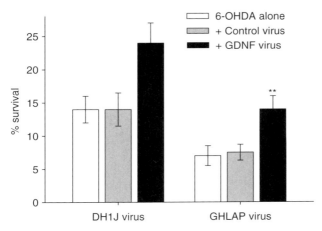

Figure 3 Survival of DA neurons in the substantia nigra following unilateral 6-OHDA lesions in control rats and rats pretreated with control of GDNF HSV viral vectors. *Abbreviation*: DA, dopamine. *Source*: From Ref. 97.

experiment we evaluated the ability of this alternative source of HSV-GDNF to protect nigral dopamine neurons against 6-OHDA toxicity using both anatomical and behavioral criteria. As with the dH1J4 vector, injection of gHLAPGDNF into the rat striatum protected against subsequent 6-OHDA lesion of the nigrostriatal dopamine neurons of the substantia nigra. However, despite the very limited attenuation of this vector compared to the DH1J-based vectors, toxicity was markedly reduced. This was apparent both in the anatomical integrity of the striatum and the absence of any rotational asymmetry in these animals associated with the initial virus injection. There was again no significant improvement in behavioral recovery associated with this. Although the changes in nigral cell survival were significant the effects were not large, as indicated by the rather limited numbers of nigral cells expressing the marker gene in the gHLAPLACZ group, which may be associated with only modest uptake and/or retrograde transport of the virus. Only few β-galactosidase expressing cells were seen in the SNc and the number of cells seen dropped off dramatically from 3 days to 4 weeks post injection. The reduction of transgene expression with time is due not to the death of infected cells, but has been shown to be the result of silencing of the non-integrating LAT promoter (100).

In theory, the more heavily deleted (DH) viruses should cause less inflammation and tissue damage, and transduce greater numbers of host cells than the gh/tk deleted vectors. Indeed that is the primary purpose of extensive gene deletion. It was something of a surprise therefore to observe that when injected into the hemi-Parkinsonian rat brain, the more deleted vector caused the most inflammation and damage. Our suspicions fell on the method of preparation and purification of the virus. The conventional method of HSV production (used by the university) was to harvest the virus from the supernatant of the complementing cells, concentrate this by centrifugation and then to purify the virus using an ultracentrifuge-based liquid (Ficoll) gradient method. By contrast, the dH1J vectors were prepared using a novel method, devised with a mind to possible future commercial scaling of virus preparation. The virus was harvested by lysing of the complementing cells in a high molarity sodium sulphate solution, which was then filtered to remove cell debris. Purification was by means of an affinity column with heparin as the binding agent. We hypothesized that the Cantab method might be co-purifying substances that were

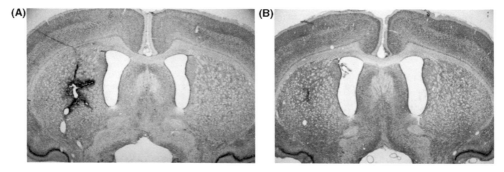

Figure 4 Comparison of the inflammation seen following injection of CS1 prepared using two different protocols. Cresyl fast violet stained sections of rat brain 4 weeks after striatal injection of 3×10^6 IU of HSV-LacZ virus (CS1). (**A**) CS1c prepared using the commercial method. There is residual inflammatory infiltrate around the injection site and in the overlying corpus callosum with enlargement of blood vessels and some perivascular cuffing. Despite this there is no obvious distension of the adjacent lateral ventricle that would indicate extensive tissue loss in the striatum. (**B**) CS1v prepared using the conventional method. A small focus of inflammation at the site of injection is all that remains. There is no evidence of a widespread inflammatory process or of striatal tissue loss.

immunogenic in the rat brain such as proteins derived form the complementing cell line or large numbers of undeveloped or dead virus particles.

In a third experiment we compared the in vivo toxicity, uptake and retrograde transport of a common LacZ vector, prepared using the two different preparation protocols. The CS1 virus was chosen for comparison, as this virus was capable of being grown on the different cell lines used by the two groups. Two batches of CS1 virus were prepared according to either the salt-harvest/affinity (CS1c) or the supernatant-harvest/centrifugation (CS1v) methods. When injected into the normal rat striatum the CS1c preparation was found to be significantly more toxic than the CSv preparation using a variety of measures. CS1c produced greater inflammation, more blood vessel enlargement and fewer transduced cells at all time points. indicating that the protocol for viral preparation was indeed the source of the toxicity seen (Figs. 4 and 5).

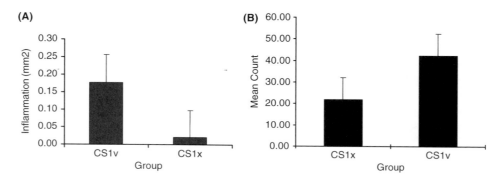

Figure 5 Comparison of the inflammation seen following injection of CS1 prepared using two different protocols. (**A**) CS1 prepared using the commercial method (CS1c) produced more inflammation than CS1 prepared using the conventional method (CS1v). (**B**) By contrast there were fewer β-galactosidase positive cells in the CS1c injected than the CS1v injected brains.

In our experiments with HSV-based vectors we were able to detect β-galactosidase expression, at least at short time points, but were not able to detect GDNF expression using immunochemistry or ELISA. In the meantime we have seen a significant effect of GDNF on dopamine cell survival in one of the two experiments, suggesting that GDNF was expressed at similar levels to that seen with β-galactosidase. Moreover, Natsume and colleagues have shown that after rats were injected with an HSV-GDNF vector, the substantia nigra exhibited a diffuse GDNF immunoreactivity around the injection site and that GDNF was released from the transduced cells (101). Another possibility is that GDNF expression was not sustained long enough for us to detect it with the methods used. In our studies, high levels of β-galactosidase expression were seen after 3 days. In a previous study, using similar HSV-based vectors, it was demonstrated that maximum levels of expression from the LAT promoter were seen two weeks post injection into rat brain (102). As a compromise, we elected to inject the virus one week before the 6-OHDA lesion in the hope of producing the maximum protection possible. HSV gene expression typically became silent 3–4 weeks post injection. This was sufficient to yield partial, but not complete, protection of TH neurons. The paradigm used involved a four site striatal lesion but just a single striatal injection of virus and this may have been a limiting factor in the extent of GDNF protection seen.

In conclusion, experiments with both of the HSV vector types tested have hinted at the potential of these vectors for PD but both have problems that need to be overcome. The LAT promoter, being non-integrating and of viral origin is being silenced in the mammalian brain and the evaluation of the multiply-deleted DH1J based vectors has been hampered by the processes used to produce and purify them. The finished preparation appears to contain pyrogenic substances that elicit a powerful immune response in rat brain resulting in severe inflammation, cytotoxicity and tissue loss. Injection of DH1J4 into the Parkinsonian brain produced an encouraging (if limited) recovery of function, despite this. Modification of the methods of virus preparation to reduce the in vivo toxicity is necessary and only then can the full potential of these vectors be properly investigated.

EX VIVO APPLICATION OF VIRAL VECTORS

The cell replacement strategy in PD has been based on the observation that restoration of dopamine in the striatum by neural grafts can lead to substantial and long-lasting functional recovery. Extensive studies in animal models have lent support to this approach and the limited data available from human transplants have been encouraging. However, the poor survival of the grafted cells (typically 5–10% of the implanted dopamine neurons) remains an issue. Much research has focussed on strategies to improve the yield of dopamine cells, principally so that the number of embryos required per treatment might be reduced. The application of factors to the dopamine grafts using gene therapy is one such strategy and we have examined the potential of the vectors being tested in our laboratory to deliver transgenes to embryonic ventral mesencephalon cells.

Suspensions of cells prepared from the ventral mesencephalon (VM) of embryos of E14 gestational age were exposed to HSV or recombinant adenoviral (RAd) vectors, each containing the LacZ transgene for 1–3 hr at a range of molarities of infection (MOI, expressed as infectious units per cell). Excess vector was removed by repeated spinning and washing of the cells. The infected cells were then resuspended in culture medium and plated onto cover slips coated with poly-lysine and allowed to differentiate. After 1 wk of incubation, the cultured cells were fixed using 4% PFA and processed for β-galactosidase immunohistochemistry. This infection protocol was seen to be efficient even at the shortest time point of 1 hr, an observation that is compatible with the requirement for the excised embryonic dopamine cells needed to be implanted as quickly as possible to maintain viability.

The HSV and RAd vectors produced very different results. Expression of β-galactosidase in cultures infected with HSV vectors was seen exclusively in neurons (Fig. 6). The HSV used in this experiment was DH1J1, with the transgene under LAT promoter control. This promoter is neuron-specific so that even if the vector had infected non-neuronal cells in the culture gene expression it would be limited to neurons. Interestingly, despite the toxicity seen in vivo with this vector there was no obvious toxicity seen in vitro even at highest molarities of infection used (250 infectious units per cell) adding weight to the hypothesis that the toxicity seen in vivo with this vector was due to an immune response of the host to some component of the injected virus preparation.

Cultures infected with RAd vectors presented a very different picture (Fig. 7). Most β-galactosidase expression was seen in cells with an astrocytic profile and only occasionally were immunoreactive neurons seen. This mirrors the in vivo appearance of these vectors in which they appear to have a primarily glial tropism. This is potentially problematic for the use of RAd vectors to deliver differentiation factors, depending on whether the transgenes concerned are expressed or have their action within the transduced cell. While diffusible factors such as GDNF and Shh should work equally well in transduced neurons or glia, other genes that might require expression within the target neurones (such as those encoding transcription factors) are likely to be ineffective.

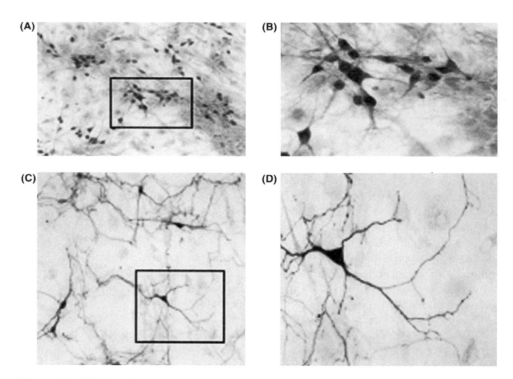

Figure 6 HSV in vitro. Photomicrographs of E14VM cultures 1 wk post infection with HSV-LacZ. (**A,B**) Immunostaining for β-galactosidase reveals numerous positive cells with a neuronal profile. (**C,D**) TH immunohistochemistry (bottom panel) shows well differentiated dopamine neurons in all cultures.

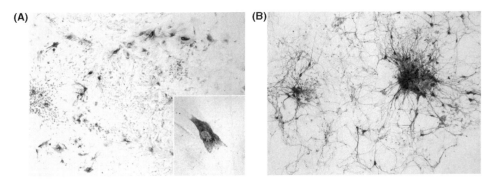

Figure 7 RAd in vitro. Photomicrographs of E14Vm cultures 1 week post infection with RAd-LacZ. (**A**) Immunostaining for β-galactosidase reveals mumerous positive cells with a glial profile (*inset*). (**B**) All cultures contain clumps of healthy well differentiated TH positive cells.

The in vitro work described here is typical of the sort of studies carried out with any vector system prior to their use in in vivo experiments. In experiments using the RAd and HSV vectors we were able to determine information regarding toxicity the efficiency of infection, levels of transgene expression and the tropism of the vectors and these data were influential in the manner in which the vectors were deployed in vivo. Following the in vitro observations we have explored the potential of ex vivo application of HSV-GDNF vectors to dopaminergic cells prior to transplantation in the rat hemi-Parkinsonian model. Rats with a unilateral lesion of the median forebrain bundle were allocated to matched groups according to their post-lesion amphetamine rotation scores. Rats then received grafts of a standard E14Vm cell suspension treated as follows: No treatment; HSV-GDNF; or HSV-LacZ. Rats were rotation tested post-graft and sacrificed at a number of time points post-lesion for postmortem analysis. In rats sacrificed 17 wk after surgery TH immunochemistry revealed grafted cells in the striatum 5 days after grafting (Fig. 8). We also observed GDNF expression in the grafted cells and in surrounding striatal tissue and adjacent globus pallidus, probably due to GDNF secretion and uptake by cells in the vicinity. We were unable to detect any expression of either β-galactosidase or GDNF.

There was no rescue of dopamine neurons in the SNc following HSV-GDNF treatment in the striatum (Fig. 9A) and counts of TH positive cells in the dopamine grafts revealed no significant differences between groups (Fig. 9B). There was amelioration of drug induced motor asymmetries induced by amphetamine (Fig. 10A) and apomorphine (Fig. 10B) in all graft groups. The improvement obtained with apomorphine was delayed in onset and weaker than that seen with amphetamine. However, no significant differences were observed between the HSV-GDNF, HSV-LacZ, and untreated graft groups. It is likely that the levels of GDNF produced by the implanted cells were too low in these experiments or that the timing of GDNF expression was delayed, issues that are discussed in more detail below.

ADENOVIRAL VECTORS AND DOPAMINE GRAFT SURVIVAL

We have explored the potential of recombinant adenoviral vectors (RAd) for improving the survival of dopaminergic grafts, in a collaboration with Pedro R. Lowenstein and

(A)

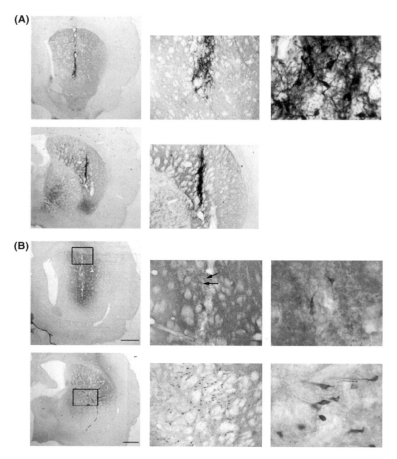

Figure 8   In vivo appearance of vector modified dopamine grafts. (**A**) TH staining of grafts treated with HSV-GDNF. While smalls the graft contain, many TH positive cells. (**B**) GDNF expression from grafted cells transduced with HSV/GDNF and implanted into rat striatum. Expression is seen within the graft and surrounding tissue as well as in surrounding areas, such as globus pallidus. Scale bar is 700 μm.

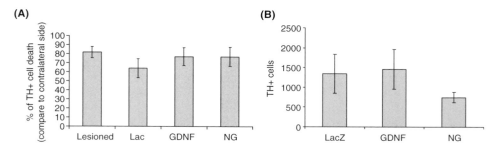

Figure 9   Postmortem analysis following ex vivo treatment of dopamine grafts with HSV vectors. (**A**) TH positive cells count in the SNc. (**B**) TH positive cells count in the graft.

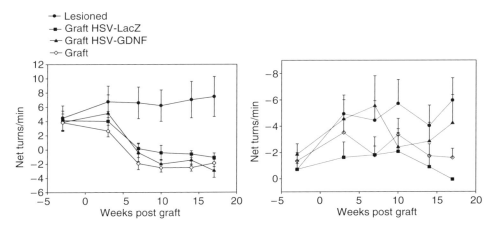

Figure 10 Drug-induced rotations. Amphetamine (*left*) and apomorphine (*right*).

Maria G. Castro. In this section we describe a number of experiments that illustrate the methods used and the problems that arise in the investigation of new gene therapy vectors.

The RAds used in this work have been described previously. They are first-generation vectors in which deletions or substitutions have been made in the E1 and E3 regions of the viral genome. The vectors are produced using a *trans*-complementing cell line established from human embryonic kidney cells. The resulting virus particles are replication deficient, but capable of infecting a wide range of cell types including non-dividing cells. Co-workers have described the expression of the LacZ recombinant AV vectors RAd35 and RAd36 in the rat brain and have suggested that RAd36 is capable of transducing striatal cells in vivo with almost 100% efficiency (that a single viral particle is capable of transducing a cell) (103). The therapeutic vectors obtained for initial consideration contained genes for either Shh or GDNF. The transgenes were driven by cytomegalovirus-derived promoters of either human or murine origin (Table 2).

Methods of Application of Viral Vectors to Dopamine Transplants

Our work using HSV and LV is aimed at treating the Parkinsonian deficit caused by a dopamine-depleting lesion and focused on direct injection of the vector into the host brain. By contrast the application of viral vectors to dopamine transplants is not so straightforward and a number of different routes of administration are possible (Fig. 11):

- First, as above, the vectors might be applied directly to the embryonic dopamine cell suspension embryo prior to implantation into the host brain.

Table 2 Summary of Adenovirus Vectors Used in These Experiments

Vector	Backbone	Transgene	Promoter[a]
RAd35	Type V/-E1,-E3	Lac Z	MIE*h*CMV/
RAd36	Type V/-E1,-E3	Lac Z	MIE*m*CMV/
RAd Shh	Type V/-E1,-E3	Shh	MIE*m*CMV/
RAdGDNF	Type V/-E1,-E3	GDNF	MIE*h*CMV/

[a] *m* = promoter derived from murine CMV, *h* = promoter derived from human CMV.

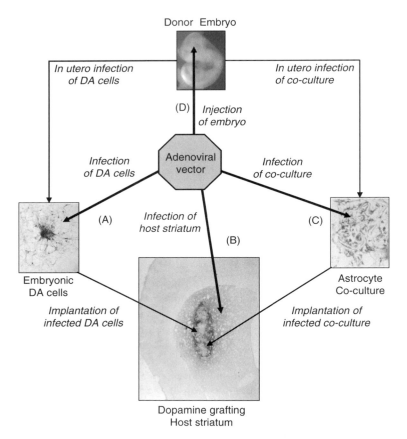

Figure 11 Diagram to show potential routes of application of AV vectors to dopamine grafts. (**A**) Transduction of primary dopamine neuron suspensions with neurotrophic genes or genes important in DA cell differentiation. (**B**) Delivery of the same transgenes to the host striatum prior to grafting. (**C**) Transduction of co-cultures of cells (e.g., astrocytes) for co-grafting with dopamine grafts. (**D**) Delivery of transgenes to the donor embryo in-utero prior to excision of graft tissue.

- Secondly, accessory cells such as astrocytes could be transduced for co-grafting together with embryonic dopamine cells, either as a mixed suspension or in separate grafts, distinct in location and/or in time from the dopaminergic grafts.
- Thirdly, as in the HSV and LV GDNF experiments, the vectors could be injected directly into the host striatum. This could be done prior to implantation of the dopaminergic graft so that the transgene product would be expressed in the region of the host brain into which the graft is to be placed.
- A final route of application might be the vectors to be injected into the donor embryos in utero, prior to excision of the ventral mesencephalic tissue used for grafting.

In Vivo Dynamics of Adenoviral Vectors in the Hemi-Parkinsonian Brain

The RAd36 vector contains a LacZ gene driven by the highly efficient, major-immediate-early promoter from the murine cytomegalovirus (MIEmCMV). The construction and purification of the vector has been described previously (104). Our initial assessment involved the direct injection of this vector into the normal rat striatum, to provide a direct comparison of these vectors with the others under consideration. In previous work by Gerdes and colleagues, RAd36 was injected into the corpus striatum of normal rats at doses from 10^4 to 10^8 IU, and was seen to transduce large numbers of cells both in the striatum and in the adjacent corpus callosum (103). Optimal transgene expression was seen following injection of 10^6–10^7 IU, which produced a cross-sectional area of transduced cells of up to 2.5 mm² at the site of injection. Only at the highest dose of 10^8 IU was there any obvious adverse reaction to the virus or tissue damage. Although cell counts were not carried out at all doses, a near 100% efficiency of transduction (i.e., nearly 1 cell transduced for every IU injected) was reported at low doses (10^1 to 10^3 IU), and the authors concluded that the mCMV promoter was 3 orders of magnitude more efficient than the hCMV promoter used in other vectors, such as RAd35 (103).

An in vivo dose response study was carried out to determine what, in our hands, would be the optimal parameters for injection using the new vectors and to observe both the volume of brain tissue and the level of gene expression at the different doses. As an example, the LacZ containing RAd36 vector was used to test the in vivo properties of the mCMV-containing vectors. Log dilutions from 1×10^4 to 1×10^6 IU/µl were prepared and 3 µl volumes were injected unilaterally into normal rat striatum. Rats were sacrificed 4 wk post-injection and the brains analyzed histologically for LacZ expression. Using this approach we determined that the volumes of transduced striatum per injection had a mean of 0.45 ± 0.13 mm³ in the lowest dose group, 2.29 ± 0.32 mm³ in the middle dose group and 3.36 ± 0.43 mm³ in the highest dose group. There was no evidence of an inflammatory reaction nor of any difference in striatal volume on the injected and uninjected sides, indicating that there was no significant cell loss due to the vector injection (Fig. 12).

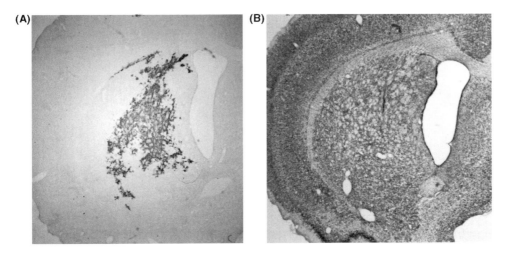

Figure 12 Histological appearance of virus injected into rat brain 4 weeks post-injection of the 3×10^5 IU of RAd36 virus. Photographs show the injected striatum from a single animal. (**A**) β-Galactosidase immunohistochemistry shows large numbers of transduced cells in the striatum around the injection site and extending to the overlying corpus callosum. (**B**) In the cresyl violet stain, the only indication of the injection is a small scar marking the site of the injection cannula. There is no indication of an inflammatory reaction. The regular spacing of the pale staining fiber bundles and the lack of tissue shrinkage indicates that little or no striatal cell loss has occurred.

At the highest dose used, some transduced cells were also seen outside the injected striatum notably in the corpus callosum. This was probably due to the spread of viral particles beyond the site of injection following local saturation of virus binding. Expression of transgenes outside the target area may or may not be desirable, depending on the therapeutic target. However it is crucial to know where transgenes are expressed when considering the parameters of the therapy itself. In our experiments, the RAds appeared not to be retrogradely transported away from the striatum after injection (or at least do not transduce cells in these areas) as no transgene expression was observed in afferent or efferent areas such as substantia nigra, neocortex or globus pallidus. This is not true of other vectors notably HSV, where retrograde transport is common, and where account needs to be taken of the possible effects of cell transduction in these areas.

One cannot assume, of course, that the levels of infection, the dynamics of dispersal, and levels of gene expression will all be the same in pathological as in a normal brain. Since the aim of our work was to use AV vectors to deliver transgenes in models of PD and transplantation-based therapies, we also investigated whether the presence of the 6-OHDA lesion might affect the in vivo properties of the vector. In a simple experiment, RAd36 virus was injected bilaterally into the striata of rats that had previously received a unilateral 6-OHDA lesion of the median forebrain bundle, the classic hemi-Parkinsonian lesion. Rats were then sacrificed at 3 days, 1 wk or 4 wk post-injection to determine the distribution of gene expression in the brain (105).

As in the normal rat brain, there was little evidence of an inflammatory reaction in any of the AV-vector injected brains at any of the time points examined (Fig. 13). Nor was there any evidence of striatal atrophy or of ventricular enlargement. Small scars, similar to those seen following injection of vehicle solutions alone were the only evidence of a striatal injection seen in the β-galactosidase immuno-stained sections. However, evident in most brains, was an asymmetry of staining in the two injected hemispheres. On the unlesioned side of the brain, β-galactosidase immunoreactivity was confined almost exclusively to the striatum in a volume of brain centred around the site of injection. In contrast, on the 6-OHDA side of the brain, many cases had staining in other structures,

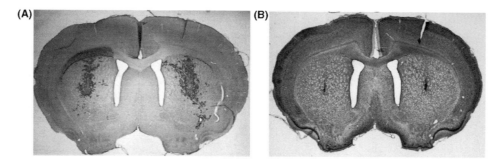

Figure 13 Histological appearance of the hemi-parkinsonian rat brain following bilateral injection of the LacZ containing AV vector RAd36. (**A**) Section stained for β-galactosidase showing transgene expression in the intact hemisphere (*right*) similar to that seen following injection into normal animals. β-galactosidase staining is seen mostly around the injection site in the striatum. However, in the dopamine-depleted hemisphere (*left*) an additional region of β-galactosidase staining is seen in the overlying corpus callosum and levels of staining in the striatum are generally lower. (**B**) Cresyl violet stained section showing that striatal morphology appears normal 1 week post-injection of the vector, apart from minor needle damage. There is little evidence of any inflammatory reaction. *Source*: From Ref. 105.

principally in the corpus callosum overlying the injection site (Fig. 13). Analysis of β-galactosidase positive cell numbers demonstrated that the 6-OHDA lesioned side of the brain contained significantly greater numbers of β-galactosidase positive cells than the unlesioned side at all of the time points observed.

There were 15% fewer β-galactosidase cells seen in the lesioned striatum than in the unlesioned striatum, although this difference was not statistically significant. By contrast, there were significantly more cells seen in the corpus callosum on the lesioned side, by nearly 40%, compared to the numbers seen on the unlesioned side of the brain. The results clearly indicated that the presence of a 6-OHDA lesion affected both the distribution of transduced cells and the levels of transgene expression, although the reason why the hemi-Parkinsonian lesion affects the in vivo dynamics of the injected vector is not known. Altered diffusion characteristics of the de-afferented striatum is one possibility, reduced numbers of vector bindings sites due to removal of the dopamine terminals is another; experiments are underway to investigate this phenomenon further. Whatever the outcome, potential gene therapy vectors will need to be tested in appropriate animal models of the disease as an essential component of determining clinical utility.

As previously, no cells expressing the transgene were seen in brain nuclei—either cortex, nigra or thalamus—that project to the striatal site of injection. This indicates either that the injected vector was not retrogradely transported from the injection site or that it was unable to transduce infected cells after transport. The significance of this observation is that, once the parameters of injection are optimized, the volume of brain infected can be limited to the site of injection, avoiding unwanted expression of transgenes in afferent areas.

The Application of Adenoviral Vectors to Dopaminergic Grafts

In 1999 Sinclair and colleagues reported differentiation in the differences of dopamine in nigral grafts compared to the time course of development in the normal embryo, using the marker for dividing cells bromo-deoxyuridine (BrdU) injected into developing embryos and dopamine grafts (106). The peak of dopamine cell neurogenesis was found to be between embryonic ages E13 and E15, in agreement with previous work done by Altman et al. using tritiated thymidine (107). They then studied dopaminergic implants derived from these embryos and determined the proportions of BrdU and TH positive cells present in the grafts. Surviving dopamine neurons in transplants from E14 rat embryos consisted almost exclusively of neurons that had undergone their final cell division prior to excision from the embryo. It was concluded that the numbers of dopamine cells in Parkinsonian grafts were low, not just because dopamine cells had failed to survive implantation. Rather, that many of the implanted cells that would have subsequently differentiated into dopaminergic neurons in situ failed to do so after transplantation, suggesting that critical developmental signals are absent in the adult host brain. Based on this hypothesis, we have reasoned that one possible strategy to improve the yield of dopamine neurons in VM grafts would be to treat the VM graft tissue suspensions prior to implantation with the factors required for dopamine differentiation.

In choosing which factors might be effective, developmental studies have suggested a number of candidates that are implicated in the development and/or differentiation of dopaminergic neurons. Glial cell-derived neurotrophic factor (GDNF) has been used both as a factor to prevent DA cell degeneration in lesion models, and had been shown to promote the growth of DA in vitro and in dopaminergic implants and is known to be involved in the normal development of the nigrostriatal dopamine system (108–111). While not a known differentiation factor this was considered to be a useful positive control that could be used to test the efficacy of the vector and promoter systems. Alternatively, the differentiation factor Shh is involved in the early neuronal specification and has been implicated directly in the development of substantia nigra (112,113). The work described here investigates the application of these two vectors to improve the survival of dopaminergic grafts.

The experiment we describe here was designed to determine whether improved survival of dopamine grafts could be achieved by transducing the host striatum with factors that might improve the survival of dopaminergic grafts. RAd vectors containing either Shh or GDNF were used. All rats first received a 6-OHDA lesion of the median forebrain bundle. After behavioral assessment of the lesion, rats were allocated to balanced groups according to their amphetamine rotation scores. Prior to grafting, the ipsilateral striatum was injected with either the Shh, GDNF or LacZ vectors. A control group received an injection of saline. Two wk post-injection of the vectors (allowing time for the transgenes to switch on and any post-surgical trauma to subside), rats received a standard E14 VM graft into the same striatum. To allow for possible effects of Shh or GDNF expression on the lesioned DA system, control groups without a dopamine graft were also included (Fig. 14).

All graft groups showed a reduction in post-lesion amphetamine rotation and showed the over compensatory rotation in the contralateral direction that are associated with good grafts (Fig. 15). Though there were no differences in the graft induced rotational response between graft groups. Conversely, non-grafted groups showed no amelioration of the rotational deficit, whether or not they had received injections of RAD/Shh or RAD/GDNF alone, indicating that neither vector was able to effect the rescue of intrinsic dopamine cells or their terminals from the effects of the lesion.

Post-mortem, histological examination of the brains revealed healthy grafts containing many TH positive cells in all graft groups. At the time of writing, in vivo levels of Shh and GDNF have yet to be determined but the protein product from all three vectors injected was easily detectable using immunohistochemistry (Figs. 16–18). Figure 16 shows the distribution of transgene expression surrounding a dopamine graft

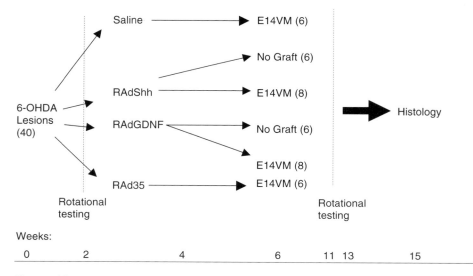

Figure 14 A schematic plan of the experiment investigating striatal delivery of AV vectors to dopamine transplants. *Abbreviation*: AV, adeno virus.

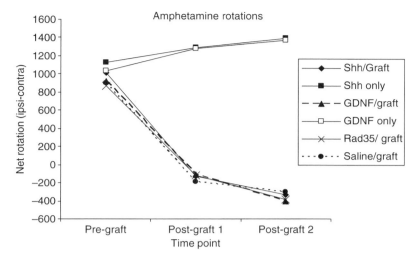

Figure 15 Rotation in rats with unilateral nigrostriatal lesions, following intrastriatal transfection with Shh or GDNF, with or without VM grafts. All grafted groups showed good recovery from the lesion-induced rotational deficit, showing over the over-compensation (rotation in the opposite direction rather than dropping to zero) that is typical of good grafts. However there were no significant differences in the graft-induced recovery between Shh-treated and GDNF-treated groups, whether grafted or not. *Abbreviations*: VM, ventral mesencephalon; GDNF, glial cell derived neurotrophic factor; Shh, sonic hedgeheg.

in an animal from the RAd35-graft group. Image analysis of the grafts revealed no significant differences between graft volume or TH cell numbers between groups.

Our results show that RAd vectors can be used to deliver transgene products to dopaminergic grafts using the method of prior transduction of the host striatum and that the transduced striatum is a permissive environment for dopamine transplantation. The

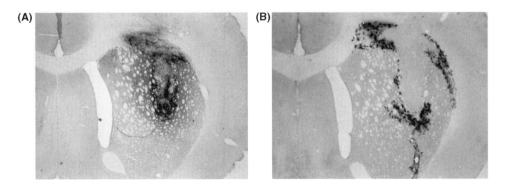

Figure 16 Adjacent sections of rat brain from the Rad35 graft group stained for TH and β-galactosidase. (**A**) TH stained section typical of the grafts seen in all groups showing numerous positive cells with processes extending within the graft and into the surrounding striatum. (**B**) β-galactosidase stained section, in which the graft is seen as a large, unstained volume mainly in the dorsal striatum and overlying corpus callosum. β-galactosidase staining can be clearly seen in both striatum and corpus callosum in close proximity with the graft. In the RAd/SHH and RAd/GDNF graft groups such an arrangement bring the grafted tissue into intimate contact with potentially beneficial transgene products. *Abbreviation*: TH, tyroisine hydroxylase.

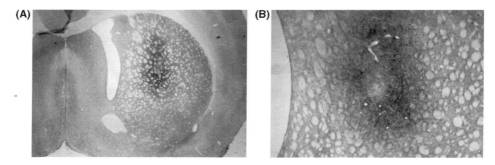

Figure 17 (**A**) GDNF expression in the striatum following RAd/GDNF injections. Dense immunoreactivity surrounds a small section of graft in a brain from the GDNF/Graft group. (**B**) Shh expression surrounding a graft in a section from an animal in the Shh/Graft group. Unlike GDNF, Shh staining shows immunoreactive cell bodies as well as diffuse staining of the striatal parenchyma. *Abbreviations*: GDNF, glial cell derived neurotrophic factor; Shh, sonic hedgehog.

diffusible factors Shh and GDNF were detectable immunohistochemically in the striatum surrounding the grafts 13 wk following vector injection indicating that the window of possible therapy is extensive. However, there was no detectable effect of any virus treatment on graft survival. A number of possible explanations could be proposed. Firstly, the levels of GDNF and Shh produced by transduction may have been insufficient. Secondly, the levels of variability in graft size within groups was large. Thirdly, the age of embryo from which dopaminergic cells were obtained may be too old. Certainly the differentiation factor Shh is likely to have its effect at a younger age of dopamine cell development. Experiments are now underway to address the levels of transgene product expression and the effects of this method of treatment on grafts of different embryonic ages.

DOPAMINE REPLACEMENT USING LENTIVIRAL VECTORS

Lentiviral (LV) vectors are derived from a group of highly pathogenic retroviruses, which includes the human immunodeficiency virus HIV. They share the useful properties of the commonly used oncoretroviral vectors, with the additional advantage that the LV vectors can infect both dividing and non-dividing cells. They have a large cloning

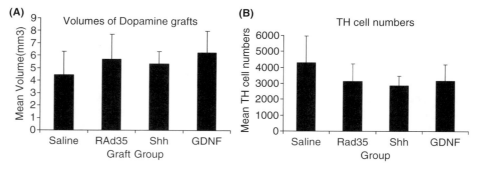

Figure 18 There were no significant differences in (**A**) mean graft volumes and (**B**) TH cell numbers between groups.

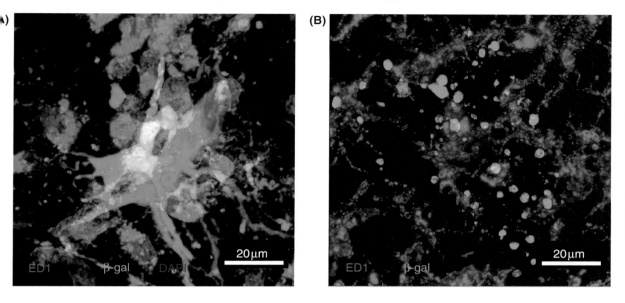

Figure 1.1 Innate immune responses. *(See p. 5)*

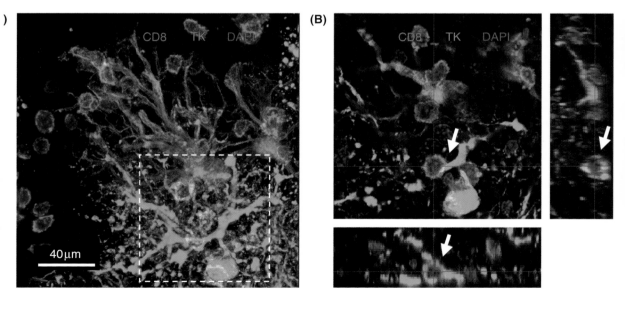

Figure 1.2 Adaptive immune responses. *(See p. 7)*

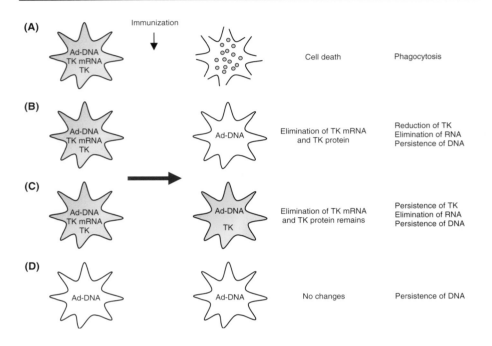

(A) Immunization → Cell death / Phagocytosis

(B) Elimination of TK mRNA and TK protein / Reduction of TK, Elimination of RNA, Persistence of DNA

(C) Elimination of TK mRNA and TK protein remains / Persistence of TK, Elimination of RNA, Persistence of DNA

(D) No changes / Persistence of DNA

Figure 1.3 The loss of transgene expression from the CNS following the systemic immunization against adenovirus. *(See p. 9)*

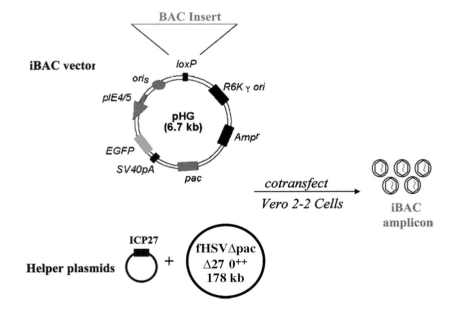

Figure 5.2 HSV-1 amplicon production scheme. *(See p. 63)*

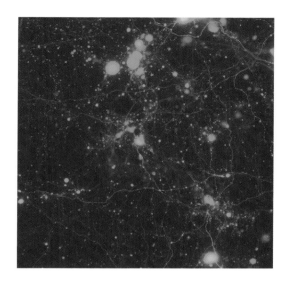

Figure 5.3 Cultured mouse cortical neurons infected with an empty iBAC vector. *(See p. 66)*

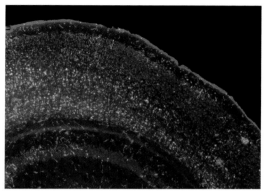

Figure 6.4 GFP expression after in utero AAV1-mediated delivery of Cre recombinase in Z/EG mice. *(See p. 87)*

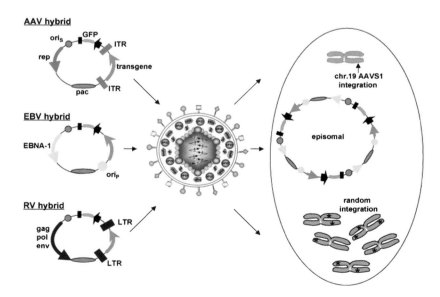

Figure 6.2 Structures and properties of HSV-1 amplicon-based hybrid vectors. *(See p. 78)*

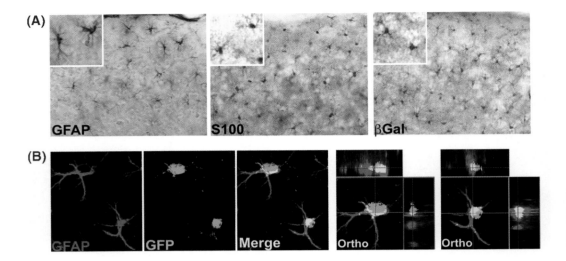

Figure 7.1 Astrocytes are effectively targeted in GFAP-Cre mice. *(See p. 107)*

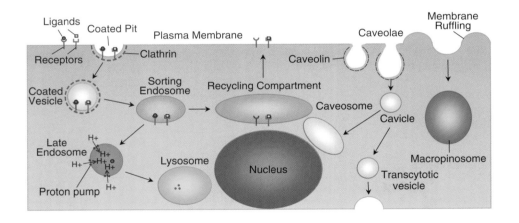

Figure 8.5 Endocytic pathways. *(See p. 122)*

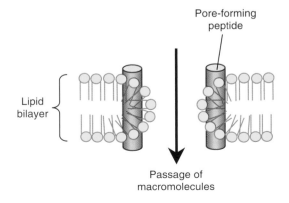

Figure 8.6 Endosomal escape via pore formation. *(See p. 125)*

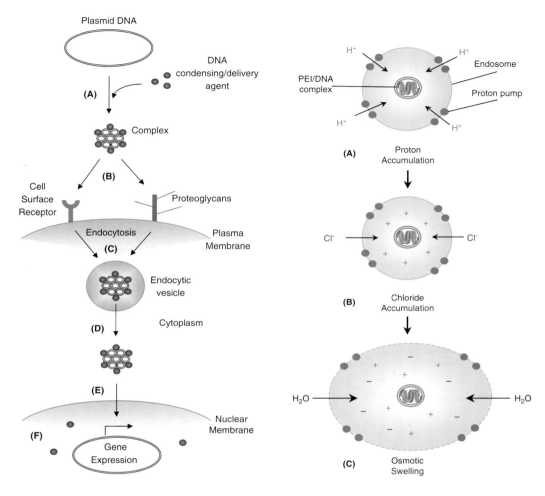

Figure 8.3 Non-viral gene transfer vector hurdles. *(See p. 118)*

Figure 8.8 Endosomolysis via proton sponge. *(See p. 127)*

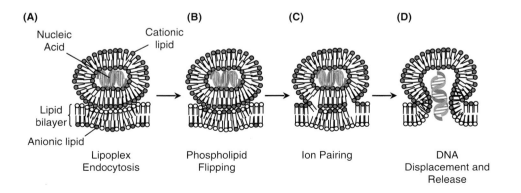

Figure 8.7 Endosomolysis via flip-flop. *(See p. 126)*

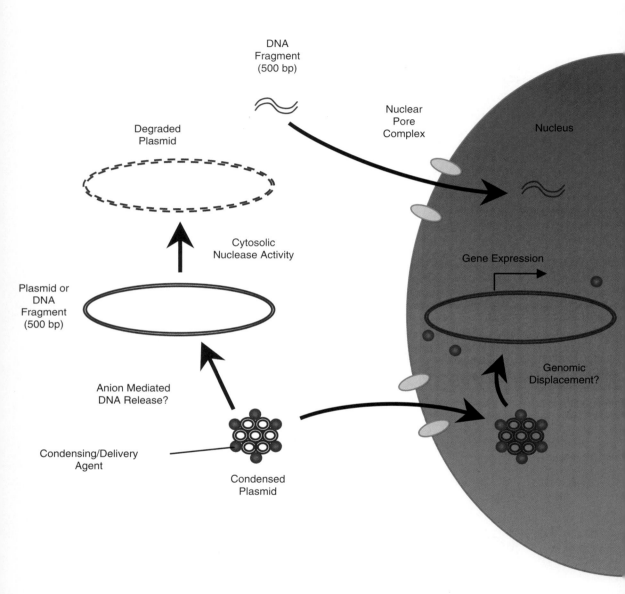

DNA
Fragment
(500 bp)

Degraded
Plasmid

Nuclear
Pore
Complex

Nucleus

Cytosolic
Nuclease Activity

Plasmid or
DNA
Fragment
(500 bp)

Gene Expression

Anion Mediated
DNA Release?

Genomic
Displacement?

Condensing/Delivery
Agent

Condensed
Plasmid

Figure 8.9 Intracellular fates of DNA after endosome escape. *(See p. 128)*

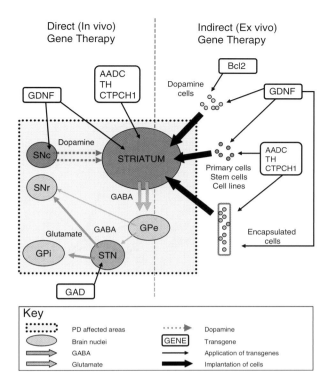

Figure 9.1 Parkinson's Disease affected brain areas and targets for gene therapeutic approaches. *(See p. 143)*

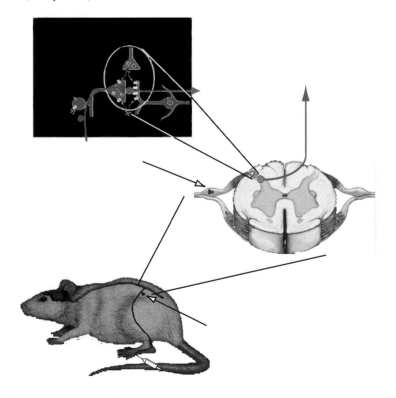

Figure 10.1 Strategy for HSV-mediated gene transfer in the treatment of chronic pain. *(See p. 188)*

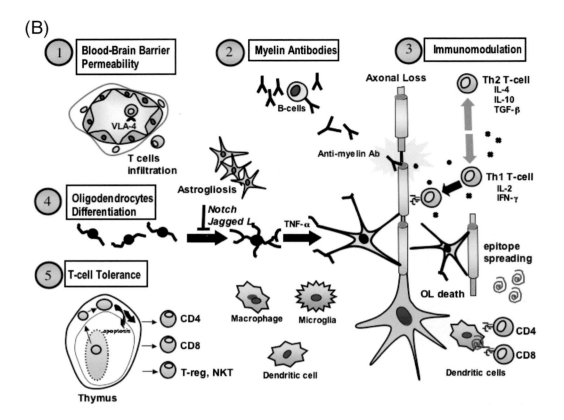

Figure 12.1B Five major targets for therapy in Multiple Sclerosis. *(See p. 217)*

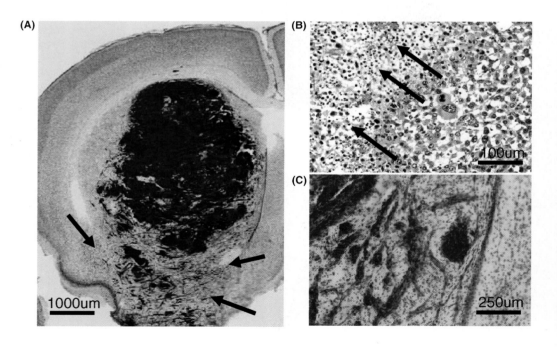

Figure 13.2 CNS–1 tumor histology. *(See p. 246)*

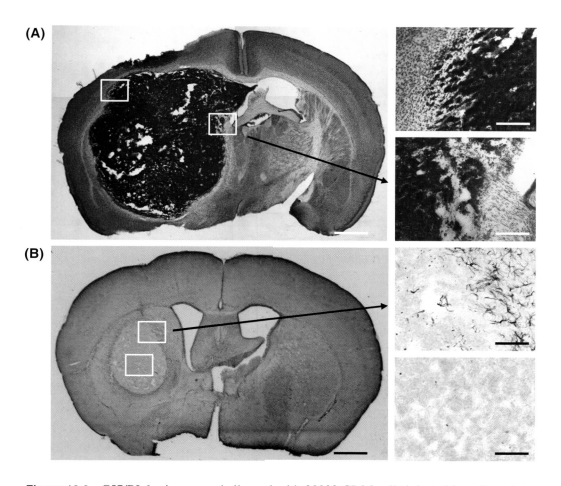

Figure 13.3 C57/BL6 mice were challenged with 20000 GL26 cells injected into the striatum. *(See p. 247)*

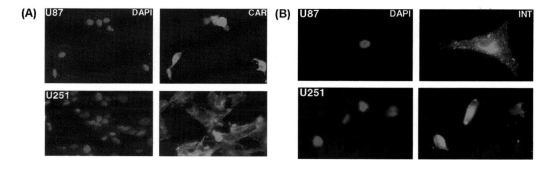

Figure 13.4 Expression of adenoviral receptors in human glioma cells. *(See p. 251)*

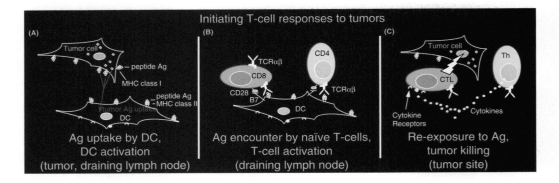

Figure 14.2 Initiating T-cell responses to tumors. *(See p. 269)*

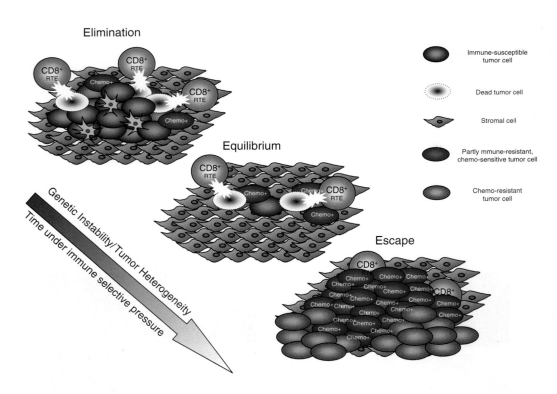

Figure 14.8 The immunoediting model in the context of glioma-immune dynamics. *(See p. 280)*

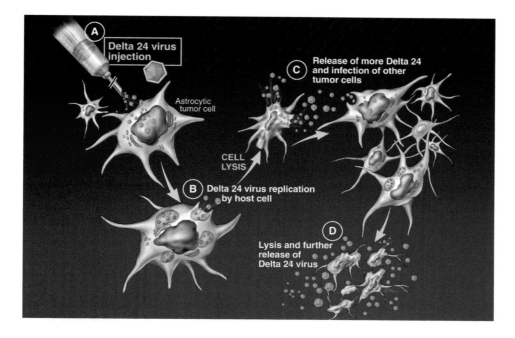

Figure 15.1 Inoculation and spread of oncolytic adenoviruses, such as Delta-24, in cancer cells. *(See p. 294)*

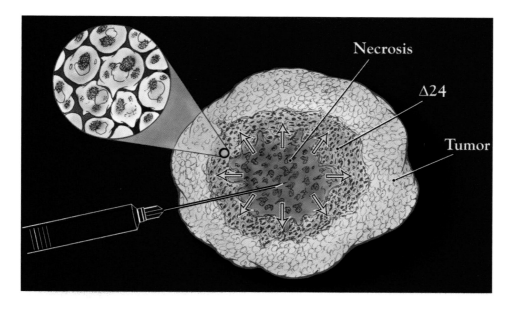

Figure 15.3 Schematic illustration of the predicted spread pattern of Delta-24 within treated gliomas. *(See p. 299)*

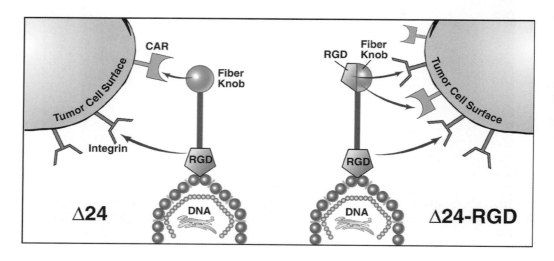

Figure 15.4 CAR-independent infection by Delta-24-RGD. (*See p. 306*)

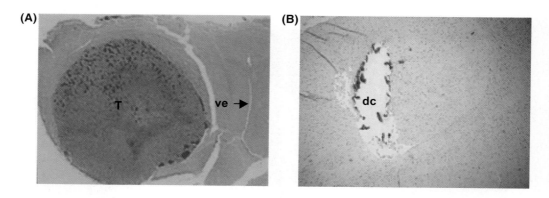

Figure 15.5 Histopathologic examination of the brains of Delta-24-RGD-treated mice. (*See p. 306*)

capacity, at least 9 kb, and are stably integrated into the genome of the target cells, properties that are favorable for long-term expression of transgenes in the nervous system (114). There are inevitable safety concerns regarding the use of lentiviral vectors, particularly those that are HIV derived. Chief among these is the possibility of reversion to replication competent forms (115). However, in this regard LV vectors are not very different from any other potential viral vector and can be attenuated to obtain replication-defective, non-pathogenic vectors. HIV-1-based lentiviral vectors have been used with success for gene transfer into the primate central nervous system (CNS). Kordower and colleagues (116) recently showed that a lentiviral vector encoding GDNF could protect TH-positive neurons and preserve dopaminergic terminals in MPTP and aged monkeys. In another study, a multiply-attenuated, self-inactivating LV vector containing a GDNF gene was successfully used to protect against the effects of a 6-OHDA lesion in a mouse model of PD (117).

Because of the concerns surrounding the use of HIV-based vectors, systems that are non-pathogenic in humans, such as those based on equine or feline LV, are particularly attractive candidates for clinical use (118–121). Our laboratory has been collaborating with Oxford Biomedica (UK) in the evaluation of an equine LV-based vector for possible use in the treatment of PD. The vector is derived from equine infectious anaemia virus (EIAV), which is non pathogenic in humans. The vector is multiply attenuated and self-inactivating. Azzouz and colleagues (2000d) have used a tricistronic self-inactivating EIAV vector (EIAV/DA) expressing TH, AADC GTPCH1 in a single transcription unit to achieve functional improvement in the rat hemi-Parkinsonian model. They showed a significant reduction in the number of turns of apomorphine-induced motor asymmetry (32). More recently they have demonstrated neuroprotection in a rat model of PD using an EIAV/GDNF vector (32). Following the demonstration of efficacy of the tricistronic dopamine replacement vector (EIAV/DA) in ameliorating drug-induced rotation, we attempted to investigate the effects of the vector using a wider range of behavioral tests for parkinsonian deficits. Rats received a unilateral 6-OHDA lesion of the median forebrain bundle and were tested post-lesion using amphetamine and apomorphine induced rotation.

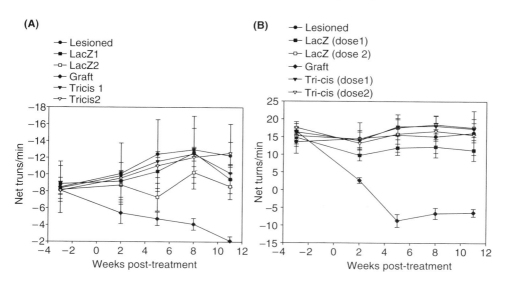

Figure 19 Drug-induced rotations. (**A**) Apomorphine-induced rotations and (**B**) amphetamine-induced rotations.

Only animals showing at least 7 net turns/min with amphetamine and 3 net turns/min with apomorphine were included in the study (38 in total). Rats were divided into 6 matched groups based on their rotation scores as follows: A lesion only group, two EIAV/DA groups (EIAV/DA1; 12×10^6 TU and EIAV/DA2; 24×10^6 TU), two matched control vector groups (EIAV/LacZ1;12×10^6 TU and EIAV/ LacZ2;24×10^6 TU) and a positive control group that received a standard E14 VM dopamine graft.

All rats underwent rotational testing at an interval of 3 wk post surgery. They were also tested on a range of motor tests including the staircase (paw-reaching), rotarod, and cylinder tests. The grafted group was the only group of animals to show an amelioration of rotational deficit (Fig. 19). EIAV/DA had no apparent effect on amphetamine-induced rotations, and neither were we able to reproduce the effect on apomorphine rotations obtained by Azzouz and colleagues. In addition, none of the treatments was able to ameliorate the lesion induced motor deficits measured using stepping and cylinder tests (data not shown).

The lack of efficacy of the EIAV/DA was puzzling. Post-mortem analysis of brain sections stained for the neuronal marker NeuN revealed no obvious damage or toxicity induced by the vectors (Fig. 20). β-galactosidase histochemistry showed that there was good expression from the EIAV/LacZ vector in the striatum, the cortex and SNr, indicating transport of either the protein or the virus in both retrograde (Fig. 21A) and anterograde (Fig. 21B) directions. TH and AADC histochemistry showed expression of transgene in brains injected with the tricistronic vector though this was weaker than that seen with for β-galactosidase (Fig. 22). Unlike the expression pattern seen with EIAV/LacZ, expression of TH and AADC in the cortex or the SNr was not seen.

The number of TH-positive cells in the groups injected with the low and high doses of the EIAV/DA vector and the grafted group are shown in Figure 23. There was a difference in cell numbers between the two doses of vectors. Perhaps the most striking result though was that the number of cells expressing TH in the high dose group and in the grafted group were in the same range. Analysis of variance confirmed that the mean number of cells in the high dose group was significantly different to that in the low dose group ($F_{2,14} = 19.98$, $P < 0.001$) but not statistically different to the number of grafted cells. The numbers of AADC-positive cells seen were slightly higher than the numbers of TH cells. Once again there was a significant difference in cell numbers between the low and the high dose groups ($F_{1,10} = 23.36$, $P < 0.001$).

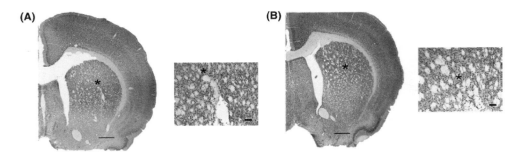

Figure 20 NeuN histochemistry. (**A**) Rat injected with EIAV/DA (high dose) shows minimal neuronal depletion at the level of the needle track. (**B**) The same animal at a more posterior level did not show any neuronal depletion or toxicity, scale bar = 1 mm. The stars show a higher magnification × 10, scale bar = 100 μm.

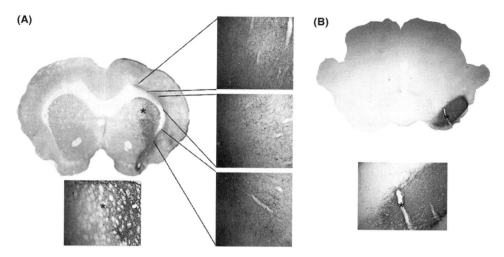

Figure 21 β-galactosidase immunohistochemistry following EIAV/LacZ. (**A**) Expression in striatum and cortex and (**B**) expression in SN pars reticulata. *Abbreviation*: SN, subthalmic nucleus.

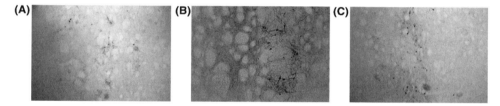

Figure 22 (**A**) TH histochemistry in rat injected with EIAV/DA (high dose). (**B**) TH histochemistry in rat grafted with E14VM. (**C**) AADC histochemistry in rat injected with EIAV/DA (high dose). *Abbreviation*: TH, tyrosine hydroxylase.

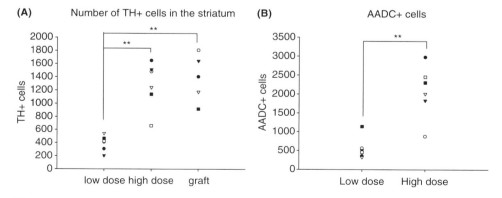

Figure 23 (**A**) Counts of TH+cells in the striatum. (**B**) Counts of AADC+cells in the striatum.

Conclusion

In our study we were able to demonstrate that EIAV vectors can produce high levels of LacZ expression in the striatum and that expression is also seen in the neocortex and anterograde (SNr) targets. Expression of genes of interest (TH and AADC) was weaker than had been reported previously by immunohistochemistry and HPLC. As a result, transgene expression was not associated with any significant improvement in behavioral recovery. This may be due to weak expression of both enzymes required for the production of DA in the striatum despite a higher titer ($\times 10$) than that used in the previous experiment. Analysis of catecholamine levels in striatal samples dissected post-mortem from animals in this study was performed using HPLC separation and electrochemical detection. Although a small increase in dopamine and DOPAC levels was observed in EIAV/DA injected animals when compared with control injected animals, this was not statistically significant. Kirik and colleagues defined a critical threshold level of L-dopa that is required to induce significant effects (122). We can only assume that in the present experiment, the levels of DA produced by the EIAV/DA vector did not reach this threshold, which might explain why no functional recovery was observed on any of the behavioral tests used. These issues are discussed in further detail in the general discussion at the end of this chapter.

GENERAL DISCUSSION

The studies carried out in our laboratory on the application of viral vector gene therapy in PD models have looked at three different viral vectors using three different therapeutic strategies and serve to illustrate both the nature of such investigations and the difficulty of the issues involved in converging on a successful therapeutic strategy.

Herpes Simplex Vectors

The HSV-based viral vectors were intended to deliver the neurotrophic factor GDNF to the hemi-Parkinsonian brain in order to protect against the effects of a subsequent 6-OHDA lesion. With one of the vectors used, a protective effect of the HSV/GDNF vector was demonstrated on the numbers of dopamine cells in the SNc, together with an associated amelioration of drug-induced turning behavior. However, the effects were variable and of relatively limited magnitude. Two major issues arise out of these experiments. First, we were unable to adequately evaluate the multiply-deleted dH1J type vectors due to the presence of toxicity, which was shown to be unrelated to viral gene expression. Second, the LAT promoter used in the HSV constructs appears to be silenced after just a few wk in vivo making it unsuitable for long term expression and sustained delivery of GDNF (97).

    The inflammation and damage caused by dH1J-HSV vectors in our studies is not typical of that seen by other workers. The method used in the production and purification of these vectors was shown to induce a level of toxicity in vivo. One theory is that the method of salt harvesting used produces virus stock containing large numbers (possibly a majority) of dead or fragmented virus particles and that, unlike the gradient purification used for the gh/tk deleted vectors, these are not removed by affinity column purification. The presence of virus-bound cellular components from the complementing cells in the preparation is also a possibility.

Despite the obvious advantages of HSV vectors in terms of tropism, transgene capacity, and the potential to establish latency, immune responses and toxicity are serious concerns that could limit the use of these vectors to treat chronic neurodegenerative disorders in humans (123,124). HSV toxicity has been linked to the host shut-off functions of some viral gene products and to the direct toxicity of others. Although recent vector modifications have made HSV vectors less toxic (125,126), the potential of the present generation of HSV vectors may be limited for gene therapy (127). Our results confirm that, under some still poorly understood conditions of vector construction, virus toxicity can be reduced into the range where therapeutic application may be acceptable. However, of greater concern, the present data also indicate that the reduction of toxicity is associated with reduction of transduction levels, which may impose an absolute limit to the feasibility of using HSV vectors for efficient gene transfer. Nevertheless, it is worth emphasizing the fact that the potential of the most deleted HSV vector may not have been seen, masked as it was by the methods of production and purification used.

The observed silencing of the LAT promoters raises the issue of which promoter will be the best to use for Parkinson's gene therapy. The processes regulating the establishment of and reactivation from latency in HSV are not well understood. Wild type infections of HSV-1 can result in the establishment of latency in neurons in which the LAT regions of the genome maintain long-term expression. It seems logical then to suppose that in an HSV-based vector, transgenes inserted into the region of the virus from which the LATs are expressed, and driven using LAT-derived promoters might effect long-term expression also. It is currently unknown which viral genes are involved in the establishment of a latent infection, but it is known that de novo viral protein synthesis is not required. Latency is related to the expression of the LAT regions of the genome, which are expressed from a promoter that is highly active in neurons. LAT expression prevents the lytic replication cycle by down-regulation of genes associated with lytic infection. Reactivation of the latent virus can be induced by different stimuli, such as stress and UV irradiation (128). Thus, it is possible that the inflammation caused by direct injection of HSV into the brain could be overriding the establishment of latency and be directing the virus down the lytic pathway, though this has yet to be demonstrated. The functions of the LATs remain unknown, although several putative roles have been suggested. These include: efficient establishment of latency (129,130), effective reactivation from latency (131–137), and prevention of apoptosis in infected neurons (138). However, it is clear that the LAT genes are not an absolute requirement for establishment, maintenance, or reactivation from latency (139–142).

The lack of a promoter that supports long-term expression in forebrain neurons has limited the utility of the HSV-based system so far. A number of viral promoters that support long-term expression in other systems do not similarly support significant levels of long-term expression from HSV-1 vectors (143). At 1 month after gene transfer into either the midbrain or striatum, HSV-1 plasmid vectors containing either the HSV-1 immediate early (IE) 4/5 promoter or the cytomegalovirus (CMV) IE promoter support expression in only a small percentage of the number of cells observed at 4 days (144–146). The Maloney murine leukaemia virus long-terminal repeat (LTR) promoter supports expression in retrovirus vectors; however, in recombinant HSV-1 vectors, this promoter supports only limited long-term expression in primary sensory neurons, and only low levels of long-term expression in forebrain neurons (147). A number of neuron-specific cellular promoters have also been examined, and the results are similar to those obtained using viral promoters. An HSV-1 plasmid vector that contains the neurofilament heavy subunit (NF-H) promoter supports high-level expression at 4 days, but expression is absent at 1 month (148). In contrast to the results with viral and neuronal-specific promoters, two promoters that are active only in specific types of neurons support significant levels of long-term expression from HSV-1 plasmid vectors (149–152). One is a vector that contains the preproenkephalin promoter and supports expression for 2 months in both the amygdala and the ventromedial hypothalamus (153). Secondly, vectors that contain either a 6.8- or a 9-kb fragment of the TH promoter can support expression for 8–10 weeks in catecholaminergic neurons of the SNc and locus coeruleus (154,155). In a very recent study, Sun and colleagues (156), have developed a helper virus-free packaging system and a promoter that supports long-term expression in forebrain neurons by adding an upstream enhancer from the TH promoter to the NF-H promoter. They have shown, in the rodent hemi-parkinsonian model, that this vector could support high-level expression of TH and AADC transgenes for up to 7 months and could improve the functional behaviour in lesioned rats.

For trophic factors such as GDNF, short-term expression may be sufficient to provide neuroprotection against acute insults (e.g., trauma, stroke, graft survival at time of implantation), including acute injection of neurotoxins such as 6-OHDA. Other studies have shown that neuroprotection could be effected in the CNS by transient HSV-mediated expression of appropriate transgenes (157–159). By contrast, protection against a chronic lesion or slowly progressive neurodegenerative disease is likely to require more long-term stability and, for clinical safety, regulated expression. So, despite their potential advantages, HSV-based vectors are still problematic for therapeutic application both in terms of levels and duration of expression and of toxicity.

Adenoviral Vectors

Our work to evaluate the potential of recombinant AV-based vectors to deliver differentiation and trophic factors to embryonic dopamine grafts used an approach aimed at improving the yield of dopamine cells within the grafts. An important issue arising from these studies was the "tropism" of the adenoviral vectors used. While the RAds were capable of transducing cells in rat striatum and of expressing a number of different transgenes, almost all the transduced cells seen were glial. In vitro, the transduction efficiency was low and the expression seen was similarly, predominantly glial. Adenoviral vectors are known to be able to infect a wide range of cell types in the CNS, including neurons (160). The restriction of gene expression to glia in our studies is probably due to preferred activation of the CMV promoters in these cells. Retrograde transport has been reported with adenoviral vectors using and Rous sarcoma virus (RSV) promoter (161). The lack of expression in neurons presents a problem for the application of these vectors directly to embryonic dopamine cells, particularly for the delivery of transcription factors that will require transduction of the target cells. On the other hand, for diffusable factors such as GDNF and Shh, glial transduction may be sufficient for the delivery of these factors to develope dopamine cells in a neural transplant. A recent study by collaborators successfully used an RAd/CMV/Shh construct to protect against the effects of a 6-OHDA lesion (162).

Initial experiments demonstrated clearly that the in vivo dynamics of AV vectors were affected by the presence of a 6-OHDA lesion, transducing greater numbers of cells than in the unlesioned brain and causing gene expression in areas outside the targeted area (105). This is an important finding, which may have implications for all directly administered gene therapies. The uptake and diffusion of any type of injected viral vector is likely to be affected by a number of different parameters. The density of the target nucleus injected and the local topography of neurons, glia, nerve terminals, axon bundles, blood vessels and ventricles, will all affect the distribution of the vectors post-injection.

That the local environment can be altered by the disease process is evident. A 6-OHDA lesion of the median forebrain bundle not only removes dopamine axons and terminals from the striatum but also induces striatal up-regulation of astrocytes and microglia for up to 4 months post-lesion (163–166). Whether this results in the striatum being more or less permissive to virus particle diffusion, or whether there are changes in the number of virus binding sites available is not known. Whatever the physical or chemical causes of altered transgene expression, it is clear that the knowledge to be gained from injections of viral vectors into normal brain is limited and pre-clinical evaluation will need to be carried out in animal models that mimic as closely as possible the pathological conditions of the disease under study.

The experiment in which host striatum was transduced with RAds prior to implantation of a dopamine graft, while demonstrating no detectable functional effects, was nonetheless highly informative. Transgene products from all three of the vectors used were detectable in the host striatum, surrounding and in intimate contact with the dopamine grafts. Following injection of the GDNF and Shh containing vectors, these diffuseable factors were also detected immunohistochemically within the graft tissue. As yet we can only hypothesize on the failure of effect on dopamine cell survival in these grafts. It is possible that the age of the donor tissue used (E14) was too old. Certainly we might expect the maximal effect of Shh to occur at younger ages (167–169). GDNF, on the other hand, has previously been shown to improve the survival of dopamine grafts derived from E14 embryos (60,170–172). It may be that the dose of GDNF needed is higher than that delivered by the RAd/GDNF.

When considering the appropriate dosage for trophic factors it is worth considering that too much GDNF may have a detrimental effect. Georgievska and colleagues used a lentiviral vector to deliver GDNF to the rat striatum 4 weeks prior to a unilateral 6-OHDA lesion (173). GDNF expression in the striatum was seen up to 9 months after injection and was successful in protecting the dopamine neurons of the SNc from the effects of the lesion. However in another experiment, long-term GDNF expression was found to be associated with a down-regulation of TH expression in the striatum, and aberrant sprouting of nerve terminals in areas afferent to the striatum (174). It is perhaps not surprising that unregulated over-expression of GDNF in the brain should have effects beyond those initially intended. Nevertheless it highlights the fact that dosage and longevity of expression of transgenes in the brain is an important issue and one which will need addressing for any potential gene therapy.

Transport of the injected vectors or their transgene product away from the site of injection into areas of the brain unaffected by the disease must also be considered. In our experience HSV-based vectors are retrogradely transported from the site of injection. For example, following striatal injection of HSV, the highest numbers of transduced cells are seen in the cortex and SNc. Thus, gene therapy using these or any other retrogradely transported vector will need to consider the effects of transgene expression in areas projecting to the site of injection as well as in the target area itself. Conversely, because of their glial tropism, the RAd vectors studied avoid the problem of retrograde effects. While it is possible that these virus particles may still be taken up into nerve terminals and transported back to the projecting nuclei, it seems that the CMV promoter used in these constructs is inactive in such circumstances and we found no evidence of transgene expression in any area of the brain outside the immediate site of injection using RAd vectors. The suitability of the CMV promoters used in the AV vectors for long term expression in vivo has yet to be assessed. We have observed expression for up to 3 months with no sign of down-regulation of the promoter elements. The present promoters are probably adequate for pre-clinical studies but, once again, regulatable promoters should be considered for human applications.

Adenovirus-based and HSV-based viral vectors were among the first considered for CNS gene therapy and it is clear that many issues pertaining to their use remain unresolved. It is likely that more recently developed vectors, such as those derived from LV or AAV, may present fewer issues of toxicity and stable expression, and in the long term may prove more tractable. Certainly, these vectors are already at a more advanced stage of development than their predecessors (175). This view has been given support from several recent studies of their utility in vivo (114,176–181).

Lentiviral Vectors

Our experiments with the tricistronic lentiviral vector demonstrated that the transduction efficiency of these vectors is high, as shown previously, and detectable levels of all three transgene products were seen. The TH, AADC, and GTPCH1 transgenes used have been proposed as minimal set necessary for replacing dopamine-production by neurons (32,182,183). However, contrary to work carried out in other laboratories and despite detectable levels of transgene expression post-mortem, no functional efficacy was demonstrated in our experiments, The precise reasons for this are unclear. One hypothesis is that the levels of striatal dopamine produced in our study were not sufficient to reduce the behavioural supersensitivity in these animals, a necessary requirement for functional recovery on the apomorphine-induced rotation test. In previous work, (32) the number of transduced cells was two or three times that seen in our study (5000 ± 700 vs 2076 ± 289 AADC-positive cells and 4800 ± 400 vs 1281 ± 145 TH-positive cells) and in a transplant of primary dopaminergic VM neurons these numbers are more than sufficient to reverse a similar rotation asymmetry (184). Another explanation could be a difference between the mechanisms of DA release i.e., regulated synaptic DA release from dopaminergic transplanted neurons versus unregulated DA release from striatal neurons that could affect efficacy (185). The tricistronic vector relies on IRES sequences to produce expression from three transgenes using a single promoter. However, gene expression from an IRES sequence is lower than that seen from the initial promoter and reduces with each IRES in the sequence (186). Thus, it may be that the sequence of transgenes is important for controlling the levels of dopamine synthesis and that the Azzouz construct (AADC/TH/GTPCH1) is simply more potent than the one used in the current work (TH/AADC/GTPCH1). In culture experiments with non-catecholaminergic cell lines DA levels were higher with latter construct. However in striatal primary neurons DA production was lower implying possible regulation of transgene expression in certain cell types. (data not shown).

Lentiviruses may yet have great potential for PD gene therapy. They have a number of advantages in being able to integrate into non-dividing cells, with a large carrying capacity and the ability for stable integration into the genome of the target cells. In the current generation of vectors, the particles are pseudotyped with the G envelope protein of the vesicular stomatitis virus (VSV-G) that gives the vector the capacity to infect a broad range of tissues, including the nervous system, and is responsible for their high affinity for fully differentiated neurons within the CNS (187–190). The level of expression in the brain may be further increased by the introduction of the woodchuck promoter regulatory element (WPRE) into the vector construct (191,192). The VSV-G pseudotyped LV vectors are highly efficient in transducing cells in both striatum and substantia nigra, and in both sites the majority of the transduced cells are neurons (32,193–197). Moreover, in the striatum, stable expression of reporter genes has been observed for up to 1 yr (198) without any signs of toxicity or adverse inflammatory reaction in the host tissue (199).

There have been a number of encouraging studies using LV vectors containing a GDNF transgene (32,117,200–204). However, there are important issues related to the level and site of expression of the transgene. It has been shown, for example, that GDNF can have a negative effect when sustained expression levels are high, resulting in down regulation of the expression of TH (205,206). So, as with other vector systems, the development of vector constructs in which transgene expression is switchable may be necessary for clinical application. For such purposes, regulatable promoters such as the tetracycline-based systems have been explored with some success (28,207–209).

The potential of LV has been further demonstrated in the CNS by their use in the creation of models of neurodegenerative disease. A lentivirus expressing mutated human huntingtin protein with extended glutamine repeats was introduced into rat striatal neurons to produce a model of Huntington's disease pathology (210). In another study a lentivirus expressing human wild-type or mutated human a-synuclein has been used to transduce rat nigral dopamine neurons as a model of PD (211,212).

CONCLUSION

The brief assessment outlined in this chapter, of the potential of gene therapy for the treatment of PD has been very much from the perspective of the neuroscientist rather than that of the virologist and the development of the optimal vector or vectors lies very firmly in the hands of the latter. From the position of the former, it would be fair to say that of the three vectors types under study in our laboratory, LV currently looks to be the most promising for clinical purposes though issues of safety remain, particularly the use of HIV derived vectors in humans. Another issue and one which is common to all vector systems, is the regulation and control of transgene expression, and those responsible for authorizing the use of gene therapies for clinical use are very likely to insist on switchable gene promoters. The strength of adenoviral vectors resides in their being non-toxic and having a proven ability to express transgenes at high levels and for long periods in the CNS. The tropism seen in the current work is almost certainly promoter related, and a new generation of "gutless" adenoviruses, containing no viral DNA coding sequences at all, holds great hope for the future for these vectors. As for HSV based vectors, their affinity for the mammalian nervous system remains a major point in their favor as does their ability to establish latent infection within the host. The problems of promoter shutdown and processing toxicity that we have experienced need to be conquered but these vectors remain firmly in contention for gene therapy purposes.

Ultimately, the choice of the vector system will depend on the genes to be delivered and the treatment strategy to be employed. Indeed, the choice of strategy may turn out to be just as difficult. For example, controlled delivery of GDNF as a preventative therapy to halt the degeneration of the dopamine system (if achievable) would seem to be a most desirable therapy. However, clinical intervention will need to be early on in the disease process, when patients are still responsive to conventional L-DOPA therapy and the ethical and regulatory issues surrounding the use of invasive treatments on such patients is likely to be a considerable hurdle. Conversely, the dopamine replacement strategy, while very much an "end stage" reparative approach and therefore seemingly the second choice therapy, may have an easier route into the clinic precisely because the balance between risk and clinical need is easier to assess.

Parkinson's gene therapy is still new and much has been learned already. Few of the problems arising seem insurmountable and as our knowledge increases, a future therapy draws ever closer. However, for the moment at least, a gene therapy for PD while not an imminent reality, remains a tantalizing prospect.

ACKNOWLEDGMENTS

The authors extend grateful thanks to our collaborators in this work:. Dr. Stacey Efstathiou and Dr. C. Scarpini at the University of Cambridge; Dr. N. Mazarakis and Dr. M. Azzouz of Oxford Biomedica and Dr. P Loudon and Dr. K Howard, formerly of Cantab Pharmaceuticals.

REFERENCES

1. Carlsson A, Lindqvist M, Magnusson T. 3,4-Dihydroxyphenylalanine and 5-hydroxytryptophan as reserpine antagonists 1. Nature 1957; 180:1200.
2. Zigmond MJ, Abercrombie ED, Stricker EM. Partial damage to nigrostriatal bundle: compensatory changes and the action of L-dopa 6. J Neural Transm 1990;217–232.
3. Marsden CD, Parkes JD. "On-off"effects in patients with Parkinson's disease on chronic levodopa therapy 152. Lancet 1976; 1:292–296.
4. Schuh LA, Bennett JP, Jr. Suppression of dyskinesias in advanced Parkinson's disease. I. Continuous intravenous levodopa shifts dose response for production of dyskinesias but not for relief of parkinsonism in patients with advanced Parkinson's disease 13. Neurology 1993; 43:1545–1550.
5. Albin RL, Young AB, Penney JB. The functional anatomy of basal ganglia disorders 20. Trends Neurosci 1989; 12:366–375.
6. Zigmond MJ, Stricker EM. Recovery of feeding and drinking by rats after intraventricular 6-hydroxydopamine or lateral hypothalamic lesions 3. Science 1973; 182:717–720.
7. Ungerstedt U. Striatal dopamine release after amphetamine or nerve degeneration revealed by rotational behaviour. Acta Physiol Scand 1971; 367:49–68.
8. Ungerstedt U. Postsynaptic supersensitivity after 6-hydroxy-dopamine induced degeneration of the nigro-striatal dopamine system 10. Acta Physiol Scand 1971; 367:69–93.
9. Hantraye P, Brownell AL, Elmaleh D, et al. Dopamine fiber detection by [11C]-CFT and PET in a primate model of parkinsonism 19. Neuroreport 1992; 3:265–268.
10. Bankiewicz KS, Oldfield EH, Chiueh CC, Doppman JL, Jacobowitz DM, Kopin IJ. Hemiparkinsonism in monkeys after unilateral internal carotid artery infusion of 1-methyl-4-phenyl-1,2,3,6-tetrahydropyridine (MPTP) 36. Life Sci 1986; 39:7–16.
11. Bergman H, Wichmann T, DeLong MR. Reversal of experimental parkinsonism by lesions of the subthalamic nucleus 7. Science 1990; 249:1436–1438.
12. Laitinen LV, Bergenheim AT, Hariz MI. Leksell's posteroventral pallidotomy in the treatment of Parkinson's disease 49. J Neurosurg 1992; 76:53–61.
13. Okun MS, Vitek JL. Lesion therapy for Parkinson's disease and other movement disorders: update and controversies 1. Mov Disord 2004; 19:375–389.
14. Limousin P, Pollak P, Benazzouz A, et al. Effect of parkinsonian signs and symptoms of bilateral subthalamic nucleus stimulation 17. Lancet 1995; 345:91–95.
15. Benabid AL. Deep brain stimulation for Parkinson's disease 2. Curr Opin Neurobiol 2003; 13:696–706.

16. Betchen SA, Kaplitt M. Future and current surgical therapies in Parkinson's disease 2. Curr Opin Neurol 2003; 16:487–493.

17. Bronte-Stewart H. Parkinson's disease: surgical options. Curr Treat Options Neurol 2003; 5:131–147.

18. Dunnett SB, Bjorklund A, Lindvall O. Cell therapy in Parkinson's disease—stop or go? Nat Rev Neurosci 2001; 2:365–369.

19. Olanow CW, Freeman TB, Kordower JH. Neural transplantation as a therapy for Parkinson's disease 2. Adv Neurol 1997; 74:249–269.

20. Lindvall O, Hagell P. Cell therapy and transplantation in Parkinson's disease. Clin Chem Lab Med 2001; 39:356–361.

21. Peschanski M. 10 yr of substitution therapy for neurodegenerative diseases using fetal neuron grafts: a positive outcome but with questions for the future. J Soc Biol 2001; 195:51–55.

22. Barker RA. Repairing the brain in Parkinson's disease: where next? 35 Mov Disord 2002; 17:233–241.

23. Bjorklund A, Dunnett SB, Brundin P, et al. Neural transplantation for the treatment of Parkinson's disease 1. Lancet Neurol 2003; 2:437–445.

24. Kang UJ, Lee WY, Chang JW. Gene therapy for Parkinson's disease: determining the genes necessary for optimal dopamine replacement in rat models. Hum Cell 2001; 14:39–48.

25. Leff SE, Spratt SK, Snyder RO, Mandel RJ. Long-term restoration of striatal L-aromatic amino acid decarboxylase activity using recombinant adeno-associated viral vector gene transfer in a rodent model of Parkinson's disease. Neuroscience 1999; 92:185–196.

26. Sanchez-Pernaute R, Harvey-White J, Cunningham J, Bankiewicz KS. Functional effect of adeno-associated virus mediated gene transfer of aromatic L-amino acid decarboxylase into the striatum of 6-OHDA-lesioned rats. Mol Ther 2001; 4:324–330.

27. Mandel RJ, Rendahl KG, Snyder RO, Leff SE. Progress in direct striatal delivery of L-dopa via gene therapy for treatment of Parkinson's disease using recombinant adeno-associated viral vectors. Exp Neurol 1999; 159:47–64.

28. Kafri T, van Praag H, Gage FH, Verma IM. Lentiviral vectors: regulated gene expression. Mol Ther 2000; 1:516–521.

29. Sun M, Zhang GR, Kong L, et al. Correction of a rat model of Parkinson's disease by coexpression of tyrosine hydroxylase and aromatic amino Acid decarboxylase from a helper virus-free herpes simplex virus type 1 vector. Hum Gene Ther 2003; 14:415–424.

30. Shen Y, Muramatsu SI, Ikeguchi K, et al. Triple transduction with adeno-associated virus vectors expressing tyrosine hydroxylase, aromatic-L-amino-acid decarboxylase, and GTP cyclohydrolase I for gene therapy of Parkinson's disease. Hum Gene Ther 2000; 11:1509–1519.

31. Muramatsu S, Fujimoto K, Ikeguchi K, et al. Behavioral recovery in a primate model of Parkinson's disease by triple transduction of striatal cells with adeno-associated viral vectors expressing dopamine-synthesizing enzymes. Hum Gene Ther 2002; 13:345–354.

32. Azzouz M, Martin-Rendon E, Barber RD, et al. Multicistronic lentiviral vector-mediated striatal gene transfer of aromatic L-amino acid decarboxylase, tyrosine hydroxylase, and GTP cyclohydrolase I induces sustained transgene expression, dopamine production, and functional improvement in a rat model of Parkinson's disease. J Neurosci 2002; 22:10302–10312.

33. Bankiewicz KS, Eberling JL, Kohutnicka M, et al. Convection-enhanced delivery of AAV vector in parkinsonian monkeys; in vivo detection of gene expression and restoration of dopaminergic function using pro-drug approach. Exp Neurol 2000; 164:2–14.

34. Bjorklund A, Rosenblad C, Winkler C, Kirik D. Studies on neuroprotective and regenerative effects of GDNF in a partial lesion model of Parkinson's disease. Neurobiol Dis 1997; 4:186–200.

35. Gash DM, Zhang Z, Ovadia A, Hoffer BJ, Gerhardt GA, et al. Functional recovery in parkinsonian monkeys treated with GDNF. Nature 1996; 380:252–255.

36. Gash DM, Gerhardt GA, Hoffer BJ. Effects of glial cell line-derived neurotrophic factor on the nigrostriatal dopamine system in rodents and nonhuman primates. Adv Pharmacol 1998; 42:911–915.

37. Gash DM, Gerhardt GA, Hoffer BJ. Effects of glial cell line-derived neurotrophic factor on the nigrostriatal dopamine system in rodents and nonhuman primates. Adv Pharmacol 1998; 42:911–915.

38. Gash DM, Zhang Z, Ovadia A, et al. Functional recovery in parkinsonian monkeys treated with GDNF. Nature 1996; 380:252–255.

39. Gill SS, Patel NK, Hotton GR, et al. Direct brain infusion of glial cell line-derived neurotrophic factor in Parkinson disease. Nat Med 2003.

40. McGrath J, Lintz E, Hoffer BJ, Gerhardt GA, Quintero EM, Granholm AC. Adeno-associated viral delivery of GDNF promotes recovery of dopaminergic phenotype following a unilateral 6-hydroxydopamine lesion. Cell Transplant 2002; 11:215–227.

41. Wang Y, Tien LT, Lapchak PA, Hoffer BJ. GDNF triggers fiber outgrowth of fetal ventral mesencephalic grafts from nigra to striatum in 6-OHDA-lesioned rats. Cell Tissue Res 1996; 286:225–233.

42. Choi-Lundberg DL, Lin Q, Schallert T, et al. Behavioral and cellular protection of rat dopaminergic neurons by an adenoviral vector encoding glial cell line-derived neurotrophic factor. Exp Neurol 1998; 154:261–275.

43. Connor B. Adenoviral vector-mediated delivery of glial cell line-derived neurotrophic factor provides neuroprotection in the aged parkinsonian rat. Clin Exp Pharmacol Physiol 2001; 28:896–900.

44. Kordower JH, Emborg ME, Bloch J, et al. Neurodegeneration prevented by lentiviral vector delivery of GDNF in primate models of Parkinson's disease. Science 2000; 290:767–773.

45. Bilang-Bleuel A, Revah F, Colin P, et al. Intrastriatal injection of an adenoviral vector expressing glial-cell-line-derived neurotrophic factor prevents dopaminergic neuron degeneration and behavioral impairment in a rat model of Parkinson disease. Proc Natl Acad Sci U S A 1997; 94:8818–8823.

46. Gerin C. Behavioral improvement and dopamine release in a Parkinsonian rat model. Neurosci Lett 2002; 330:5–8.

47. Chen X, Liu W, Guoyuan Y, et al. Protective effects of intracerebral adenoviral-mediated GDNF gene transfer in a rat model of Parkinson's disease 6. Parkinsonism Relat Disord 2003; 10:1–7.

48. Natsume A, Mata M, Goss J, et al. Bcl-2 and GDNF delivered by HSV-mediated gene transfer act additively to protect dopaminergic neurons from 6-OHDA-induced degeneration 2. Exp Neurol 2001; 169:231–238.

49. Luo J, Kaplitt MG, Fitzsimons HL, et al. Subthalamic GAD gene therapy in a Parkinson's disease rat model. Science 2002; 298:425–429.

50. Lindner MD, Winn SR, Baetge EE, et al. Implantation of encapsulated catecholamine and GDNF-producing cells in rats with unilateral dopamine depletions and parkinsonian symptoms 3. Exp Neurol 1995; 132:62–76.

51. Date I, Shingo T, Yoshida H, et al. Grafting of encapsulated genetically modified cells secreting GDNF into the striatum of parkinsonian model rats 2. Cell Transplant 2001; 10:397–401.

52. Shingo T, Date I, Yoshida H, Ohmoto T. Neuroprotective and restorative effects of intrastriatal grafting of encapsulated GDNF-producing cells in a rat model of Parkinson's disease 1. J Neurosci Res 2002; 69:946–954.

53. Tseng JL, Baetge EE, Zurn AD, Aebischer P. GDNF reduces drug-induced rotational behavior after medial forebrain bundle transection by a mechanism not involving striatal dopamine. J Neurosci 1997; 17:325–333.

54. Bencsics C, Wachtel SR, Milstien S, Hatakeyama K, Becker JB, Kang UJ. Double transduction with GTP cyclohydrolase I and tyrosine hydroxylase is necessary for spontaneous synthesis of L-DOPA by primary fibroblasts. J Neurosci 1996; 16:4449–4456.

55. Chen S, Xianwen C, Dehua X, et al. Behavioral correction of Parkinsonian rats following the transplantation of immortalized fibroblasts genetically modified with TH and GCH genes 4 Parkinsonism. Relat Disord 2003; 9:S91–S97.

56. Schwarz EJ, Reger RL, Alexander GM, Class R, Azizi SA, Prockop DJ. Rat marrow stromal cells rapidly transduced with a self-inactivating retrovirus synthesize L-DOPA in vitro. Gene Ther 2001; 8:1214–1223.

57. Espejo EF, Gonzalez-Albo MC, Moraes JP, El Banoua F, Flores JA, Caraballo I. Functional regeneration in a rat Parkinson's model after intrastriatal grafts of glial cell line-derived neurotrophic factor and transforming growth factor beta1-expressing extra-adrenal chromaffin cells of the Zuckerkandl's organ. J Neurosci 2001; 21:9888–9895.

58. Cunningham LA, Su C. Astrocyte delivery of glial cell line-derived neurotrophic factor in a mouse model of Parkinson's disease. Exp Neurol 2002; 174:230–242.

59. Akerud P, Canals JM, Snyder EY, Arenas E. Neuroprotection through delivery of glial cell line-derived neurotrophic factor by neural stem cells in a mouse model of Parkinson's disease. J Neurosci 2001; 21:8108–8118.

60. Brundin P, Karlsson J, Emgard M, et al. Improving the survival of grafted dopaminergic neurons: a review over current approaches. Cell Transplant 2000; 9:179–195.

61. Kordower JH, Goetz CG, Freeman TB, Olanow CW. Dopaminergic transplants in patients with Parkinson's disease: neuroanatomical correlates of clinical recovery. Exp Neurol 1997; 144:41–46.

62. Lindvall O, Sawle G, Widner H, et al. Evidence for long-term survival and function of dopaminergic grafts in progressive Parkinson's disease. Ann Neurol 1994; 35:172–180.

63. Olanow CW, Kordower JH, Freeman TB. Fetal nigral transplantation as a therapy for Parkinson's disease. Trends Neurosci 1996; 19:102–109.

64. Dunnett SB, Hernandez TD, Summerfield A, Jones GH, Arbuthnott G. Graft-derived recovery from 6-OHDA lesions: specificity of ventral mesencephalic graft tissues. Exp Brain Res 1988; 71:411–424.

65. Lindvall O. Neural transplantation in Parkinson's disease. Novartis Found Symp 2000; 231:110–123.

66. Hagell P, Brundin P. Cell survival and clinical outcome following intrastriatal transplantation in Parkinson disease. J Neuropathol Exp Neurol 2001; 60:741–752.

67. Armstrong RJ, Hurelbrink CB, Tyers P, et al. The potential for circuit reconstruction by expanded neural precursor cells explored through porcine xenografts in a rat model of Parkinson's disease. Exp Neurol 2002; 175:98–111.

68. Jacoby DB, Lindberg C, Ratliff J, Wetzel K, Stewart GR, Dinsmore J. Comparison of fresh and cryopreserved porcine ventral mesencephalon cells transplanted in A rat model of Parkinson's disease 11. J Neurosci Res 2002; 69:382–396.

69. Lindvall O. Stem cells for cell therapy in Parkinson's disease. Pharmacol Res 2003; 47:279–287.

70. Kim JH, Auerbach JM, Rodriguez-Gomez JA, et al. Dopamine neurons derived from embryonic stem cells function in an animal model of Parkinson's disease. Nature 2002; 418:50–56.

71. Bjorklund LM, Sanchez-Pernaute R, Chung S, et al. Embryonic stem cells develop into functional dopaminergic neurons after transplantation in a Parkinson rat model. Proc Natl Acad Sci USA 2002; 99:2344–2349.

72. Kawasaki H, Mizuseki K, Sasai Y. Selective neural induction from ES cells by stromal cell-derived inducing activity and its potential therapeutic application in Parkinson's disease 23. Methods Mol Biol 2002; 185:217–227.

73. Morizane A, Takahashi J, Takagi Y, Sasai Y, Hashimoto N. Optimal conditions for in vivo induction of dopaminergic neurons from embryonic stem cells through stromal cell-derived inducing activity. J Neurosci Res 2002; 69:934–939.

74. Fawcett J, Rosser AE, Dunnet SB. Brain damage. Brain Repair. Oxford: Oxford University Press, 2001.

75. Vogel R, Amar L, Thi AD, Saillour P, Mallet J. A single lentivirus vector mediates doxycycline-regulated expression of transgenes in the brain 3. Hum Gene Ther 2004; 15:157–165.

76. Kafri T, van Praag H, Gage FH, Verma IM. Lentiviral vectors: regulated gene expression 4. Mol Ther 2000; 1:516–521.

77. Chtarto A, Bender HU, Hanemann CO, et al. Tetracycline-inducible transgene expression mediated by a single AAV vector 16. Gene Ther 2003; 10:84–94.

78. Kirik D, Rosenblad C, Bjorklund A. Characterization of behavioral and neurodegenerative changes following partial lesions of the nigrostriatal dopamine system induced by intrastriatal 6-hydroxydopamine in the rat. Exp Neurol 1998; 152:259–277.

79. Fricker RA, Barker RA, Fawcett JW, Dunnett SB. A comparative study of preparation techniques for improving the viability of striatal grafts using vital stains, in vitro cultures, and in vivo grafts. Cell Transplant 1996; 5:599–611.

80. Latchman DS, Coffin RS. Viral vectors for gene therapy in Parkinson's disease. Rev Neurosci 2001; 12:69–78.

81. Fink DJ, Glorioso J, Mata M. Therapeutic gene transfer with herpes-based vectors: studies in Parkinson's disease and motor nerve regeneration. Exp Neurol 2003; 184:S19–S24.

82. Hobbs WE, DeLuca NA. Perturbation of cell cycle progression and cellular gene expression as a function of herpes simplex virus ICP0. J Virol 1999; 73:8245–8255.

83. Krisky DM, Wolfe D, Goins WF, et al. Deletion of multiple immediate-early genes from herpes simplex virus reduces cytotoxicity and permits long-term gene expression in neurons. Gene Ther 1998; 5:1593–1603.

84. Samaniego LA, Wu N, DeLuca NA. The herpes simplex virus immediate-early protein ICP0 affects transcription from the viral genome and infected-cell survival in the absence of ICP4 and ICP27. J Virol 1997; 71:4614–4625.

85. Wu N, Watkins SC, Schaffer PA, DeLuca NA. Prolonged gene expression and cell survival after infection by a herpes simplex virus mutant defective in the immediate-early genes encoding ICP4, ICP27, and ICP22. J Virol 1996; 70:6358–6369.

86. Ozuer A, Wechuck JB, Russell B, et al. Evaluation of infection parameters in the production of replication-defective HSV-1 viral vectors. Biotechnol Prog 2002; 18:476–482.

87. Yeung SN, Tufaro F. Replicating herpes simplex virus vectors for cancer gene therapy. Expert Opin Pharmacother 2000; 1:623–631.

88. Markert JM, Parker JN, Gillespie GY, Whitley RJ. Genetically engineered human herpes simplex virus in the treatment of brain tumours. Herpes 2001; 8:17–22.

89. Cavazzana-Calvo M, Hacein-Bey S, de Saint BG, et al. Gene therapy of human severe combined immunodeficiency (SCID)-X1 disease. Science 2000; 288:669–672.

90. Check E. Regulators split on gene therapy as patient shows signs of cancer. Nature 2002; 419:545–546.

91. Nakai H, Montini E, Fuess S, Storm TA, Grompe M, Kay MA. AAV serotype 2 vectors preferentially integrate into active genes in mice. Nat Genet 2003; 34:297–302.

92. Forrester A, Farrell H, Wilkinson G, Kaye J, Davis-Poynter N, Minson T. Construction and properties of a mutant of herpes simplex virus type 1 with glycoprotein H coding sequences deleted. J Virol 1992; 66:341–348.

93. Lachmann RH, Efstathiou S. Utilization of the herpes simplex virus type 1 latency-associated regulatory region to drive stable reporter gene expression in the nervous system. J Virol 1997; 71:3197–3207.

94. Marshall KR, Lachmann RH, Efstathiou S, Rinaldi A, Preston CM. Long-term transgene expression in mice infected with a herpes simplex virus type 1 mutant severely impaired for immediate-early gene expression. J Virol 2000; 74:956–964.

95. Efstathiou S, Kemp S, Darby G, Minson AC. The role of herpes simplex virus type 1 thymidine kinase in pathogenesis. J Gen Virol 1989; 70:869–879.

96. Latchman DS, Coffin RS. Viral vectors for gene therapy in Parkinson's disease. Rev Neurosci 2001; 12:69–78.

97. Monville C, Torres E, Thomas E, et al. HSV vector-delivery of GDNF in a rat model of PD: partial efficacy obscured by vector toxicity. Brain Res 2004; 1024:1–15.

98. Barker R, Dunnett SB. Ibotenic acid lesions of the striatum reduce drug-induced rotation in the 6-hydroxydopamine-lesioned rat. Exp Brain Res 1994; 101:365–374.

99. Scarpini CG, May J, Lachmann RH, et al. Latency associated promoter transgene expression in the central nervous system after stereotaxic delivery of replication-defective HSV-1-based vectors. Gene Ther 2001; 8:1057–1071.

100. Scarpini CG, May J, Lachmann RH, et al. Latency associated promoter transgene expression in the central nervous system after stereotaxic delivery of replication-defective HSV-1-based vectors. Gene Ther 2001; 8:1057–1071.

101. Natsume A, Mata M, Goss J, et al. Bcl-2 and GDNF delivered by HSV-mediated gene transfer act additively to protect dopaminergic neurons from 6-OHDA-induced degeneration. Exp. Neurol. 2001; 169:231–238.

102. Scarpini CG, May J, Lachmann RH, et al. Latency associated promoter transgene expression in the central nervous system after stereotaxic delivery of replication-defective HSV-1-based vectors. Gene Ther 2001; 8:1057–1071.

103. Gerdes CA, Castro MG, Lowenstein PR. Strong promoters are the key to highly efficient, noninflammatory and noncytotoxic adenoviral-mediated transgene delivery into the brain in vivo. Mol Ther 2000; 2:330–338.

104. Thomas CE, Schiedner G, Kochanek S, Castro MG, Lowenstein PR. Peripheral infection with adenovirus causes unexpected long-term brain inflammation in animals injected intracranially with first-generation, but not with high-capacity, adenovirus vectors: toward realistic long-term neurological gene therapy for chronic diseases. Proc Natl Acad Sci USA 2000; 97:7482–7487.

105. Torres EM, Monville C, Lowenstein PR, Castro MG, Dunnet SB. In vivo transgene expression from an adenoviral vector is altered following a 6-OHDA lesion of the dopamine sytem. Brain Res Mol. Brain Res. 137, 1–2, 1–10.

106. Sinclair SR, Fawcett JW, Dunnett SB. Dopamine cells in nigral grafts differentiate prior to implantation. Eur J Neurosci 1999; 11:4341–4348.

107. Altman J, Bayer SA. Development of the brain stem in the rat. V. Thymidine-radiographic study of the time of origin of neurons in the midbrain tegmentum 1. J Comp Neurol 1981; 198:677–716.

108. Espejo M, Cutillas B, Arenas TE, Ambrosio S. Increased survival of dopaminergic neurons in striatal grafts of fetal ventral mesencephalic cells exposed to neurotrophin-3 or glial cell line-derived neurotrophic factor. Cell Transplant 2000; 9:45–53.

109. Mehta V, Hong M, Spears J, Mendez I. Enhancement of graft survival and sensorimotor behavioral recovery in rats undergoing transplantation with dopaminergic cells exposed to glial cell line-derived neurotrophic factor. J. Neurosurg 1998; 88:1088–1095.

110. Rosenblad C, Martinez-Serrano A, Bjorklund A. Glial cell line-derived neurotrophic factor increases survival, growth and function of intrastriatal fetal nigral dopaminergic grafts. Neuroscience 1996; 75:979–985.

111. Yurek DM. Glial cell line-dervied neurotrophic factor improves survival of dopaminergic neurons in transplants of fetal ventral mesencephalic tissue. Exp. Neurol 1998; 153:195–202.

112. Hynes M, Rosenthal A. Specification of dopaminergic and serotonergic neurons in the vertebrate CNS. Curr Opin Neurobiol 1999; 9:26–36.

113. Ye W, Shimamura K, Rubenstein JL, Hynes MA, Rosenthal A. FGF and Shh signals control dopaminergic and serotonergic cell fate in the anterior neural plate. Cell 1998; 93:755–766.

114. Bjorklund A, Kirik D, Rosenblad C, Georgievska B, Lundberg C, Mandel RJ. Towards a neuroprotective gene therapy for Parkinson's disease: use of adenovirus, AAV and lentivirus vectors for gene transfer of GDNF to the nigrostriatal system in the rat Parkinson model. Brain Res 2000; 886:82–98.

115. Castro MG, David A, Hurtado-Lorenzo A, et al. Gene therapy for Parkinson's disease: recent achievements and remaining challenges. Histol Histopathol 2001; 16:1225–1238.

116. Kordower JH, Emborg ME, Bloch J, et al. Neurodegeneration prevented by lentiviral vector delivery of GDNF in primate models of Parkinson's disease. Science 2000; 290:767–773.

117. Bensadoun JC, Deglon N, Tseng JL, Ridet JL, Zurn AD, Aebischer P. Lentiviral vectors as a gene delivery system in the mouse midbrain: cellular and behavioral improvements in a 6-OHDA model of Parkinson's disease using GDNF. Exp Neurol 2000; 164:15–24.

118. Poeschla EM, Wong-Staal F, Looney DJ. Efficient transduction of nondividing human cells by feline immunodeficiency virus lentiviral vectors. Nat Med 1998; 4:354–357.

119. Mitrophanous K, Yoon S, Rohll J, et al. Stable gene transfer to the nervous system using a non-primate lentiviral vector. Gene Ther 1999; 6:1808–1818.

120. Johnston JC, Gasmi M, Lim LE, et al. Minimum requirements for efficient transduction of dividing and nondividing cells by feline immunodeficiency virus vectors. J Virol 1999; 73:4991–5000.

121. Curran MA, Kaiser SM, Achacoso PL, Nolan GP. Efficient transduction of nondividing cells by optimized feline immunodeficiency virus vectors. Mol Ther 2000; 1:31–38.

122. Kirik D, Georgievska B, Burger C, et al. Reversal of motor impairments in parkinsonian rats by continuous intrastriatal delivery of L-dopa using rAAV-mediated gene transfer. Proc Natl Acad Sci USA 2002; 99:4708–4713.

123. Lowenstein PR, Morrison EE, Bain D, et al. Use of recombinant vectors derived from herpes simplex virus 1 mutant tsK for short-term expression of transgenes encoding cytoplasmic and membrane anchored proteins in postmitotic polarized cortical neurons and glial cells in vitro. Neuroscience 1994; 60:1059–1077.

124. Laquerre S, Goins WF, Motiuchi S, et al. Gene-transfer tool: herpes simplex virus vectors. In: Friedman T, ed. The Development of Human Gene Therapy. New York: Cold Spring Harbor Laboratory Press, 1999:173–208.

125. Glorioso JC, Goins WF, DeLuca N, Fink DJ. Development of herpes simplex virus as a gene transfer vector for the nervous system. Gene Ther 1994; 1:S39.

126. Krisky DM, Wolfe D, Goins WF, et al. Deletion of multiple immediate-early genes from herpes simplex virus reduces cytotoxicity and permits long-term gene expression in neurons. Gene Ther 1998; 5:1593–1603.

127. Samaniego LA, Neiderhiser L, DeLuca NA. Persistence and expression of the herpes simplex virus genome in the absence of immediate-early proteins. J Virol 1998; 72:3307–3320.

128. Kootstra NA, Verma IM. Gene therapy with viral vectors. Annu Rev Pharmacol Toxicol 2003; 43:413–439.

129. Perng GC, Slanina SM, Yukht A, Ghiasi H, Nesburn AB, Wechsler SL. The latency-associated transcript gene enhances establishment of herpes simplex virus type 1 latency in rabbits. J Virol 2000; 74:1885–1891.

130. Thompson RL, Sawtell NM. The herpes simplex virus type 1 latency-associated transcript gene regulates the establishment of latency. J Virol 1997; 71:5432–5440.

131. Perng GC, Zwaagstra JC, Ghiasi H, et al. Similarities in regulation of the HSV-1 LAT promoter in corneal and neuronal cells. Invest Ophthalmol Vis Sci 1994; 35:2981–2989.

132. Block TM, Deshmane S, Masonis J, Maggioncalda J, Valyi-Nagi T, Fraser NW. An HSV LAT null mutant reactivates slowly from latent infection and makes small plaques on CV-1 monolayers. Virology 1993; 192:618–630.

133. Perng GC, Ghiasi H, Slanina SM, Nesburn AB, Wechsler SL. The spontaneous reactivation function of the herpes simplex virus type 1 LAT gene resides completely within the first 1.5 kilobases of the 8.3-kilobase primary transcript. J Virol 1996; 70:976–984.

134. Drolet BS, Perng GC, Villosis RJ, Slanina SM, Nesburn AB, Wechsler SL. Expression of the first 811 nucleotides of the herpes simplex virus type 1 latency-associated transcript (LAT) partially restores wild-type spontaneous reactivation to a LAT-null mutant. Virology 1999; 253:96–106.

135. Perng GC, Slanina SM, Yukht A, et al. A herpes simplex virus type 1 latency-associated transcript mutant with increased virulence and reduced spontaneous reactivation. J Virol 1999; 73:920–929.

136. Loutsch JM, Perng GC, Hill JM, et al. Identical 371-base-pair deletion mutations in the LAT genes of herpes simplex virus type 1 McKrae and 17syn+ result in different in vivo reactivation phenotypes. J Virol 1999; 73:767–771.

137. Perng GC, Slanina SM, Ghiasi H, Nesburn AB, Wechsler SL. A 371-nucleotide region between the herpes simplex virus type 1 (HSV-1) LAT promoter and the 2-kilobase LAT is not essential for efficient spontaneous reactivation of latent HSV-1. J Virol 1996; 70:2014–2018.

138. Perng GC, Jones C, Ciacci-Zanella J, et al. Virus-induced neuronal apoptosis blocked by the herpes simplex virus latency-associated transcript. Science 2000; 287:1500–1503.

139. Ho DY, Mocarski ES. Herpes simplex virus latent RNA (LAT) is not required for latent infection in the mouse. Proc Natl Acad Sci USA 1989; 86:7596–7600.

140. Javier RT, Stevens JG, Dissette VB, Wagner EK. A herpes simplex virus transcript abundant in latently infected neurons is dispensable for establishment of the latent state. Virology 1988; 166:254–257.

141. Sedarati F, Izumi KM, Wagner EK, Stevens JG. Herpes simplex virus type 1 latency-associated transcription plays no role in establishment or maintenance of a latent infection in murine sensory neurons. J Virol 1989; 63:4455–4458.

142. Steiner I, Spivack JG, Lirette RP, et al. Herpes simplex virus type 1 latency-associated transcripts are evidently not essential for latent infection. EMBO J 1989; 8:505–511.

143. Zhang GR, Wang X, Yang T, et al. A tyrosine hydroxylase-neurofilament chimeric promoter enhances long-term expression in rat forebrain neurons from helper virus-free HSV-1 vectors. Brain Res Mol Brain Res 2000; 84:17–31.

144. During MJ, Naegele JR, O'Malley KL, Geller AI. Long-term behavioral recovery in parkinsonian rats by an HSV vector expressing tyrosine hydroxylase. Science 1994; 266:1399–1403.

145. Song S, Wang Y, Bak SY, et al. An HSV-1 vector containing the rat tyrosine hydroxylase promoter enhances both long-term and cell type-specific expression in the midbrain. J Neurochem 1997; 68:1792–1803.

146. Fraefel C, Song S, Lim F, et al. Helper virus-free transfer of herpes simplex virus type 1 plasmid vectors into neural cells. J Virol 1996; 70:7190–7197.

147. Dobson AT, Margolis TP, Sedarati F, Stevens JG, Feldman LT. A latent, nonpathogenic HSV-1-derived vector stably expresses beta-galactosidase in mouse neurons. Neuron 1990; 5:353–360.

148. Wang Y, Yu L, Geller AI. Diverse stabilities of expression in the rat brain from different cellular promoters in a helper virus-free herpes simplex virus type 1 vector system. Hum Gene Ther 1999; 10:1763–1771.

149. Kaplitt MG, Leone P, Samulski RJ, et al. Long-term gene expression and phenotypic correction using adeno-associated virus vectors in the mammalian brain. Nat Genet 1994; 8:148–154.

150. Song S, Wang Y, Bak SY, et al. An HSV-1 vector containing the rat tyrosine hydroxylase promoter enhances both longyterm and cell type-specific expression in the midbrain. J Neurochem 1997; 68:1792–1803.

151. Wang Y, Yu L, Geller AI. Diverse stabilities of expression in the rat brain from different cellular promoters in a helper virus-free herpes simplex virus type 1 vector system. Hum Gene Ther 1999; 10:1763–1771.

152. Jin BK, Belloni M, Conti B, et al. Prolonged in vivo gene expression driven by a tyrosine hydroxylase promoter in a defective herpes simplex virus amplicon vector. Hum Gene Ther 1996; 7:2015–2024.

153. Kaplitt MG, Leone P, Samulski RJ, et al. Long-term gene expression and phenotypic correction using adeno-associated virus vectors in the mammalian brain. Nat Genet 1994; 8:148–154.

154. Jin BK, Belloni M, Conti B, et al. Prolonged in vivo gene expression driven by a tyrosine hydroxylase promoter in a defective herpes simplex virus amplicon vector. Hum Gene Ther 1996; 7:2015–2024.

155. Song S, Wang Y, Bak SY, et al. An HSV-1 vector containing the rat tyrosine hydroxylase promoter enhances both long-term and cell type-specific expression in the midbrain. J Neurochem 1997; 68:1792–1803.

156. Sun M, Zhang GR, Kong L, et al. Correction of a rat model of Parkinson's disease by coexpression of tyrosine hydroxylase and aromatic amino Acid decarboxylase from a helper virus-free herpes simplex virus type 1 vector. Hum Gene Ther 2003; 14:415–424.

157. During MJ, Naegele JR, O'Malley KL, Geller AI. Long-term behavioral recovery in parkinsonian rats by an HSV vector expressing tyrosine hydroxylase. Science 1994; 266:1399–1403.

158. Natsume A, Mata M, Goss J, et al. Bcl-2 and GDNF delivered by HSV-mediated gene transfer act additively to protect dopaminergic neurons from 6-OHDA-induced degeneration. Exp Neurol 2001; 169:231–238.

159. Sun M, Zhang GR, Kong L, et al. Correction of a rat model of Parkinson's disease by coexpression of tyrosine hydroxylase and aromatic amino Acid decarboxylase from a helper virus-free herpes simplex virus type 1 vector. Hum Gene Ther 2003; 14:415–424.

160. Davidson BL, Bohn MC. Recombinant adenovirus: a gene transfer vector for study and treatment of CNS diseases. Exp Neurol 1997; 144:125–130.

161. Perng GC, Slanina SM, Ghiasi H, Nesburn AB, Wechsler SL. A 371-nucleotide region between the herpes simplex virus type 1 (HSV-1) LAT promoter and the 2-kilobase LAT is not essential for efficient spontaneous reactivation of latent HSV-1. J Virol 1996; 70:2014–2018.

162. Hurtado-Lorenzo A, Millan E, Gonzalez-Nicolini V, Suwelack D, Castro MG, Lowenstein PR. Differentiation and transcription factor gene therapy in experimental parkinson's disease: sonic hedgehog and gli-1, but not Nurr-1, protect nigrostriatal cell bodies from 6-OHDA-induced neurodegeneration 1. Mol Ther 2004; 10:507–524.

163. Pasinetti GM, Hassler M, Stone D, Finch CE. Glial gene expression during aging in rat striatum and in long-term responses to 6-OHDA lesions 35. Synapse 1999; 31:278–284.

164. Rataboul P, Vernier P, Biguet NF, Mallet J, Poulat P, Privat A. Modulation of GFAP mRNA levels following toxic lesions in the basal ganglia of the rat 4. Brain Res Bull 1989; 22:155–161.

165. Sheng JG, Shirabe S, Nishiyama N, Schwartz JP. Alterations in striatal glial fibrillary acidic protein expression in response to 6-hydroxydopamine-induced denervation 34. Exp Brain Res 1993; 95:450–456.

166. Stromberg I, Bjorklund H, Dahl D, Jonsson G, Sundstrom E, Olson L. Astrocyte responses to dopaminergic denervations by 6-hydroxydopamine and 1-methyl-4-phenyl-1,2,3,6-tetrahy-dropyridine as evidenced by glial fibrillary acidic protein immunohistochemistry. Brain Res Bull 1986; 17:225–236.

167. Briscoe J, Ericson J. Specification of neuronal fates in the ventral neural tube. Curr Opin Neurobiol 2001; 11:43–49.

168. Goetz JA, Suber LM, Zeng X, Robbins DJ. Sonic Hedgehog as a mediator of long-range signaling. Bioessays 2002; 24:157–165.

169. Matsuura N, Lie DC, Hoshimaru M, et al. Sonic hedgehog facilitates dopamine differentiation in the presence of a mesencephalic glial cell line. J Neurosci 2001; 21:4326–4335.

170. Apostolides C, Sanford E, Hong E, Mendez I. Glial cell line-derived neurotrophic factor improves intrastriatal graft survival of stored dopaminergic cells. Neuroscience 1998; 83:363–372.

171. Helt CE, Hoernig GR, Albeck DS, et al. Neuroprotection of grafted neurons with a GDNF/caspase inhibitor cocktail. Exp Neurol 2001; 170:258–269.

172. Yurek DM, Fletcher-Turner A. GDNF partially protects grafted fetal dopaminergic neurons against 6-hydroxydopamine neurotoxicity. Brain Res 1999; 845:21–27.

173. Georgievska B, Kirik D, Rosenblad C, Lundberg C, Bjorklund A. Neuroprotection in the rat Parkinson model by intrastriatal GDNF gene transfer using a lentiviral vector. Neuroreport 2002; 13:75–82.

174. Georgievska B, Kirik D, Bjorklund A. Aberrant sprouting and downregulation of tyrosine hydroxylase in lesioned nigrostriatal dopamine neurons induced by long-lasting over-expression of glial cell line derived neurotrophic factor in the striatum by lentiviral gene transfer. Exp Neurol 2002; 177:461–474.

175. Finkelstein R, Baughman RW, Steele FR. Harvesting the neural gene therapy fruit. Mol Ther 2001; 3:3–7.
176. Kirik D, Rosenblad C, Bjorklund A, Mandel RJ. Long-term rAAV-mediated gene transfer of GDNF in the rat Parkinson's model: intrastriatal but not intranigral transduction promotes functional regeneration in the lesioned nigrostriatal system. J Neurosci 2000; 20:4686–4700.
177. Kirik D, Georgievska B, Burger C, et al. Reversal of motor impairments in parkinsonian rats by continuous intrastriatal delivery of L-dopa using rAAV-mediated gene transfer. Proc Natl Acad Sci USA 2002; 99:4708–4713.
178. Palfi S, Leventhal L, Chu Y, et al. Lentivirally delivered glial cell line-derived neurotrophic factor increases the number of striatal dopaminergic neurons in primate models of nigrostriatal degeneration. J Neurosci 2002; 22:4942–4954.
179. Wang L, Muramatsu S, Lu Y, et al. Delayed delivery of AAV-GDNF prevents nigral neurodegeneration and promotes functional recovery in a rat model of Parkinson's disease. Gene Ther 2002; 9:381–389.
180. Palfi S, Leventhal L, Chu Y, et al. Lentivirally delivered glial cell line-derived neurotrophic factor increases the number of striatal dopaminergic neurons in primate models of nigrostriatal degeneration. J Neurosci 2002; 22:4942–4954.
181. Kirik D, Georgievska B, Burger C, et al. Reversal of motor impairments in parkinsonian rats by continuous intrastriatal delivery of L-dopa using rAAV-mediated gene transfer. Proc Natl Acad Sci USA 2002; 99:4708–4713.
182. Kang UJ. Potential of gene therapy for Parkinson's disease: neurobiologic issues and new developments in gene transfer methodologies. Mov Disord 1998; 13:59–72.
183. Kang UJ, Lee WY, Chang JW. Gene therapy for Parkinson's disease: determining the genes necessary for optimal dopamine replacement in rat models. Hum Cell 2001; 14:39–48.
184. Brundin P, Petersen A, Hansson O. Graft survival. J Neurosurg 1999; 90:804–806.
185. Cragg SJ, Clarke DJ, Greenfield SA. Read time dynamics of of dopamine released from neuronal transplant in experimental parkinson's disease. Experimental Neurology 2000; 164(1):145–153.
186. Metz MZ, Pichler A, Kuchler K, Kane SE. Construction and characterization of single-transcript tricistronic retroviral vectors using two internal ribosome entry sites. Somat Cell Mol Genet 1998; 24:53–69.
187. Blomer U, Naldini L, Kafri T, Trono D, Verma IM, Gage FH. Highly efficient and sustained gene transfer in adult neurons with a lentivirus vector. J Virol 1997; 71:6641–6649.
188. Miyoshi H, Blomer U, Takahashi M, Gage FH, Verma IM. Development of a self-inactivating lentivirus vector. J Virol 1998; 72:8150–8157.
189. Naldini L, Blomer U, Gage FH, Trono D, Verma IM. Efficient transfer, integration, and sustained long-term expression of the transgene in adult rat brains injected with a lentiviral vector. Proc Natl Acad Sci U S A 1996; 93:11382–11388.
190. Naldini L, Blomer U, Gallay P, et al. In vivo gene delivery and stable transduction of nondividing cells by a lentiviral vector. Science 1996; 272:263–267.
191. Deglon N, Tseng JL, Bensadoun JC, et al. Self-inactivating lentiviral vectors with enhanced transgene expression as potential gene transfer system in Parkinson's disease. Hum Gene Ther 2000; 11:179–190.
192. Zufferey R, Dull T, Mandel RJ, et al. Self-inactivating lentivirus vector for safe and efficient in vivo gene delivery. J Virol 1998; 72:9873–9880.
193. Blomer U, Naldini L, Kafri T, Trono D, Verma IM, Gage FH. Highly efficient and sustained gene transfer in adult neurons with a lentivirus vector. J Virol 1997; 71:6641–6649.
194. Deglon N, Tseng JL, Bensadoun JC, et al. Self-inactivating lentiviral vectors with enhanced transgene expression as potential gene transfer system in Parkinson's disease. Hum Gene Ther 2000; 11:179–190.
195. Kordower JH, Bloch J, Ma SY, et al. Lentiviral gene transfer to the nonhuman primate brain. Exp Neurol 1999; 160:1–16.

196. Naldini L, Blomer U, Gallay P, et al. In vivo gene delivery and stable transduction of nondividing cells by a lentiviral vector. Science 1996; 272:263–267.

197. Mazarakis ND, Azzouz M, Rohll JB, et al. Rabies virus glycoprotein pseudotyping of lentiviral vectors enables retrograde axonal transport and access to the nervous system after peripheral delivery. Hum Mol Genet 2001; 10:2109–2121.

198. Bienemann AS, Martin-Rendon E, Cosgrave AS, et al. Long-term replacement of a mulated nonfunctional CNS gene: reversal of hypothalamic diabetes insipidus using an EIAU-based lentivival vector expressing arginine vasopressin. Molecular Therapy 2003; 7:588–596.

199. Blomer U, Naldini L, Kafri T, Trono D, Verma IM, Gage FH. Highly efficient and sustained gene transfer in adult neurons with a lentivirus vector. J Virol 1997; 71:6641–6649.

200. Sun B, Hui GZ, Guo LH, Reiser J. Dopaminergic trophism after intrastriatal injection of lentivirus-transferred GDNF in Parkinson rat model. Sheng Wu Hua Xue. Yu Sheng Wu Wu Li Xue. Bao. (Shanghai) 2003; 35:937–940.

201. Palfi S, Leventhal L, Chu Y, et al. Lentivirally delivered glial cell line-derived neurotrophic factor increases the number of striatal dopaminergic neurons in primate models of nigrostriatal degeneration. J Neurosci 2002; 22:4942–4954.

202. Ostenfeld T, Tai YT, Martin P, Deglon N, Aebischer P, Svendsen CN. Neurospheres modified to produce glial cell line-derived neurotrophic factor increase the survival of transplanted dopamine neurons. J Neurosci Res 2002; 69:955–965.

203. Kordower JH, Emborg ME, Bloch J, et al. Neurodegeneration prevented by lentiviral vector delivery of GDNF in primate models of Parkinson's disease. Science 2000; 290:767–773.

204. Georgievska B, Kirik D, Rosenblad C, Lundberg C, Bjorklund A. Neuroprotection in the rat Parkinson model by intrastriatal GDNF gene transfer using a lentiviral vector. Neuroreport 2002; 13:75–82.

205. Rosenblad C, Georgievska B, Kirik D. Long-term striatal overexpression of GDNF selectively downregulates tyrosine hydroxylase in the intact nigrostriatal dopamine system. Eur J Neurosci 2003; 17:260–270.

206. Georgievska B, Kirik D, Bjorklund A. Aberrant sprouting and downregulation of tyrosine hydroxylase in lesioned nigrostriatal dopamine neurons induced by long-lasting over-expression of glial cell line derived neurotrophic factor in the striatum by lentiviral gene transfer. Exp Neurol 2002; 177:461–474.

207. Kafri T. Lentivirus vectors: difficulties and hopes before clinical trials. Curr Opin Mol Ther 2001; 3:316–326.

208. Regulier E, Pereira dA, Sommer B, Aebischer P, Deglon N. Dose-dependent neuroprotective effect of ciliary neurotrophic factor delivered via tetracycline-regulated lentiviral vectors in the quinolinic acid rat model of Huntington's disease. Hum Gene Ther 2002; 13:1981–1990.

209. Regulier E, Trottier Y, Perrin V, Aebischer P, Deglon N. Early and reversible neuropathology induced by tetracycline-regulated lentiviral overexpression of mutant huntingtin in rat striatum. Hum Mol Genet 2003; 12:2827–2836.

210. de Almeida LP, Ross CA, Zala D, Aebischer P, Deglon N. Lentiviral-mediated delivery of mutant huntingtin in the striatum of rats induces a selective neuropathology modulated by polyglutamine repeat size, huntingtin expression levels, and protein length. J Neurosci 2002; 22:3473–3483.

211. Lauwers E, Debyser Z, Van Dorpe J, De Strooper B, Nuttin B, Baekelandt V. Neuropathology and neurodegeneration in rodent brain induced by lentiviral vector-mediated overexpression of alpha-synuclein. Brain Pathol 2003; 13:364–372.

212. Lo BC, Ridet JL, Schneider BL, Deglon N, Aebischer P. Alpha-Synucleinopathy and selective dopaminergic neuron loss in a rat lentiviral-based model of Parkinson's disease. Proc Natl Acad Sci USA 2002; 99:10813–10818.

10

HSV-Mediated Gene Transfer in the Treatment of Chronic Pain

Marina Mata
Department of Neurology, University of Michigan and Neurology Service, Ann Arbor VA Healthcare System, Ann Arbor, Michigan, U.S.A.

Joseph C. Glorioso
Department of Molecular Genetics and Biochemistry, University of Pittsburgh, Pittsburgh, Pennsylvania, U.S.A.

David J. Fink
Department of Neurology, University of Michigan and Neurology Service, Ann Arbor VA Healthcare System, Ann Arbor, Michigan, U.S.A.

INTRODUCTION

Acute pain, a phenomenon with which we are all familiar, is an experience with sensory and affective components that serves to warn the individual about potentially harmful stimuli in the environment. The sensory component of pain allows the individual to localize the sensation to a site on the body and identify to some extent the nature of the inciting insult. The affective component of pain, mediated by structures in the brainstem and limbic lobes of the brain, lends pain the unpleasant emotional content that is so important in making individuals withdraw from and avoid painful stimuli. Chronic pain is defined as pain persisting more than one month beyond the resolution of an acute tissue injury, or pain that persists or recurs for more than three months associated with a tissue injury that is expected to continue or progress. Unlike acute pain, chronic pain has few redeeming features. Chronic pain has been estimated to affect more than 60 million people in the United States, and the cost, to individuals in terms of suffering and lost income, and the cost to society in terms of lost productivity and requirement of care is enormous.

The anatomy of acute pain perception is well defined. Small thinly myelinated fibers and unmyelinated fibers in the peripheral nerve that serve as the primary pain sensors project from the skin and tissues to synapse in the dorsal horn of spinal cord. The principal neurotransmitter between the primary nociceptor and second order neurons in dorsal horn is glutamate. Projection neurons of the dorsal horn project ascend to sensory nuclei in the thalamus and other subcortical structures. Projections from there to sensory cortex mediate the discriminative aspects of pain perception, while projections to limbic structures mediate the affective component of the pain experience.

185

Advances over the last two decades have lead to the recognition that while many of the same neuroanatomic pathways involved in the transmission of acute pain are also involved in chronic pain, the biology of chronic pain is complex. Continuing pain over time leads to alterations in gene expression, protein composition, and distribution of receptors in primary sensory afferents, in second order neurons of dorsal horn of spinal cord, and ultimately in the organization of cortex. At each of these levels there is a possibility that selective intervention to alter sensory neurotransmission and treat chronic pain. But because a limited repertoire of neurotransmitters and second order signaling mechanisms are involved in a wide array of central and peripheral neural processes not only in nociceptive neurotransmission but in other functions as well, selective alteration of nociceptive processing by systemic administration of pharmacologic agents has proven difficult. Vector-mediated gene transfer to selected locations in nociceptive pathways provides the opportunity to selectively modulate pain processing using well-characterized peptides as therapeutic mediators.

Two major categories of chronic pain can be distinguished, on the basis of pathogenesis. Inflammatory (also referred to as nociceptive) pain occurs in response to tissue damage; release of substances in the vicinity of nociceptor nerve terminals activate the primary nociceptors and the continuous acting of these primary afferents ultimately results in the changes characteristic of chronic pain. Common examples of inflammatory pain include the pain that accompanies infection, arthritis, or bone fracture. Neuropathic pain results from damage to nerve structures in the absence of any appreciable damage to the tissue from which these nerve project. Peripheral neuropathic pain occurs in situations of injury to peripheral nerve; the most common cause of peripheral neuropathic pain in the U.S. is diabetic neuropathy, although peripheral neuropathic pain also occurs after physical damage to peripheral nerves caused by trauma, or resulting from anatomic abnormalities. Central neuropathic pain occurs after damage to central neural structures, like that after spinal cord injury or the chronic hemibody pain following thalamic stroke. Like peripheral neuropathic pain, central neuropathic pain continues in the absence of appreciable tissue damage.

Available approaches to the treatment of pain, although largely developed prior to the modern understanding of the pathogenesis of chronic pain, intervene at several levels in the pain pathway. Inflammatory pain is often effectively treated through the use of nonsteroidal anti-inflammatory drugs that act at both the periphery, to reduce peripheral inflammation, as well as in the dorsal horn of spinal cord to reduce inflammatory mediators that are released in dorsal horn and that exacerbate increased nociceptive neurotrans-mission. The electrical hyperexcitability of peripheral nerve characteristic of neuropathic pain may be ameliorated through the use of drugs that stabilize the electrical activity of neurons such as anticonvulsants (phenytoin, carbamazepine, gabapentin). Neurotrans-mission of pain impulses from the primary afferent to the second order neuron in the spinal cord may also be blocked by drugs that act as the receptors for inhibitory neurotransmitters located there. The paradigmatic example of drugs that act at inhibitory neurotransmitters are opiate drugs that, acting at endogenous opiate receptors located presynaptically on primary sensory afferents and post-synaptically on second order neurons of the spinal cord, selectively block nociceptive neurotransmission at the spinal level. In all of these cases, the action of the drug is not limited to the peripheral nerve or spinal cord, so that side effects resulting from action of the drugs on neurons in the brain or brainstem, or in non-neural tissues such as gut or bladder may cause unrelated adverse effects that limit the dose and ultimately the therapeutic efficacy of these drugs.

There are few identified genetic causes of chronic pain. Nonetheless gene transfer provides a potentially attractive alternative for the treatment of chronic pain; gene transfer vectors may be used to express short-lived peptides to modulate the transmission of painful impulses in a local fashion, while avoiding systemic side effects that oral or intrathecal delivery of the same drugs might cause. Because many of the substances that one might want to use to achieve analgesic effects are peptides with very short half-lives, so that systemic administration may not be possible while local release from transduced cells may be effective. In this chapter we will review studies of the last several years that have applied a gene transfer methodology for the treatment of chronic pain with a focus on the use of herpes simplex virus (HSV) based vectors.

ANIMAL MODELS OF CHRONIC PAIN

Animal models have been developed that recapitulate essential features of chronic inflammatory and chronic neuropathic pain. Inflammatory pain can be modeled by the injection of irritating substances such as formalin, carrageenan, or complete Freund's adjuvant (CFA) (1). The resulting pain lasts from one hour for formalin to several weeks after injection of CFA. Other models including the establishment of a mono-articular or poly-articular arthritis have also been developed. Peripheral neuropathic pain can be created by partial nerve injury produced either by a selective spinal nerve ligation, chronic constriction of the sciatic nerve, ligation of one peripheral branch of the nerve, or injection of inflammatory substances into the nerve (2). Central neuropathic pain resulting from spinal cord injury is best modeled by partial in the section of the spinal cord (3). In all of these models expression of pain can be assessed by spontaneous pain behavior, abnormal sensitivity to normally innocuous mechanical stimuli (mechanical allodynia), a lowered threshold to painful mechanical stimuli (mechanical hyperalgesia), and a lowered threshold to painful thermal stimuli (thermal hyperalgesia), all of which occur to different degrees in the different models.

CELL TRANSPLANTATION IN THE TREATMENT OF PAIN

The first studies to use gene transfer in the treatment of pain relied on an ex vivo model of gene transfer. Chromaffin cells, which naturally express and release a number of neuroactive substances involved in the pain processing pathway at the spinal level (4,5), transplanted into the lumbar subarachnoid space, reduce pain-related behavior in models of neuropathic and inflammatory pain (6,7). Other studies demonstrated that cells modified by gene transfer to secrete enkephalin, galanin, gamma amino butyric acid (GABA) or brain derived neurotrophic factor (BDNF) are able to provide an analgesic effect in a variety of relevant animal models (8–11). While this approach has the advantage that the bioactive peptide is released in the natural conformation in and does not require the hardware associated with an intrathecal pump, an inflammatory reaction to the transplanted cells and the inability to control the release of the peptides make it unlikely that this approach will be transferred into the clinic.

The same end can be achieved, without the use of cells, though in vivo gene transfer to ependymal cells. Iadarola and colleagues demonstrated that a first generation replication deficient adenoviral vector contained the coding sequence for human beta-endorphin, injected to the subarachnoid space, effectively transduces cells of the pia mater to release beta-endorphin into the CSF, resulting in an attenuation of inflammatory hyperalgesia measured as an increase in the thermal withdrawal latency in the carrageenan model of inflammatory pain in the rodent (12). Using a similar approach Watkins and coworkers more recently reported that intrathecal injection of either an adenoviral or adeno-associated viral vector coding for the anti-inflammatory cytokine IL10 reduces pain and reverses hyperalgesia in models of peripheral neuropathic pain caused by sciatic nerve inflammation or chronic constriction injury (13). This approach has obvious heuristic appeal compared to systemic administration of anti-inflammatory drugs, but the duration of the transgene-mediated effect has yet to be established, and it is not known if the long-term release of cytokines into CSF will be tolerated without difficulty.

HERPES SIMPLEX VIRUS VECTORS

An alternative to the transduction of ependymal cells is the transduction of primary sensory neuron in the DRG to achieve release of substances from the axonal terminals in the dorsal spinal cord. An advantage of this approach is that release of the bioactive substance occurs in directly in the parenchyma of the spinal cord and can be limited in rostocaudal extent by selection of the site of injection (Fig. 1). For this purpose, HSV has many characteristics that make it particularly suitable as a gene transfer vector to DRG

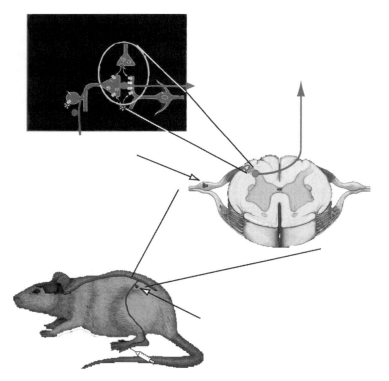

Figure 1 (*See color insert*) Strategy for HSV-mediated gene transfer in the treatment of chronic pain. Nonreplicating HSV vectors injected subcutaneously (syringe) are taken up by nerve terminals and transported to the dorsal root ganglia projecting to that site (*open arrows*). Transgene products produced by the vector may be transported to nerve terminals in the dorsal horn of spinal cord (*slice schematic*) where these peptides may act to inhibit nociceptive neurotransmission (*inset*) between the first order nociceptor and the second order neuron in the spinal cord that projects rostrally (*curved arrow*). *Source*: From Ref. 15.

(14,15). HSV is a neurotropic virus that naturally infects skin and mucous membranes, but following the initial epithelial infection viral particles are taken up by nerve terminals in the skin and carried by retrograde axonal transport to the DRG (16). Uptake and transport of the virus is a highly selective process that relies on specific interactions between viral coat glycoproteins and high affinity receptors in the nerve terminals in the skin (17,18); retrograde transport require specific interactions of capsid and tegument proteins with dynein molecules in the axoplasm to mediate the retrograde transport along microtubules to the cell body (19). The wild type virus naturally establishes a lifelong latent state in neurons of the DRG as an intranuclear but episomal element. The HSV genome does not integrate into the host chromosome, so that insertional mutagenesis is not an issue.

HSV is a double-stranded DNA virus with a very large genome (152 KB) containing more than 88 open reading frames, but in the process of lytic infection the HSV genes are expressed in a rigid temporal cascade. Thus a small subset of only five immediate early (IE) genes that do not require viral protein synthesis are expressed immediately on entry of the HSV genome into the nucleus (16,20). The remainder of the viral genes require activation by either IE gene products, early (E) gene products and/or DNA replication for expression. Deletion of a single essential IE gene from the HSV genome results in a recombinant that is incapable of replicating, except in a complementing cell line that provide the IE gene product in trans (21). Vectors deleted for one or more IE genes are appropriate for use in human trials (22,23). Deletion of the HSV thymidine kinase (TK) gene from the viral genome results in the recombinant that has impaired replication and is unable to reactivate from latency in neurons (24,25). TK⁻ vectors have been used in a number of animal studies, although it is unlikely that they will be approved for use in humans.

The first demonstration of pain modulation using herpes vectors employed a TK⁻ recombinant HSV vector defective in the HSV thyoridinekinare (tk) gene containing the human proenkephalin (PE) gene, coding for five copies of met-enkephalin and one copy of leu-enkephalin. Enkephalin binds to the delta opioid receptor in the spinal cord to act presynaptically and postsynaptically at the terminals of primary nociceptors in dorsal horn to reduce transmission of nociceptive impulses in the dorsal horn of spinal cord. Delta opioid receptors are present at many other sites in the nervous system including nuclei in brainstem and in brain, as well as in organs outside the neuroaxis. A TK⁻ recombinant HSV vector expressing PE delivered to the DRG by subcutaneous inoculation into the dorsum of the foot reduces thermal hyperalgesic responses to noxious radiant heat without altering normal foot withdrawal to the same stimulus (26). Similarly in mice with polyarthritis induced by the intradermal injection of CFA, subcutaneous inoculation of a PE expressing TK minus HSV vector into the foot reduces both spontaneous and evoked pain responses (27). In the CFA arthritis model release of enkephalin from the peripheral terminals of the transduced neurons also significantly reduced arthritic destruction of the joint space and bone, presumably related to opiate effects on inflammatory cells in the periphery (27). The production and intracellular transport of the transgene product has been characterized in detail by Pohl and co-workers (28,29).

Because they could be potentially used in treatment of patients with chronic pain our laboratories have extensively studied replication incompetent HSV recombinant deleted for one or more essential IE genes in a number of models of inflammatory and neuropathic pain (15,30,31). A PE expressing replication incompetent HSV vector injected subcutaneously in the plantar surface of the foot establishes a latent state in DRG and expresses PE mRNA in the DRG. In the formalin test of inflammatory pain injection of the PE expressing replication incompetent HSV vector one week prior to testing reduces spontaneous pain (Fig. 2) during the delayed phase of the formalin test (32). The analgesic effect of vector inoculation is limited to the injected limb, is reversed by intraperitoneal

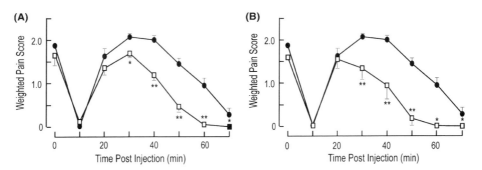

Figure 2 Rats inoculated with the PE-expressing HSV vector SHPE (*open boxes*) show a reduction in spontaneous pain in the delayed phase (20–60 minutes after injection) of the formalin test. (**A**) The effect is maximal 1 week after vector inoculation and wanes over the subsequent 3 weeks. (**B**) Reinoculation of the vector at 4 weeks re-establishes the analgesic effect in animals tested one week after reinoculation. *Source*: From Ref. 32.

naloxone or intrathecal naltrexone, and lasts for several weeks. By 4 wk after vector inoculation the analgesic effect of vector-mediated PE production is no longer present, but reinoculation of the vector at that time point re-establishes the analgesic effect. The time course of the effect follows the well-known kinetics of transgene expression driven by the HCMV IEp. The observation that re-inoculation re-establishes the analgesic effect provides additional evidence that the loss of effect over several weeks is not a manifestation of the development of tolerance to vector-mediated peptide release. We have found a similar effect of the nonreplicating PE expressing HSV vector in the CFA model of inflammatory pain induced by injection of CFA into the plantar surface of the foot. In this model untreated pain results over the course of three weeks but vector inoculation provided an analgesic effect over the entire time course (Hao et al. unpublished data).

In the spinal nerve ligation model of neuropathic pain mechanical allodynia begins one week after spinal nerve ligation and persists for at least three months. Subcutaneous inoculation of the PE-expressing HSV vector into the foot one week after spinal nerve ligation produces an anti-allodynic effect that is maximal 2.5 wk after inoculation (Fig. 3), lasts about 4 wk, and like the effect of the same vector in the formalin test of inflammatory pain. Like the effect seen in the formalin test of inflammatory pain, the effect of vector-mediated transgene expression is re-established by reinoculation of the vector 6 wk after

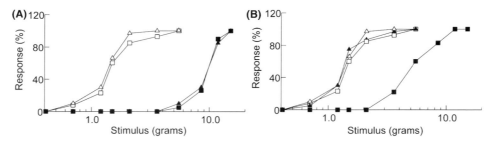

Figure 3 (**A**) In the selective spinal nerve ligation model of neuropathic pain, the threshold to mechanical stimulus of normal animals (*black symbols*) is substantially reduced after spinal nerve ligation (*open symbols*). (**B**) Subcutaneous inoculation of SHPE results in a significant increase in this threshold in treated animals (*black squares*), not seen in animals injected with a control vector (*black triangles*). *Source*: From Ref. 33.

the initial inoculation. The second inoculation results in an anti-allodynic effect that is greater in magnitude and appears to last longer than the initial effect. Other characteristics of HSV mediated analgesia have been evaluated in the neuropathic pain model. The effect of vector mediated enkephalin release is less than that of a maximum dose of morphine, but in contrast to the effect of morphine the vector mediated effect is continuous over time (while the effect of morphine alone lasts for only 1 to 2 hr). Twice daily inoculation of morphine at a maximal dose results in the development of tolerance by one week, and after that time continued twice-daily administration of morphine has no appreciable effect of pain measurements. In contrast, animals inoculated with the PE-expressing HSV vector continue to show an anti-allodynic effect despite the development of tolerance to morphine. The effect of the vector and of morphine are additive. The ED_{50} of morphine is 1.8 mg per kg in animals with neuropathic pain from spinal nerve ligation but 0.15 mg per kg in animals with neuropathic pain inoculated with the PE-expressing HSV vector (33).

Pain resulting from cancer metastatic to bone is a particularly vexing problem that impacts adversely on the quality of life at the end-of-life in patients with cancer. This form of chronic pain has characteristics of both of neuropathic pain as well as inflammatory pain as well as some unique features (34). Importantly for the current consideration, patients with pain from cancer represent an appropriate group for phase one trials of gene therapy for pain. We examined the effect of the PE expressing vector in rodent model of pain resulting from cancer in bone created by implantation of NCTCP 2472 osteogenic sarcoma cells into the distal femur (35). Subcutaneous inoculation of the PE expressing replication incompetent HSV vector into the plantar surface of the foot one week after the establishment of the tumor resulted in a significant reduction in ambulatory pain score in tumor bearing animals.

OTHER INHIBITORY NEUROTRANSMITTERS

Enkephalin is only one of several endogenous inhibitory neurotransmitters that are present in the dorsal horn of spinal cord and may modulate nociceptive neurotransmission. Endomorphin -1 and -2 are amidated tetrapeptides that have been identified as the endogenous ligands of the mu opioid receptor (36,37), and both glycine and GABA are important inhibitory neurotransmitters with a widespread distribution throughout the central nervous system and specific effects on nociceptive neurotransmission in the dorsal horn (38). GABA is particularly interesting because of the evidence that GABAergic neurotransmission may be reduced in neuropathic pain (39,40) and the clinical observation that GABAergic agonists (e.g., baclofen) have analgesic effects in central neuropathic pain syndromes although the dose of baclofen that can be administered a severe the limited by central effects of the drug.

We constructed a nonreplicating HSV vector (QHGAD67) defective in expression for the HSV IE genes ICP4, ICP22, and ICP47 and containing the human glutamic acid decarboxylase (GAD67) gene under the control of the HCMV IEp. Transduction of primary DRG neurons in culture with this vector resulted in the production of Glutamic Acid Decarboxylase (GAD) and the release of GABA from the transduced neurons (41). Subcutaneous inoculation of the vector in the foot resulted in transduction of DRG neurons in vivo and constitutive release of GABA from the central terminals of those neurons that could be measured in a microdialysate of the dorsal horn (Fig. 4) (41). We examined the analgesic effect of QHGAD67 in the T-13 spinal hemisection model of central neuropathic pain resulting from spinal cord injury. Inoculation of QHGAD67 subcutaneously in the plantar surface of the hind feet bilaterally one week after hemisection significantly reduced

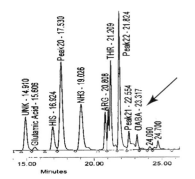 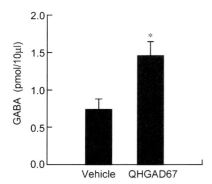

Figure 4 An HSV vector constructed to express GAD (QHGAD67) injected subcutaneously in the foot causes transduced DRG neurons to constitutively release GABA (indicated by arrow in HPLC trace) into dorsal horn (*left*). The amount of GABA released was determined by microdialysis of spinal cord (*right*). *Abbreviations*: HSV, herpes simplex virus; GAD, glutamic acid decarboxylase; GABA, gamma aminobutyric acid; HPLC, high performance liquid chromatography. *Source*: From Ref. 41.

mechanical allodynia and thermal hyperalgesia resulting from the spinal cord injury (41). The analgesic effect of GABA release was partially reversed by intrathecal bicuculline and phaclofen, indicating that the effect was mediated through both $GABA_A$ and $GABA_B$ receptors in the spinal cord. Vector mediated GABA release also attenuated the increase in spinal calcitonin gene related peptide (CGRP) immunoreactivity caused by spinal cord hemisection (42). Like the effect of the PE expressing vector the effect of GABA release was transient disappearing after about six weeks. However like the PE expressing vector reinoculation of QHGAD67 resulted in reestablishment of the analgesic effect.

GLIAL CELL DERIVED NEUROTROPHIC FACTOR

A substantial fraction of the primary nociceptors in DRG express the GDNF receptor GFRα1, and a recent study demonstrated that intrathecal administration of GDNF can produce a substantial anti-nociceptive effect in the spinal nerve ligation model of neuropathic pain in rodents (43). The dose of GDNF requires, when compared to the limits

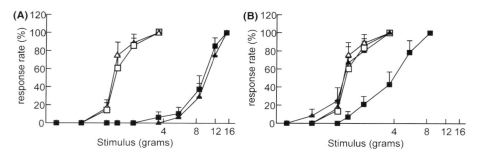

Figure 5 Subcutaneous inoculation of the GDNF-expressing vector DHGD provides an antiallodynic effect. (**A**) Spinal nerve ligation shifts the mechanical threshold curve to the left (similar to Fig. 3). (**B**) Injection of DHGD results in a significant increase in threshold in treated animals (*black squares*) not seen in animals injected with control vector (*black triangles*). *Source*: From Ref. 44.

in the amount of GDNF that human subjects tolerate by intraventricular administration, indicated an alternate mode delivery of this neurotrophic peptide would be required were it to be considered for the treatment of neuropathic pain. Accordingly we constructed a GDNF expressing HSV vector (DHGD) and tested subcutaneous inoculation of the vector in the spinal nerve ligation of neuropathic pain. Inoculation of DHGD one week after spinal nerve ligation resulted in a significant elevation in mechanical threshold that lasted for about five weeks reinoculation of the vector re-established the effect (Fig. 5) (44). Like the PE expressing vector, DHGD blocks non-noxious touch induced c-fos expression in the dorsal horn of spinal cord.

HUMAN TRIAL

Based on the preclinical animal data, we have proposed human trial of HSV mediated gene transfer in the treatment of intractable pain. Because this would be the first gene therapy trial for pain we have selected the population of patients with cancer metastatic to a vertebral body and pain unresponsive to maximal conventional therapy. These patients have a limited life expectancy that makes them appropriate candidates for such an experimental phase one trial to test safety and dose finding.

Patients with severe pain in a radicular distribution will receive the vector intradermally in the dermatome corresponding to the radicular distribution of the pain. Three patients in each dose level will be examined the dose increased by half like intervals from 10^6 to 10^9 plaque forming units. This study has been reviewed by the recombinant DNA advisory committee (RAC) of the NIH and discussions have been initiated with the FDA to obtain an investigational new drug (IND) waiver. Replication competent HSV has already been established to be safe in a phase one trial in which the compromised virus was inoculated directly into glioblastoma. Based on that evidence in the preclinical data it seems highly likely that the PE expressing vector will be safe for intradermal administration in humans. Successful completion of this phase one trial could then be followed by further trials of the same vector in other types of regional pain, and of HSV vectors expressing other gene products and specific for other types of pain.

ACKNOWLEDGMENTS

This work was supported by grants from the NIH (MM, JCG and DJF) and the Department of Veterans Affairs (MM and DJF).

REFERENCES

1. Yaksh TL. Spinal systems and pain processing: development of novel analgesic drugs with mechanistically defined models. Trends Pharmacol Sci 1999; 20:329–337.
2. Gazda LS, Milligan ED, Hansen MK, et al. Sciatic inflammatory neuritis (SIN): behavioral allodynia is paralleled by peri-sciatic proinflammatory cytokine and superoxide production. J Peripher Nerv Syst 2001; 6:111–129.
3. Christensen MD, Hulsebosch CE. Chronic central pain after spinal cord injury. J Neurotrauma 1997; 14:517–537.
4. Wilson SP, Chang KJ, Viveros OH. Opioid peptide synthesis in bovine and human adrenal chromaffin cells. Peptides 1981; 2:83–88.

5. Unsicker K. The trophic cocktail made by adrenal chromaffin cells. Exp Neurol 1993; 123:167–173.
6. Hama AT, Sagen J. Alleviation of neuropathic pain symptoms by xenogeneic chromaffin cell grafts in the spinal subarachnoid space. Brain Res 1994; 651:183–193.
7. Siegan JB, Sagen J. Attenuation of formalin pain responses in the rat by adrenal medullary transplants in the spinal subarachnoid space. Pain 1997; 70:279–285.
8. Wu HH, Wilcox GL, McLoon SC. Implantation of AtT-20 or genetically modified AtT-20/hENK cells in mouse spinal cord induced antinociception and opioid tolerance. J Neurosci 1994; 14:4806–4814.
9. Eaton MJ, Karmally S, Martinez MA, Plunkett JA, Lopez T, Cejas PJ. Lumbar transplant of neurons genetically modified to secrete galanin reverse pain-like behaviors after partial sciatic nerve injury. J Peripher Nerv Syst 1999; 4:245–257.
10. Eaton MJ, Plunkett JA, Martinez MA, et al. Transplants of neuronal cells bioengineered to synthesize GABA alleviate chronic neuropathic pain. Cell Transplant 1999; 8:87–101.
11. Cejas PJ, Martinez M, Karmally S, et al. Lumbar transplant of neurons genetically modified to secrete brain-derived neurotrophic factor attenuates allodynia and hyperalgesia after sciatic nerve constriction. Pain 2000; 86:195–210.
12. Finegold AA, Mannes AJ, Iadarola MJ. A paracrine paradigm for in vivo gene therapy in the central nervous system: treatment of chronic pain. Hum Gene Ther 1999; 10:1251–1257.
13. Milligan ED, Langer SJ, Sloane EM, et al. Inflammatory and chronic constriction injury-induced pain states are controlled by spinal delivery of viral and non-viral vectors encoding the anti-inflammatory gene, interleukin-10 (IL-10). Soc Neurosci 2003; 909:15. Abstract Viewer/Itinerary Planner.
14. Davar G, Bebrin WR, Day R, Breakefield XO. Gene delivery to mouse sensory neurons with herpes simplex virus: a model for postherpetic neuralgia and its treatment? Neurology 1995; 45:S69.
15. Mata M, Glorioso J, Fink DJ. Development of HSV-mediated gene transfer for the treatment of chronic pain. Exp Neurol 2003; 184:25–29.
16. Roizman B, Sears A. Herpes simplex viruses and their replication. In: Fields BN et al, eds. Fields Virology. Philadelphia, PA: Lippincott-Raven, 1996:2231–2295.
17. Spear PG, Eisenberg RJ, Cohen GH. Three classes of cell surface receptors for alpha-herpesvirus entry. Virology 2000; 275:1–8.
18. Kwong AD, Frenkel N. The herpes simplex virus virion host shutoff function. J Virol 1989; 63:4834–4839.
19. Smith GA, Enquist LW. Breaks ins and break outs: viral interactions with the cytoskeleton of mammalian cells. Annu Rev Cell Dev Biol 2002; 18:135–161.
20. Glorioso JC, Fink DJ. Herpes vector-mediated gene transfer in treatment of diseases of the nervous system. Annu Rev Microbiol 2004; 58:253–271.
21. DeLuca NA, McCarthy AM, Schaffer PA. Isolation and characterization of deletion mutants of herpes simplex virus type 1 in the gene encoding immediate-early regulatory protein ICP4. J Virol 1985; 56:558–570.
22. Krisky DM, Wolfe D, Goins WF, et al. Deletion of multiple immediate-early genes from herpes simplex virus reduces cytotoxicity and permits long-term gene expression in neurons. Gene Ther 1998; 5:1593–1603.
23. Wolfe D, Goins WF, Yamada M, et al. Engineering herpes simplex virus vectors for CNS applications. Exp Neurol 1999; 159:34–46.
24. Price RW, Khan A. Resistance of peripheral autonomic neurons to in vivo productive infection by herpes simplex virus mutants deficient in thymidine kinase activity. Infect Immun 1981; 34:571–580.
25. Tenser RB, Hay KA, Edris WA. Latency-associated transcript but not reactivatable virus is present in sensory ganglion neurons after inoculation of thymidine kinase-negative mutants of Herpes Simplex Virus Type 1. J Virol 1989; 63:2861–2865.
26. Wilson SP, Yeomans DC, Bender MA, Lu Y, Goins WF, Glorioso JC. Antihyperalgesic effects of infection with a preproenkephalin-encoding herpes virus. Proc Natl Acad Sci USA 1999; 96:3211–3216.

27. Braz J, Beaufour C, Coutaux A, et al. Therapeutic efficacy in experimental polyarthritis of viral-driven enkephalin overproduction in sensory neurons. J Neurosci 2001; 21:7881–7888.

28. Antunes Bras JM, Epstein AL, Bourgoin S, Hamon M, Cesselin F, Pohl M. Herpes simplex virus 1-mediated transfer of preproenkephalin A in rat dorsal root ganglia. J Neurochem 1998; 70:1299–1303.

29. Antunes Bras J, Becker C, Bourgoin S, et al. Met-enkephalin is preferentially transported into the peripheral processes of primary afferent fibres in both control and HSV1-driven proenkephalin A overexpressing rats. Neuroscience 2001; 103:1073–1083.

30. Glorioso JC, Mata M, Fink DJ. Gene therapy for chronic pain. Curr Opin Mol Ther 2003; 5:483–488.

31. Glorioso JC, Mata M, Fink DJ. Exploiting the neurotherapeutic potential of peptides: targeted delivery using HSV vectors. Expert Opin Biol Ther 2003; 3:1233–1239.

32. Goss JR, Mata M, Goins WF, Wu HH, Glorioso JC, Fink DJ. Antinociceptive effect of a genomic herpes simplex virus-based vector expressing human proenkephalin in rat dorsal root ganglion. Gene Ther 2001; 8:551–556.

33. Honore P, Rogers SD, Schwei MJ, Salak-Johnson JL, Luger NM, Sabino MC, Clohisy DR, Mantyh PW. Transgene-mediated enkephalin release enhances the effect of morphine and evades tolerance to produce a sustained antiallodynic effect. Pain 2003; 102:135–142.

34. Honore P, Rogers SD, Schwei MJ, et al. Murine models of inflammatory, neuropathic and cancer pain each generates a unique set of neurochemical changes in the spinal cord and sensory neurons. Neuroscience 2000; 98:585–598.

35. Schwei MJ, Honore P, Rogers SD, et al. Neurochemical and cellular reorganization of the spinal cord in a murine model of bone cancer pain. J Neurosci 1999; 19:10886–10897.

36. Zadina JE, Hackler L, Ge LJ, Kastin AJ. A potent and selective endogenous agonist for the mu-opiate receptor. Nature 1997; 386:499–502.

37. Przewlocki R, Labuz D, Mika J, Przewlocka B, Tomboly C, Toth G. Pain inhibition by endomorphins. Ann NY Acad Sci 1999; 897:154–164.

38. Sawynok J. GABAergic mechanisms of analgesia: an update. Pharmacol Biochem Behav 1987; 26:463–474.

39. Sivilotti L, Woolf CJ. The contribution of GABAA and glycine receptors to central sensitization: disinhibition and touch-evoked allodynia in the spinal cord. J Neurophysiol 1994; 72:169–179.

40. Moore KA, Kohno T, Karchewski LA, Scholz J, Baba H, Woolf CJ. Partial peripheral nerve injury promotes a selective loss of GABAergic inhibition in the superficial dorsal horn of the spinal cord. J Neurosci 2002; 22:6724–6731.

41. Liu J, Wolfe D, Hao S, et al. Peripherally delivered glutamic acid decarboxylase gene therapy for spinal cord injury pain. Mol Ther 2004; 10:57–66.

42. Natsume A, Wolfe D, Hu J, et al. Enhanced functional recovery after proximal nerve root injury by vector-mediated gene transfer. Exp Neurol 2003; 184:878–886.

43. Boucher TJ, Okuse K, Bennett DL, Munson JB, Wood JN, McMahon SB. Potent analgesic effects of GDNF in neuropathic pain states. Science 2000; 290:124–127.

44. Hao S, Mata M, Wolfe D, Huang S, Glorioso J, Fink DJ. HSV-mediated gene transfer of the glial cell derived neurotrophic factor (GDNF) provides an anti-allodynic effect in neuropathic pain. Mol Ther 2003; 8:367–375.

11

Immunotherapeutic Approaches for Alzheimer's Disease

William J. Bowers
Department of Neurology, Center for Aging and Developmental Biology, University of Rochester School of Medicine and Dentistry, Rochester, New York, U.S.A.

Howard J. Federoff
Departments of Neurology, Microbiology and Immunology, Center for Aging and Developmental Biology, University of Rochester School of Medicine and Dentistry, Rochester, New York, U.S.A.

Alzheimer's disease (AD) is an age-related neurodegenerative disorder associated with progressive functional decline, dementia, and neuronal loss. Demographics make evident that the prevalence of AD will increase substantially. The pervasive societal burden wrought by this debilitating disease should provide sufficient impetus for the development of new natural history modifying therapeutic approaches. However, because the mechanistic underpinnings of AD are incompletely understood, the clinical disease spectrum broad, and the neuropathological features of its initiation and progression limited, the development of such potential disease modifying therapies has been impeded. Herein, we review AD pathophysiology and currently employed therapies, and subsequently discuss experimental therapeutics predicated upon recent concepts of immune modulation to attenuate disease progression.

OVERVIEW OF ALZHEIMER'S DISEASE

The pathological hallmarks of AD brain include extracellular proteinaceous deposits (plaques), composed largely of amyloid beta (Aβ) peptides, and intraneuronal neurofibrillary tangles (NFTs), which are characterized by excessive phosphorylation of tau protein. Other AD-related histopathologic features are astrogliosis, microglial activation, and reduction of synaptic markers. These features appear to arise in a region- and time-dependent manner (1). Amyloid pathology evolves in stages: early involvement is anatomically circumscribed to the basal neocortex, most often within poorly myelinated temporal areas; progression involves adjacent neocortical areas, the hippocampal formation, perforant path inclusive of its coursing through the subiculum and termination within the molecular layers of the dentate gyrus, and; finally the process involves all cortical areas (2). NFT pathology is also progressive: Initially involving projection neurons with somata in the transenthorhinal region, tangles then extend to the entrohinal region proper typically in the absence of amyloid depostion. Subsequent progression to the hippocampus and temporal proneocortex, and then association neocortex, followed by superiolateral spread and ultimately extending to primary neocortical areas (2).

Numerous studies have demonstrated that the proteins comprising AD-associated pathological hallmarks contribute to pathogenesis. Aβ peptides (Aβ1–39, Aβ1–40, and Aβ1–42) are proteolytic cleavage products of the amyloid precursor protein (APP), the derivation of which is consequent to extracellular and intramembraneous cleavages by β and γ-secretase proteases, respectively (3,4). Recently, Aβ has been shown in hippocampal neurons to both dampen excitatory neurotransmission and inhibit its own production by feedback onto the β-secretase (5). The Aβ peptides, particularly Aβ1–42, when released extraneuronally undergo sequential conformation changes. This process, referred to as fibrillization, results in the assembly of higher order oligomeric, protofibrillar and fibrillar forms of Aβ (6). The most neurotoxic Aβ species appears to an oligomer of $\sim$8–12 subunits that adopts a unique conformation capable of preventing induction of long-term potentiation (LTP), inducing cell death and forming pores in artificial lipid bilayers (7–12).

Tau, a microtubule-associated protein, is involved in the stabilization and promotion of the polymerization of microtubules in neurons (13–16). While mutations in the tau gene account for some frontotemporal dementia (FTD), another neurodegenerative disease, the protein is not mutated in the vastly more prevalent late onset AD. Rather, pathologic activation of neuronal kinases such as GSK-3β, Cdk5, and MARCKS appears to mediate hyperphosphorylation of tau rendering it dysfunctional. Consequently, microtubule dynamics are destabilized resulting in disruption of intraneuronal transport of organelles and proteins (17–19). Efforts are underway to formally test the "amyloid cascade hypothesis" by investigating how Aβ peptides may modulate tau phosphorylation and hence, lead to the formation of NFTs and neuronal synaptic dysfunction in AD (20). The sequence of pathophysiological events encompassed by this hypothesis is depicted in Figure 1.

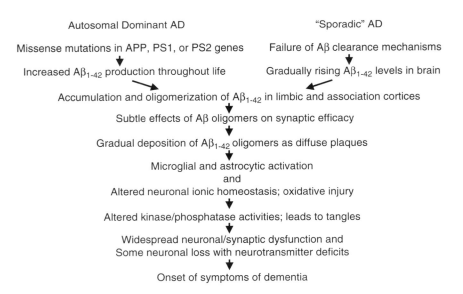

Figure 1   Amyloid cascade hypothesis. *Source*: Adapted from http://www.alzforum.org and Ref. 89.

AD is categorized by age of disease onset and etiology: early-onset familial (genetic) and late-onset (idiopathic) (Fig. 1). Three genetic loci have been implicated in autosomal dominant familial AD cases: *APP* on human chromosome 21, presenilin 1 (*PS1*) on chromosome 14, and presenilin 2 (*PS2*) on chromosome 1. Although these autosomal dominant cases are rare, they produce disease onset as early as the third decade of life. Mutations in the APP gene appear fully penetrant, while the penetrance of PS gene mutations remains complex due to the existence of multiple missense mutations and the lack of longitudinal studies assessing the contribution of each genetic change to disease onset (21). Functional characterization of these mutations has led to the development of numerous animal models that mimic the amyloid pathology observed in human AD, thus providing experimental models in which to test novel therapeutics targeted towards prevention and/or disruption of Aβ deposition.

The vast majority of late-onset AD cases arise sporadically with age being the most influential risk factor; approximately 40 percent of individuals over age 85 are affected. Other risk factors are environmental influences, including diet, heavy metal exposure, viral and bacterial infections, and prior head trauma (22–25). A genetic susceptibility locus on chromosome 19q, which encodes for the apolipoprotein E (ApoE) gene product, has been implicated in sporadic AD (26,27). The three alleles (E2, E3, and E4) encode different isoforms of the ApoE protein that are believed to play a chaperone-like whereby they assist in Aβ folding and clearance from the interstitial space. Individuals carrying the ApoE4 allele have a significantly higher risk of developing late-onset AD (28). Other genes that may be associated with an increased risk for AD have been identified (29–35), but further study is required to establish their respective contributions.

CURRENT THERAPEUTICS FOR AD

Presently available therapeutic agents employed to treat AD are designed to alleviate cognitive and emotional symptoms of the disease (36). The cholinergic system exhibits decreased functioning in AD patients due to impaired synaptic integrity and progressive neuronal loss. This observation suggests that inhibiting the activities of enzymes responsible for the degradation of neurotransmitters could prolong neurotransmission and, thus, enhance cognitive function. Cholinesterases, such as acetylcholinesterase and butrylcholinesterase, represent suitable therapeutic targets. Cholinesterase inhibitors, including tacrine, donepezil, rivastigmine, and galantamine, exhibit generally acceptable tolerability profiles and have been shown to preserve cognitive function in some patients depending upon the specific therapeutic outcome assessed (37–43).

Excitotoxicity can occur under pathologic conditions in the brain, including AD, due to excessive activation of the primary excitatory amino acid, glutamate. Glutamate signaling occurs through metabotropic and ionotropic receptors. Hyperexcitation via glutamate has been shown to enhance appearance of pathological forms of tau and Aβ, and Aβ itself has been demonstrated to exacerbate glutamate toxicity (44). Memantine, an uncompetitive *N*-methyl-D-aspartate (NMDA) ionotropic receptor antagonist, is used to block glutamate excitotoxicity in AD patients. Several clinical trials evaluating memantine have demonstrated a slowing in the rate of cognitive and functional decline (45,46). Targeting of ionotropic receptor classes, α-amino-3-hydroxy-5-methyl-4-isoxalone propionic acid (AMPA) glutamate receptor modulators have been developed but, at present, have only been reported in limited numbers of studies (47).

EXPERIMENTAL THERAPEUTICS FOR AD

One of the affected brain regions consistently affected in AD is the basal forebrain cholinergic complex; accounting for correlation between the cholinergic deficit and both the magnitude of pathological severity and degree of dementia (48–52). Nerve growth factor (NGF) stimulates expression of choline acetyltransferase (ChAT), the rate-limiting biosynthetic enzyme for acetylcholine (53), and through its trophic actions promotes survival and maintenance of the cholinergic septohippocampal pathway that is a major pathway for memory and learning (54). Grafting of fibroblasts genetically modified to produce NGF via a retrovirus vector-mediated gene transfer promotes restoration and survival of the septohippocampal pathway (55–59). A Phase I trial of autologous NGF-gene modified fibroblasts has been recently completed. Other modalities such as adeno-associated virus (AAV)-mediated gene transfer for increasing NGF concentration in specific brain regions are currently being tested by California-based Ceregene in human Phase I clinical trials (ClinicalTrials.gov Identifier: NCT00087789). While NGF clearly has therapeutic potential, it is not capable of modifying the underlying pathogenic mechanisms causing AD, thus its utility is limited to potential symptomatic therapy. Further clinical trials are needed to evaluate its efficacy in ameliorating symptoms of AD.

Other foci for therapeutic intervention in AD are inflammation and oxidative stress. A number of inflammatory mediators have been detected in AD brain (60). Whether inflammation is a primary or secondary phenomenon in the AD brain is unclear. Formally, inflammation may trigger plaque or tangles or be consequent to their pathophysiologic actions. In addition, the source of proinflammatory molecules is still unresolved. Some data suggest that the inflammatory response is produced by glia that results in neuronal demise (60). Retrospective studies with antioxidants and non-steroidal anti-inflammatory drugs suggest that decreasing free radicals and inhibiting inflammatory processes may confer protection against AD and/or slow the rate of cognitive decline seen in AD (61). A study was designed to address whether selective or non-selective cyclooxygenase (COX) inhibitors would delay the emergence of AD in individuals over 65 yr and who have a first degree relative with the disease (ClinicalTrials.gov Identifier: NCT00009230). However, because of safety concerns relating to prolonged usage of non-steroidal anti-inflammatory drugs (NSAIDS), this trial has been put on hold (62). Novel gene therapeutics are also being evaluated preclinically; these are intended to scavenge free radicals and block inflammatory processes.

The amyloid cascade hypothesis suggests therapeutics that will abrogate the proteolytic generation of Aβ peptides, prevent Aβ fibrillogenesis and/or amyloid deposition would impact the onset and/or severity of AD. To this end, β- and γ-secretase inhibitors are being tested pre-clinically and in early stage clinical trials for their abilities to impede the generation of Aβ1–42 peptide. One potential drawback of this approach relates to the multiple substrates of the secretase complexes. For example, γ-secretase proteolytically processes APP as well as the vitally important developmental regulatory protein, Notch, thus, creating the potential for untoward effects resulting from γ-secretase inhibitor administration (63). At least one γ-secretase inhibitor has in preclinical dose escalation paradigms demonstrated substantial gastrointestinal toxicity (64).

A promising, yet inherently complex, means of inhibiting Aβ fibrillogenesis and/or deposition relates to the use of the host immune system to mount specific immune responses against the self-peptide, Aβ. The findings from a variety of immune-based strategies speak to the promise of this approach, but also reveal the potential for morbid complications of AD immunotherapy. The remainder of this discourse describes this approach and its future viability for preventing or treating AD.

Aβ-BASED IMMUNOTHERAPEUTICS

Recent publications have highlighted the potential of Aβ peptide immunization in the treatment of AD (65–67). Schenk et al. used a transgenic model that overexpresses a mutant APP (V717F) mini-gene driven by the platelet-derived growth factor promoter (PDAPP) (68). PDAPP mice immunized and boosted with $A\beta_{1-42}$ peptide with complete and incomplete Freund's adjuvant, respectively, before the onset of AD-like pathology, were protected from development of plaque formation, neuritic dystrophy, and astrogliosis. Treatment of older PDAPP animals (11 mo) with existing pathology resulted in reduced plaque burden and slower progression of AD-like neuropathology. Two other laboratories have also demonstrated the effectiveness of Aβ peptide vaccination. Janus et al. utilized a triple mutation model of AD (65). This TgCRND8 model of AD expresses a mutant human βAPP_{695} (K670N/M671L; Swedish mutation) and the V717F mutation under the regulation of the Syrian hamster prion promoter. In this model there is an increase in fibrillogenic Aβ and an increase in amyloid plaques. Additionally, spatial learning deficits are detectable at 3 mo of age. Immunization of TgCRND8 mice with Aβ reduces fibrillar Aβ deposits and cognitive dysfunction as measured by a reference memory version of the Morris water maze test. However, total Aβ levels in the brain were unchanged. Aβ-directed vaccination was also assessed in a model of AD that overexpresses mutant human βAPP_{695} (K670N/M671L; Swedish mutation) and PS1 mutations under the control of the hamster prion promoter (PSAPP) (66,68). Neuropathologically, these animals demonstrate compact amyloid plaques but no dramatic neuronal loss in either the hippocampus or association cortices. Behaviorally, PSAPP mice exhibit learning and age-related memory deficits as amyloid accumulates. Following vaccination with Aβ, PSAPP mice were protected from learning and age-related deficits as well as a partial reduction in amyloid burden. There were no apparent deleterious effects of the vaccination. A listing of previously published reports on the use of active vaccination strategies is shown in Table 1.

Passive immunization achieved by administration of Aβ-specific antibodies may provide an alternative to the active vaccine strategies described above. The laboratories of Holtzman and Ashe have independently reported the benefits of systemic delivery of Aβ-specific antibodies to AD mice (69,70). Treated mice exhibited a marked reduction in amyloid accumulation and a significant improvement in memory-oriented behavioral tests. Using a similar passive immunization approach, Bard et al. showed that peripherally administered monoclonal antibodies against the amyloid β-peptide enter the CNS of PDAPP mice (71). Additionally, these passively administered antibodies promoted the clearance of pre-existing amyloid, thus reducing the plaque burden. A series of passive vaccination studies have been conducted and are summarized in Table 2. Prophylaxis against amyloid pathology required multiple injections of high-titer antibody in all studies. Approaches that provide for the stable production of Aβ-specific antibody in situ may represent a more viable therapeutic option.

The biological mechanism(s) by which these anti-Aβ immunotherapeutics act remain controversial. However, three non-mutually exclusive hypotheses have emerged (72): (1) Aβ-specific antibodies whether elicited or passively administered act at the blood-brain-barrier (BBB) to alter the equilibrium of soluble $A\beta_{1-42}$ concentrations to enhance its clearance from the brain. This "peripheral sink mechanism" is posited to prevent additional Aβ peptide deposition and perhaps promote aggregate dissolution.

Table 1 Previously Reported Preclinical Active Vaccination Studies

Antigen(s)	Antigen form/dose	Adjuvant	Model	Age	Route	Injection regimen	Reference
$A\beta_{1-42}$	Unknown/100 μg	CFA/IFA	PDAPP mice	1.5 mo	IP	Twice bi-weekly, thereafter monthly until 13 mo of age	(67)
				11 mo		Twice bi-weekly, thereafter monthly until 18 mo of age	
$A\beta_{1-42}$	Protofillar/100 μg	CFA/IFA	TgCRND8 mice	1.5 mo	IP	Twice bi-weekly, thereafter monthly until 5 mo of age	(65)
$A\beta_{1-42}$	Unknown/100 μg	CFA/IFA	APP/PS1 mice	7.5 mo	SQ	Twice bi-weekly, thereafter monthly until 10 mo of age	(66)
$A\beta_{1-42}$	Unknown/10–100 μg	None	PDAPP mice	5	Oral	Daily for 5 days, thereafter once weekly for 7 mo	(91)
	Unknown/5–10 μg			>	IN	Days 1, 3, and 5, thereafter once weekly for 7 mo	
$A\beta_{1-40}$	Non-fibrillar/100 μg	CFA/IFA	Tg2576 mice	~12 mo	SQ	Twice bi-weekly, thereafter monthly until 16 mo of age	(92)
$A\beta_{1-42}$ $A\beta_{1-30}NH_2$ $K6A\beta_{1-30}NH_2$							
$A\beta_{1-40}$	Unknown/100 μg	CFA/IFA	C57BL/6 mice	1 mo	IP	Once	(93)
$A\beta_{1-42}$				2 mo	IP	Thrice bi-weekly, once at 12 wk / Twice bi-weekly, thereafter monthly until 16 mo of age	
$A\beta_{1-15}$ $A\beta_{1-40/42}$	Unknown/100 μg	LT or LT(R192G)	B6D2F1 mice	1.5 mo	IN / IN / IP	Twice weekly for 6 wk / Twice weekly for 8 wk / Twice weekly for 8 wk	(94)
$A\beta_{3-6}$	Phage-displayed/10^{11} TU	None	APP(V717I) mice	16 mo	IP	Twice bi-weekly then twice monthly	(95)
$A\beta_{1-5}$	Unknown/100 μg	OVA (aa323–339) fusion peptide w/CFA/IFA	PDAPP mice	~12 mo	IP	Twice bi-weekly, thereafter monthly until 18 mo of age	(96)

Aβ$_{3-9}$
Aβ$_{5-11}$
Aβ$_{15-24}$

Aβ$_{1-42}$	rAAV vector/5×10^{10} TU	None or fused cholera tox B	PDAPP mice	1 or 12 mo	Oral, IN, IM	Once	(82)
Aβ$_{1-42}$	Aggregated/10 mg	CFA/IFA	Rhesus monkeys	15–20 yr	IP	Twice bi-weekly, thereafter monthly for 6 mo	(97)
Aβ$_{1-42}$	HSV amplicon/1×10^5 TU	None or fused TtxFC	Tg2576 mice	1.5 mo	SQ	Once monthly for 3 mo	(75)

Abbreviations: CFA, complete Freund's adjuvant; IFA, incomplete Freund's adjuvant; IP, intraperitoneal; IN, intranasal; SQ, subcutaneous; LT, lymphotoxin; TU, transduction units; IM, intramuscular.

Table 2 Previously Reported Preclinical Passive Vaccination Studies

Antibody	Dose	Model	Age	Route	Injection regimen	Reference
AMY-33 6F/3D	N/A	In vitro	N/A	N/A	N/A	(98)
6C6 1C2 14C2	N/A	In vitro	N/A	N/A	N/A	(99)
3D6	Not provided	PDAPP mice	8–10 mo	IP	Once weekly for 6 mo	(71)
10D5			12 mo			
m266	500 μg	PDAPP mice	4 mo	IP	Once every other week for 5 mo	(73)
m266	360 μg	PDAPP mice	11 mo	IP	Once weekly for 6 mo	(69)
			24 mo			
6C6	10 mg/kg	PDAPP mice	12 mo	IP	Once weekly for 6 mo	(96)
10D5 2C1 12B4 3A3 12A11						
AMY-33	10 μg	Tg2576 mice	10 mo	ICV	Once	(100)

Abbreviations: IP, intraperitoneal; PDAPP, Alzheimer's disease mouse model harboring human platelet derived growth factor promoter-driven human amyloid precursor protein transgene with the valine at residue 717 substituted by phenylalanine; ICV, intracerebroventricular.

Long-term peripheral administration of the m266 anti-Aβ monoclonal antibody led to a significant elevation in plasma Aβ levels and concomitant reduction in cerebrospinal fluid Aβ levels as well as a subsequent diminution in amyloid deposition (73); (2) Aβ-specific antibodies cross a compromised BBB and bind to Aβ within the brain parenchyma where antibody-Aβ complexes are postulated to bind microglia which then phagocytose amyloid deposits. Bard and colleagues demonstrated in ex vivo assays that microglia internalize Aβ following incubation with anti-Aβ antibodies and brain tissue samples (71). Moreover, microglial activation has been documented in areas of amyloid plaque clearance following immunization (73); (3) N-terminal anti-Aβ specific antibodies have been shown to inhibit Aβ fibrillogenesis in vitro, and thereby hypothesized to prevent oligomeric assembly of Aβ. An antibody specific to residues 4–10 has been demonstrated to reduce Aβ-induced neuronal toxicity in cell culture, and when administered to AD transgenic mice resulted in diminished amyloid burden and synaptic degeneration (74).

The mechanisms of Aβ vaccine action, if not properly regulated, can lead to possibly harmful side effects. Figure 2 depicts the potential brain specific immunological outcomes that can attend active or passive Aβ immunotherapy. Immunization with Aβ peptide could stimulate the T-helper 2 (TH$_2$; humoral) arm of the immune response resulting in antibodies that act by one or multiple mechanisms discussed above. However, if the antibodies elicited in situ or those passively administered target endogenous APP,

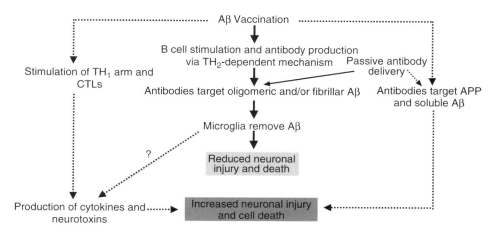

Figure 2 Immunological outcomes arising from Aβ-based vaccination for AD. Immunization with Aβ peptide could stimulate the T-helper 2 (TH₂; humoral) arm of the immune response resulting in antibodies that act by the "peripheral sink" mechanism, Fc receptor-mediated phagocytosis, and/or inhibition of Aβ fibrillogenesis. This would lead to reduced Aβ-induced neurotoxicity and improved cognitive functioning. However, if the antibodies elicited in situ or those passively administered target endogenous APP or soluble Aβ, a deleterious anti-self response may occur leading to destruction of neurons expressing APP or disruption of normal APP/soluble Aβ physiological function. In addition, activation of the TH₁ or cellular arm of the immune response could trigger T-cell migration and enhanced inflammatory conditions in the brain ultimately leading to increased neuronal injury and cell death. *Abbrevations*: APP, amyloid precursor protein; AD, Alzheimer's disease. *Source*: From Ref. 90.

a deleterious autoimmune response may occur leading to destruction of cells expressing APP (primarily neurons) or disruption of normal APP physiological functioning. Moreover, if the TH₁ or cellular arm of the immune response is triggered, T-cell migration and enhanced inflammation could arise in the brain ultimately leading to increased neuronal injury and cell death.

The latter scenario may have occurred in a clinical trial conducted in Europe (76,77). In a Phase I study that was co-sponsored by Elan Pharmaceuticals and Wyeth-Ayerst Laboratories, the observations indicated that the amyloid peptide-based vaccine, AN-1792, was well-tolerated in human subjects, and induced the formation of anti-Aβ amyloid antibodies in a subset of trial participants. These promising results propelled a Phase IIA study in 2001 in which 375 people with mild to moderate AD were enrolled at study sites in Europe and the United States to assess vaccine efficacy, optimal dosage, and safety. However, by mid-January 2002, Elan and Wyeth-Ayerst suspended the Phase IIA study due to the development of CNS inflammation in four of the study participants in France. Subsequently, an additional 14 patients also developed clinical evidence for meningoencephalitis (78). At present, study investigators and governmental health agencies are determining the genesis of the inflammatory response. Hock and colleagues demonstrated that a subset of immunized subjects harbored antibodies that recognized pathogenic structures of Aβ-containing plaque-like deposits and did not bind to full-length APP or to soluble Aβ$_{1-42}$, leading to the inference that the TH₁ arm was more likely responsible for the meningoencephalytic condition. The antisera were tested on tissue from AD mice (APP^{Sw}/PS1M146L double transgenic) and on post-mortem tissue isolated from human AD brains and indicated that the antibodies recognized similar pathogenic, aggregated forms of Aβ$_{1-42}$

(79). Interestingly, this group demonstrated in a follow-up study that a subset of vaccinated patients exhibited attenuated cognitive decline (80). The neuropathology of a single study subject who had presented with meningoencephalitis showed an uncharacteristic patchy amyloid plaque pattern, suggesting that the Aβ vaccine led to heterogeneous clearing of amyloid burden (81). Given these mixed clinical results, the viability but safety profile of Aβ-directed immunotherapy warrants further study particularly if an optimal immune response/antibody can be developed. Although presently untested in human clinical trials, virus vaccination technology (due to its inherent versatility) may allow for greater precision in antigen presentation and immunomodulation that could lead to safer and more efficacious vaccines for AD.

VIRUS VACCINE-BASED Aβ IMMUNOTHERAPY

Implementation of virus vaccine-based methodologies for AD immunotherapy may potentially provide vigorous and prolonged antigen-specific immune responses. Moreover, these approaches are amenable to molecular genetic manipulation and can allow for the co-introduction of immunomodulatory genes along with sequences encoding the Aβ antigen to finely tune the antigen-specific response. A variety of gene-based vaccines exist, including adenovirus (Ad), lentivirus, AAV, Herpes simplex virus (HSV), and plasmid-based vectors. Each vector platform has been shown to efficiently deliver heterologous genetic material to cells in vivo, while only a subset of these vectors possess the ability to serve as viable vaccine platforms due to their inherent capability to deliver genes to antigen presenting cells (APCs) and the relatively minimal anti-vector immune response elaborated. Zhang and colleagues employed rAAV vectors to express $A\beta_{1-42}$ as a fusion protein with the non-TH_1 molecular adjuvant protein, cholera toxin B subunit (AAV-CB-Aβ42) (82). $PDAPP^{V717I}$ transgenic mice, which overexpress $A\beta_{1-42}$ derived from the harbored the human APP751 London mutation (V717I), were given a single inoculation (5×10^{10} viral particles) of AAV-CB-Aβ42, an AAV vector expressing $A\beta_{1-42}$ alone (AAV-Aβ42), or a control vector expressing green fluorescent protein (AAV–GFP) via the intranasal, intramuscular, or oral route. Serum anti-Aβ IgG titer was detectable only in mice receiving AAV-CB-Aβ42, suggesting that the fused cholera toxin B subunit facilitated humoral responses against the vectored $A\beta_{1-42}$ immunogen. Moreover, brain Aβ plaque burden and memory/learning behavior was significantly improved in only $PDAPP^{V717I}$ transgenic mice injected with AAV-CB-Aβ42.

More recently, our laboratory employed the HSV-derived amplicons to elicit distinctive immune responses against Aβ. Two vaccine vectors were constructed: one expressing $A\beta_{1-42}$ alone (HSVAβ), and a second expressing $A\beta_{1-42}$ fused with the molecular adjuvant tetanus toxin Fragment C (HSVAβ/TtxFC). Peripheral administration of these vaccines augmented humoral responses to Aβ and reduced CNS Aβ deposition in Tg2576 AD mice. Interestingly and unexpectedly, HSVAβ vaccination was uniquely toxic and incited the expression of pro-inflammatory molecule transcripts within the hippocampi of Tg2576 mice, suggesting that this paradigm may serve as a relevant approach to study Aβ vaccine-elicited CNS inflammatory syndromes.

The HSV-1 amplicon possesses a number of advantages over other gene delivery platforms. First, the amplicon is not a live virus (as are vaccinia, canarypox, etc.) and therefore, has an inherently safer in vivo profile. Second, compared to DNA delivery systems or most virus-based vectors, expression is directed from multiple episomal copies within each transduced cell, and the genome is maintained in non-dividing cells such as APCs. Third, the transgene size limit is larger (≤ 130 kb) (83–86) than many other viral vectors affording an opportunity to co-express factors with known immunomodulating activity. Lastly, the lack of encoded viral genes avoids the effects that wild-type herpesviruses typically use to evade the immune system, such as downregulation of MHC expression and antigen processing, and inhibition of dendritic cell maturation (87,88).

CONCLUDING REMARKS

The goal of ongoing Aβ-directed immunotherapeutic studies is to determine the relationship between Aβ antigen structure/context and the elicitation of protective immune responses that attenuate Aβ toxicity, prevent amyloid plaque deposition and/or lead to dissolution of pre-existing amyloid. Development of an immunotherapeutic approach for AD is a challenging endeavor given the extant inflammatory state within the AD brain. Employing various virus-based vaccines to elicit antigen specific responses devoid of autoimmune reaction will require systematic assessment of immune responses achieved through different routes of inoculation, co-expression of various immunomodulating factors, and design of Aβ pathogenic peptides with varying structural characteristics. This newer approach will not only enable the development of novel AD immunotherapeutics, but will contribute to the mechanistic dissection of AD pathogenesis and the immune responses required to mediate protection.

REFERENCES

1. Nestor PJ, Scheltens P, Hodges JR. Advances in the early detection of Alzheimer's disease. Nat Med 2004; 10:S34–S41.
2. Braak H, Braak E. Neuropathological staging of Alzheimer-related changes. Acta Neuropathol (Berl) 1991; 82:239–259.
3. Selkoe DJ. Alzheimer's disease: genotypes, phenotypes, and treatments. Science 1997; 275:630–631.
4. Selkoe DJ. The cell biology of beta-amyloid precursor protein and presenilin in Alzheimer's disease. Trends Cell Biol 1998; 8:447–453.
5. Kamenetz F, Tomita T, Hsieh H, Seabrook G, Borchelt D, Iwatsubo T, Sisodia S, Malinow R. APP processing and synaptic function. Neuron 2003; 37:925–937.
6. Gorman PM, Chakrabartty A. Alzheimer beta-amyloid peptides: structures of amyloid fibrils and alternate aggregation products. Biopolymers 2001; 60:381–394.
7. Mobley DL, Cox DL, Singh RR, Maddox MW, Longo ML. Modeling amyloid beta-peptide insertion into lipid bilayers. Biophys J 2004; 86:3585–3597.
8. Kayed R, Sokolov Y, Edmonds B, et al. Permeabilization of lipid bilayers is a common conformation-dependent activity of soluble amyloid oligomers in protein misfolding diseases. J Biol Chem 2004; 279:46363–46366.
9. Torok M, Huwyler J, Gutmann H, Fricker G, Drewe J. Modulation of transendothelial permeability and expression of ATP-binding cassette transporters in cultured brain capillary endothelial cells by astrocytic factors and cell-culture conditions. Exp Brain Res 2003; 153:356–365.
10. Lansbury PT, Jr. Consequences of the molecular mechanism of amyloid formation for the understanding of the pathogenesis of Alzheimer's disease and the development of therapeutic strategies. Arzneimittelforschung 1995; 45:432–434.
11. Lansbury PT, Jr., Costa PR, Griffiths JM, et al. Structural model for the beta-amyloid fibril based on interstrand alignment of an antiparallel-sheet comprising a C-terminal peptide. Nat Struct Biol 1995; 2:990–998.

12. Harper JD, Lansbury PT, Jr. Models of amyloid seeding in Alzheimer's disease and scrapie: mechanistic truths and physiological consequences of the time-dependent solubility of amyloid proteins. Annu Rev Biochem 1997; 66:385–407.

13. Gustke N, Trinczek B, Biernat J, Mandelkow EM, Mandelkow E. Domains of tau protein and interactions with microtubules. Biochemistry 1994; 33:9511–9522.

14. Kosik KS, McConlogue L. Microtubule-associated protein function: lessons from expression in Spodoptera frugiperda cells. Cell Motil Cytoskeleton 1994; 28:195–198.

15. Drubin DG, Kirschner MW. Tau protein function in living cells. J Cell Biol 1986; 103:2739–2746.

16. Weingarten MD, Lockwood AH, Hwo SY, Kirschner MW. A protein factor essential for microtubule assembly. Proc Natl Acad Sci USA 1975; 72:1858–1862.

17. Ksiezak-Reding H, Binder LI, Yen SH. Alzheimer disease proteins (A68) share epitopes with tau but show distinct biochemical properties. J Neurosci Res 1990; 25:420–430.

18. Kosik KS, Orecchio LD, Binder L, Trojanowski JQ, Lee VM, Lee G. Epitopes that span the tau molecule are shared with paired helical filaments. Neuron 1988; 1:817–825.

19. Greenberg SG, Davies P. A preparation of Alzheimer paired helical filaments that displays distinct tau proteins by polyacrylamide gel electrophoresis. Proc Natl Acad Sci USA 1990; 87:5827–5831.

20. Cedazo-Minguez A, Popescu BO, Blanco-Millan JM, et al. Apolipoprotein E and beta-amyloid (1–42) regulation of glycogen synthase kinase-3beta. J Neurochem 2003; 87:1152–1164.

21. Lovestone S. Early diagnosis and the clinical genetics of Alzheimer's disease. J Neurol 1999; 246:69–72.

22. Mattson MP. Gene-diet interactions in brain aging and neurodegenerative disorders. Ann Intern Med 2003; 139:441–444.

23. Mattson MP. Metal-catalyzed disruption of membrane protein and lipid signaling in the pathogenesis of neurodegenerative disorders. Ann NY Acad Sci 2004; 1012:37–50.

24. Fleminger S, Oliver DL, Lovestone S, Rabe-Hesketh S, Giora A. Head injury as a risk factor for Alzheimer's disease: the evidence 10 years on; a partial replication. J Neurol Neurosurg Psychiatry 2003; 74:857–862.

25. Itzhaki RF, Ling W-R, Shang D, Wilcock GK, Faragher B, Jamieson GA. Herpes simplex virus type 1 in brain and risk of Alzheimer's disease. Lancet 1997; 349:241–244.

26. Corder EH, Saunders AM, Risch NJ, et al. Protective effect of apolipoprotein E type 2 allele for late onset Alzheimer disease. Nat Genet 1994; 7:180–184.

27. Strittmatter WJ, Roses AD. Apolipoprotein E and Alzheimer disease. Proc Natl Acad Sci USA 1995; 92:4725–4727.

28. Van Broeckhoven C. Alzheimer's disease: identification of genes and genetic risk factors. Prog Brain Res 1998; 117:315–325.

29. Kamboh MI, Sanghera DK, Ferrell RE, DeKosky ST. APOE*4-associated Alzheimer's disease risk is modified by alpha 1-antichymotrypsin polymorphism. Nat Genet 1995; 10:486–488 [published erratum appears in Nat Genet Sep;11(1):104].

30. Okuizumi K, Onodera O, Namba Y, et al. Genetic association of the very low density lipoprotein (VLDL) receptor gene with sporadic Alzheimer's disease. Nat Genet 1995; 11:207–209.

31. Xia Y, Rohan de Silva HA, Rosi BL, et al. Genetic studies in Alzheimer's disease with an NACP/alpha-synuclein polymorphism. Ann Neurol 1996; 40:207–215.

32. Saitoh T, Xia Y, Chen X, et al. The CYP2D6B mutant allele is overrepresented in the Lewy body variant of Alzheimer's disease. Ann Neurol 1995; 37:110–112.

33. Tycko B, Feng L, Nguyen L, et al. Polymorphisms in the human apolipoprotein-J/clusterin gene: ethnic variation and distribution in Alzheimer's disease. Hum Genet 1996; 98:430–436 [published erratum appears in Hum Genet 1998 Apr;102(4):496].

34. Li T, Holmes C, Sham PC, et al. Allelic functional variation of serotonin transporter expression is a susceptibility factor for late onset Alzheimer's disease. Neuroreport 1997; 8:683–686.

35. Curran M, Middleton D, Edwardson J, et al. HLA-DR antigens associated with major genetic risk for late-onset Alzheimer's disease. Neuroreport 1997; 8:1467–1469.
36. Tariot PN, Federoff HJ. Current treatment for Alzheimer disease and future prospects. Alzheimer Dis Assoc Disord 2003; 17:S105–S113.
37. Tariot PN, Cummings JL, Katz IR, et al. A randomized, double-blind, placebo-controlled study of the efficacy and safety of donepezil in patients with Alzheimer's disease in the nursing home setting. J Am Geriatr Soc 2001; 49:1590–1599.
38. Tariot P, Solomon P, Morris J, Kershaw P, Lilienfeld S, Ding C. A 5-month, randomized, placebo-controlled trial of galantamine in AD. Neurology 2000; 54:2269–2276.
39. Raskind MA, Peskind ER, Wessel T, Yuan W. Galantamine in AD: a 6-month randomized, placebo-controlled trial with a 6-month extension. The Galantamine USA-1 Study Group. Neurology 2000; 54:2261–2268.
40. Knopman D, Schneider L, Davis K, et al. Long-term tacrine (Cognex) treatment: effects on nursing home placement and mortality. Tacrine Study Group. Neurology 1996; 47:166–177.
41. Feldman H, Gauthier S, Hecker J, Vellas B, Subbiah P, Whalen E. A 24-week, randomized, double-blind study of donepezil in moderate to severe Alzheimer's disease. Neurology 2001; 57:613–620.
42. Mohs RC, Doody RS, Morris JC, et al. A 1-year, placebo-controlled preservation of function survival study of donepezil in AD patients. Neurology 2001; 57:481–488.
43. Winblad B, Engedal K, Soininen H, et al. A 1-year, randomized, placebo-controlled study of donepezil in patients with mild to moderate AD. Neurology 2001; 57:489–495.
44. Butterfield DA. Amyloid beta-peptide (1–42)-induced oxidative stress and neurotoxicity: implications for neurodegeneration in Alzheimer's disease brain. A review. Free Radic Res 2002; 36:1307–1313.
45. Reisberg B, Doody R, Stoffler A, Schmitt F, Ferris S, Mobius HJ. Memantine in moderate-to-severe Alzheimer's disease. N Engl J Med 2003; 348:1333–1341.
46. Winblad B, Poritis N. Memantine in severe dementia: results of the 9M-Best study (benefit and efficacy in severely demented patients during treatment with memantine). Int J Geriatr Psychiatry 1999; 14:135–146.
47. Lynch G, Granger R, Ambros-Ingerson J, Davis CM, Kessler M, Schehr R. Evidence that a positive modulator of AMPA-type glutamate receptors improves delayed recall in aged humans. Exp Neurol 1997; 145:89–92.
48. Bartus RT, Dean RL, 3rd, Beer B, Lippa AS. The cholinergic hypothesis of geriatric memory dysfunction. Science 1982; 217:408–414.
49. Coyle JT, Price DL, DeLong MR. Alzheimer's disease: a disorder of cortical cholinergic innervation. Science 1983; 219:1184–1190.
50. Masliah E, Terry RD, Alford M, DeTeresa R, Hansen LA. Cortical and subcortical patterns of synaptophysinlike immunoreactivity in Alzheimer's disease. Am J Pathol 1991; 138:235–246.
51. Perry EK, Perry RH, Blessed G, Tomlinson BE. Changes in brain cholinesterases in senile dementia of Alzheimer type. Neuropathol Appl Neurobiol 1978; 4:273–277.
52. Perry EK, Tomlinson BE, Blessed G, Bergmann K, Gibson PH, Perry RH. Correlation of cholinergic abnormalities with senile plaques and mental test scores in senile dementia. Br Med J 1978; 2:1457–1459.
53. Hefti F, Dravid A, Hartikka J. Chronic intraventricular injections of nerve growth factor elevate hippocampal choline acetyltransferase activity in adult rats with partial septo-hippocampal lesions. Brain Res 1984; 293:305–311.
54. Dutar P, Bassant MH, Senut MC, Lamour Y. The septohippocampal pathway: structure and function of a central cholinergic system. Physiol Rev 1995; 75:393–427.
55. Blesch A, Tuszynski M. Ex vivo gene therapy for Alzheimer's disease and spinal cord injury. Clin Neurosci 1995; 3:268–274.
56. Tuszynski MH, Gage FH. Bridging grafts and transient nerve growth factor infusions promote long-term central nervous system neuronal rescue and partial functional recovery. Proc Natl Acad Sci USA 1995; 92:4621–4625.

57. Tuszynski MH, Gage FH. Potential use of neurotrophic agents in the treatment of neurodegenerative disorders. Acta Neurobiol Exp (Warsz) 1990; 50:311–322.

58. Tuszynski MH, Senut MC, Ray J, Roberts J. Somatic gene transfer to the adult primate central nervous system: in vitro and in vivo characterization of cells genetically modified to secrete nerve growth factor. Neurobiol Dis 1994; 1:67–78.

59. Rosenberg MB, Friedmann T, Robertson RC, et al. Grafting genetically modified cells to the damaged brain: restorative effects of NGF expression. Science 1988; 242:1575–1578.

60. Akiyama H, Barger S, Barnum S, et al. Inflammation and Alzheimer's disease. Neurobiol Aging 2000; 21:383–421.

61. Behl C. Alzheimer's disease and oxidative stress: implications for novel therapeutic approaches. Prog Neurobiol 1999; 57:301–323.

62. Caporali R, Montecucco C. Cardiovascular effects of coxibs. Lupus 2005; 14:785–788.

63. Tarassishin L, Yin YI, Bassit B, Li YM. Processing of Notch and amyloid precursor protein by {gamma}-secretase is spatially distinct. Proc Natl Acad Sci USA 2004; 101:17050–17055.

64. Searfoss GH, Jordan WH, Calligaro DO, et al. Adipsin, a biomarker of gastrointestinal toxicity mediated by a functional gamma-secretase inhibitor. J Biol Chem 2003; 278:46107–46116.

65. Janus C, Pearson J, McLaurin J, et al. A beta peptide immunization reduces behavioural impairment and plaques in a model of Alzheimer's disease. Nature 2000; 408:979–982.

66. Morgan D, Diamond DM, Gottschall PE, et al. A beta peptide vaccination prevents memory loss in an animal model of Alzheimer's disease. Nature 2000; 408:982–985.

67. Schenk D, Barbour R, Dunn W, et al. Immunization with amyloid-beta attenuates Alzheimer-disease-like pathology in the PDAPP mouse. Nature 1999; 400:173–177.

68. Takeuchi A, Irizarry MC, Duff K, et al. Age-related amyloid beta deposition in transgenic mice overexpressing both Alzheimer mutant presenilin 1 and amyloid beta precursor protein Swedish mutant is not associated with global neuronal loss. Am J Pathol 2000; 157:331–339.

69. Dodart JC, Bales KR, Gannon KS, et al. Immunization reverses memory deficits without reducing brain Abeta burden in Alzheimer's disease model. Nat Neurosci 2002; 5:452–457.

70. Kotilinek LA, Bacskai B, Westerman M, et al. Reversible memory loss in a mouse transgenic model of Alzheimer's disease. J Neurosci 2002; 22:6331–6335.

71. Bard F, Cannon C, Barbour R, et al. Peripherally administered antibodies against amyloid beta-peptide enter the central nervous system and reduce pathology in a mouse model of Alzheimer disease. Nat Med 2000; 6:916–919.

72. Gelinas DS, DaSilva K, Fenili D, George-Hyslop P, St, McLaurin J. Immunotherapy for Alzheimer's disease. Proc Natl Acad Sci USA 2004; 101:14657–14662.

73. DeMattos RB, Bales KR, Cummins DJ, Dodart JC, Paul SM, Holtzman DM. Peripheral anti-A beta antibody alters CNS and plasma A beta clearance and decreases brain A beta burden in a mouse model of Alzheimer's disease. Proc Natl Acad Sci USA 2001; 98:8850–8855.

74. McLaurin J, Cecal R, Kierstead ME, et al. Therapeutically effective antibodies against amyloid-beta peptide target amyloid-beta residues 4–10 and inhibit cytotoxicity and fibrillogenesis. Nat Med 2002; 15:15.

75. Bowers WJ, Mastrangelo MA, Stanley HA, Casey AE, Milo LJ, Jr, Federoff HJ. HSV amplicon-mediated Abeta vaccination in Tg2576 mice: differential antigen-specific immune responses. Neurobiol Aging 2005; 26:393–407.

76. Bowers WJ, Federoff HJ. Amyloid immunotherapy-engendered CNS inflammation. Neurobiol Aging 2002; 23:675–676 discussion 674–683.

77. Imbimbo BP. Toxicity of beta-amyloid vaccination in patients with Alzheimer's disease. Ann Neurol 2002; 51:794.

78. Orgogozo JM, Gilman S, Dartigues JF, et al. Subacute meningoencephalitis in a subset of patients with AD after Abeta42 immunization. Neurology 2003; 61:46–54.

79. Hock C, Konietzko U, Papassotiropoulos A, et al. Generation of antibodies specific for beta-amyloid by vaccination of patients with Alzheimer disease. Nat Med 2002; 8:1270–1275.

80. Hock C, Konietzko U, Streffer JR, et al. Antibodies against beta-amyloid slow cognitive decline in Alzheimer's disease. Neuron 2003; 38:547–554.

81. Nicoll JA, Wilkinson D, Holmes C, Steart P, Markham H, Weller RO. Neuropathology of human Alzheimer disease after immunization with amyloid-beta peptide: a case report. Nat Med 2003; 9:448–452.

82. Zhang J, Wu X, Qin C, et al. A novel recombinant adeno-associated virus vaccine reduces behavioral impairment and beta-amyloid plaques in a mouse model of Alzheimer's disease. Neurobiol Dis 2003; 14:365–379.

83. Wade-Martins R, Smith ER, Tyminski E, Chiocca EA, Saeki Y. An infectious transfer and expression system for genomic DNA loci in human and mouse cells. Nat Biotechnol 2001; 19:1067–1070.

84. Wade-Martins R, Saeki Y, Antonio Chiocca E. Infectious delivery of a 135-kb LDLR genomic locus leads to regulated complementation of low-density lipoprotein receptor deficiency in human cells. Mol Ther 2003; 7:604–612.

85. White RE, Wade-Martins R, James MR. Infectious delivery of 120-kilobase genomic DNA by an epstein-barr virus amplicon vector. Mol Ther 2002; 5:427–435.

86. Wade-Martins R, Frampton J, James MR. Long-term stability of large insert genomic DNA episomal shuttle vectors in human cells. Nucleic Acids Res 1999; 27:1674–1682.

87. Salio M, Cella M, Suter M, Lanzavecchia A. Inhibition of dendritic cell maturation by herpes simplex virus. Eur J Immunol 1999; 29:3245–3253.

88. Thomas J, Rouse BT. Immunopathogenesis of herpetic ocular disease. Immunol Res 1997; 16:375–386.

89. Hardy J, Selkoe DJ. The amyloid hypothesis of Alzheimer's disease: progress and problems on the road to therapeutics. Science 2002; 297:353–356.

90. Munch G, Robinson SR. Potential neurotoxic inflammatory responses to Abeta vaccination in humans. J Neural Transm 2002; 109:1081–1087.

91. Weiner HL, Lemere CA, Maron R, et al. Nasal administration of amyloid-beta peptide decreases cerebral amyloid burden in a mouse model of Alzheimer's disease. Ann Neurol 2000; 48:567–579.

92. Sigurdsson EM, Scholtzova H, Mehta PD, Frangione B, Wisniewski T. Immunization with a nontoxic/nonfibrillar amyloid-beta homologous peptide reduces Alzheimer's disease-associated pathology in transgenic mice. Am J Pathol 2001; 159:439–447.

93. Town T, Vendrame M, Patel A, et al. Reduced Th1 and enhanced Th2 immunity after immunization with Alzheimer's beta-amyloid(1–42). J Neuroimmunol 2002; 132:49–59.

94. Leverone JF, Spooner ET, Lehman HK, Clements JD, Lemere CA. Abeta1–15 is less immunogenic than Abeta1–40/42 for intranasal immunization of wild-type mice but may be effective for "boosting". Vaccine 2003; 21:2197–2206.

95. Frenkel D, Dewachter I, Van Leuven F, Solomon B. Reduction of beta-amyloid plaques in brain of transgenic mouse model of Alzheimer's disease by EFRH-phage immunization. Vaccine 2003; 21:1060–1065.

96. Bard F, Barbour R, Cannon C, et al. Epitope and isotype specificities of antibodies to beta-amyloid peptide for protection against Alzheimer's disease-like neuropathology. Proc Natl Acad Sci USA 2003; 100:2023–2028.

97. Gandy S, DeMattos RB, Lemere CA, et al. Alzheimer's Abeta vaccination of rhesus monkeys (Macaca mulatta). Mech Ageing Dev 2004; 125:149–151.

98. Solomon B, Koppel R, Hanan E, Katzav T. Monoclonal antibodies inhibit in vitro fibrillar aggregation of the Alzheimer beta-amyloid peptide. Proc Natl Acad Sci USA 1996; 93:452–455.

99. Solomon B, Koppel R, Frankel D, Hanan-Aharon E. Disaggregation of Alzheimer beta-amyloid by site-directed mAb. Proc Natl Acad Sci USA 1997; 94:4109–4112.

100. Chauhan NB, Siegel GJ. Intracerebroventricular passive immunization with anti-Abeta antibody in Tg2576. J Neurosci Res 2003; 74:142–147.

12

Gene Therapy of Multiple Sclerosis and in CNS Autoimmune Mouse Models

Daniel Larocque, Josée Bergeron, Maria G. Castro, and Pedro R. Lowenstein
Gene Therapeutics Research Institute, Cedars-Sinai Medical Center, and Departments of Medicine, and Medical and Molecular Pharmacology, David Geffen School of Medicine, University of California Los Angeles, Los Angeles, California, U.S.A.

ABSTRACT

Multiple Sclerosis (MS) and its animal model, experimental autoimmune encephalitis (EAE), are autoimmune disease of the central nervous system (CNS) characterized by inflammation and demyelination. Neurological gene therapy strategies involving the use of therapeutic transgenes expressed by viral vectors, DNA vectors, recombinant proteins or myelin-expressing cells have shown indications of inhibiting autoimmune-mediated inflammation in the brain. Here we review currently used pharmacological approaches for treating MS and we describe the currently used gene and cell therapy approaches for treating MS and his rodent model (EAE). Moreover, we summarize the advantage and disadvantages of these methodology and clinical studies. Also, we will propose five different avenues that could be pursued with the objective of developing gene therapy to treat MS, e.g., The inhibition of leukocyte migration into the CNS by targeting the blood-brain barrier; Reducing the production of anti-myelin antibodies; Expressing immune-modulating molecules within the affected CNS; Target differentiation factors to oligodendrocytes precursors to repair damaged myelin, and the abrogation of the myelin specific T-cell tolerance in the thymus and in the periphery. This will enable us to design specific and new therapeutic strategy for the treatment of autoimmune disease such as MS.

INTRODUCTION

One of the most important and well studied demyelinating diseases is MS, affecting at least 350,000 individuals in the United States alone and more than 1.1 million people worldwide (1,2). MS appears mainly in young adults between the ages of 20–40 and women are affected at least twice as often as men. MS is an autoimmune CNS demyelinating disease that causes relapsing and chronic CNS inflammation. Common symptoms of MS are incoordination, sensory disturbances, visual impairment and paralysis, which usually worsen as the disease progresses. The disease usually starts suddenly with an acute attack which lasts for a few days to weeks, followed by stabilization of the disease or remission. This relapsing remitting phase can last for many years. About 30% of individuals with relapsing-remitting MS develop a secondary chronic progressive state. In the chronic progressive phase distinct attacks are infrequent and the disease worsens at a constant rate, without recovery of functions. In rare instances, clinical disability begins with this progressive phase, and in this case the disease is called primary progressive MS. Although several clinical patterns of disease have been described, these do not correlate precisely with CNS pathology or MRI (magnetic resonance imaging) studies. Thus, it is difficult to predict disease progression in individual patients.

Pathological changes that underlie clinical MS include inflammation, demyelination, oligodendrocyte death, and axonal degeneration (3,4). Variation in disease pathology correlates with heterogeneous MRI appearance, unpredictable clinical progression and different responses to treatment. Disease variability also correlates with very different pathological processes thought to underlie clinical MS. Autoimmunity or virus infection have been proposed to induce MS-like inflammatory demyelinating plaques in the CNS. Experimentally, immunization against myelin proteins or Theiler's virus infection are used to model MS. An international effort using over one hundred biopsies from pathology samples of MS, collected in three international centers, resulted in a new pathological classification of MS based on careful neuropathological and immunological analysis (5,6). Four fundamentally different patterns of neuropathology were found. Characteristics of classification were based on: the type of myelin protein loss, the patterns of oligodendrocyte destruction, the localization and the extension of plaques, and the immunopathological evidence of complement activation (Table 1).

Interestingly, these four patterns of neuropathology are homogenous within lesions from the same patient, but differ from patient to patient. This suggests that each pattern represents a different disease entity. By combining technology such as MRI, blood analysis and biopsies, this classification may have fundamental implications for the future diagnosis of subtypes of MS in the future. If so, treatments will target individual disease types.

Apart from oligodendrocytes, lesions in MS target axons and other brain cells such as astrocytes and microglia that provide neuronal support and protection (7). In addition, inflammatory cells, such as Th1 (pro-inflammatory) T-cells and macrophages contribute to lesion formation. In chronic lesions, the lost axons and myelin are eventually replaced by dense, "sclerotic" astrocytic scar tissue, hence the name MS. Overall, MS is a chronic

Table 1 Pathological Subtypes of Multiple Sclerosis

Pathological patterns	Characteristics
I	Presence of T-cells and macrophages, and effector molecules including TNF-α, IFN-γ, and free radical species molecules in the demyelinated area
II	Antibody and complement deposition. MBP and MOG-specific antibodies are present
III	Lesions characterized by preferential loss of MAG and oligodendrocytes. Primary oligodendrocyte dystrophy, focal cerebral ischemia and heat shock proteins specific immunoreactivity
IV	Characterized by non-apoptotic oligodendrocyte degeneration

inflammatory disease in which patients exhibit high levels of circulating pro-inflammatory cytokines (8). The presence of pro-inflammatory cytokines skews the immune response toward a Th1 bias, an imbalance that is thought to be characteristic of many autoimmune diseases, such as MS, rheumatoid arthritis and autoimmune diabetes. One of the major focuses of MS therapies since the last decade has therefore focused on restoring the Th1 vs. Th2 T-cells balance to ameliorate the disease (Table 2).

Several studies suggest that susceptibility to MS has a genetic component (9). MS has been associated with the HLA-DR2 haplotype. Haplotypes most frequently linked to MS are DRB1*1501, DRB5*0101, DQA1*01012, DQB1*0602. However, the linkage with several alleles suggests a polygenic influence on MS, and several major histocompatibility complex (MHC) genes could be implicated in the disease.

In the last few years, the management of patients with MS has improved significantly with the introduction of immune-modulators such as interferon-β (IFN-β), glatiramer acetate (GA) or copaxone (10). Many patients respond favorably to these drugs, however some have a less than an ideal response (11). The treatment with these compounds has frequently resulted in side effects such as toxicity, increased oncogenic risk, or hypertension. In addition, the efficacy of MS treatment with anti-inflammatory drugs is limited by their poor entry into the CNS or their short half lives.

The current treatments for MS consist of anti-inflammatory and/or neuroprotective molecules such as IFN-β and immunosuppressors such as azathioprine, cyclophosphamide,

Table 2   Treatment Currently Used or in Development for Treating Chronic MS

Treatment	Postulated modes of action
Interferon β-1a (Avonex^{TM} and Rebif$^{\circledR}$) Interferon β-1b (Betaferon)	General suppression of T helper 1 (Th1) and Th2 cytokines; Prevention of T-cells from entering the CNS by decreasing metalloproteinase production (gelatinase) and adhesion molecule expression (70). Complete mechanism of action unknown
Glatiramer acetate (Copaxone$^{\circledR}$)	Synthetic oligopeptide similar to the sequence of a myelin epitope from MBP. Generation of glatiramer acetate-reactive Th2 lymphocytes; production of brain-derived neutrophic factor (71,72) Proposed mechanism of action: competition for MBP 82-100 binding to the MHC-class II, and therefore reducing anti-myelin immune responses
$\alpha4\beta1$ integrin antibody (Natalizumab$^{\circledR}$)	Inhibits lymphocyte entry into the brain, T-cell migration and homing inhibitor (22). Mechanism of action: binds to $\alpha4\beta1$ integrin receptor on infiltrating T-cell
Statins (HMGCoA reductase inhibitor)	Statins competitively inhibit HMG CoA reductase. The enzyme product (L-mevalonate) is an intermediate in cholesterol synthesis, several of its metabolites are involved in post-translational modification of specific proteins involved in cell proliferation and differentiation. Statins have anti-inflammatory and neuroprotective properties by triggering activation of Th2 T-cells (73). Detailed mechanism of action is unknown
Immunosuppressors (Cyclosporin A and FK506)	Both cause reduction of IL-2 production. FK506 binds to FK506 binding protein-12 (FKBP-12) in lymphocytes and inhibiting calcineurin activation, resulting in a marked reduction in interleukin IL-2 production (74)
Minocycline	Inhibition of nitric oxide synthase, attenuate microglia activation and glutamate excitotoxicity (10). Complete mechanism of action: unknown

and cyclosporine (12). However, the treatment with these compounds is only partially effective, does not halt disease progression and has frequently resulted in side effects such as toxicity, increased oncogenic risk, or hypertension. For these reasons, new therapeutic approaches including the transfer of genes into the CNS using viral vectors, stem cells or other gene therapy methods are being developed as potential new treatments. Much of the treatment of MS continues to be limited by our difficulties in disentangling the mechanisms underlying immune responses in the CNS, and the fact that within the brain itself, two different immune compartments, with individualized afferent and efferent immune response, are present (13).

New medications and the rational combination of existing therapies may lead to improved therapeutic outcomes in MS. Systemic administration of IFN-β is one of the currently approved therapies for MS. IFN-β has potent activity at the blood-brain barrier (BBB) and impairs the trafficking of inflammatory cells into the CNS. In contrast, GA, another existing therapy, has negligible effect at the BBB, but it is thought to allow GA specific Th2 lymphocytes to enter the CNS to decrease inflammation by producing anti-inflammatory cytokines IL-10 and transforming growth factor beta (TGF-β). The mode of action of GA is through its high avidity binding to MHC molecules and consequent competition with various endogenous myelin antigens for their presentation to T-cells (11). One characteristic of MS is the increased production of metallo-proteinases (MMPs), such as MMP-9, also called Gelatinase B. MMP-9 is capable of damaging components of the BBB, and of cleaving myelin basic protein into immunodominant and encephalitogenic fragments, thus playing a functional role in

Figure 1 (*Figure on facing page*) (*See color insert*) (**A**) Important steps in disease progression during Multiple Sclerosis. Both cellular and humoral immune mechanisms are involved. (**B**) Five majors targets for therapy in Multiple Sclerosis. 1. In MS and EAE, the BBB is affected by pro-inflammatory cytokines released by infiltrating T-cells and glial cells in the brain. Cytokines such as IFN-γ, TNF-α, IL-1 and/or Chemokines (MCP-1), MMPs and adhesion molecules are expressed by CNS endothelium and infiltrating T-cells that increase BBB permeability. 2. Demyelinating antibodies are often present in the blood of MS patients. Increased incidence of antibodies against myelin proteins such as MOG and MBP in CSF and sera of MS patients suggest a pathogenic role for these antibodies in MS. A gene therapy approach using immunoglobulins fused to myelin antigen could trigger immune tolerance for myelin antigens and thus reverse the myelin autoimmune disease. 3. In MS, T helper 1 (Th1)-cytokines are overexpressed and dominate over Th2-cytokines. Immunomodulation strategy could be to trigger anti-inflamatory cytokines. A gene therapy approach is to express Th2 cytokines (IL-4. Il-10, TGF-β, IFN-β). 4. Oligodendrocyte (OL) differentiation is blocked in MS plaques by a Notch dependent pathway. A barrier to myelin repair, astrocytic gliosis, increases the secretion of Jagged Ligands which block oligodendrocyte differentiation and remyelination in MS plaques. The use of transgenes promoting oligodendrocyte differentiation might be considered. 5. In MS and EAE, central and peripheral tolerance mechanisms fail. Self-reactive T-cells recognizing myelin-MHC molecules escape the selection in the thymus and in the periphery. A gene therapy strategy could be directed to the thymus by injecting vectors coding for myelin antigens, and triggering deletion of the T-cell recognizing myelin-MHC molecules, thereby inducing tolerance to specific antigens or inducing regulatory T-cells (T-reg) specific for myelin antigens. *Abbreviations*: MS, multiple sclerosis; BBB, blood-brain barrier; MOG, myelin oligodendrocyte glycoprotein; MBP, myelin basic protein; CSF, cerebrospinal fluid; IL, TGF, transforming growth factor; IFN, EAE, experimental autoimmune encephalitis; CNS, central nervous system; MHC, major histocompatibility complex; MMPs, metalloproteinase.

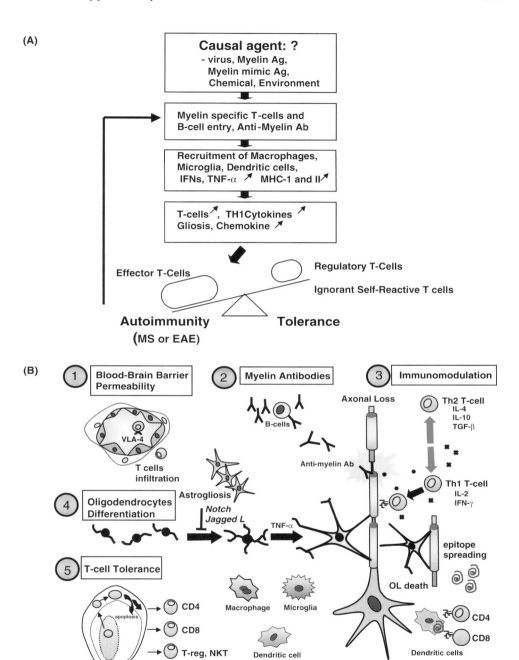

Figure 1 (*Caption on facing page*)

disease progression and being a novel therapeutic target amenable to pharmacological inhibition (15).

Strategies involving the use of therapeutic transgenes expressed by viral vectors, DNA vectors or cells have shown indications of inhibiting autoimmune-mediated inflammation in the brain (14,15). For designing an efficient gene therapy, an important condition is that the transgene has to be expressed long term, and has to be under regulated expression. Novel developments in gene delivery methods offer the possibility of long-term expression and site-directed expression of therapeutic transgenes. In animal model of MS, e.g., experimental allergic encephalomyelitis (EAE), gene therapy experiments are currently being investigated, and important examples will be described below. While some immune effectors may be targeted systemically using DNA vaccination, strategies for both viral and non-viral gene delivery are being developed to target agents into the CNS either via direct delivery or using the trafficking properties of cell-carrier systems.

We propose five different avenues that could be pursued with the aim of developing gene therapy to treat MS: (1) The inhibition of leukocyte migration into the CNS by targeting the BBB; (2) Reducing the production of anti-myelin antibodies; (3) Expressing immune-modulating molecules within the affected CNS; (4) Target differentiation factors to oligodendrocytes precursors to repair damaged myelin; (5) Abrogation of the myelin specific T-cell tolerance in the thymus and in the periphery (Fig. 1).

The Inhibition of Leukocyte Migration Through the Blood-Brain Barrier

Among the earliest cerebrovascular abnormalities seen in MS is the deregulation of the BBB and entry of activated leukocytes into the brain parenchyma. This leukocyte infiltration eventually leads to the release of inflammatory cytokines/chemokines. Mechanisms for breakdown of the BBB in MS are incompletely understood, but appear to involve cytokines/ chemokines, metalloproteinases (MMPs), adhesion molecules expressed by the endothelium cells and glia at the BBB (8). Integrins are heterodimeric adhesion molecules that play key roles in leukocyte trafficking and activation (16). One of the major integrin proteins in the brain is VLA-4, which consists of an $\alpha4$ chain noncovalently linked to the $\beta1$ molecule. In fact, VLA-4 may bind to adhesion molecules on the surface of inflamed endothelium and allow penetration of the endothelium that forms the BBB. Blockade of VLA-4 reverses clinical paralysis in acute experimental autoimmune encephalomyelitis (EAE), and prevents further relapses in the chronic model of this disease (17,18). Thus, a gene delivery approach using a vector expressing VLA-4 might saturate the receptors and thus block the infiltration of leukocytes into the endothelium of the brain.

For targeting the BBB, studies performed in the EAE model suggested that VLA-4 blockade could benefit MS patients since monoclonal antibodies targeting VLA-4 can moderate or reverse signs of paralysis in mouse and guinea pig models of EAE (19,20). A gene therapy approach using antisense oligonucleotide specific for VLA-4 mRNA has been used. Mice immunized to develop EAE were injected subcutaneously with the VLA-4 antisense oligonucleotides. The effect of the anitisense molecules was effective at inhibiting paralysis in EAE mice when administered either before or after clinical symptoms were apparent (21).

Another strategy targeting the BBB consists of blocking the lymphocyte migration into the brain by blocking the $\alpha4\beta1$ integrin interaction with its ligand VCAM1 (20). Those proteins are present at high levels in the brain endothelium and on perivascular macrophages. A monoclonal antibody produced in mice against human $\alpha4\beta1$ integrin was humanized and placed on an IgG4 framework (22). This was done to reduce its immunogenicity, to increase its half-life and to avoid complement fixation. This antibody was named natalizumab (Tysabri®).

However, in early 2005, only 3 mo after FDA approval of nataluzimab, its manufacturers, Biogen-IDEC and Elan, suspended all clinical trials with nataluzimab, and stopped marketing the drug. Two cases of progressive multifocal leukoencephalopathy (PML), one fatal, were reported in patients on nataluzimab, which also received IFN-β (Avonex). This decision by the FDA was made after confirmation of one fatal case and one additional case of PML in patients receiving nataluzimab for MS. Both patients were enrolled in a long-term clinical trial and had been taking nataluzimab for more than two years. After that clinical incident, the hypothesis has been brought that the combination of nataluzimab and Avonex have led to the activation of JC virus, a polyoma virus normally latent in the CNS, and whose reactivation causes PML (23). It is noteworthy to know that polyoma viruses have receptors in their genome for α4β1 integrin. Thus, the usage of α4β1 integrin antibody might have caused the activation of JC virus by blocking the ability of T-cells to enter the CNS and control virus therein. Additionally, the addition of IFN-β (Avonex), which blocks the lymphocyte homing in the brain, had down-regulated the anti-JC immune response. However, a clinical trial of nataluzimab for Crohn's disease has demonstrated that nataluzimab therapy by itself caused PML (24). At present the risk and prevalence of PML and other opportunistic infections following the use of α4β1 integrin antibody in human is unknown. The FDA, Elan and Biogen-IDEC are reviewing the cases of all individuals who received nataluzimab.

Targeting Anti-Myelin Antibody Production

MS and the mouse model EAE are T-cell-mediated diseases; however B cells and demyelinating antibodies are also important for the onset of the MS disease (25). Immunoglobulin therapy has been touted as a potential treatment for triggering immune cell tolerance against auto-antigens such as myelin antigens. Interestingly, B-cells could be modified into a gene delivery vehicle for the induction of tolerance against myelin in MS. B-cell therapy in EAE models has shown that peripheral tolerance of both Th1 and Th2 compartments can be induced using B cells transduced by a retrovirus that expresses MBP or myelin oligodendrocyte glycoprotein (MOG) inserted into IgG heavy chain (26). The phenotype of EAE can even be blocked by genetically modified B-cells expressing MOG-IgG. Moreover, the production of anti-myelin antibodies such as anti-MOG has been inhibited and the chronic EAE has been suppressed by this B-cell treatment. This study demonstrates the feasibility of allowing a specific humoral immune response against myelin antigens without knowing the specific antigen or epitope. In general, the ultimate goal is to specify deleting or tolerizing (anergizing) myelin-specific T-cells, so they no longer respond to myelin antigens. Studies performed by McMillan's group consisting of the continuous exposing of a low level of PLP antigen secreted by gene modified fibroblast demonstrated that a cell-based gene therapy for EAE is possible to ameliorate the disease (27).

However, this approach of expressing autoantigen systemically to induce tolerance should be taken with caution. In fact, vaccination experiments in EAE using a DNA construct encoding the MOG developed an exacerbated form of EAE when challenged with either proteolipid protein (PLP) or MOG myelins antigens. This has been explained by the inability of DNA vaccination to tolerize the MOG-specific T-cell response.

Moreover, cytopathic MOG-specific autoantibody response has been induced and this promoting a demyelination phenotype in the CNS of DNA-vaccinated mice (28). Similar difficulties of inducing tolerance once immunity has been activated, has also been encountered in the development of treatments for other autoimmune diseases such as type 1 diabetes (29).

The Targeting of Immune-Modulating Molecules to the CNS

It has been demonstrated that CNS inflammation and clinical disease in myelin-induced EAE could be prevented completely by a replication-defective adenovirus vector expressing the anti-inflammatory cytokine IL-10 injected into the CNS (30). Another study using the anti-inflammatory Th2 cytokine, i.e., IL-10, expressed by a replication-defective adenovirus vector into the lateral ventricles of the EAE mouse brain has shown the inhibition of the progression and even accelerated disease remission (30). However, the systemic (intravascular) injection of adenoviruses expressing human IL-10 was ineffective; quite a surprising result since IL-10 is known to promote the Th2 general anti-inflammatory response in other mice autoimmune models such as arthritis (31). In a relapsing-remitting EAE disease model, IL-10 gene transfer during remission prevented subsequent relapses. These experiments have demonstrated that IL-10 must access the CNS from the peripheral circulation or be delivered directly to the brain to be effective in autoimmune demyelinating diseases such as EAE.

A gene therapy strategy in EAE using herpes simplex virus-based vectors expressing the Th2 cytokine IL-4 has previously shown a significant inhibition of disease symptoms by the virus expressing IL-4 in the brain (32,33). The HSV-IL-4 injection into the brain of myelin-induced EAE in BALB/c and AB/H mice affected by a relapsing-remitting form of myelin-induced EAE promoted the in situ production of IL-4 by CNS-resident cells facing the cerebrospinal fluid (CSF) spaces and reduced the disease-related deaths. HSV-IL-4 treated mice also showed a shorter duration of the first EAE attack, a longer inter-relapse period and a reduction in the severity and duration of the first relapse. These results demonstrate that IL-4 gene delivery using HSV-1 vectors could protect from EAE by modulating the cytokine/chemokine expression and are promoting the expression of Th2 type of anti-inflammatory cytokines.

Another study reported the use of a recombinant adenovirus vector to induce regulatory responses for the prevention of autoimmune diseases through transient expression of a T-cell receptor (TCR) β chain expressed by most MBP-specific T-cells (34). It is established that T-cells which react to the N-terminal determinant, MBPAc1-9, are predominant and they use the Vβ8.2 TCR chain. Immunization of B10.PL mice with a recombinant adenovirus expressing the TCR Vβ8.2 chain demonstrated an up-regulation of type 1 regulatory CD4 T-cells, directed against the framework region 3 determinant within the B5 peptide (aa 76–101) of the Vβ8.2 chain. Adenovirus delivery to the brain of the TCR Vβ8.2 chain protected mice from MBP-induced EAE. However, when the adenovirus expressing TCR Vβ8.2 was co-administered with either an IL-4- or IL-10-expressing vector, regulation was disrupted and disease was exacerbated. These results highlight the importance of the Th1-like cytokine requirement necessary for the generation and activity of effective regulatory T-cells in this model of EAE.

Another interesting gene therapy approach is the induction of tolerance by suppressing co-stimulatory signals from the TCR-CD3 complex. Among the TCR complex, an important protein is the ligand CTLA4 (CD152). In fact, the co-stimulatory molecule CTLA4, expressed on the surface of T-cells following activation, has a much higher affinity for B7 molecules compared with CD28 and is a negative regulator of T-cell activation (35). In contrast to some of the stimulating/agonist capabilities of CTLA4-specific monoclonal antibodies, CTLA4-Ig fusion proteins (CTLA4-Ig) appear to act as CD28 antagonists and prevent co-stimulation in vitro and in vivo (36,37). Delivering a non-replicative adenovirus expressing CTLA4-human Ig into the CNS of the AB/H mouse myelin-induced EAE model resulted in significant protection from seizures and CNS inflammation. Moreover, an injection of recombinant adenovirus in the brain has been shown to be more effective than a single injection of CTLA4-human Ig protein systemically. Thus, local gene delivery of CTLA4-Ig may thus be an important target for immunotherapy of MS.

Targeting of Stem Cells or Differentiation Factors to Repair the Damaged Myelin

Spontaneous remyelination does occur in MS lesions, but it cannot prevent irreversible axonal damage in the long term (38,39). In fact, the major consequence of CNS damage is the secretion of inhibitory molecules for oligodendrocyte differentiation by reactive astrocytes. Inflammatory cells and astrocytes create an environment in which surviving endogenous oligodendrocyte progenitor cells (OPCs) are unable to differentiate and myelinate. Interestingly, Brosnan's group demonstrated that the binding of Jagged-1 ligand secreted from the astrocytic scar activates the Notch pathway in OPCs, leading to an inhibition of oligodendrocyte differentiation and myelination (40). Therefore, blocking Notch, an inhibitory factor for oligodendrocyte differentiation, or the expression of oligodendrocyte differentiation factors could lead to the development of new gene therapies for treating MS.

A therapeutic approach could consist of repairing the damaged myelin in the CNS by using vectors coding for oligodendrocyte differentiation factors. The discovery of proteins that activate myelination such as PDGF, Olig1, Olig2, Nkx, QKI and others are just starting to be elucidated (41). A gene therapy approach using retrovirus and adenovirus coding for the RNA binding protein QKI demonstrated an activation of oligodendrocyte differentiation and myelination in the brain (42). Even though this approach has never been tried in a MS model such as EAE, the use of genes coding for oligodendrocyte differentiation factors might be envisaged as a strategy for targeting oligodendrocyte progenitors and thus remyelinating damaged axons in MS or EAE brains.

The growing evidence that stem cells could be used in neurological diseases such as spinal cord injury, Parkinson, Alzheimer and Huntington's diseases (43–47) leads us to investigate whether a therapy using neural stem cells or gene-modified neural stem cells could be amenable. A cell therapy approach has been successfully implemented by by using neural precursor cells (neurospheres) from the periventricular zone of the brain to attenuate paralysis and oligodendrocytes and neuronal death in EAE (48). Similar approaches have been tried in EAE and other demyelinating diseases (49,50). Although the exact nature of the therapeutically effective cells is still unknown, Martino and collaborators found that the neural precursor cells express $\alpha 4$ integrin, like the myelin specific T-cell in EAE and MS (51). Once injected, neural precursor cells were able to move to the points of inflammation within the brain and spinal cord of mice with EAE. There they somehow became involved in processes that decrease the levels of inflammatory molecules, such as TNF-α and metalloproteases.

Macrophages arise from circulating monocyte precursors from the bone marrow. The CNS contains several macrophage populations, some of which are long-term residents while others have faster turnover times (52,53). Among the resident macrophages in CNS, there are perivascular macrophages that are continuously replenished from circulating monocyte precursors and have thus a fast turnover. In contrast, the resident brain macrophages, the microglial cells, arrive in the CNS before birth and persist for very long periods with little turnover from the bone marrow. Moreover, it has been shown that perivascular macrophages actually regulate T-cell responses in the CNS and may govern the ability of T-cells to enter the neural parenchyma (54). During brain inflammation, large increases of monocyte-derived macrophages could be detected in the CNS. Bone marrow transplantation (BMT) following a myelo-ablation is a current treatment to treat MS during the chronic progression phase, usually as a last resort treatment (55–59). The expectation is that the replacement of autoaggressive lymphocytes by naive precursors should arrest autoimmunity, and potentially induce tolerance; equally BMT-derived cells will exchange the population of perivascular macrophages, but not microglia (60). Unfortunately, in practice these clinical trials results were not conclusive (61). It is speculated that the high level of IFN-γ in MS patient and the low level of CD25+ regulatory T-cells might play a role in this failure (62,63). A gene therapy approach causing the downregulation of IFN-γ and the upregulation of regulatory T-cells might increase the efficiency of the BMT treatment for MS.

We expect that the usage of combinatory approach using gene therapy and stem cell technology together will allow to modify glial and neuronal precursors cells to repair the myelin damage in EAE and MS. However, to apply such cell and gene therapy based strategies in MS, it will be imperative to reduce the risk that newly formed myelin-producing cells will be targeted in another round of inflammatory and relapsing or chronic phase of MS. Those strategies can perhaps be combined with established drugs for MS to suppress the autoimmunity.

Induction of T-Cell Tolerance

More recently, gene therapy strategy delivered directly to the thymus have been investigated for autoimmune diseases (64–66). The thymus is the primary site for T-cell development and induction of self-tolerance. During the thymic selection process, the TCR-mediated positive and negative selection of T-cells allows the selection of a diverse TCR repertoire able to react with foreign peptide presented by autologous MHC molecules, but tolerant to self-antigens. This property renders the thymus an attractive site for manipulation of T-cell tolerance. Since lentiviral vectors have unique ability to integrate into the genome of quiescent cells, it is thought that it could be a convenient choice of vector for targeting stromal cells in the thymus and may be best suited for long-term expression of a transgene in the thymus. David Klatzmann and collaborators have used adult mice and injected them in the thymus with lentiviral vectors expressing EGFP or the neo-antigen hemagglutinin of the Influenza virus under the control of the ubiquitous promoter (68–70). Thereafter, thymi were examined 5 to 90 days directly under a UV-light microscope and by flow cytometry. Intrathymic injection of lentiviral vectors predominantly resulted in infection of stromal cells that could be detected for at least 3 mo. Importantly, hemagglutinin expression by thymic stromal cells mediated negative selection of thymocytes expressing the cognate TCR. This study demonstrated that intrathymic delivery of a lentiviral vector could be useful to induce tolerance to a specific antigen. Proof of principle using myelin antigens still has to be performed in EAE model before envisaging this approach to treat MS or others autoimmune diseases.

CONCLUSION

Since MS is an autoimmune disease, new immunotherapies will have to target the "Tolerance and Auto-immunity equilibrium" that is affected in MS and other auto-immune diseases such as systemic lupus erythematosus, rheumatoid arthritis and type 1 insulin-dependent diabetes. In fact, the central and peripheral tolerance is not efficient at eliminating self-reactive T-cells for myelin. Recent indications suggest that the tolerance mechanism in the thymus and in the periphery for self-antigens such as myelin proteins for MS is affected (67). So far, no gene therapy approach has been envisaged to target regulatory T-cells, which inhibit self-reactive T-cells that were aberrantly activated. In a near future, gene therapy approaches up-regulating CD25 + regulatory T-cells should be investigated. By such treatments, regulatory T-cells might inhibit cytokine production by myelin specific T-cells and then down-regulate inflammation in the brain, which has been previously postulated in others experimental neuro-degenarative models such as optic nerve injury (68,69).

Before moving forward into clinical trials using gene therapy approaches, safety validations will have to be assessed. Primary concern is the immunogenicity of the vector itself, which will have to be tested prior to injection. Another key question remains to be addressed: we will need to be careful to avoid gene therapy viral vectors or DNA plasmids vectors mimicking myelin antigens, and thereby potentially worsening MS. This will have to be addressed before starting any MS gene therapy clinical trial. What therapeutic genes should be used? How long an expression period is necessary to provide therapeutic effect systemically as well as in the brain? What are the consequences of prolonged expression of a myelin antigen? Is there a danger disrupting healthy regions of the brain during the delivery of the vector? Furthermore, advances in the vectorology will provide new tools to researchers to counteract MS. In the near future, the usage of combination of therapies such as IFN-β or cytokines with oligodendrocytes differentiation factors could be promising for more specific therapies in MS. Such therapies will have a dual effect of blocking the immune response as well as repairing the damaged myelin in CNS. Since gene therapy is still in its infancy, exhaustive research will have to be performed in the future to overcome gene delivery side effects. More specific and expression-controlled vectors designed for CNS auto-immunity pathology are currently ongoing to further help in the treatment of MS by gene therapy.

ACKNOWLEDGMENTS

For space constraints, we apologize to the authors who have made important contributions to the field but could not be cited. We are grateful to Kurt Kroeger for helping in the preparation of this manuscript and Guillermina Almazan and Von Wee Yong for their helpful discussions. Daniel Larocque held a postdoctoral fellowship from the MS Society of Canada and Human Frontier Science Program (HFSP). This work was supported by grants from the NIH/ National Institute of Neurological Disorders and Stroke to P.R.L. and M.G.C. (R01 NS44556.01, NS 42893.01) and the Bram and Elaine Kane Fellowship. We also thank the generous funding our Institute receives from the Board of Governors at Cedars-Sinai Medical Center.

REFERENCES

1. Steinman L, Martin R, Bernard C, Conlon P, Oksenberg JR. Multiple sclerosis: deeper understanding of its pathogenesis reveals new targets for therapy. Annu Rev Neurosci 2002; 25:491.
2. Sospedra M, Martin R. Immunology of multiple sclerosis. Annu Rev Immunol 2004.
3. Steinman L. Multiple approaches to multiple sclerosis. Nat Med 2000; 6:15.
4. Lassmann H. Comparative neuropathology of chronic experimental allergic encephalomyelitis and multiple sclerosis. Schriftenr Neurol 1983; 25:1.
5. Bruck W, Lucchinetti C, Lassmann H. The pathology of primary progressive multiple sclerosis. Mult Scler 2002; 8:93.
6. Lassmann H, Bruck W, Lucchinetti C. Heterogeneity of multiple sclerosis pathogenesis: implications for diagnosis and therapy. Trends Mol Med 2001; 7:115.
7. Bjartmar C, Yin X, Trapp BD. Axonal pathology in myelin disorders. J Neurocytol 1999; 28:383.
8. Owens T. The enigma of multiple sclerosis: inflammation and neurodegeneration cause heterogeneous dysfunction and damage. Curr Opin Neurol 2003; 16:259.
9. Dyment DA, Herrera BM, Cader MZ, et al. Complex interactions among MHC haplotypes in multiple sclerosis: susceptibility and resistance. Hum Mol Genet 2005; 14:2019.
10. Yong VW. Prospects for neuroprotection in multiple sclerosis. Front Biosci 2004; 9:864.
11. Sela M, Teitelbaum D. Glatiramer acetate in the treatment of multiple sclerosis. Expert Opin Pharmacother 2001; 2:1149.
12. Kappos L, Patzold U, Dommasch D, et al. Cyclosporine versus azathioprine in the long-term treatment of multiple sclerosis—results of the German multicenter study. Ann Neurol 1988; 23:56.
13. Lowenstein PR. Immunology of viral-vector-mediated gene transfer into the brain: an evolutionary and developmental perspective. Trends Immunol 2002; 23:23.
14. Chernajovsky Y, Gould DJ, Podhajcer OL. Gene therapy for autoimmune diseases: quo vadis? Nat Rev Immunol 2004; 4:800.
15. Baker D, Hankey DJ. Gene therapy in autoimmune, demyelinating disease of the central nervous system. Gene Ther 2003; 10:844.
16. Hynes RO. Integrins: versatility, modulation, and signaling in cell adhesion. Cell 1992; 69:11.
17. Theien BE, Vanderlugt LC, Nickerson-Nutter C, et al. Differential effects of treatment with a small-molecule VLA-4 antagonist before and after onset of relapsing EAE. Blood 2003; 102:4464.
18. Cannella B, Gaupp S, Tilton RG, Raine CS. Differential efficacy of a synthetic antagonist of VLA-4 during the course of chronic relapsing experimental autoimmune encephalomyelitis. J Neurosci Res 2003; 71:407.
19. Kent SJ, Karlik JS, Cannon C, et al. A monoclonal antibody to alpha 4 integrin suppresses and reverses active experimental allergic encephalomyelitis. J Neuroimmunol 1995; 58:1.
20. Yednock TA, Cannon C, Fritz LC, Sanchez-Madrid F, Steinman L, Karin N. Prevention of experimental autoimmune encephalomyelitis by antibodies against alpha 4 beta 1 integrin. Nature 1992; 356:63.
21. Myers KJ, Witchell DR, Graham MJ, Koo S, Butler M, Condon TP. Antisense oligonucleotide blockade of alpha 4 integrin prevents and reverses clinical symptoms in murine experimental autoimmune encephalomyelitis. J Neuroimmunol 2005; 160:12.
22. Leger OJ, Yednock TA, Tanner L, et al. Humanization of a mouse antibody against human alpha-4 integrin: a potential therapeutic for the treatment of multiple sclerosis. Hum Antibodies 1997; 8:3.
23. Caruso M, Belloni L, Sthandier O, Amati P, Garcia MI. Alpha4beta1 integrin acts as a cell receptor for murine polyomavirus at the postattachment level. J Virol 2003; 77:3913.
24. Steinman L. Blocking adhesion molecules as therapy for multiple sclerosis: natalizumab. Nat Rev Drug Discov 2005; 4:510.

25. Bar-Or A, Oliveira EM, Anderson DE, Hafler DA. Molecular pathogenesis of multiple sclerosis. J Neuroimmunol 1999; 100:252.

26. Xu B, Scott DW. A novel retroviral gene therapy approach to inhibit specific antibody production and suppress experimental autoimmune encephalomyelitis induced by MOG and MBP. Clin Immunol 2004; 111:47.

27. Louie KA, Weiner LP, Du J, et al. Cell-based gene therapy experiments in murine experimental autoimmune encephalomyelitis. Gene Ther 2005; 12:1145.

28. Bourquin C, Iglesias A, Berger T, Wekerle H, Linington C. Myelin oligodendrocyte glycoprotein-DNA vaccination induces antibody-mediated autoaggression in experimental autoimmune encephalomyelitis. Eur J Immunol 2000; 30:3663.

29. Bach JF, Chatenoud L. Tolerance to islet autoantigens in type 1 diabetes. Annu Rev Immunol 2001; 19:131.

30. Cua DJ, Hutchins B, LaFace DM, Stohlman SA, Coffman RL. Central nervous system expression of IL-10 inhibits autoimmune encephalomyelitis. J Immunol 2001; 166:602.

31. Setoguchi K, Misaki Y, Araki Y, et al. Antigen-specific T-cells transduced with IL-10 ameliorate experimentally induced arthritis without impairing the systemic immune response to the antigen. J Immunol 2000; 165:5980.

32. Furlan R, Poliani PL, Marconi PC, et al. Central nervous system gene therapy with interleukin-4 inhibits progression of ongoing relapsing-remitting autoimmune encephalomyelitis in Biozzi AB/H mice. Gene Ther 2001; 8:13.

33. Broberg EK, Salmi AA, Hukkanen V. IL-4 is the key regulator in herpes simplex virus-based gene therapy of BALB/c experimental autoimmune encephalomyelitis. Neurosci Lett 2004; 364:173.

34. Braciak TA, Pedersen B, Chin J, et al. Protection against experimental autoimmune encephalomyelitis generated by a recombinant adenovirus vector expressing the V beta 8.2 TCR is disrupted by coadministration with vectors expressing either IL-4 or -10. J Immunol 2003; 170:765.

35. Karandikar NJ, Vanderlugt CL, Walunas TL, Miller SD, Bluestone JA. CTLA-4: a negative regulator of autoimmune disease. J Exp Med 1996; 184:783.

36. Croxford JL, O'Neill JK, Ali RR, et al. Local gene therapy with CTLA4-immunoglobulin fusion protein in experimental allergic encephalomyelitis. Eur J Immunol 1998; 28:3904.

37. Croxford JL, Feldmann M, Chernajovsky Y, Baker D. Different therapeutic outcomes in experimental allergic encephalomyelitis dependent upon the mode of delivery of IL-10: a comparison of the effects of protein, adenoviral or retroviral IL-10 delivery into the central nervous system. J Immunol 2001; 166:4124.

38. Raine CS, Wu. E. Multiple sclerosis: remyelination in acute lesions. J Neuropathol Exp Neurol 1993; 52:199.

39. Keirstead HS, Blakemore WF. Identification of post-mitotic oligodendrocytes incapable of remyelination within the demyelinated adult spinal cord. J Neuropathol Exp Neurol 1997; 56:1191.

40. John GR, Shankar SL, Shafit-Zagardo B, et al. Multiple sclerosis: re-expression of a developmental pathway that restricts oligodendrocyte maturation. Nat Med 2002; 8:1115.

41. Rowitch DH. Glial specification in the vertebrate neural tube. Nat Rev Neurosci 2004; 5:409.

42. Larocque D, Galarneau A, Liu HN, Scott M, Almazan G, Richard S. Protection of p27(Kip1) mRNA by quaking RNA binding proteins promotes oligodendrocyte differentiation. Nat Neurosci 2005; 8:27.

43. McDonald JW, Liu XZ, Qu Y, et al. Transplanted embryonic stem cells survive, differentiate and promote recovery in injured rat spinal cord. Nat Med 1999; 5:1410.

44. Snyder EY, Macklis JD. Multipotent neural progenitor or stem-like cells may be uniquely suited for therapy for some neurodegenerative conditions. Clin Neurosci 1995; 3:310.

45. Cao QL, Zhang YP, Howard RM, Walters WM, Tsoulfas P, Whittemore SR. Pluripotent stem cells engrafted into the normal or lesioned adult rat spinal cord are restricted to a glial lineage. Exp Neurol 2001; 167:48.

46. Gage FH. Mammalian neural stem cells. Science 2000; 287:1433.

47. Johansson CB. Mechanism of stem cells in the central nervous system. J Cell Physiol 2003; 196:409.
48. Pluchino S, Zanotti L, Ross B, et al. Neurosphere-derived multipotent precursors promote neuroprotection by an immunomodulatory mechanism. Nature 2005; 436:266.
49. Archer DR, Cuddon PA, Lipsitz D, Duncan ID. Myelination of the canine central nervous system by glial cell transplantation: a model for repair of human myelin disease. Nat Med 1997; 3:54.
50. Imaizumi T, Lankford KL, Burton WV, Fodor WL, Kocsis JD. Xenotransplantation of transgenic pig olfactory ensheathing cells promotes axonal regeneration in rat spinal cord. Nat Biotechnol 2000; 18:949.
51. Sobel RA, Hinojoza JR, Maeda A, Chen M. Endothelial cell integrin laminin receptor expression in multiple sclerosis lesions. Am J Pathol 1998; 153:405.
52. Hickey WF. Migration of hematogenous cells through the blood-brain barrier and the initiation of CNS inflammation. Brain Pathol 1991; 1:97.
53. Hickey WF. Basic principles of immunological surveillance of the normal central nervous system. Glia 2001; 36:118.
54. Aloisi F, Ria F, Adorini L. Regulation of T-cell responses by CNS antigen-presenting cells: different roles for microglia and astrocytes. Immunol Today 2000; 21:141.
55. Burt RK, Burns W, Hess A. Bone marrow transplantation for multiple sclerosis. Bone Marrow Transplant 1995; 16:1.
56. Mandalfino P, Rice G, Smith A, Klein JL, Rystedt L, Ebers GC. Bone marrow transplantation in multiple sclerosis. J Neurol 2000; 247:691.
57. McAllister LD, Beatty PG, Rose J. Allogeneic bone marrow transplant for chronic myelogenous leukemia in a patient with multiple sclerosis. Bone Marrow Transplant 1997; 19:395.
58. Burt RK, Burns WH, Miller SD. Bone marrow transplantation for multiple sclerosis: returning to Pandora's box. Immunol Today 1997; 18:559.
59. Haase CG, Hohlfeld R. Bone marrow and stem cell transplantation in multiple sclerosis? Nervenarzt 1999; 70:178.
60. Flugel A, Bradl M, Kreutzberg GW, Graeber MB. Transformation of donor-derived bone marrow precursors into host microglia during autoimmune CNS inflammation and during the retrograde response to axotomy. J Neurosci Res 2001; 66:74.
61. Fassas A, Passweg JR, Anagnostopoulos A, et al. Hematopoietic stem cell transplantation for multiple sclerosis. A retrospective multicenter study. J Neurol 2002; 249:1088.
62. Hassan-Zahraee M, Tran EH, Bourbonniere L, Owens T. Elevated interferon-gamma in CNS inflammatory disease: a potential complication for bone marrow reconstitution in MS. J Neuroimmunol 2000; 108:40.
63. Herrmann MM, Gaertner S, Stadelmann C, et al. Tolerance induction by bone marrow transplantation in a multiple sclerosis model. Blood 2005; 106:1875.
64. Adjali O, Marodon G, Steinberg M, et al. In vivo correction of ZAP-70 immunodeficiency by intrathymic gene transfer. J Clin Invest 2005; 115:2287.
65. Darrasse-Jeze G, Marodon G, Salomon BL, Catala M, Klatzmann D. Ontogeny of CD4+ CD25+ regulatory/suppressor T-cells in human fetuses. Blood 2005; 105:4715.
66. Marodon G, Klatzmann D. In situ transduction of stromal cells and thymocytes upon intrathymic injection of lentiviral vectors. BMC Immunol 2004; 5:18.
67. Goverman J, Perchellet A, Huseby ES. The role of CD8(+) T-cells in multiple sclerosis and its animal models. Curr Drug Targets Inflamm Allergy 2005; 4:239.
68. Kipnis J, Mizrahi T, Hauben E, Shaked I, Shevach E, Schwartz M. Neuroprotective autoimmunity: naturally occurring CD4+CD25+ regulatory T-cells suppress the ability to withstand injury to the central nervous system. Proc Natl Acad Sci USA 2002; 99:15620.
69. Schwartz M, Kipnis J. Autoimmunity on alert: naturally occurring regulatory CD4(+)CD25(+) T-cells as part of the evolutionary compromise between a 'need' and a 'risk'. Trends Immunol 2002; 23:530.

70. Van Weyenbergh J, Wietzerbin J, Rouillard D, Barral-Netto M, Liblau R. Treatment of multiple sclerosis patients with interferon-beta primes monocyte-derived macrophages for apoptotic cell death. J Leukoc Biol 2001; 70:745.
71. Teitelbaum D, Sela M, Arnon R. Copolymer 1 from the laboratory to FDA. Isr J Med Sci 1997; 33:280.
72. Arnon R, Aharoni R. Mechanism of action of glatiramer acetate in multiple sclerosis and its potential for the development of new applications. Proc Natl Acad Sci USA 2004; 101:14593.
73. Stuve O, Youssef S, Steinman L, Zamvil SS. Statins as potential therapeutic agents in neuroinflammatory disorders. Curr Opin Neurol 2003; 16:393.
74. Hohlfeld R. Current therapy of multiple sclerosis: value of cyclosporin A and FK 506. Nervenarzt 1991; 62:136.

13

Novel Gene Therapeutic Approaches to Brain Cancer

Maria G. Castro, James F. Curtin, Gwendalyn D. King, Marianela Candolfi, Peter Czer, Sandra A. Sciascia, Kurt Kroeger, Tamer Fakhouri, Sarah Honig, William Kuoy, Terry Kang, Stephen Johnson, and Pedro R. Lowenstein
Gene Therapeutics Research Institute, Cedars-Sinai Medical Center, and Departments of Medicine, and Medical and Molecular Pharmacology, David Geffen School of Medicine, University of California Los Angeles, Los Angeles, California, U.S.A.

INTRODUCTION

In the United States, approximately 17,000 people per year are diagnosed with brain tumors, the leading cause of death from cancers in children ages 1–15 year (1,2). Gliomas are the most prevalent type of brain tumors in adults, affecting 3.2/100,000 persons/yr in the United States (www.CBTRUS.org). In spite of advances in surgery, chemotherapy, and radiotherapy, the mean survival time of patients post-diagnosis remains approximately 9–12 months.

The nervous system is comprised of neurons supported and nourished by glial cells. There are four different types of glial cells: astrocytes, oligodendroctyes, microglia, and ependymal cells. Technically, a glioma is defined as "any neoplasm [an uncontrolled growth of abnormal tissue] derived from one of the various types of cells that form the interstitial tissue [glial cells] of the brain, spinal cord, pineal gland, posterior pituitary gland, and retina"(3), and they can also be found in nasal lobes, peripheral, and cranial nerves. In general, gliomas rarely metastasize beyond the central nervous system (CNS); however, tumors from other parts of the body can metastasize to the CNS. Gliomas may be found in many different regions of the CNS and are usually comprised of a heterogenous cellular population.

There are many different types of gliomas each with its own characteristic features. For example, there are brainstem gliomas, gigantocellular gliomas, mixed gliomas, nasal gliomas, gliomas of the optic chasm, optic nerve gliomas, gliomas of the spinal cord, telangiectactic gliomas (4). However, we will only discuss the main types: astrocytomas and mixed gliomas. Astrocytomas are located anywhere in the CNS, grow slowly, are invasive and are believed to originate from astrocytes. The most devastating type of astrocytoma, grade-four astrocytoma, is more commonly known as glioblastoma multiforme. It is located mostly in the cerebral hemisphere, is highly invasive, malignant, and probably originates from mature astrocytes. Glioblastomas are the most common type of brain tumors diagnosed in middle aged adults, accounting for about 30% of all primary brain tumors. They are the most malignant of all brain tumors and the most difficult to treat with mean survival of less than 1 year following diagnosis (4). Astrocytoma is also the most common pediatric tumor diagnosed, accounting for just over 50% of all newly diagnosed tumors in children (5). The diagnosis of gliomas includes recognition of its symptoms, performing physical tests and assigning a grade to the tumor. Symptoms of gliomas can include headaches (where pain increases especially when one lies down), nausea, vomiting seizures, dizziness, personality changes, sudden vision loss, memory loss, speech problems, sensory changes, mental impairment, weakness, and perhaps paralysis (6). A physician may utilize CT scans, MRIs, EEGs, X-rays, angiography, myelography, and/or a lumbar puncture to diagnose gliomas. If a glioma is found, it is given a grade between one and four. A low grade glioma is a tumor with a well-defined border that grows slowly. A mid or high grade number is assigned to a tumor that grows more rapidly, is pathologically malignant and is difficult to remove due to invasion in normal tissue. High grade tumors typically recur within 1–2 year post treatment.

The current treatment for gliomas includes surgery, radiation, and chemotherapy. The first step in treatment for a glioma is resection or biopsy. With resection, as much of the tumor is removed as possible. A resection may also establish a pathological diagnosis as the results from a biopsy might not be conclusive. Unfortunately, the lack of a clearly defined tumor border makes it difficult to discern whether or not the entire tumor was removed by resection. Also, if the glioma is close to critical areas within the brain, there is a high risk of normal tissue damage during resections. In this case, partial resections can be of some value. A partial resection can improve neurological functions, relieve pressure, and increase tumor sensitivity to chemotherapeutic drugs. During surgery, shunts may also be placed near the tumor to relieve pressure and to drain excess fluid. A biopsy is useful when the tumor is inoperable and when imaging is difficult. Another therapeutic option is radiation therapy (maximum dose of 60 Gy) which is typically confined to tumor mass and 2 cm of surrounding tissue. Hyper-fractionated radiation is an exposure to more frequent fractions of a smaller dose of radiation over a smaller area of the brain. Stereotactic radiosurgery is an increased dose of radiation to tumors less than 1.5 inches in diameter that minimizes exposure of normal brain tissue by guiding the radiation with computer assisted imaging. In interstital radiation therapy (brachytherapy), radioactive pellets are implanted in tumor mass. Physicians also induce hyperthermia or use radiosensitizers, such as tirapazamine, to increase the response of a tumor to radiation. Chemotherapeutic drugs such as carmustine, lomustine, procarbazine, and vincristine are administered in six week cycles (6). The drawbacks of chemotherapy against brain tumors include the increase of chemoresistant cells, inadequate drug delivery and the problems posed by the blood-brain barrier resulting in only limited success, with an 80% relapse in glioblastoma patients. In summary, current treatments for malignant or high-grade gliomas rarely achieve long-term tumor control with frequent recurrence of the tumor (4,7) and death quite probable in the near future for those patients diagnosed with gliomas. Therefore, there is a critical need to develop novel therapeutic approaches to treat this devastating cancer. Gene therapy constitutes a very attractive treatment option and in this chapter will discuss some of the most promising gene therapeutic targets and precinical model systems. We will also review the clincal implementation of these therapies in GBM patients.

CANCER GENE THERAPY APPROACHES

Correcting the Primary Genetic Defect in Cancer Using Gene Therapy

Cancerous cells usually harbor harmful mutations in genes that regulate proliferation and/or apoptosis. It is widely accepted that tumorigenesis is a multi-step process that requires mutations in many different genes in the DNA of an individual cell. Although the exact nature and order of these mutations varies between different types of cancer and even between cancers classified as the same type, a common theme is often evident during cancer progression. Mutations in genes that promote cell cycle progression, growth factor independence, angiogenesis, increased motility, anchorage independence, decreased levels of apoptosis and reduced sensitivity to chemotherapeutic agents are commonly reported in many different cancers and often correlate with progression of the cancer from benign to malignant. The genetics of gliomagenesis is well characterized in comparison with other cancers and this information can be used to develop gene therapy strategies that address these genetic aberrations. Mutations in four pathways involved in cell cycle regulation are commonly associated with glioma formation in humans; the p53/ARF/human MDM2 pathway, the p16/Rb/cyclinD/CDK4 pathway, the receptor tyrosine kinase (RTK)/Ras pathway and the pI3K/PTEN/Akt pathway (8). Viral vectors have been designed that express transgenes commonly mutated in glioma in an attempt to correct the genetic lesions in gliomagenesis. Below we outline the progress in developing therapies for the two most commonly mutated pathways in glioma, p53, and Rb.

P53/ARF/HumanMDM2 Pathway

P53 is often referred to as "the guardian of the genome" and is mutated or absent in over 50% of all human tumors. The principle role of p53 as a tumor suppressor is to detect gross genetic abnormalities during DNA synthesis. Active p53 is absent in quiescent cells but its activation is induced in cells during cell cycle progression or in response to genotoxic insults. Once a genetic abnormality has been detected, p53 arrests cell cycle progression and monitors the DNA repair process. If the DNA damage is too great, p53 activates the apoptotic pathway reducing the frequency of tumor formation. This pivotal role played by p53 in tumor suppression is perhaps most striking in humans with Li-Fraumeni syndrome. Mutations in the p53 gene have been identified in over 70% of all these individuals and family members have an exceptionally high risk of developing multiple primary carcinomas and sarcomas during their lifetime (9). These patients are known to have a particularly high predisposition to developing glioblastoma and other tumors of the CNS (10). Other proteins known to regulate p53 expression and stability in cells include the transcription factor c-Jun, the ubiquitin-binding molecule MDM2 and downstream effectors of p53 including p21 and E2F1, all of which are frequently mutated in cancer as well. In fact, mutations in components of the p53 pathway are believed to occur in >90% of all human tumors, including human gliomas. Allelic loss of chromosome 17p or mutations in p53 gene are observed with equal frequency in low grade gliomas and high grade glioblastomas (11). This suggests that inactivation of p53 is an early event during gliomagenesis and may be an important target for gene therapy. Re-introduction of wild-type p53 into glioma cells with p53 mutations has been the subject of intense scientific research. Early results suggested that the re-introduction of p53 reduced the proliferation of glioma cells in vitro and suppressed tumor formation when implanted into nude mice (12). Adenovirus with the p53 transgene was subsequently demonstrated to reduce tumor volume by 40% over 14 days in rats, demonstrating significant anti-tumor activity (13,14). p53 is known to regulate cell cycle progression, but mutations in p53 are also associated with a variety of other functions including multi-drug resistant cancer cells. P53 overexpression increased the sensitivity of drug and radiation resistant glioma cell lines to cisplatin and radiotherapy in vitro (15) and adenovirus expressing p53 restored the sensitivity of 9L glioblastoma cells to cisplatin (16) and radiotherapy (17) in a rat model of glioblastoma. Overexpression of p53 using viral vectors was also observed to improve survival in animal models inoculated with wild type p53 expressing glioma cell lines, indicating a versatile function for this transgene in treating all forms of glioma (18). Overexpression of p53 in cells increases the expression of numerous apoptotic proteins including BAX activators, Bim, DP5, and the death receptor ligand FasL. In a recent study, adenoviral vectors expressing p53 under the control of the CMV promoter were demonstrated to induce significant levels of apoptosis as measured by DNA fragmentation when injected intracranially into the tumor. Furthermore, a 100% survival rate was observed in these animals 100 days following viral injection (19). The success of these pre-clinical studies has led to Phase I clinical trials designed to assess the toxicity of p53 gene therapy in human patients. The results of one trial have been recently published to show the maximum tolerated dose was not reached and transgene expression was evident in all patients in the nucleus of astrocytic tumor cells. Although expression was limited to within 5 mm from the site of injection, it is hoped that higher doses of virus may improve the distribution in subsequent studies (20).

A number of downstream pathways of p53 have also been tested and the overexpression of two of these have shown promising results in controlling glioma in pre-clinical animal models (21,22). Comparison between p53, p21, and p16-based therapies suggests that vectors expressing p16 and p21 are even more potent tumor suppressors than p53 (23). However, these transgenes have not yet been tested in clinical models of glioma.

An alternative strategy was originally conceived by Bischoff JR and others, which takes advantage of the anti-viral properties of p53. The human AdE1B gene is expressed during adenovirus infection and codes for a 55 kDa protein that binds with and inactivates p53. AdE1B is essential for a successful replication cycle within the host cell and adenoviral vectors lacking the AdE1B gene are unable to replicate inside cells expressing normal p53. These recombinant viral particles were cytopathic against p53-deficient human tumor cell lines both in vitro and also in flank tumors in nude mice. Furthermore, these viruses increased the efficacy of other viral vector therapies expressing cytotoxic transgene products (24,25). In a recent report, combined therapy using this virus and conventional radiotherapy was significantly more effective than either therapy alone in improving the long term survival of nude mice with both p53 positive and p53 negative glioma (26). These results highlight a common trend with viral vectors as useful therapies when combined with more conventional chemotherapy or radiotherapy.

P16/Rb/CyclinD/CDK4 Pathway

The p16/Rb/cyclinD/CDK4 pathway is the most frequently mutated pathway in glioma, and its mutations generally characterize a transition from low-grade tumors with relatively slow rate of proliferation to intermediate-grade gliomas with dramatically increased cell proliferation (27). In normal quiescent cells, Rb is present in a hypophosphorylated form and is bound by the transcription factor E2F1. This prevents transcription of genes important for mitosis and prevents progression of the cell cycle through the G1/S phase restriction point (28). In general, mutations targeting the Rb pathway often inactivate Rb directly through decreased affinity for E2F1 or reduced expression. Alternatively, mutations that induce constitutive phosphorylation of Rb by CDK2, CDK4 or CDK6 can all contribute to reducing the affinity of Rb for E2F1 and subsequent increases in proliferation (28). In gliomagenesis, allelic losses on chromosome 9q or 13q, or amplification of 12q usually accompany transition of glioma from low grade to intermediate grade (29,30). This was later found to correspond with loss of Rb (13q14) loss of INK4A and ARF (9p21), or amplification of CDK4 (12q13–14). Adenovirus mediated Rb gene therapy has been successfully used in pre-clinical models of various cancers including bladder cancer, where constitutively active truncated Rb delivered by adenovirus produced marked growth inhibition, cytotoxicity, caspase-dependent apoptosis, and G2/M block in the human RB-negative, telomerase-positive bladder cancer cell line UM-UC14 (31). In an animal model, Rb was found to decrease the proliferation of spontaneous pituitary tumors in $Rb^{+/-}$ mice and prolonged survival of animals (32). In a similar strategy to the oncolytic virus targeting p53, recombinant adenovirus lacking AdE1A (Delta24) can only replicate in cells expressing phospho-RB and is preferentially cytotoxic to glioma cells. A single injection of Delta24 reduced growth of flank tumors by 66%, and multiple injections reduced tumor growth by 84% (33). These data clearly highlight the fundamental role played by Rb in pathogenesis of glioma.

More recently, substantial research has also investigated the potential of Rb regulators and effectors in treating glioma. In particular, therapies that target p16[INK4A] have successfully reduced tumor proliferation and improved survival in rodent models of glioma. P16[INK4A] reduces Rb phosphorylation by inhibiting CDK4 and CDK6 activity and is the most frequently mutated gene in human cancer after p53 and is mutated in more than 50% of glioblastomas (34). Initial in vitro experiments demonstrated that adenoviral vectors expressing p16[INK4A] induced cell cycle arrest of glioma cell lines (35). Results in vivo corroborated these initial observations and p16[INK4A] delivery was demonstrated to improve survival in animal models of glioma, even when compared with p53 expressing vectors (23).

In spite of these promising results, caution is warranted with all therapies designed to repair common genetic lesions in glioma. In a recent report, p16[INK4A] was expressed in glioma cell lines under the control of the Tet repressor system (36). Elevated p16[INK4A] reduced tumor proliferation in vivo initially, supporting work published by others (36). However, long term transgene expression induced a decrease in the expression of Rb suggesting that gene therapy approaches involving p16[INK4A] may ultimately lead to the selection of Rb deficient tumors (36). In fact, this is a potential problem of all approaches designed to correct genetic lesions in cancer. Tumor cells are genetically unstable and undergo accelerating genetic mutation. Unfortunately, this accelerates natural selection and will select for tumor cells that overcome this transgene insertion. The possibility of tumor cells compensating for transgene insertion through one or more subsequent mutations must be explored in all promising therapies that repair the primary genetic lesion in cancer.

Suppressing Angiogenesis

Microscopic tumors are composed of populations of cells with altered characteristics to the surrounding tissue that contribute to growth factor independence and elevated rates of proliferation. In tumors, the rate of proliferation exceeds the rate of cell death and tumors increase in size. Oxygen and nutrients required to fuel this expansion in tumor volume are scavenged from surrounding tissue vasculature. However, diffusion of oxygen and nutrients from neovascularure limits the absolute size of the tumor to about 2 mm^3. Angiogenesis is required to supply sufficient oxygen and nutrients to sustain further growth. Angiogenesis involves the rapid proliferation of endothelial vascular cells and is tightly regulated in adults. This regulation is coordinated by the expression of activators and inhibitors of angiogenesis. Tumors that acquire the ability to alter the expression of promoters or inhibitors of angiogenesis stimulate the development of new vasculature and subsequently increase in size. In fact, promotion of angiogenesis appears to be a critical step in the progression of glioma from a benign, microscopic lesion to a malignant macroscopic cancer (37). Consequently, angiogenesis has received much attention as a target of potential therapies. Angiogenesis in adult humans usually only occurs in response to pathophysiological stimuli from wounds or hypoxia and angiogenic inhibitors generally have few side effects (38). Several of these angiogenic inhibitors have been shown to reduce tumor growth in vitro and in vivo and of these, thalidomide has been most successfully used to treat glioma to date (39–42). However, a number of disadvantages limit the potential of angiogenic inhibitors in clinical setting. Firstly, production of sufficient quantities of angiogenic inhibitors is problematic and has limited the availability of these drugs in clinical trials. Synthetic small molecule inhibitors of angiogenesis are being developed to overcome this problem but the side effects of these drugs are currently unknown. Secondly, angiogenic inhibitors are believed to be cytostatic, not cytotoxic and this requires long-term treatment strategies to control and ultimately reduce tumor size. Thirdly, toxic side effects have been observed with systemic delivery of some angiogenic inhibitors (43). Gene therapy offers distinct advantages over conventional chemotherapy in the safe delivery of clinically effective doses of angiogenic inhibitors to the tumor and has been successfully employed in the treatment of a variety of tumors in preclinical studies (44). This section will explore the various strategies employed by gene therapy in treating brain tumors targeting both promoters and inhibitors of angiogenesis.

Promoters of Angiogenesis

The first growth factor identified as a positive regulator of angiogenesis was basic fibroblast growth factor (bFGF) (45). Glioblastoma is among the most highly vascularized of all tumors and increased expression of bFGF correlates with progression of a wide variety of solid tumors (46). Adenoviral gene transfer of bFGF was found to promote angiogenesis in rat brains (47). However, a clear correlation between increased bFGF expression and glioma progression has not been demonstrated in glioma suggesting that bFGF is not the principle mediator of angiogenesis (48). Another promoter of angiogenesis called vascular endothelial growth factor (VEGF) was found to be overexpressed in high grade gliomas (49). Expression of the receptors for VEGF, Flt-1 (VEGFR-1) and Flk-1 (VEGFR-2), are also elevated in glioblastoma in comparison with surrounding normal tissue and Flk-1 in particular is believed to promote angiogenesis in response to VEGF (50). VEGF was one of the first proteins identified to play a key role in angiogenesis (51,52) and has since been the target of numerous gene therapy strategies designed to reduce tumor burden. Early studies utilized anti-sense RNA to reduce expression of VEGF in tumor cells. It was found that transfection of anti-sense VEGF cDNA into rat glioma C6 cells in vitro impaired C6 tumor cells growth in vivo when implanted into nude mice (53). More recently, recombinant virus has been used as a vehicle for the transfer of antisense sequences in pre-clinical models of brain tumors. Retrovirus encoding antisense VEGF cDNA sequence showed a statistically significant improvement in survival of rats with intracranial neoplasms (54). An alternative strategy for interfering with VEGF function has also been explored. A VEGF-R2 mutant has been constructed that lacks normal kinase activity. This receptor displays dominant negative function when overexpressed in cells that also express the wild type VEGF-R2 and a retrovirus encoding this mutant VEGF2 receptor successfully prolonged survival of rats with intracranial tumors. These tumors displayed many classical signs of impaired angiogenesis including reduced vascular density and elevated necrosis (55).

Inhibitors of Angiogenesis

The relatively low percentage of cells transduced by recombinant viral vectors is a limiting factor in reducing promoters of angiogenesis, and indeed in every gene therapy strategy that aims to reduce the expression or activity of target proteins. Inhibitors of angiogenesis overcome this problem and have been the subject of numerous pre-clinical studies. Many naturally occurring inhibitors of angiogenesis are derived from proteolytic degradation of the extracellular matrix. Endostatin and angiostatin are generated following the proteolytic cleavage of plasminogen and collagen respectively and are potent inhibitors of angiogenesis (56,57). These peptides are difficult to generate in sufficient quantities in vitro and are ideal candidates as transgenes for gene therapy. Recombinant viral vectors that express endostatin (58,59) or angiostatin (60,61) have been developed and tested in preclinical models of glioma. Improved survival of animals with intracranial neoplasms was observed in all cases and tumor growth rates were reduced by as much as 90%. Other anti-angiogenic protein fragments have also been studied for effectiveness in animal models of glioma and these include soluble human platelet factor four and the N-terminal fragment of rat prolactin. However, it appears that these transgenes are not as effective as endostatin and angiostatin in significantly improving survival (62,63). A number of proteins associated with immune system function have also anti-angiogenic properties. IL-4 and Interferon gamma have been studied in rat models of glioma (64,65). Improved survival and reduced angiogenesis and tumor growth rates were also observed in these studies. However, the principle function of these transgenes is in recruiting and modulating various cellular and humoral aspects of the immune response and will be dealt with in the appropriate section.

Activating the Immune Response

Histological analysis of tumors reveals that an immune response is often elicited against the tumor. Inflammation, and even tumor-specific lymphocytes are often evident, and in some rare cases, tumor regression spontaneously occurs in response to autoimmune paraneoplastic syndromes (66,67). This is believed to be caused by tumor specific antigen expression and underscores a role for the immune system in cancer immunosurveillance and control of disease. Unfortunately, most tumors develop countermeasures that hamper an effective immune response developing against the growing tumor. In pancreatic β-cell tumors for example, it has been demonstrated that the immune system was incapable of either developing or maintaining an effective anti-immune response (68,69). More recent studies in sarcoma suggest that tumor antigens fail to reach the lymph nodes and consequently an effective cytotoxic T lymphocyte response is not evident (70). Consequently, there is significant interest in developing an immunotherapy to improve the response of the immune system to the tumor. Since the immunosuppression state associated with gliomas appears to be mediated by an increase in autocrine secretion of transforming growth factor-beta (TGF-beta), a TGF-beta inhibitor, decorin has been delivered to intracranial CNS-1 gliomas in vivo using adenoviral vectors, which prolonged the survival of experimental tumor bearing rats, slowing glioma progression (71). Recent progress in understanding the mechanisms of an immune response has led to a renaissance in immunotherapy and over 100 Phase II clinical trials studying the effectiveness of various cancer vaccines are currently underway in the United States.

Many of these are already showing promising results with minor, limited side effects (73). Gene therapy offers numerous different mechanisms to stimulate an immune response against the proliferating tumor. We shall briefly outline progress in the four most promising mechanisms below.

Tumor Antigen Delivered Through Adenoviral Transgene Expression

Most if not all tumors express proteins that are recognized by the immune system and are called tumor antigens. Adenoviral vectors can be engineered to express these antigens as transgenes and subsequently used to prime an immune response against that target antigen if injected systemically. Promising results from preclinical trials have been reported for renal cell carcinoma among others, where adenovirus expresses the tumor antigen carbonic anhydrase IX protein (73). However, it is unclear whether this approach would be effective reducing glioma in an immune-privileged organ as the brain.

Enhancement of the Anti-Tumor Immune Response Using Cytokines

Cytokines are a diverse collection of secreted and membrane bound proteins involved in immunity and inflammation. Interferon β, an immunomodulatory and anti-tumor cytokine has been demonstrated to provide systemic anti-tumor immunity against GL261 cells when delivered intracranially in lysosomes. This cytokine reduces tumor growth and improves survival in C57/BL6 mice through a combination of anti-proliferative effects and also activation of $CD8^+$ but not $CD4^+$ cells (74). In another report, tumor growth was suppressed when mice were treated with a combination of IFN-β gene via cationic liposomes and dendritic cells. This was mediated by a highly effective cytotoxic lymphocyte (CTL) response against the tumor and was far more efficient that either therapy alone (75). Adeno-associated virus designed to deliver the transgene IFNβ has also been developed and completely inhibits growth of exogenous human tumor xenografts when delivered intratumorally in nude mice, further supporting the potential of IFN-β as a novel therapy for treating human glioma (76). Phase I clinical trials have recently begun using a replication deficient adenovirus expressing IFN-β in human subjects with the primary aim of assessing the maximum tolerated dose (77).

Enhancing T-Cell Activation

A number of cytokines are believed to activate various subclasses of T lymphocytes. For example, IL-12 is required for anti-tumor T_{H1} type pattern of differentiation in naïve mature T lymphocytes. An adenovirus expressing the transgene IL-12 has been reported to enhance the immune response against brain tumors and improve survival in mice inoculated with GL26 glioma cells intracranially. At the tumor site an increased number of $CD4^+$ and $CD8^+$T cells were identified (78). Recently, allogenic cells genetically engineered to secrete IL-2 were found to significantly improve survival in a mouse glioma carcinoma model. The immune response was found to be predominantly mediated by $CD8^+$ and natural killer cells (NK) and was highly specific for the glioma cells above non-neoplastic cells (79).

Enhancing Dendritic Cells Activation

It is believed that dendritic cells are the principle antigen presenting cells of the immune system and are required for the development of an antigen-dependent immune response. However, dendritic cells are absent from the brain except under conditions of inflammation and it is believed that this is a major reason behind immune privilege in the brain (80–85). Dendritic cells differentiate from precursor cells in response to Flt3L through a STAT3 dependent mechanism (86). Expression of Flt3L by daily administration of purified, recombinant Flt3L has been demonstrated to induce complete tumor regression and significantly improve survival (87). Furthermore, dendritic cells are highly effective inducers of tumor specific killer and helper T lymphocyte generation in animal models of tumors (88). Therefore, a lot of interest has been generated recently surrounding the use of dendritic cells and Flt3L in immunotherapy. The use of dendritic cell based vaccines is currently ongoing in about 20 Phase II and at least one Phase III clinical trial in the U.S.A., many of which are showing promising results. In addition, early studies have indicated that toxicity of dendritic cell vaccination is mild and limited to local reactions at the site of injection (72). In a stringent glioma model, in which RAdTK/ganciclovir administration is ineffective, we have demonstrated that recombinant adenovirus expressing RAdFlt3L eliminates intracranial neoplasms and significantly improves survival when co-delivered with the tumoricidal agent RAdTK/ganciclovir (89,90). This data highlight the promise of immunotherapies in greatly enhancing the efficacy of current therapies and the potential of curing glioma.

Harnessing Death Receptor Ligand Interactions

Apoptosis, also known as programmed cell death, is a universal feature of multi-cellular eukaryotes and plays a fundamental role in controlling many diverse physiological processes including tissue sculpting during development and tissue homeostasis in adults. Defects in apoptosis are responsible for numerous pathologies including tumor initiation and progression (91,92). For these reasons, apoptosis is tightly regulated and studies in vertebrates have identified a number of signal transduction pathways that can either induce or inhibit apoptosis. A number of studies have investigated the potential selectively activate tumor cell death by inducing pro-apototic genes using gene therapy (93). In particular, focus has centered on components of a family of receptors called death receptors.

Death receptors are present on the plasma membrane and their activation can induce apoptosis in cells following engagement of receptors with extracellular ligands. In mammals, death receptors belong to a large family of membrane bound receptors called the tumor necrosis factor receptor superfamily (TNFRSF), which include at least nine death receptors. TNFRSF members regulate various aspects of cell proliferation, differentiation, and apoptosis and all members of this family contain between one and four short cysteine-rich extracellular domains. These repeats usually contain six conserved cysteine residues that form three disulphide bonds and these subdomains adopt conserved tertiary folds. It is believed that the order of cysteine rich repeats determines the affinity and specificity of receptor for ligand. The ligands that bind with these receptors belong to another large family of transmembrane proteins called the tumor necrosis factor superfamily. Ligands bind with receptors and induce trimerisation of receptors at the plasma membrane, which in turn permits the recruitment of initiator caspases to the death domain, propagating the apoptosis inducing signal transduction cascades (94,95). Initiator procaspases cleave effector caspase which, once activated, inactivate target proteins and thereby promoting the ordered degradation of nucleic acids, enzymes, and structural proteins (96).

The Fas receptor is perhaps the most widely studied death receptor and ligand system. Viral vectors expressing Fas ligand have been demonstrated to possess potent anti-glioma activity both in vitro and in vivo (97–99). Furthermore, these vectors enhance the anti-tumor activity of virus expressing p53 and Thymidine kinase (TK) (100,101). TRAIL, the ligand for TRAILR1 and TRAILR2, has also been assessed as a potential therapeutic transgene for gene therapy. The anti-tumor activity of recombinant virus expressing TRAIL is more controversial, although this transgene is not effective alone in glioma cell lines (102), co-delivery of TRAIL and Fas ligand expressing viral vectors enhances apoptosis induction compared to either virus alone (103). In addition, intracranial injection of virus expressing TRAIL significantly improves survival in a rat model of glioma (104).

Providing Drug Resistance to Hematopoietic Cells

Gene therapy vectors can not only be used to kill tumoral cells, but also be engineered to confer survival advantages on normal cells. A limiting factor with conventional radiotherapy and chemotherapy is the toxicity to normal cells. Many of these therapies are toxic to proliferating cells, including but not limited to tumor cells, and relatively non-toxic to non-proliferating cells. Although the majority of cells in adults are non-proliferating, a small but important proportion of these are rapidly dividing. Hematopoietic stem cells are rapidly dividing cells that are often decimated in response to radiotherapy and chemotherapy. Bone marrow transplants are often required, increasing the risk of anemia, infection, and further complications in cancer patients. Stem cells can be transduced in vitro where drug resistant stem cells can be selected and amplified in vivo (105). A number of Phase I clinical trials have been undertaken with various chemotherapy drug resistant genes including 0-6-methylguanine-DNA methyltransferase gene and MDR-1 (106). Although many of these approaches have not been very successful, in part due to poor transduction efficiencies, recent improvements in vector design may increase the efficacy of these agents in promoting drug resistance in vivo (107). Many of these vectors are retroviral in origin and may result in the accidental transfer of the drug resistance gene to cancer cells via retroviral integration into cancer genomes. Therefore safety checks including replication deficiency and inefficient repackaging of the multi-drug resistance gene are also being developed in these vectors.

Enzyme/Prodrug Gene Therapy

While radiotherapy and surgery succeed in treating confined malignancies, the majority of cancers require systemic therapies that target tumor cells but, unfortunately their low specificity also produces toxicity to normal cells. Current research is attempting to identify more specific ways to directly target tumor cells and reduce treatment toxicity to normal cells. The use of enzyme/prodrug combinations directly targeting therapeutics to the tumor mass through the use of antibody or viral vectors has emerged as a potentially viable option.

Prodrugs are chemicals that are non-cytotoxic over a wide range of dosages however upon conversion by a specific activating enzyme, become a toxic molecule capable of triggering cell death. The ideal prodrug should (1) be freely diffusible throughout the tumor (2) remain chemically stable under physiological conditions, (3) possess suitable pharmacological and pharmacokinetic properties, (4) convert into a chemical that is at least 100-fold more toxic than the prodrug, and (5) induce cytotoxicity that is cell cycle phase independent. In addition to the prodrug characteristics, dynamics of the enzyme are also crucial to successful cancer treatment. Ideal enzymes should be of low molecular weight with high catalytic activity under physiological conditions such that even at low concentrations of prodrug, efficient catalysis can occur. Expression of the enzyme should not alone lead to cytotoxicity. Additionally the reaction pathway for conversion of the prodrug into a toxin should be unique from pathways utilized by endogenous enzymes to avoid cytotoxcicity in normal tissue (108).

Initial investigations sought to exploit prodrug activation using endogenous enzymes expressed at higher levels in tumor cells (109,110). However, clinical application was limited since such enzymes were expressed in normal cells and only a small number of human cancers had high enough levels of activating enzymes for efficacy. To overcome these problems, identification of non-mammalian enzyme/prodrug combinations were identified. Usage of antibodies and viral vectors to specifically target enzyme to tumor tissue has produced promising results in vitro and in vivo.

Antibody-Directed Enzyme Prodrug Therapy

Antibodies have been used to target tumor antigens or growth factors in attempts to specifically deliver cytotoxic drugs, toxins, and radionucleotides (111,112). Likewise conjugation of prodrugs to monoclonal antibodies may also be used for specific targeting (113–115). In antibody-directed enzyme prodrug therapy (ADEPT); the catalytic enzyme is covalently linked to an antibody, which recognizes tumor-specific antigen and binds to this specific surface antigen, causing its internalization together with the activating enzyme. Upon prodrug administration a large number of toxic molecules can be produced in the local tumor area. Since internalization of the complex is not required for catalysis, diffusion of the toxin into nearby tumor cells may result in tumor cell death. Likewise, transfer of toxin after its internalization to adjacent cells via gap junctions further enhances the bystander effect of ADEPT. In order to minimize death of normal cells, administration of the enzyme used to convert the prodrug can be time delayed to allow removal of unbound enzyme-antibody conjugates.

There are several disadvantages to ADEPT that limit its clinical applications. One limitation is the low number of tumor-specific antigens that have been identified thus far for use as targets; however ADEPT strategies have been used to treat colorectal, breast, and choriocarcinoma tumors. In addition, most monoclonal antibodies are of murine origin and elicit a significant immunogenic response in a human patient that requires use of immunosuppressive drugs. Humanized antibodies have been constructed that retain the mouse antibody determining region and its high affinity binding but within a human antibody framework (116–118). Last, monoclonal antibodies are large molecular weight molecules with slow rates of diffusion that may limit the total tumor area able to be treated (119,120). Use of recombinant antibodies engineered to be smaller while retaining a high specificity and affinity may overcome this limitation (121–126).

Gene-Directed and Virus-Directed Enzyme Prodrug Therapy

To further extend ADEPT while overcoming some of its limitations, utilization of vectors other than monoclonal antibodies were developed. Gene-directed enzyme prodrug therapy (GDEPT) seeks to introduce a gene encoding a prodrug-activating enzyme directly into tumor cells. Once inside the cell transcription of the gene produces an active but non-cytotoxic enzyme. Upon systemic administration of the prodrug, cells transduced with the enzyme will convert the prodrug into its toxic metabolite triggering cell death. For GDEPT to be successful the enzyme must be expressed exclusively within the tumor cells and its catalytic activity must be high enough compared to normal tissue for clinical benefit. Since expression will not occur in all tumor cells, a significant bystander effect is essential in this strategy. Bystander effects occur when the cytotoxic metabolite is transmitted to cells not originally transduced with the enzyme. This may occur via transport through gap junctions or by diffusion through the extracellular space. In addition to delivery of the enzyme, administration of the prodrug must be delayed sufficiently to allow expression of the enzyme in target cells. The majority of GDEPT strategies have exploited viral-mediated delivery systems. These systems exploit the ability of viruses to enter cells and express the transgenes they carry. Use of viruses as the delivery agent has been termed virus directed enzyme prodrug therapy or VDEPT.

Enzyme/Prodrug Combinations

A large number of enzyme/prodrug combinations have been discovered and characterized. While the ideal characteristics for enzymes and prodrugs used in ADEPT/GDEPT strategies was outlined above, none of the enzyme/prodrug combinations are perfect, each has its advantages and disadvantages. The most well characterized enzyme/prodrug combinations are herpes simplex virus type 1 - thymidine kinase (HSV1-TK)/ganciclovir (GCV) and cytosine deaminase (CD)/ 5-fluorocytosine (5-FC). Each of these pairings has been used in numerous gene therapy GDEPT clinical trials. The bacterial enzyme carboxypeptidase G2 (CPG2)/CMDA is the only ADEPT combination to reach clinical trial stage. In addition to these well characterized pairings *E. coli* guanine phosphoribosyl transferase/6-thioxanthine, cytochrome P450/CPA, *E. coli* purine nucleoside phosphorylase/6-methyl-purine-2$'$-deoxynucleoside, *E. coli* nitroreductase/CB1954, cytochrome P450 4B1/4-IM and 2AA, horseradish peroxidase/indole-3-acetic acid and carboxypeptidase/methotrexate-α-phenylalanine have all been under investigation (108,127).

Herpes Simplex Virus Type 1: Thymidine Kinase/Ganciclovir

HSV1-TK was first developed as a prodrug-activating enzyme by Moolten and has been studied intensively in preclinical and clinical studies to treat a wide range of solid tumors (128,129). HSV1-TK delivery to tumor cells has been accomplished using both adeno- and retroviral vector systems (130–137). HSV1-TK is nearly 1000-fold more efficient at mono-phosphorylation of GCV than any mammalian HSV1-TK (138). GCV, acyclic analog of the nucleoside 2-deoxyguanosine, is an anti-herpetic agent with a known toxicity profile (138–141). When HSV1-TK phosphorylates GCV it is converted to GCV-monophosphate that is further converted by other cellular kinases to di- and triphosphorylated forms. GCV-triphosphate is the most toxic of these forms (138–141). GCV-triphosphate is structurally similar to 2-deoxyguanosine triphosphate and thus can be incorporated into DNA chains by DNA polymerase (138–141). GCV-triphosphate may inhibit DNA polymerase or upon incorporation into the DNA chain, trigger chain termination which induces cell death (139–141).

HSV1-TK/GCV pairing was the first in which bystander effects were described (142). In murine glioma studies, total tumor regression was observed when only 10% of tumor cells were transduced with HSV1-TK (130,142,143). HSV1-TK/GCVs bystander effect requires cell to cell contact. GCV-triphosphates are highly charged molecules that are insoluble in lipid membranes and thus cannot diffuse freely in the extracellular space. Instead, GCV-triphosphates move between cells via gap junctions (144–147). In addition to movement through gap junctions the bystander effect of HSV1-TK/GCV may be enhanced by the host immune response to the tumor following treatment. Treatment was observed to trigger infiltration of CD4 + and CD8 + T cells and macrophages as well as increased expression of a host of cytokines (148). Induction of the immune system resulted in tumor regression locally at the site of HSV1-TK/GCV action and at distant sites in both normal and immunocompromised animals (136,149–151).

Based on positive preclinical tumor regression data, HSV1-TK/GCV studies have been conducted as Phase I and Phase II clinical trials. In the initials trials undertaken, survival of patients treated with HSV1-TK/GCV after surgical resection were similar to patients who had not received the GDEPT therapy (152,153). Several theories exist for the disparity between preclinical and clinical trial data. First, an insufficient number of tumor cells may have been transduced for therapeutic benefit. Second, the growth rate of the tumor cells may play an important role in HSV1-TK/GCV action and would be different between experimental tumors and those spontaneously arising in humans. Third, the dosages of GCV used preclinically were much higher than those used in the clinical trials indicating that the lack of GCV substrate may have precluded therapeutic benefit. Increased tumor transduction efficiency, exploitation of bystander effects, and further engineering of HSV1-TK to be more efficient and/or GCV to be less toxic will be required for clinically relevant therapeutic benefits from HSV1-TK/GCV prodrug therapy.

Cytosine Deaminase/5-Fluorocytosine

As with HSV1-TK, CD produces a toxic nucleotide analog that triggers cell death. CD is an enzyme expressed in bacteria and fungi and absent in in mammalian cells catalyzes the conversion of cytosine to uracil (154,155). When combined with the prodrug 5-FC, deamination generates 5-fluorouracil (5-FU). CD/5-FD kills cells via both proliferation-dependent and independent means. Metabolites of 5-FU cause cell death through inhibition of thymidylate synthase, resulting in nicked DNA and inhibition of RNA processing. CD/5-FC results in a strong bystander effect that, unlike HSV1-TK/GCV, does not require cell to cell contact (156). Transduction of only 2–4% of cells resulted in significant regression of tumor as toxic metabolites freely diffuse cells (157,158). This effect is not restricted to tumor cells and damage to normal tissue may result. In addition to bystander effects caused by diffusion of the toxin, as with HSV1-TK, immune mediated bystander effects also occur as NK infiltrate tumors treated with CD/5-FC therapy (159). The species of origin for CD may produce more catalytically active forms as observed with *S. cerevisiae* CD compared to *E. coli* CD (160,161). Currently Phase I trials of adenovirally delivered CD in patients with metastatic liver disease are ongoing (162–164).

Carboxypeptidase G2/4-Benzoyl-L-Glutamic Acid

CPG2 is found in bacteria but not humans and removes glutamic acid moieties from folic acid, inhibiting cell growth. When combined with the prodrug 4-benzoyl-L-glutamic acid (CMDA), a DNA-crosslinking mustard drug is released (165). Unlike HSV1-TK and CD, catalysis of the prodrug with CPG2 does not require further enzymatic processing to become the final toxic compound. Mustard-alkylating agents are not cell-cycle dependent enabling the killing of proliferating and non-proliferating cells (166). As with other enzyme/prodrugs, CPG2/CMDA produces a robust bystander effect. Only 10–12% transduction resulted in 50–100% killing in vitro and in vivo (167–169). Immune mediated bystander effects are currently unreported. CPG2/CMDA was first used in ADEPT Phase I clinical trial and did not show toxicity related to the enzyme or prodrug (162,163). GDEPT usages of CPG2 have not reached clinical trial stage yet.

Targeted Toxins for Glioma Therapy

Over the past several years, research efforts have focused on the utilization of cellular receptors exclusively over-expressed in brain tumor cells for targeted therapy. It has been reported that human tumors, including established glioma cell lines, primary glioblastoma cell cultures and surgical glioma biopsies express a variant of the IL-13 receptor. This receptor (IL13Rα2) is different from its physiological counterpart, i.e., IL13/IL4R (170–174). The urokinase-type plasminogen activator (uPA) receptor is also overexpressed in glioblastomas (170–173,175), as well as receptors for growth factors, such as epidermal growth factor (EGF) receptor (176,177). Importantly, since these receptors are virtually absent in the normal brain, they are very attractive targets for targeted therapeutic approaches in glioma, minimizing any putative adverse side effects to normal brain tissue. Thus, ligands of these receptors, such as IL-13, uPA, EGF, and transforming growth factor α (TGF-α) have been fused to the catalytic and translocation domains of highly cytotoxic bacterial products, including *Pseudomonas* (174,177,178) and Diphteria toxins (78,173,175,176), in order to selectively kill glioma cells, but preserving surrounding normal brain tissue. These fusion toxins have shown promising results in in vitro and in vivo experiments using murine glioma models and clinical trials have shown that direct interstitial infusion can be used to successfully distribute chimeric toxins in tumors in the CNS, achieving anti-tumor responses without systemic toxicity in patients with malignant brain tumors (179). The chimeric toxin composed of IL-13 and truncated *Pseudomonas* exotoxin, also termed IL-13 toxin, is currently being used in several clinical trials that recruit patients throughout the country as well as Canada, Germany, Israel, and the Netherlands. The IL-13 toxin has been shown to exert a potent cytotoxic effect in most human glioblastoma cells tested in culture (174,178,180) and in vivo, in human xenografts consisting of glioma cells implanted in the flank of nude mice (181). Moreover, the intratumoral administration of IL13-PE toxin into intracranial human glioma xenografts in mice showed highly cytotoxic effects without undesirable side effects (182). To optimize the targeting of GBM associated IL-13α2 receptor, human IL-13 (hIL-13) gene has been engineered leading to a mutated form of hIL-13 that exhibits 50 fold higher affinity for the IL-13α2 receptor present in human glioma cells when compared to the wild type IL-13 (183,184). Fusion of this muIL-13 to PE resulted in an even more active cytotoxin in glioma tumors both in vitro and in vivo (183). Importantly, the muIL13 no longer interacts with the principal chain of IL4R, thus becoming ineffective in its binding to this receptor and signaling through the physiological IL13/IL4R of normal cells. This in turn decreases the already low toxicity of the chimeric toxin to normal cells (183). Thus, although this mutant has negligible affinity by IL-13 receptor of normal cells, it exerts an enhanced cytotoxic effect towards glioma cells. We are currently developing a gene therapy approach based on IL-13R-targeting, in which a high capacity adenoviral vector encodes for muIL-13 fused to the truncated PE toxin and a mutated IL-4 that functions as antagonist of the IL13R present in normal cells without interacting with IL13α2R for an enhanced safety profile (Fig. 1) (185). The fact that IL13Rα2 is over expressed not only in glioma cells, but also in other malignancies, including renal cell carcinoma (186), ovarian carcinoma (187), colon adenocarcinoma (178), epidermoid carcinoma (178), AIDS-associated Kaposi's sarcoma (188), prostate carcinoma (189) and pancreatic cancer (190), makes IL13Rα2 a unique target for anticancer therapy. Gene therapy offers the possibility of making the targeted toxins approach more efficacious and less toxic for GBM therapy, by expressing the genetically engineered toxin under a regulatable promoter, within a viral vector, it would eliminate the need of

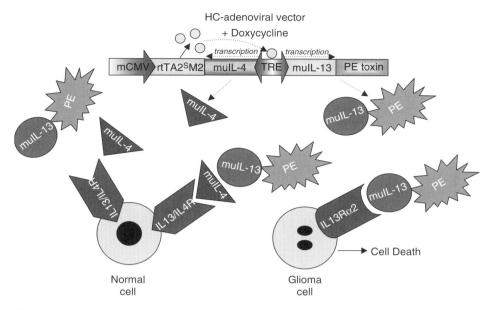

Figure 1 Targeted toxins for glioma gene therapy. Structure of a high capacity adenoviral vectors encoding muIL-13 fused to the truncated PE toxin, which binds and kills glioma cells without affecting normal brain cells. For further safety, this vector includes a mutated IL-4 (muIL-4), which functions as antagonist of the IL13R present in normal cells, without interacting with IL13Rα2, thus it prevents muIL-13-PE to interact with normal cells, protecting them from the detrimental effect of the toxin, while it does not affect muIL-13-PE binding to glioma cells. Therapeutic trangenes are encoded under the control of the TRE promoter, which is activated by a transactivator (rtTA2SM2) only in the presence of the antibiotic doxycycline, further increasing the safety of this approach. *Abbreviations*: PE, pseudomonas exotoxin; TRE, tetracycline response element.

repeated treatment due to the short half-life of the therapy, it will also allow the fine regulation of the levels of toxin expressed in case the therapy is no longer needed or to obviate adverse side effects.

VALIDATION OF CANCER GENE THERAPY STRATEGIES IN VITRO AND IN VIVO

An Overview of Commonly Used Glioma Models

Accurate experimental models are of paramount importance in developing effective therapies against diseases. A clinically relevant model helps establish the effectiveness of new therapies, such as gene therapy in a pre-clinical setting. In addition, genetic, and biochemical studies of these experimental models may shed light on defects that contribute to the development of brain tumors in humans. Table 1 shows the requirements that an ideal experimental model for glioma should meet (191).

Rodents are routinely used in preclinical studies of glioma and offer many advantages over other vertebrate models, invertebrate models or cell culture models. Unlike many larger mammals, mice, and rats have a high reproductive rate and are easy to handle and maintain. In addition, mice, and rats have been extensively studied in scientific literature and consequently have well-defined genetics, biochemistry, and physiology.

Table 1 Features of Cell Implantation and Genetic Glioma Models

Desired features of glioma animal models	Cell implantation models	Genetic models
Glial origin	☑	☑
Biological similarity to human gliomas		☑
Hystological similarity to human gliomas (invasion, neovascularization)	±	☑
Intact tumor-host interactions	☑	☑
Allow detection of antitumoral immune responses	☑	☑
Non-immunogenic in syngeneic animals	☑	☑
Allow study of human glioma tumors	☑	
Allow non-invasive techniques of tumor progression diagnosis	☑	
Accurate knowledge of tumor location	☑	
Predictable and reproducible tumor growth rates	☑	
Similar time to death of animals	☑	
Enough survival time to test therapy	☑	☑
Tumor progression	Fast	Slow
Technically easy and not expensive	☑	
Available for rat and mice	☑	Only mice

Genomics has further endorsed the use of mice and rats as models for human disease. Most human genes have homologues in rats and mice that share significant sequence homology with their human counterparts. Moreover, the mouse genome is very pliable, and a large number of genetically modified strains have been created, characterized, and maintained either by selectively breeding mice with spontaneous genetic mutations or by using transgenics. Transgenics in particular has established mice as the most commonly used laboratory mammal for studying human disease. Transgenic rats have also been recently created and as this technology progresses, the rat may offer attractive models for GBM preclinical studies.

Early Models of Glioma

Prior to 1970, research in glioma was limited by the lack of suitable pre-clinical models to design and test new therapies. DNA alkylating agents, including N-methyl-N-nitrosourea (NMU), generate point mutations in DNA and were found to promote gliomagenesis when injected *i.v.* into rabbits (192). This observation quickly led to the development of rat models of glioma involving repeated injection of NMU *i.v.* and subsequent observations for neurological symptoms to appear (193). Although these models are labor intensive and not particularly suited to pre-clinical studies, cell lines were developed from rats and mice injected with NMU. Many of these cell lines grow in vitro and in vivo and quickly gave rise to a more versatile pre-clinical model of glioma, using GBM cell lines to develop implantation models in xenogeneic or syngeneic hosts.

Xenograft Models of Glioma

Many models of glioma currently inoculate mice and rats with exogenous glioma cell lines grown in vitro. These cell lines can either be injected in the periphery giving rise to flank tumors, or alternatively injected directly into the brain of animals. Injection of cells directly into the brain requires a stereotactic device to ensure accurate and reproducible results and is clinically more relevant than flank tumors. However, some experimental designs require the convenient access of flank tumors and consequently researchers utilize both models. In these cases, data should be corroborated using intracranial models to account for differences in the extracellular environments. Exogenous glioma xenografts offer several advantages over other glioma models including highly efficient gliomagenesis, reproducible growth rates, similar time to death for different animals and an accurate knowledge of the site of the tumor. This last point is particularly advantageous in intracranial models of glioma where injection sites must be carefully chosen to overlap with the site of the tumor. Furthermore, xenograft models of glioma have been widely used and are well characterized in the literature. However, these models also have a number of important limitations that must be considered when choosing a suitable model for gliomagenesis. Paramount of these is that the majority of exogenous glioma xenografts utilize cell lines originally derived from human glioma. Consequently, immune rejection of the implanted tumor can alter the progression of the disease and decrease the clinical accuracy of the model. To limit this problem, human GBM models have been developed in immune-deficient mice and/or rats. Most models currently use cell lines originally derived from the same animal strain; these syngeneic xenografts generally have minimal non-specific immune reactivity. Another limiting factor with these models is the absence of developing stages of glioma. Therefore, while these models are useful to estimate the clinical effectiveness of various transgenes in gene therapy, they are not well designed to understand initial events that occur during gliomagenesis. In addition, promising results should be verified in more stringent models of glioma before progressing to clinical trials in human patients.

Rat Intracranial Glioma Cell Implantation Models

Intracranial injection of cell lines into rats has been used as to model glioma since the early 1970s (194). A wide diversity of cell lines have been developed for this purpose. Some of the most widely used rat brain tumor models include 9L gliosarcoma, CNS-1 glioma, C6 glioma, F98 glioma, RG2 glioma, and RT-2 induced glioma (195). The most widely used intracranial glioma model has been the 9L gliosarcoma model. This model uses 9L gliosarcoma cells originally derived from CD Fischer rats injected *i.v.* with methylnitrosourea to promote spontaneous gliomagenesis. Early studies in gene therapy primarily used this model and some spectacular results were observed (196), (Nam M, Brain Res 1996). However, this model is highly immunogenic and it has since been demonstrated that an immune response against the 9L gliosarcoma is the principal means by which non-transduced cells are killed by HSV1-TK/ganciclover treatment. Consequently this model is not optimal for studies involving gene therapy, especially approaches that aim to harness immunotherapeutic targets (197,198). Another cell line derived from rats injected with methylnitrosourea (MNU) (C6) was developed.

Unfortunately, the C6 glioma cell line was originally developed in an outbred Wistar rat and consequently there is no syngeneic host that can be used to propragate it. Consequently, C6 is immunogenic in most hosts and like 9L gliosarcoma cells this severely limits the usefulness of C6 glioma models in gene therapy (195). Recently, the CNS-1 glioma cell line was derived from an inbred Lewis rat that had been injected with MNU in a similar fashion to both 9L and C6 glioma cells. However, unlike 9L cells the CNS-1 glioma stains positive for GFAP and S-100. CNS-1 cells have in vivo growth rates and histology that more closely resemble human glioma than 9L cells. Furthermore, CNS-1 cells are not immunogenic in vivo in Lewis rats and therefore are ideally suited for pre-clinical testing (Fig. 2) (199).

An alternative approach was utilized in the development of F98 and RG2 cell lines. The mutagen of choice was not MNU but instead was ethylnitrosourea (ENU) in both cases. Both of these glioma cell lines are non-immunogenic. F98 glioma cells were originally from offspring of a pregnant CD Fisher rat and are remarkably similar to human glioma in many ways. They are very weakly immunogenic, they display an infiltrative pattern of growth similar to human glioma and as few as 10 cells invariably kill animals when inoculated intracranially in vivo. RG2 cells were produced in a similar fashion and are non-immunogenic in syngeneic Fischer rats (200). The invasive pattern of growth and refractory nature to chemotherapeutic agents are advantages to using this model in assessing the effectiveness of novel gene therapeutic agents.

Mouse Intracranial Glioma Cell Implantation Models

Historically, the rat was the rodent of choice for pre-clinical models of glioma due to its larger size and well documented physiology and anatomy. However, in the genomic era with the advent of transgenics, the mouse has superseded the rat as the most popular model of human diseases. Many of these models seek to explore the early events of gliomagenesis by mutating key regulatory genes using transgenics and in doing so develop more accurate

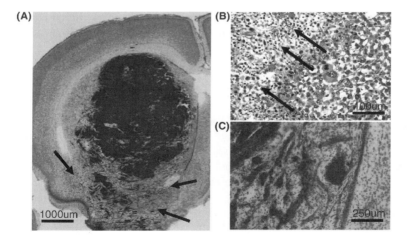

Figure 2 (*See color insert*) CNS-1 tumor histology. 5000 CNS-1 glioma cells were implanted in the striatum of syngeneic Lewis rats. Animals become moribund within 3 weeks of implantation. (**A**) Nissl staining of a brain section showing a CNS-1 tumor from an untreated moribund animal. Note areas of infiltration (*arrows*). (**B**) Hematoxilin/eosin stained brain section showing a CNS-1 tumor from an untreated moribund animal. The arrow indicates an area of cell death within the tumor. (**C**) Nissl stained brain section showing areas of tumoral cell infiltration in the same animal pictured in **A**.

pre-clinical models of human glioma. Also number of intracranial xenograft models have also been developed to accelerate the discovery of novel promising therapies. Unfortunately many of the earlier models often used human glioma xenografts (i.e., SF-9o295, U-251 or D54) or rat glioma xenografts (primarily C6) transplanted into immunocompromised mice. Immune-mediated events before, during, and after therapy cannot be observed in these models, limiting their usefulness. A number of syngeneic models have been developed. The first model used was glioma 26 (GL-26). These cells were found to be non-immunogenic when injected either subcutaneously or intracranially into C57/BL6 mice and this model is still commonly used today (Fig. 3) (201). Another mouse glioma cell line called GL261, also derived from C57/BL6 mice, has similar characteristics to GL26 cells and both these cell lines are useful for studying the response of brain tumors to immunotherapy (202). More recently, other models have been developed, including a syngeneic glioma cell line derived from spontaneous tumor in a transgenic mouse model called 4C8. These cells express GFAP and the histology was densely cellular, and developed a pseudopallisading pattern of necrosis. All these features are commonly found in human glioblastoma, making this a very useful model for testing and developing novel gene therapeutic agents (203). Although these models are useful in pre-clinical studies of anti-tumor therapies, the main focus has centered on understanding the molecular pattern of gliomagenesis by altering genes believed to play

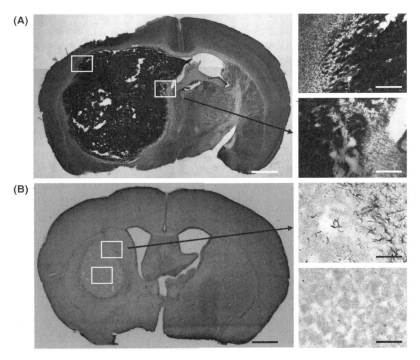

Figure 3 (*See color insert*) C57/BL6 mice were challenged with 20000 GL26 cells injected into the striatum. The animals were moribund after 25–30 days. (**A**) Nissel staining of a brain section showing a GL26 tumor from an untreated moribund animal. Scale bars: 1000 μm in low magnification shots, 250 μm in higher magnification shots. (**B**) GFAP immunostaining of a brain section from an untreated moribund animal shows activated astrocytes. A higher magnification picture shows infiltration of tumor cells into the surrounding CNS tissue. Scale bars: 1000 μm in low magnification shots; 100 μm in higher magnification shots.

an important role. Transgenics in particular have led to the development of a wide variety of mouse models of glioma that are closer approximations of human disease.

Genetic Modelling of Glioma Formation

Researchers have aspired to develop mouse glioma models by deleting (knockout) or inserting (transgenic) genes commonly mutated in human disease. The aim of this approach is twofold. Firstly, a greater insight into the key factors contributing to gliomagenesis and disease progression can be elucidated from these studies. This may lead to the identification of key targets for gene therapy or more conventional drugs. Secondly, more accurate pre-clinical models of the human disease should improve the process of drug testing and development for treating glioma. Recently, a number of mouse strains have been developed that mimic many of the histological and pathological features of human gliomas. Furthermore, many of these models consistently give rise to brain tumors that strongly resemble particular classes or types of human glioma. These models have enormous potential for understanding the different genetic alterations and cellular precursors of glioma tumors and in refining novel therapies, including gene therapy, in a relevant pre-clinical model. In this section we will discuss the recently developed and most promising models of glioma.

Transgenic Mouse Models of Glioma

Two transgenic mice in particular have proved very useful in the study of gliomagenesis and have also been used to evaluate glioma therapies. In these mice, the oncogenes v-src and ^{v12}H-Ras have been introduced into murine germlines under the control of the GFAP promoter. GFAP expression is confined to cells of the astroglial lineage and this regulation is under control of the highly specific GFAP promoter. Consequently, the oncogenic potential of v-src or ^{v12}H-Ras is also confined to astroglial cells in this model. One line derived from ^{v12}H-Ras transgenic mice develop solitary tumors that closely resemble low grade astrocytoma (grade II), whereas animals homozygous for the transgene develop multifocal tumors that represent anaplastic astrocytoma (grade III). Similarly transgenic mice expressing v-src under the control of GFAP promoter also develop tumors that resemble human astrocytomas (grade II) (204). Tumors in these models further develop into grade III tumors and ultimately to glioblastoma (grade IV). This order of events closely follows progression of glioma in humans. Furthermore, tumors in ^{v12}H-Ras transgenic mice displayed many molecular changes commonly associated with glioblastoma in humans including elevated EGFR and MDM2 and CDK4 expression, elevated AKT activity, and decreased levels of INK4A, ARF, and PTEN expression (205,206). Additional mutations in tumor suppressor genes and proto-oncogenes have also been developed and these in general accelerate the development of glioblastoma (206). Consequently, these mice closely model glioma progression in humans and may be more accurate indicators of gene therapeutic agents in pre-clinical studies.

Knockout Mouse Models of Glioma

In general, mutations in signal transduction pathways regulating the cell cycle or RTK activity are evident in many if not all gliomas and play a fundamental role in the progression of the disease. Of the many mouse strains developed with mutations in genes commonly altered in human glioma, only germline deletion of the tumor suppressor genes p53 and NF1 alone was found to increase the susceptibility of mice to astrocytoma and glioblastoma (207). This supports the work of others suggesting that p53 mutation or deletion is a very early event in gliomagenesis (11). INK4A and ARF have also been studied as regulators of gliomagenesis. Although deletion of either or both gene products alone is not sufficient to induce glioma formation in mice, somatic transfer of the RTK PDGF into astrocytes and nestin-producing CNS progenitor cells greatly enhances the appearance of mixed oligoastrocytomas and oligodendrogliomas, respectively (208). This supports the conclusions of others that disregulation of the cell cycle induces a change in phenotype of glioma from slowly proliferating grade II to rapidly proliferating grade III tumors. However, initial growth factor independence is required to promote gliomagenesis (27).

CLINICAL TRIALS

Clinical trials are scientifically designed experiments to determine how efficient new treatment modalities would affect disease outcome and progression in human patients. Many therapeutic formulations can be used in clinical trials such as chemotherapeutic drugs, surgical procedures or gene therapy. The majority of brain tumor clinical trials involve radiation therapy or chemotherapy. There are three different phases (Phase I, II, III) that clinical trials must encompass in order to answer all the needed research and therapeutic questions. Phase I trials determine the best treatment schedule and the best dose of treatment and importantly the safety of the proposed treatment. The effect of the treatment on the actual brain tumor is not the primary issue while safety, dosage, and side effects are. A small trial size is used due to the uncertainties. Phase II trials determine the effect of the treatment on the brain tumor (i.e., does the tumor size shrink?). A safe dosage has been established in Phase I so investigating the anticancer effect is the primary goal. Phase III trials compare the new treatment to already existing treatments. A much larger trial size is used in phase III trials because these are proposed as established treatments that will help reduce the tumor size and prolong patients' life span. There are definite benefits to being a part of a clinical trial. Even if patients do not get selected for receiving the new treatment, they will still receive the best possible treatments for brain cancer available.

Table 2 summarizes the advantages and benefits of gene therapy vectors that already tested in clinical trials. One of the main gene therapy approaches that have been implemented in clinical trials is the use of the herpes simplex virus gene for HSV1-TK as a conditional cytotoxic strategy. The gene is expressed in all infected cells, but it will only cause cytotoxicity in the presence of the prodrug, GCV, in dividing, tumor cells and it will not affect non-dividing, normal brain cells. After patients are administered the HSV1-TK gene encoded withing a viral vector, they are given the antiviral drug, GCV. The HSV1-TK gene product phosphorylates GCV and intracellular kinases convert it to GCV triphosphate that intercalates in replicating DNA causing cell death. Most of the clinical trials using HSV1-TK and GCV have provided positive data for the outcome of brain tumor patients (209–211). The intratumoral injection of retrovirus-packaging cells as well as adenoviruses encoding HSV1-TK followed by GCV administration has been tested for glioma treatment in Phase I/II clinical trials (213,214). Human glioma cells express CAR and integrin αV on their cell surface, which mediate adenoviral attachment and internalization, therefore making Ad attractive vectors for GBM gene therapy approaches (Fig. 4). Both therapies were well tolerated and safe (152,212,213), with adenoviral vectors encoding TK observed to be more efficient than retrovirus vectors, based on tumor re-growth three months after gene therapy and extended glioma-bearing patients' survival (212). Also, since delivery of retrovirus vectors is achieved by implantation of xenograft

Table 2 Gene Therapy Vectors Tested in Clinical Trials for Glioma Treatment

Viral vectors	Therapeutic effect	Advantages	Disadvantages
• Retrovirus (Virus producing cells)	• HSV1-TK: apoptosis	• Antitumor effect	• Low bystander effect
	• IL-2/HSV1-TK: apoptosis and antitumor immune response	• Survival rate increase	• Low tumor transduction
		• Low immune response against the vector	
		• No systemic/local adverse effects	
• Adenovirus (replication-defective)	• HSV1-TK: apoptosis	• High transduction efficiency	• Low diffusibility
	• p53: apoptosis	• Antitumor effect	• Immune response against the vector
		• Survival rate increase	
		• No systemic/local adverse effects	
• Replicating vectors ONYX-015 (adenovirus) G207, HSV1716 (Herpesvirus) Newcastle disease virus	• Replication in tumoral cells selective cell lysis	• Antitumor effect	• Immune response against vectors
		• Low recurrence	
		• Survival rate increase	
		• No systemic/local adverse effects	

virus-producing cells rather than the retrovirus (152), this approach adds the hazards of xenogeneic transplant rejection, absent in adenoviral-based therapies. A recent Phase III clinical trial compared the efficacy of HSV1-TK delivery using adenoviral gene therapy with standard care of glioma patients, consisting of radical excision followed by radiotherapy (214). The intracranial injection of the adenoviral vector encoding HSV1-TK followed by the intravenous administration of ganciclovir (GCV) increased the survival time of glioma from 40 to 70 weeks, without adverse side effects (214). In summary, intratumoral adenoviral delivery of TK, combined with GCV is a potential new treatment for operable primary or recurrent high-grade glioma.

Phase I trials consisting in the intratumoral injection of an adenoviral vector to deliver the p53 gene in glioma cells have also led to interesting results. The toxicity of this treatment was minimal and there was no evidence of systemic viral dissemination. The adenoviral p53 trial showed that exogenous p53 was expressed in the nuclei of glioma

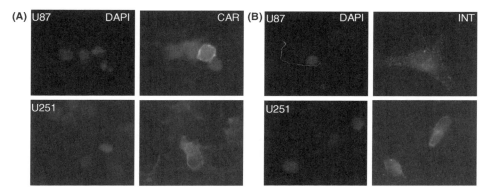

Figure 4 (*See color insert*) Expression of adenoviral receptors in human glioma cells. (**A**) The coxsackie-adenoviral receptor (CAR) and (**B**) Integrine αV [INT] expression were detected in U251 and U87 cells by immunofluorescence. Left panels show nuclei stained with DAPI and right panels show the expression of the receptors using indirect immunofluorescence.

cells and activated a downstream pathway that induces apoptosis and prevents the tumor from expanding (20). The only downfall of this therapy was that the transgene expression was not widespread and therefore only the tumor cells close to the injection site were killed. Further work to enhance the distribution of the therapeutic gene will increase the possibilities of this therapy considerably.

A recent phase I clinical trial has been conducted to determine the safety of ONYX-015, a mutated adenovirus that is able to replicate selectively in and kill tumor cells, but not normal cells (215,216). The dose-escalation trial showed intra-cerebral injections of ONYX-015 to be very well tolerated by glioma-bearing patients without any adverse side effects attributable to the viral vector, even at doses as high as 10^{10} pfu (217). Although therapeutic efficacy of all these novel gene therapy approaches will have to await larger trials, they provide a solid scientific rationale for additional studies of adenoviral-based gene therapy for brain tumors.

Replicating herpes simplex viral (HSV) vectors have also been used as replication competent vectors to treat brain tumors in clinical trials. HSV-G207 vector contains two mutations within the virus that confer specificity of G207 for dividing in tumoral cells, while intact HSV1-TK gene provides a mechanism to control any herpetic infection that may arise from use of these replicating vectors. In phase one clinical trials with G207 was intratumorally injected in patients with progressive or recurrent glioma (218). MTD was not established as the highest level 3×10^9 pfu was well tolerated and no herpetic, encephalic or inflammatory effects were observed. Although one patient seroconverted, exhibiting serum antibodies anti-HSV1 after treatment, no systemic toxicity attributable to G207 treatment was observed. Four patients survived at the end of the trial, while the mean survival from diagnosis to death increased to 15.9 months.

Another replicating HSV vector, HSV1716, showed to be unable to replicate in neurons while replicates and lyses glioma cells. In a phase one clinical trial, HSV1716 was intratumorally injected in glioma patients. The MTD for this vector was not determined as up to 1×10^5 pfu were tolerated well with no encephalitis or herpetic complications, all patients remaining seronegative for HSV-1 (219). In an additional trial, recurrent patient tumors were examined after injection of HSV1716 and virus was detectable by semiquantitative PCR (220). Even in inoculated tumors for which virus was not detectible, reinfection in vitro triggered low level HSV1716 viral shedding indicating persistent long-term effects may be possible (221). HSV1716 was also intracranially injected after glioma resection to eliminate residual tumor cells (222). Of 12 patients, three survived, one died of non related events, and eight died after tumor progression. No treatment related toxicities were observed. Further clinical trials are ongoing.

Replication-competent Newcastle disease virus (NDV) has also been used in clinical trials. Glioma tumor cells taken from patients were infected with NDV, irradiated, and used to vaccinate the patient, who survived significantly longer than non-vaccinated controls and the therapy was well tolerated (223,224).

Several clinical trials have been testing the potential of chimeric toxins targeting receptor that are overexpressed in human gliomas. Clinical trials testing the antitumoral potential of the intratumoral administration of IL-13 toxin, consisting in IL-13 fused to *Pseudomonas* exotoxin, are currently being developed in the United States, Canada, Germany, Israel, and the Netherlands. In a PhaseI/II clinical trial, patients with glioblastoma multiforme were intratumorally injected with IL-13 toxin eight days before surgical resection (225). Necrotic areas were found in the tumors from half the patients, suggesting that the toxin successfully induced tumoral cell death.

The chimeric toxin composed of IL-4 and Pseudomonas exotoxin was intracranially administered to patients with recurrent glioblastoma multiforme in Phase I and Phase I/II clinical trials. The intratumoral administration of IL-4 cytotoxin showed an acceptable safety profile, being well tolerated at low doses (226). These studies suggested that this cytotoxin has anti-tumor activity, inducing necrosis in the tumor parenchyma, without histological evidence of toxicity to normal brain tissues (227). Although local toxicity, such as intracranial edema, was reported, it seems to be due to tumor necrosis or occasionally to the volume of infusion.

Transferrin-diptheria toxin was locally administered by high-flow interstitial microinfusion to patients with recurrent malignant brain tumors, which were refractory to conventional therapy (179). Although episodes of local toxicity in some of the patients were reported, direct interstitial infusion was shown to successfully distribute the toxin in the tumor and infiltrated brain areas, achieving anti-tumor responses without severe neurologic or systemic toxicity (228).

A chimeric toxin consisting of TGF and *Pseudomonas* toxin was tested in a Phase I trial to determine its dose limiting toxicity. The chimeric toxin was determined by convection-enhanced delivery in 20 patients with recurrent malignant brain tumors. In this trial the maximal tolerated dose could not be established, being the overall median survival 23 weeks after intracranial administration of the toxin (229).

ACKNOWLEDGMENTS

Gene therapy projects for neurological diseases are funded by the National Institutes of Health/National Institute of Neurological Disorders and Stroke Grant 1R01 NS44556.01, National Institute of Diabetes and Digestive and Kidney Diseases 1 RO3 TW006273-01 to M.G.C.; National Institutes of Health/National Institute of Neurological Disorders and Stroke Grant 1 RO1 NS 42893.01, U54 NS045309-01, and 1R21 NS047298-01 and Bram and Elaine Goldsmith Chair In Gene Therapeutics to P.R.L.; and The Linda Tallen & David Paul Kane Annual Fellowship to M.G.C and P.R.L. We also thank the generous funding our Institute receives from the Board of Governors at Cedars-Sinai Medical

Center. We thank the support and academic leadership of S. Melmed, R. Katzman, and D. Meyer for their superb administrative and organizational support.

REFERENCES

1. Baldwin RT, Preston-Martin S. Epidemiology of brain tumors in childhood-a review. Toxicol Appl Pharmacol 2004; 199:118–131.
2. McCance KL, Huether SE. 3rd ed. Pathophysiology: The Biologic Basis for Disease in Adults and Children. St. Louis: Mosby, 1998.
3. Stedman TL. Stedman's medical dictionary. 27th ed. Philadelphia: Lippincott Williams & Wilkins, 2000.
4. Castro MG, Cowen R, Williamson IK, David A, Jimenez-Dalmaroni MJ, Yuan X, Bigliari A, Williams JC, Hu J, Lowenstein PR. Current and future strategies for the treatment of malignant brain tumors. Pharmacol Ther 2003; 98:71–108.
5. Halperin EC. Pediatric radiation oncology. 3rd ed. Philadelphia: Lippincott Williams & Wilkins, 1999.
6. Kaba SE, Kyritsis AP. Recognition and management of gliomas. Drugs 1997; 53:235–244.
7. Grossman SA, Batara JF. Current management of glioblastoma multiforme. Semin Oncol 2004; 31:635–644.
8. Merlo A. Genes and pathways driving glioblastomas in humans and murine disease models. Neurosurg Rev 2003; 26:145–158.
9. Hisada M, Garber JE, Fung CY, Fraumeni JF, Jr., Li FP. Multiple primary cancers in families with Li-Fraumeni syndrome. J Natl Cancer Inst 1998; 90:606–611.
10. Watkins D, Rouleau GA. Genetics, prognosis and therapy of central nervous system tumors. Cancer Detect Prev 1994; 18:139–144.
11. Louis DN. The p53 gene and protein in human brain tumors. J Neuropathol Exp Neurol 1994; 53:11–21.
12. Asai A, Miyagi Y, Sugiyama A, Gamanuma M, Hong SH, Takamoto S, Nomura K, Matsutani M, Takakura K, Kuchino Y. Negative effects of wild-type p53 and s-Myc on cellular growth and tumorigenicity of glioma cells. Implication of the tumor suppressor genes for gene therapy. J Neurooncol 1994; 19:259–268.
13. Badie B, Drazan KE, Kramar MH, Shaked A, Black KL. Adenovirus-mediated p53 gene delivery inhibits 9L glioma growth in rats. Neurol Res 1995; 17:209–216.
14. Kock H, Harris MP, Anderson SC, et al. Adenovirus-mediated p53 gene transfer suppresses growth of human glioblastoma cells in vitro and in vivo. Int J Cancer 1996; 67:808–815.
15. Gjerset RA, Turla ST, Sobol RE, et al. Use of wild-type p53 to achieve complete treatment sensitization of tumor cells expressing endogenous mutant p53. Mol Carcinog 1995; 14:275–285.
16. Dorigo O, Turla ST, Lebedeva S, Gjerset RA. Sensitization of rat glioblastoma multiforme to cisplatin in vivo following restoration of wild-type p53 function. J Neurosurg 1998; 88:535–540.
17. Badie B, Kramar MH, Lau R, Boothman DA, Economou JS, Black KL. Adenovirus-mediated p53 gene delivery potentiates the radiation-induced growth inhibition of experimental brain tumors. J Neurooncol 1998; 37:217–222.
18. Li H, Alonso-Vanegas M, Colicos MA, et al. Intracerebral adenovirus-mediated p53 tumor suppressor gene therapy for experimental human glioma. Clin Cancer Res 1999; 5:637–642.
19. Cirielli C, Inyaku K, Capogrossi MC, Yuan X, Williams JA. Adenovirus-mediated wild-type p53 expression induces apoptosis and suppresses tumorigenesis of experimental intracranial human malignant glioma. J Neurooncol 1999; 43:99–108.
20. Lang FF, Bruner JM, Fuller GN, et al. Phase I trial of adenovirus-mediated p53 gene therapy for recurrent glioma: biological and clinical results. J Clin Oncol 2003; 21:2508–2518.

21. Chen J, Willingham T, Shuford M, et al. Effects of ectopic overexpression of p21(WAF1/CIP1) on aneuploidy and the malignant phenotype of human brain tumor cells. Oncogene 1996; 13:1395–1403.
22. Fueyo J, Gomez-Manzano C, Yung WK, et al. Overexpression of E2F-1 in glioma triggers apoptosis and suppresses tumor growth in vitro and in vivo. Nat Med 1998; 4:685–690.
23. Wang TJ, Huang MS, Hong CY, Tse V, Silverberg GD. Comparisons of tumor suppressor p53, p21, and p16 gene therapy effects on glioblastoma tumorigenicity in situ. Biochem Biophys Res Commun 2001; 287:173–180.
24. Bischoff JR, Kirn DH, Williams A, et al. An adenovirus mutant that replicates selectively in p53-deficient human tumor cells. Science 1996; 274:373–376.
25. Heise C, Sampson-Johannes A, Williams A, McCormick F, Von Hoff DD, Kirn DH. ONYX-015, an E1B gene-attenuated adenovirus, causes tumor-specific cytolysis and antitumoral efficacy that can be augmented by standard chemotherapeutic agents. Nat Med 1997; 3:639–645.
26. Geoerger B, Grill J, Opolon P, et al. Potentiation of radiation therapy by the oncolytic adenovirus dl1520 (ONYX-015) in human malignant glioma xenografts. Br J Cancer 2003; 89:577–584.
27. Maher EA, Furnari FB, Bachoo RM, et al. Malignant glioma: genetics and biology of a grave matter. Genes Dev 2001; 15:1311–1333.
28. Sherr CJ. Cancer cell cycles. Science 1996; 274:1672–1677.
29. Schmidt EE, Ichimura K, Reifenberger G, Collins VP. CDKN2 (p16/MTS1) gene deletion or CDK4 amplification occurs in the majority of glioblastomas. Cancer Res 1994; 54:6321–6324.
30. Ueki K, Ono Y, Henson JW, Efird JT, Von Deimling A, Louis DN. CDKN2/p16 or RB alterations occur in the majority of glioblastomas and are inversely correlated. Cancer Res 1996; 56:150–153.
31. Zhang X, Multani AS, Zhou JH, et al. Adenoviral-mediated retinoblastoma 94 produces rapid telomere erosion, chromosomal crisis, and caspase-dependent apoptosis in bladder cancer and immortalized human urothelial cells but not in normal urothelial cells. Cancer Res 2003; 63:760–765.
32. Riley DJ, Nikitin AY, Lee WH. Adenovirus-mediated retinoblastoma gene therapy suppresses spontaneous pituitary melanotroph tumors in Rb+/− mice. Nat Med 1996; 2:1316–1321.
33. Fueyo J, Gomez-Manzano C, Alemany R, et al. A mutant oncolytic adenovirus targeting the Rb pathway produces anti-glioma effect in vivo. Oncogene 2000; 19:2–12.
34. Lee SH, Kim MS, Kwon HC, et al. Growth inhibitory effect on glioma cells of adenovirus-mediated p16/INK4a gene transfer in vitro and in vivo. Int J Mol Med 2000; 6:559–563.
35. Fueyo J, Gomez-Manzano C, Yung WK, et al. Adenovirus-mediated p16/CDKN2 gene transfer induces growth arrest and modifies the transformed phenotype of glioma cells. Oncogene 1996; 12:103–110.
36. Simon M, Simon C, Koster G, Hans VH, Schramm J. Conditional expression of the tumor suppressor p16 in a heterotopic glioblastoma model results in loss of pRB expression. J Neurooncol 2002; 60:1–12.
37. Garkavtsev I, Kozin SV, Chernova O, et al. The candidate tumour suppressor protein ING4 regulates brain tumour growth and angiogenesis. Nature 2004; 428:328–332.
38. Rege TA, Fears CY, Gladson CL. Endogenous inhibitors of angiogenesis in malignant gliomas: nature's antiangiogenic therapy. Neuro-oncol 2005; 7:106–121.
39. Chang SM, Lamborn KR, Malec M, et al. Phase II study of temozolomide and thalidomide with radiation therapy for newly diagnosed glioblastoma multiforme. Int J Radiat Oncol Biol Phys 2004; 60:353–357.
40. Baumann F, Bjeljac M, Kollias SS, et al. Combined thalidomide and temozolomide treatment in patients with glioblastoma multiforme. J Neurooncol 2004; 67:191–200.
41. Morabito A, Fanelli M, Carillio G, Gattuso D, Sarmiento R, Gasparini G. Thalidomide prolongs disease stabilization after conventional therapy in patients with recurrent glioblastoma. Oncol Rep 2004; 11:93–95.

42. Fine HA, Wen PY, Maher EA, et al. Phase II trial of thalidomide and carmustine for patients with recurrent high-grade gliomas. J Clin Oncol 2003; 21:2299–2304.

43. Puduvalli VK, Sawaya R. Antiangiogenesis—therapeutic strategies and clinical implications for brain tumors. J Neurooncol 2000; 50:189–200.

44. Chen QR, Zhang L, Gasper W, Mixson AJ. Targeting tumor angiogenesis with gene therapy. Mol Genet Metab 2001; 74:120–127.

45. Montesano R, Vassalli JD, Baird A, Guillemin R, Orci L. Basic fibroblast growth factor induces angiogenesis in vitro. Proc Natl Acad Sci USA 1986; 83:7297–7301.

46. Szabo S, Sandor Z. The diagnostic and prognostic value of tumor angiogenesis. Eur J Surg Suppl 1998;99–103.

47. Yukawa H, Takahashi JC, Miyatake SI, et al. Adenoviral gene transfer of basic fibroblast growth factor promotes angiogenesis in rat brain. Gene Ther 2000; 7:942–949.

48. Ke LD, Shi YX, Im SA, Chen X, Yung WK. The relevance of cell proliferation, vascular endothelial growth factor, and basic fibroblast growth factor production to angiogenesis and tumorigenicity in human glioma cell lines. Clin Cancer Res 2000; 6:2562–2572.

49. Plate KH, Risau W. Angiogenesis in malignant gliomas. Glia 1995; 15:339–347.

50. Stratmann A, Machein MR, Plate KH. Anti-angiogenic gene therapy of malignant glioma. Acta Neurochir Suppl (Wien) 1997; 68:105–110.

51. Leung DW, Cachianes G, Kuang WJ, Goeddel DV, Ferrara N. Vascular endothelial growth factor is a secreted angiogenic mitogen. Science 1989; 246:1306–1309.

52. Keck PJ, Hauser SD, Krivi G, et al. Vascular permeability factor, an endothelial cell mitogen related to PDGF. Science 1989; 246:1309–1312.

53. Saleh M, Stacker SA, Wilks AF. Inhibition of growth of C6 glioma cells in vivo by expression of antisense vascular endothelial growth factor sequence. Cancer Res 1996; 56:393–401.

54. Sasaki M, Wizigmann-Voos S, Risau W, Plate KH. Retrovirus producer cells encoding antisense VEGF prolong survival of rats with intracranial GS9L gliomas. Int J Dev Neurosci 1999; 17:579–591.

55. Machein MR, Risau W, Plate KH. Antiangiogenic gene therapy in a rat glioma model using a dominant-negative vascular endothelial growth factor receptor 2. Hum Gene Ther 1999; 10:1117–1128.

56. O'Reilly MS, Boehm T, Shing Y, et al. Endostatin: an endogenous inhibitor of angiogenesis and tumor growth. Cell 1997; 88:277–285.

57. O'Reilly MS, Holmgren L, Shing Y, et al. Angiostatin: a novel angiogenesis inhibitor that mediates the suppression of metastases by a Lewis lung carcinoma. Cell 1994; 79:315–328.

58. Peroulis I, Jonas N, Saleh M. Antiangiogenic activity of endostatin inhibits C6 glioma growth. Int J Cancer 2002; 97:839–845.

59. Yamanaka R, Zullo SA, Ramsey J, et al. Induction of therapeutic antitumor antiangiogenesis by intratumoral injection of genetically engineered endostatin-producing. Semliki Forest virus. Cancer Gene Ther 2001; 8:796–802.

60. Ma HI, Lin SZ, Chiang YH, et al. Intratumoral gene therapy of malignant brain tumor in a rat model with angiostatin delivered by adeno-associated viral (AAV) vector. Gene Ther 2002; 9:2–11.

61. Tanaka T, Cao Y, Folkman J, Fine HA. Viral vector-targeted antiangiogenic gene therapy utilizing an angiostatin complementary DNA. Cancer Res 1998; 58:3362–3369.

62. Tanaka T, Manome Y, Wen P, Kufe DW, Fine HA. Viral vector-mediated transduction of a modified platelet factor 4 cDNA inhibits angiogenesis and tumor growth. Nat Med 1997; 3:437–442.

63. Witte JS, Palmer LJ, O'Connor RD, Hopkins PJ, Hall JM. Relation between tumour necrosis factor polymorphism TNFalpha-308 and risk of asthma. Eur J Hum Genet 2002; 10:82–85.

64. Saleh M, Jonas NK, Wiegmans A, Stylli SS. The treatment of established intracranial tumors by in situ retroviral IFN-gamma transfer. Gene Ther 2000; 7:1715–1724.

65. Saleh M, Wiegmans A, Malone Q, Stylli SS, Kaye AH. Effect of in situ retroviral interleukin-4 transfer on established intracranial tumors. J Natl Cancer Inst 1999; 91:438–445.

66. Nagel GA, Piessens WF, Stilmant MM. Lejeune F Evidence for tumor-specific immunity in human malignant melanoma. Eur J Cancer 1971; 7:41–47.
67. Darnell RB, DeAngelis LM. Regression of small-cell lung carcinoma in patients with paraneoplastic neuronal antibodies. Lancet 1993; 341:21–22.
68. Speiser DE, Miranda R, Zakarian A, et al. Self antigens expressed by solid tumors. Do not efficiently stimulate naive or activated T cells: implications for immunotherapy. J Exp Med 1997; 186:645–653.
69. Marincola FM, Wang E, Herlyn M, Seliger B, Ferrone S. Tumors as elusive targets of T-cell-based active immunotherapy. Trends Immunol 2003; 24:335–342.
70. Ochsenbein AF, Klenerman P, Karrer U, et al. Immune surveillance against a solid tumor fails because of immunological ignorance. Proc Natl Acad Sci USA 1999; 96:2233–2238.
71. Biglari A, Bataille D, Naumann U, et al. Effects of ectopic decorin in modulating intracranial glioma progression in vivo, in a rat syngeneic model. Cancer Gene Ther 2004; 11:721–732.
72. Svane IM, Soot ML, Buus S, Johnsen HE. Clinical application of dendritic cells in cancer vaccination therapy. Apmis 2003; 111:818–834.
73. Jongmans W, van den Oudenalder K, Tiemessen DM, et al. Targeting of adenovirus to human renal cell carcinoma cells. Urology 2003; 62:559–565.
74. Natsume A, Tsujimura K, Mizuno M, Takahashi T, Yoshida J. IFN-beta gene therapy induces systemic antitumor immunity against malignant glioma. J Neurooncol 2000; 47:117–124.
75. Nakahara N, Pollack IF, Storkus WJ, Wakabayashi T, Yoshida J, Okada H. Effective induction of antiglioma cytotoxic T cells by coadministration of interferon-beta gene vector and dendritic cells. Cancer Gene Ther 2003; 10:549–558.
76. Yoshida J, Mizuno M, Nakahara N, Colosi P. Antitumor effect of an adeno-associated virus vector containing the human interferon-beta gene on experimental intracranial human glioma. Jpn J Cancer Res 2002; 93:223–228.
77. Eck SL, Alavi JB, Judy K, et al. Treatment of recurrent or progressive malignant glioma with a recombinant adenovirus expressing human interferon-beta (H5.010CMVhIFN-beta): a phase I trial. Hum Gene Ther 2001; 12:97–113.
78. Liu Y, Ehtesham M, Samoto K, et al. In situ adenoviral interleukin 12 gene transfer confers potent and long-lasting cytotoxic immunity in glioma. Cancer Gene Ther 2002; 9:9–15.
79. Lichtor T, Glick RP. Cytokine immuno-gene therapy for treatment of brain tumors. J Neurooncol 2003; 65:247–259.
80. Lowenstein PR. Immunology of viral-vector-mediated gene transfer into the brain: an evolutionary and developmental perspective. Trends Immunol 2002; 23:23–30.
81. McMenamin PG. Distribution and phenotype of dendritic cells and resident tissue macrophages in the dura mater, leptomeninges, and choroid plexus of the rat brain as demonstrated in wholemount preparations. J Comp Neurol 1999; 405:553–562.
82. Fischer HG, Reichmann G. Brain dendritic cells and macrophages/microglia in central nervous system inflammation. J Immunol 2001; 166:2717–2726.
83. Fischer HG, Bonifas U, Reichmann G. Phenotype and functions of brain dendritic cells emerging during chronic infection of mice with Toxoplasma gondii. J Immunol 2000; 164:4826–4834.
84. Santambrogio L, Belyanskaya SL, Fischer FR, et al. Developmental plasticity of CNS microglia. Proc Natl Acad Sci USA 2001; 98:6295–6300.
85. Serafini B, Columba-Cabezas S, Di Rosa F, Aloisi F. Intracerebral recruitment and maturation of dendritic cells in the onset and progression of experimental autoimmune encephalomyelitis. Am J Pathol 2000; 157:1991–2002.
86. Laouar Y, Crispe IN. Functional flexibility in T cells: independent regulation of CD4 + T cell proliferation and effector function in vivo. Immunity 2000; 13:291–301.
87. Lynch DH, Andreasen A, Maraskovsky E, Whitmore J, Miller RE, Schuh JC. Flt3 ligand induces tumor regression and antitumor immune responses in vivo. Nat Med 1997; 3:625–631.

88. Schuler G, Schuler-Thurner B, Steinman RM. The use of dendritic cells in cancer immunotherapy. Curr Opin Immunol 2003; 15:138–147.

89. Ali S, King GD, Curtin JF, et al. Combined immunostimulation and conditional cytotoxic gene therapy provide long-term survival in a large glioma model. Cancer Res 2005; 65:7194–7204.

90. Ali S, Curtin JF, Zirger J, et al. Inflammatory and anti-glioma effects of an adenovirus expressing human soluble fms-like tyrosine kinase 3-lignad (hsFlt3L): treatment with hsFlt3L inhibits intracranial glioma progression. Mol Ther 2004; 10.

91. Reed JC. Apoptosis-based therapies. Nat Rev Drug Discov 2002; 1:111–121.

92. Townson JL, Naumov GN, Chambers AF. The role of apoptosis in tumor progression and metastasis. Curr Mol Med 2003; 3:631–642.

93. Shinoura N, Hamada H. Gene therapy using an adenovirus vector for apoptosis-related genes is a highly effective therapeutic modality for killing glioma cells. Curr Gene Ther 2003; 3:147–153.

94. Naismith JH, Sprang SR. Modularity in the TNF-receptor family. Trends Biochem Sci 1998; 23:74–79.

95. Bodmer JL, Schneider P, Tschopp J. The molecular architecture of the TNF superfamily. Trends Biochem Sci 2002; 27:19–26.

96. Curtin JF, Cotter TG. Live and let die: regulatory mechanisms in Fas-mediated apoptosis. Cell Signal 2003; 15:983–992.

97. Maleniak TC, Darling JL, Lowenstein PR, Castro MG. Adenovirus-mediated expression of HSV1-TK or Fas ligand induces cell death in primary human glioma-derived cell cultures that are resistant to the chemotherapeutic agent CCNU. Cancer Gene Ther 2001; 8:589–598.

98. Morelli AE, Larregina AT, Smith-Arica J, et al. Neuronal and glial cell type-specific promoters within adenovirus recombinants restrict the expression of the apoptosis-inducing molecule Fas ligand to predetermined brain cell types, and abolish peripheral liver toxicity. J Gen Virol 1999; 80:571–583.

99. Ambar BB, Frei K, Malipiero U, et al. Treatment of experimental glioma by administration of adenoviral vectors expressing Fas ligand. Hum Gene Ther 1999; 10:1641–1648.

100. Nafe C, Cao YJ, Quinones A, Dobberstein KU, Kramm CM, Rainov NG. Expression of mutant non-cleavable Fas ligand on retrovirus packaging cells causes apoptosis of immunocompetent cells and improves prodrug activation gene therapy in a malignant glioma model. Life Sci 2003; 73:1847–1860.

101. Shinoura N, Yoshida Y, Asai A, Kirino T, Hamada H. Adenovirus-mediated transfer of p53 and Fas ligand drastically enhances apoptosis in gliomas. Cancer Gene Ther 2000; 7:732–738.

102. Naumann U, Waltereit R, Schulz JB, Weller M. Adenoviral (full-length) Apo2L/TRAIL gene transfer is an ineffective treatment strategy for malignant glioma. J Neurooncol 2003; 61:7–15.

103. Rubinchik S, Yu H, Woraratanadharm J, Voelkel-Johnson C, Norris JS, Dong JY. Enhanced apoptosis of glioma cell lines is achieved by co-delivering FasL-GFP and TRAIL with a complex Ad5 vector. Cancer Gene Ther 2003; 10:814–822.

104. Lee J, Hampl M, Albert P, Fine HA. Antitumor activity and prolonged expression from a TRAIL-expressing adenoviral vector. Neoplasia 2002; 4:312–323.

105. Banerjee D, Bertino JR. Myeloprotection with drug-resistance genes. Lancet Oncol 2002; 3:154–158.

106. Cowan KH, Moscow JA, Huang H, et al. Paclitaxel chemotherapy after autologous stem-cell transplantation and engraftment of hematopoietic cells transduced with a retrovirus containing the multidrug resistance complementary DNA (MDR1) in metastatic breast cancer patients. Clin Cancer Res 1999; 5:1619–1628.

107. Flasshove M, Moritz T, Bardenheuer W, Seeber S. Hematoprotection by transfer of drug-resistance genes. Acta Haematol 2003; 110:93–106.

108. Greco O, Dachs GU. Gene directed enzyme/prodrug therapy of cancer: historical appraisal and future prospectives. J Cell Physiol 2001; 187:22–36.

109. Cobb LM, Connors TA, Elson LA, et al. 2, 4-dinitro-5-ethyleneiminobenzamide (CB 1954): a potent and selective inhibitor of the growth of the Walker carcinoma 256. Biochem Pharmacol 1969; 18:1519–1527.

110. Connors TA, Whisson ME. Cure of mice bearing advanced plasma cell tumours with aniline mustard: the relationship between glucuronidase activity and tumour sensitivity. Nature 1966; 210:866–867.

111. Waldmann TA, White JD, Carrasquillo JA, et al. Radioimmunotherapy of interleukin-2R alpha-expressing adult T-cell leukemia with Yttrium-90-labeled anti-Tac. Blood 1995; 86:4063–4075.

112. Cairns J. The evolution of cancer research. Cancer Cells 1989; 1:1–8.

113. Huennekens FM. Tumor targeting: activation of prodrugs by enzyme-monoclonal antibody conjugates. Trends Biotechnol 1994; 12:234–239.

114. Senter PD, Wallace PM, Svensson HP, et al. Generation of cytotoxic agents by targeted enzymes. Bioconjug Chem 1993; 4:3–9.

115. Bagshawe KD. Antibody-directed enzyme prodrug therapy. Clin Pharmacokinet 1994; 27:368–376.

116. Benhar I, Padlan EA, Jung SH, Lee B, Pastan I. Rapid humanization of the Fv of monoclonal antibody B3 by using framework exchange of the recombinant immunotoxin B3(Fv)-PE38. Proc Natl Acad Sci USA 1994; 91:12051–12055.

117. Co MS, Queen C. Humanized antibodies for therapy. Nature 1991; 351:501–502.

118. Riechmann L, Clark M, Waldmann H, Winter G. Reshaping human antibodies for therapy. Nature 1988; 332:323–327.

119. Jain RK. Delivery of molecular medicine to solid tumors. Science 1996; 271:1079–1080.

120. Paulie S, Ehlin-Henriksson B, Mellstedt H, Koho H, Ben-Aissa H, Perlmann P. A p50 surface antigen restricted to human urinary bladder carcinomas and B lymphocytes. Cancer Immunol Immunother 1985; 20:23–28.

121. Brinkmann U, Reiter Y, Jung SH, Lee B, Pastan I. A recombinant immunotoxin containing a disulfide-stabilized Fv fragment. Proc Natl Acad Sci USA 1993; 90:7538–7542.

122. Reiter Y, Brinkmann U, Webber KO, Jung SH, Lee B, Pastan I. Engineering interchain disulfide bonds into conserved framework regions of Fv fragments: improved biochemical characteristics of recombinant immunotoxins containing disulfide-stabilized Fv. Protein Eng 1994; 7:697–704.

123. Reiter Y, Brinkmann U, Lee B, Pastan I. Engineering antibody Fv fragments for cancer detection and therapy: disulfide-stabilized Fv fragments. Nat Biotechnol 1996; 14:1239–1245.

124. Ward ES, Gussow D, Griffiths AD, Jones PT, Winter G. Binding activities of a repertoire of single immunoglobulin variable domains secreted from Escherichia coli. Nature 1989; 341:544–546.

125. Davies J, Riechmann L. "Camelising" human antibody fragments: NMR studies on VH domains. FEBS Lett 1994; 339:285–290.

126. Davies J, Riechmann L. Single antibody domains as small recognition units: design and in vitro antigen selection of camelized, human VH domains with improved protein stability. Protein Eng 1996; 9:531–537.

127. Aghi M, Hochberg F, Breakefield XO. Prodrug activation enzymes in cancer gene therapy. J Gene Med 2000; 2:148–164.

128. Ram Z, Culver KW, Oshiro EM, et al. Therapy of malignant brain tumors by intratumoral implantation of retroviral vector-producing cells. Nat Med 1997; 3:1354–1361.

129. Moolten FL. Tumor chemosensitivity conferred by inserted herpes thymidine kinase genes: paradigm for a prospective cancer control strategy. Cancer Res 1986; 46:5276–5281.

130. Caruso M, Panis Y, Gagandeep S, Houssin D, Salzmann JL, Klatzmann D. Regression of established macroscopic liver metastases after in situ transduction of a suicide gene. Proc Natl Acad Sci USA 1993; 90:7024–7028.

131. Culver KW, Ram Z, Wallbridge S, Ishii H, Oldfield EH, Blaese RM. In vivo gene transfer with retroviral vector-producer cells for treatment of experimental brain tumors. Science 1992; 256:1550–1552.

132. Kuriyama S, Mitoro A, Yamazaki M, et al. Comparison of gene therapy with the herpes simplex virus thymidine kinase gene and the bacterial cytosine deaminase gene for the treatment of hepatocellular carcinoma. Scand J Gastroenterol 1999; 34:1033–1041.

133. O'Malley BW, Jr., Chen SH, Schwartz MR, Woo SL. Adenovirus-mediated gene therapy for human head and neck squamous cell cancer in a nude mouse model. Cancer Res 1995; 55:1080–1085.

134. Short MP, Choi BC, Lee JK, Malick A, Breakefield XO, Martuza RL. Gene delivery to glioma cells in rat brain by grafting of a retrovirus packaging cell line. J Neurosci Res 1990; 27:427–439.

135. Smythe WR, Hwang HC, Elshami AA, et al. Treatment of experimental human mesothelioma using adenovirus transfer of the herpes simplex thymidine kinase gene. Ann Surg 1995; 222:78–86.

136. Dewey RA, Morrissey G, Cowsill CM, et al. Chronic brain inflammation and persistent herpes simplex virus 1 thymidine kinase expression in survivors of syngeneic glioma treated by adenovirus-mediated gene therapy: implications for clinical trials. Nat Med 1999; 5:1256–1263.

137. Solly SK, Trajcevski S, Frisen C, et al. Replicative retroviral vectors for cancer gene therapy. Cancer Gene Ther 2003; 10:30–39.

138. Elion GB, Furman PA, Fyfe JA, de Miranda P, Beauchamp L, Schaeffer HJ. Selectivity of action of an antiherpetic agent, 9-(2-hydroxyethoxymethyl) guanine. Proc Natl Acad Sci USA 1977; 74:5716–5720.

139. Davidson RL, Kaufman ER, Crumpacker CS, Schnipper LE. Inhibition of herpes simplex virus transformed and nontransformed cells by acycloguanosine: mechanisms of uptake and toxicity. Virology 1981; 113:9–19.

140. Elion GB. The chemotherapeutic exploitation of virus-specified enzymes. Adv Enzyme Regul 1980; 18:53–66.

141. Mar EC, Chiou JF, Cheng YC, Huang ES. Inhibition of cellular DNA polymerase alpha and human cytomegalovirus-induced DNA polymerase by the triphosphates of 9-(2-hydroxy-ethoxymethyl)guanine and 9-(1,3-dihydroxy-2-propoxymethyl)guanine. J Virol 1985; 53:776–780.

142. Freeman SM, Abboud CN, Whartenby KA, et al. The "bystander effect": tumor regression when a fraction of the tumor mass is genetically modified. Cancer Res 1993; 53:5274–5283.

143. Chen CY, Chang YN, Ryan P, Linscott M, McGarrity GJ, Chiang YL. Effect of herpes simplex virus thymidine kinase expression levels on ganciclovir-mediated cytotoxicity and the "bystander effect". Hum Gene Ther 1995; 6:1467–1476.

144. Elshami AA, Saavedra A, Zhang H, et al. Gap junctions play a role in the "bystander effect" of the herpes simplex virus thymidine kinase/ganciclovir system in vitro. Gene Ther 1996; 3:85–92.

145. Dilber MS, Abedi MR, Christensson B, et al. Gap junctions promote the bystander effect of herpes simplex virus thymidine kinase in vivo. Cancer Res 1997; 57:1523–1528.

146. Mesnil M, Piccoli C, Tiraby G, Willecke K, Yamasaki H. Bystander killing of cancer cells by herpes simplex virus thymidine kinase gene is mediated by connexins. Proc Natl Acad Sci USA 1996; 93:1831–1835.

147. Touraine RL, Vahanian N, Ramsey WJ, Blaese RM. Enhancement of the herpes simplex virus thymidine kinase/ganciclovir bystander effect and its antitumor efficacy in vivo by pharmacologic manipulation of gap junctions. Hum Gene Ther 1998; 9:2385–2391.

148. Vile RG, Castleden S, Marshall J, Camplejohn R, Upton C, Chong H. Generation of an anti-tumour immune response in a non-immunogenic tumour: HSVtk killing in vivo stimulates a mononuclear cell infiltrate and a Th1-like profile of intratumoural cytokine expression. Int J Cancer 1997; 71:267–274.

149. Wilson KM, Stambrook PJ, Bi WL, Pavelic ZP, Pavelic L, Gluckman JL. HSV-tk gene therapy in head and neck squamous cell carcinoma. Enhancement by the local and distant bystander effect. Arch Otolaryngol Head Neck Surg 1996; 122:746–749.

150. Bi W, Kim YG, Feliciano ES, et al. An HSVtk-mediated local and distant antitumor bystander effect in tumors of head and neck origin in athymic mice. Cancer Gene Ther 1997; 4:246–252.

151. Dilber MS, Abedi MR, Bjorkstrand B, et al. Suicide gene therapy for plasma cell tumors. Blood 1996; 88:2192–2200.

152. Klatzmann D, Valery CA, Bensimon G, et al. A phase I/II study of herpes simplex virus type 1 thymidine kinase "suicide" gene therapy for recurrent glioblastoma. Study Group on Gene Therapy for Glioblastoma. Hum Gene Ther 1998; 9:2595–2604.

153. Shand N, Weber F, Mariani L, et al. A phase 1-2 clinical trial of gene therapy for recurrent glioblastoma multiforme by tumor transduction with the herpes simplex thymidine kinase gene followed by ganciclovir. GLI328 European-Canadian Study Group. Hum Gene Ther 1999; 10:2325–2335.

154. Moolten FL. Drug sensitivity ("suicide") genes for selective cancer chemotherapy. Cancer Gene Ther 1994; 1:279–287.

155. Yazawa K, Fisher WE, Brunicardi FC. Current progress in suicide gene therapy for cancer. World J Surg 2002; 26:783–789.

156. Domin BA, Mahony WB, Zimmerman TP. Transport of 5-fluorouracil and uracil into human erythrocytes. Biochem Pharmacol 1993; 46:503–510.

157. Huber BE, Austin EA, Richards CA, Davis ST, Good SS. Metabolism of 5-FC to 5-fluorouracil in human colorectal tumor cells transduced with the cytosine deaminase gene: significant antitumor effects when only a small percentage of tumor cells express cytosine deaminase. Proc Natl Acad Sci USA 1994; 91:8302–8306.

158. Trinh QT, Austin EA, Murray DM, Knick VC, Huber BE. Enzyme/prodrug gene therapy: comparison of cytosine deaminase/5-fluorocytosine versus thymidine kinase/ganciclovir enzyme/prodrug systems in a human colorectal carcinoma cell line. Cancer Res 1995; 55:4808–4812.

159. Pierrefite-Carle V, Baque P, Gavelli A, et al. Cytosine deaminase/5-fluorocytosine-based vaccination against liver tumors: evidence of distant bystander effect. J Natl Cancer Inst 1999; 91:2014–2019.

160. Kievit E, Bershad E, Ng E, et al. Superiority of yeast over bacterial cytosine deaminase for enzyme/prodrug gene therapy in colon cancer xenografts. Cancer Res 1999; 59:1417–1421.

161. Hamstra DA, Rice DJ, Fahmy S, Ross BD, Rehemtulla A. Enzyme/prodrug therapy for head and neck cancer using a catalytically superior cytosine deaminase. Hum Gene Ther 1999; 10:1993–2003.

162. Martin J, Stribbling SM, Poon GK, et al. Antibody-directed enzyme prodrug therapy: pharmacokinetics and plasma levels of prodrug and drug in a phase I clinical trial. Cancer Chemother Pharmacol 1997; 40:189–201.

163. Napier MP, Sharma SK, Springer CJ, et al. Antibody-directed enzyme prodrug therapy: efficacy and mechanism of action in colorectal carcinoma. Clin Cancer Res 2000; 6:765–772.

164. Crystal RG, Hirschowitz E, Lieberman M, et al. Phase I study of direct administration of a replication deficient adenovirus vector containing the E. coli cytosine deaminase gene to metastatic colon carcinoma of the liver in association with the oral administration of the prodrug 5-fluorocytosine. Hum Gene Ther 1997; 8:985–1001.

165. Springer CJ, Antoniw P, Bagshawe KD, Searle F, Bisset GM, Jarman M. Novel prodrugs which are activated to cytotoxic alkylating agents by carboxypeptidase G2. J Med Chem 1990; 33:677–681.

166. Springer CJ, Niculescu-Duvaz I. Prodrug-activating systems in suicide gene therapy. J Clin Invest 2000; 105:1161–1167.

167. Stribbling SM, Friedlos F, Martin J, et al. Regressions of established breast carcinoma xenografts by carboxypeptidase G2 suicide gene therapy and the prodrug CMDA are due to a bystander effect. Hum Gene Ther 2000; 11:285–292.

168. Marais R, Spooner RA, Light Y, Martin J, Springer CJ. Gene-directed enzyme prodrug therapy with a mustard prodrug/carboxypeptidase G2 combination. Cancer Res 1996; 56:4735–4742.

169. Cowen RL, Williams JC, Emery S, et al. Adenovirus vector-mediated delivery of the prodrug-converting enzyme carboxypeptidase G2 in a secreted or GPI-anchored form: High-level expression of this active conditional cytotoxic enzyme at the plasma membrane. Cancer Gene Ther 2002; 9:897–907.

170. Debinski W, Gibo DM. Molecular expression analysis of restrictive receptor for interleukin 13, a brain tumor-associated cancer/testis antigen. Mol Med 2000; 6:440–449.

171. Debinski W, Gibo DM, Hulet SW, Connor JR, Gillespie GY. Receptor for interleukin 13 is a marker and therapeutic target for human high-grade gliomas. Clin Cancer Res 1999; 5:985–990.

172. Li C, Hall WA, Jin N, Todhunter DA, Panoskaltsis-Mortari A, Vallera DA. Targeting glioblastoma multiforme with an IL-13/diphtheria toxin fusion protein in vitro and in vivo in nude mice. Protein Eng 2002; 15:419–427.

173. Todhunter DA, Hall WA, Rustamzadeh E, Shu Y, Doumbia SO, Vallera DA. A bispecific immunotoxin (DTAT13) targeting human IL-13 receptor (IL-13R) and urokinase-type plasminogen activator receptor (uPAR) in a mouse xenograft model. Protein Eng Des Sel 2004; 17:157–164.

174. Debinski W, Obiri NI, Powers SK, Pastan I, Puri RK. Human glioma cells overexpress receptors for interleukin 13 and are extremely sensitive to a novel chimeric protein composed of interleukin 13 and pseudomonas exotoxin. Clin Cancer Res 1995; 1:1253–1258.

175. Mori T, Abe T, Wakabayashi Y, et al. Up-regulation of urokinase-type plasminogen activator and its receptor correlates with enhanced invasion activity of human glioma cells mediated by transforming growth factor-alpha or basic fibroblast growth factor. J Neurooncol 2000; 46:115–123.

176. Liu TF, Hall PD, Cohen KA, et al. Interstitial diphtheria toxin-epidermal growth factor fusion protein therapy produces regressions of subcutaneous human glioblastoma multiforme tumors in athymic nude mice. Clin Cancer Res 2005; 11:329–334.

177. Phillips PC, Levow C, Catterall M, Colvin OM, Pastan I, Brem H. Transforming growth factor-alpha-Pseudomonas exotoxin fusion protein (TGF-alpha-PE38) treatment of subcutaneous and intracranial human glioma and medulloblastoma xenografts in athymic mice. Cancer Res 1994; 54:1008–1015.

178. Debinski W, Obiri NI, Pastan I, Puri RK. A novel chimeric protein composed of interleukin 13 and Pseudomonas exotoxin is highly cytotoxic to human carcinoma cells expressing receptors for interleukin 13 and interleukin 4. J Biol Chem 1995; 270:16775–16780.

179. Laske DW, Youle RJ, Oldfield EH. Tumor regression with regional distribution of the targeted toxin TF-CRM107 in patients with malignant brain tumors. Nat Med 1997; 3:1362–1368.

180. Liu TF, Willingham MC, Tatter SB, et al. Diphtheria toxin-epidermal growth factor fusion protein and Pseudomonas exotoxin-interleukin 13 fusion protein exert synergistic toxicity against human glioblastoma multiforme cells. Bioconjug Chem 2003; 14:1107–1114.

181. Husain SR, Joshi BH, Puri RK. Interleukin-13 receptor as a unique target for anti-glioblastoma therapy. Int J Cancer 2001; 92:168–175.

182. Kawakami K, Kawakami M, Kioi M, Husain SR, Puri RK. Distribution kinetics of targeted cytotoxin in glioma by bolus or convection-enhanced delivery in a murine model. J Neurosurg 2004; 101:1004–1011.

183. Debinski W, Gibo DM, Obiri NI, Kealiher A, Puri RK. Novel anti-brain tumor cytotoxins specific for cancer cells. Nat Biotechnol 1998; 16:449–453.

184. Madhankumar AB, Mintz A, Debinski W. Interleukin 13 mutants of enhanced avidity toward the glioma-associated receptor, IL13Ralpha2. Neoplasia 2004; 6:15–22.

185. Debinski W, Gibo DM, Puri RK. Novel way to increase targeting specificity to a human glioblastoma-associated receptor for interleukin 13. Int J Cancer 1998; 76:547–551.

186. Obiri NI, Debinski W, Leonard WJ, Puri RK. Receptor for interleukin 13. Interaction with interleukin 4 by a mechanism that does not involve the common gamma chain shared by receptors for interleukins 2, 4, 7, 9, and 15. J Biol Chem 1995; 270:8797–8804.

187. Cicuttini FM, Hurley SF, Forbes A, et al. Association of adult glioma with medical conditions, family and reproductive history. Int J Cancer 1997; 71:203–207.

188. Obiri NI, Leland P, Murata T, Debinski W, Puri RK. The IL-13 receptor structure differs on various cell types and may share more than one component with IL-4 receptor. J Immunol 1997; 158:756–764.

189. Maini A, Hillman G, Haas GP, et al. Interleukin-13 receptors on human prostate carcinoma cell lines represent a novel target for a chimeric protein composed of IL-13 and a mutated form of Pseudomonas exotoxin. J Urol 1997; 158:948–953.

190. Kornmann M, Kleeff J, Debinski W, Korc M. Pancreatic cancer cells express interleukin-13 and -4 receptors, and their growth is inhibited by Pseudomonas exotoxin coupled to interleukin-13 and -4. Anticancer Res 1999; 19:125–131.

191. Castro MG, Cowen R, Smith-Arica J, et al. Gene therapy strategies for intracranial tumours: glioma and pituitary adenomas. Histol Histopathol 2000; 15:1233–1252.

192. Kleihues P, Zulch KJ, Matsumoto S, Radke U. Morphology of malignant gliomas induced in rabbits by systemic application of N-methyl-N-nitrosourea. Z Neurol 1970; 198:65–78.

193. Grossi-Paoletti E, Paoletti P, Schiffer D, Fabiani A. Experimental brain tumours induced in rats by nitrosourea derivatives. II. Morphological aspects of nitrosoethylurea tumours obtained by transplacental induction. J Neurol Sci 1970; 11:573–581.

194. Barker M, Hoshino T, Gurcay O, et al. Development of an animal brain tumor model and its response to therapy with 1,3-bis(2-chloroethyl)-1-nitrosourea. Cancer Res 1973; 33:976–986.

195. Barth RF. Rat brain tumor models in experimental neuro-oncology: the 9L, C6, T9, F98, RG2 (D74), RT-2 and CNS-1 gliomas. J Neurooncol 1998; 36:91–102.

196. Boviatsis EJ, Park JS, Sena-Esteves M, et al. Long-term survival of rats harboring brain neoplasms treated with ganciclovir and a herpes simplex virus vector that retains an intact thymidine kinase gene. Cancer Res 1994; 54:5745–5751.

197. Barba D, Hardin J, Sadelain M, Gage FH. Development of anti-tumor immunity following thymidine kinase-mediated killing of experimental brain tumors. Proc Natl Acad Sci USA 1994; 91:4348–4352.

198. Tapscott SJ, Miller AD, Olson JM, Berger MS, Groudine M, Spence AM. Gene therapy of rat 9L gliosarcoma tumors by transduction with selectable genes does not require drug selection. Proc Natl Acad Sci USA 1994; 91:8185–8189.

199. Kruse CA, Molleston MC, Parks EP, Schiltz PM, Kleinschmidt-DeMasters BK, Hickey WF. A rat glioma model, CNS-1, with invasive characteristics similar to those of human gliomas: a comparison to 9L gliosarcoma. J Neurooncol 1994; 22:191–200.

200. Tzeng JJ, Barth RF, Orosz CG, James SM. Phenotype and functional activity of tumor-infiltrating lymphocytes isolated from immunogenic and nonimmunogenic rat brain tumors. Cancer Res 1991; 51:2373–2378.

201. Albright L, Madigan JC, Gaston MR, Houchens DP. Therapy in an intracerebral murine glioma model, using Bacillus Calmette-Guerin, neuraminidase-treated tumor cells, and 1-(2-chloroethyl)-3-cyclohexyl-1-nitrosourea. Cancer Res 1975; 35:658–665.

202. Akbasak A, Oldfield EH, Saris SC. Expression and modulation of major histocompatibility antigens on murine primary brain tumor in vitro. J Neurosurg 1991; 75:922–929.

203. Weiner NE, Pyles RB, Chalk CL, et al. A syngeneic mouse glioma model for study of glioblastoma therapy. J Neuropathol Exp Neurol 1999; 58:54–60.

204. Weissenberger J, Steinbach JP, Malin G, Spada S, Rulicke T, Aguzzi A. Development and malignant progression of astrocytomas in GFAP-v-src transgenic mice. Oncogene 1997; 14:2005–2013.

205. Ding H, Roncari L, Shannon P, et al. Astrocyte-specific expression of activated p21-ras results in malignant astrocytoma formation in a transgenic mouse model of human gliomas. Cancer Res 2001; 61:3826–3836.

206. Begemann M, Fuller GN, Holland EC. Genetic modeling of glioma formation in mice. Brain Pathol 2002; 12:117–132.

207. Reilly KM, Loisel DA, Bronson RT, McLaughlin ME. Nf1;Trp53 mutant mice develop glioblastoma with evidence of strain-specific effects. Nat Genet 2000; 26:109–113.

208. Dai C, Celestino JC, Okada Y, Louis DN, Fuller GN, Holland EC. PDGF autocrine stimulation dedifferentiates cultured astrocytes and induces oligodendrogliomas and oligoastrocytomas from neural progenitors and astrocytes in vivo. Genes Dev 2001; 15:1913–1925.

209. Germano IM, Fable J, Gultekin SH, Silvers A. Adenovirus/herpes simplex-thymidine kinase/ganciclovir complex: preliminary results of a phase I trial in patients with recurrent malignant gliomas. J Neurooncol 2003; 65:279–289.

210. Prados MD, McDermott M, Chang SM, et al. Treatment of progressive or recurrent glioblastoma multiforme in adults with herpes simplex virus thymidine kinase gene vector-producer cells followed by intravenous ganciclovir administration: a phase I/II multi-institutional trial. J Neurooncol 2003; 65:269–278.

211. Smitt PS, Driesse M, Wolbers J, Kros M, Avezaat C. Treatment of relapsed malignant glioma with an adenoviral vector containing the herpes simplex thymidine kinase gene followed by ganciclovir. Mol Ther 2003; 7:851–858.

212. Sandmair AM, Loimas S, Puranen P, et al. Thymidine kinase gene therapy for human malignant glioma, using replication-deficient retroviruses or adenoviruses. Hum Gene Ther 2000; 11:2197–2205.

213. Trask TW, Trask RP, Aguilar-Cordova E, et al. Phase I study of adenoviral delivery of the HSV-tk gene and ganciclovir administration in patients with current malignant brain tumors. Mol Ther 2000; 1:195–203.

214. Immonen A, Vapalahti M, Tyynela K, et al. AdvHSV-tk gene therapy with intravenous ganciclovir improves survival in human malignant glioma: a randomised, controlled study. Mol Ther 2004; 10:967–972.

215. Madara J, Krewet JA, Shah M. Heat shock protein 72 expression allows permissive replication of oncolytic adenovirus dl1520 (ONYX-015) in rat glioblastoma cells. Mol Cancer 2005; 4:12.

216. O'Shea CC, Johnson L, Bagus B, et al. Late viral RNA export, rather than p53 inactivation, determines ONYX-015 tumor selectivity. Cancer Cell 2004; 6:611–623.

217. Chiocca EA, Abbed KM, Tatter S, et al. A phase I open-label, dose-escalation, multi-institutional trial of injection with an E1B-Attenuated adenovirus, ONYX-015, into the peritumoral region of recurrent malignant gliomas, in the adjuvant setting. Mol Ther 2004; 10:958–966.

218. Markert JM, Medlock MD, Rabkin SD, et al. Conditionally replicating herpes simplex virus mutant, G207 for the treatment of malignant glioma: results of a phase I trial. Gene Ther 2000; 7:867–874.

219. Rampling R, Cruickshank G, Papanastassiou V, et al. Toxicity evaluation of replication-competent herpes simplex virus (ICP 34.5 null mutant 1716) in patients with recurrent malignant glioma. Gene Ther 2000; 7:859–866.

220. Papanastassiou V, Rampling R, Fraser M, et al. The potential for efficacy of the modified (ICP 34.5(-)) herpes simplex virus HSV1716 following intratumoural injection into human malignant glioma: a proof of principle study. Gene Ther 2002; 9:398–406.

221. Harland J, Papanastassiou V, Brown SM. HSV1716 persistence in primary human glioma cells in vitro. Gene Ther 2002; 9:1194–1198.

222. Harrow S, Papanastassiou V, Harland J, et al. HSV1716 injection into the brain adjacent to tumour following surgical resection of high-grade glioma: safety data and long-term survival. Gene Ther 2004; 11:1648–1658.

223. Schneider T, Gerhards R, Kirches E, Firsching R. Preliminary results of active specific immunization with modified tumor cell vaccine in glioblastoma multiforme. J Neurooncol 2001; 53:39–46.

224. Steiner HH, Bonsanto MM, Beckhove P, et al. Antitumor vaccination of patients with glioblastoma multiforme: a pilot study to assess feasibility, safety, and clinical benefit. J Clin Oncol 2004; 22:4272–4281.

225. Hall WA, Rustamzadeh E, Asher AL. Convection-enhanced delivery in clinical trials. Neurosurg Focus 2003; 14:e2.
226. Weber F, Asher A, Bucholz R, et al. Safety, tolerability, and tumor response of IL4-Pseudomonas exotoxin (NBI-3001) in patients with recurrent malignant glioma. J Neurooncol 2003; 64:125–137.
227. Rand RW, Kreitman RJ, Patronas N, Varricchio F, Pastan I, Puri RK. Intratumoral administration of recombinant circularly permuted interleukin-4-Pseudomonas exotoxin in patients with high-grade glioma. Clin Cancer Res 2000; 6:2157–2165.
228. Weaver M, Laske DW. Transferrin receptor ligand-targeted toxin conjugate (Tf-CRM107) for therapy of malignant gliomas. J Neurooncol 2003; 65:3–13.
229. Sampson JH, Akabani G, Archer GE, et al. Progress report of a Phase I study of the intracerebral microinfusion of a recombinant chimeric protein composed of transforming growth factor (TGF)-alpha and a mutated form of the Pseudomonas exotoxin termed PE-38 (TP-38) for the treatment of malignant brain tumors. J Neurooncol 2003; 65:27–35.

14

Vaccines and Beneficial Immunity in Glioma Patients

Christopher J. Wheeler and Keith L. Black
Maxine Dunite Neurosurgical Institute, Cedars-Sinai Medical Center, Los Angeles, California, U.S.A.

ABSTRACT

The dismal prognoses suffered by malignant primary brain tumor (glioma) patients remain unchanged over the past two decades despite significant improvements in the treatment of distinct tumors. Immunotherapy, and vaccine therapy in particular, represents a promising experimental approach to treat malignant gliomas, but major challenges still remain to render vaccination clinically effective. These challenges include diminishing the risk of pathologic autoimmunity, identifying the cellular basis of clinical vaccine benefits, and increasing the proportion of patients experiencing such benefits. Recent studies in glioma patients have characterized tumor antigens on human gliomas, identified some of the immune cells involved in beneficial anti-glioma immunity, and examined how gliomas may be altered by sub-lethal immune influences, providing a glimpse of the strength to which immunity influences glioma clinical outcome, and hope that clinically effective vaccines to treat these tumors are within reach. Insight into the complex dynamics of immune-tumor interactions promises to extend this reach by delineating mechanisms of immune synergy with other forms of treatment.

INTRODUCTION

Malignant brain tumors are among the gravest forms of cancer. The most common of these incurable tumors, glioblastoma multiforme (GBM), is responsible for 50% of all intracranial gliomas and 25% of intracranial tumors in adults (1,2). GBM diagnosis carries with it an average survival between 12 and 18 months (with 90–95% patients surviving less than 2 years), without the possibility of spontaneous remission or effective treatment (1–3). The consistently short survival and absence of spontaneous remission that makes GBM such a devastating disease also renders the evaluation of new therapies for GBM relatively rapid and unequivocal. Overall survival represents the standard by which therapies for GBM are evaluated, in part because tumor mass reduction (i.e., surgically) does not necessarily correlate with prolonged survival (4–6).

Treatment for Malignant Gliomas

Unfortunately, conventional therapies are remarkably ineffective at improving GBM clinical outcome despite their ability to confer significant benefits to patients with non-glioma tumors (3,7,8). Even the few treatments effective against GBM typically either exhibit small increases in survival that are evident only from large population studies, or primarily benefit certain (i.e., young) patient subpopulations (9,10). Thus, novel therapies for GBM are needed.

Cancer vaccines represent one novel therapy for GBM (11–13). The clinical efficacy of therapeutic vaccination for any human tumor, however, remains controversial because consistent tumor destruction or extended lifespan is not observed in most vaccinated cancer patients (14–16). In contrast, current cancer vaccines do reliably elicit tumor-reactive cytotoxic T lymphocytes (CTL) in most patients (14,15,17). The improvement of vaccine therapy for GBM and other cancer patients is contingent upon identifying and overcoming the mechanisms underlying the general clinical failure of cancer vaccines in light of their experimental and apparent immunological success.

Cancer Vaccines: Historical Overview

An immunological influence on tumor rejection has long been recognized. Even before the advent of inbred strains of mice, it was discovered that transplants of tumors originating in white mice would grow in other white mice, but were rejected when transplanted into nondescript wild mice (18). This ultimately led to the concept of tumor antigens (19) that can initiate immune responses that lead to the destruction of susceptible tumors (20). It was not until the late 20th century, however, that it was demonstrated that immune effector cells (CD8$^+$ cytotoxic T-cells or CTL) could kill tumors by recognizing tumor antigens bound to MHC I molecules (21–23).

Tumor immunotherapy, and indeed any immune response against tumors, requires the expression of a target antigen on neoplastic cells. The derivation of tumor antigens was long presumed to be from self molecules altered within neoplastic cells so as to appear "foreign" to the host immune system. It was somewhat surprising, then, that many antigens mediating the rejection of human tumors were found to be essentially unaltered self molecules involved in routine functioning of the affected tissue (24,25). This paradox was partially resolved by the realization that tumor cells themselves were not the exclusive in vivo presenters of MHC I-restricted antigen to immune cells, but that this was a function of a specialized group of professional antigen-presenting cells, dendritic cells (DCs), that could process self antigens for presentation on MHC I (26).

Therapeutic vaccination of cancer patients has enjoyed a surge in popularity as an experimental clinical platform with the demonstration that ex vivo-generated, antigen-presenting (DCs) can potently stimulate anti-tumor T-cell responses that effectively treat established tumors in experimental rodents (26–28). In these model systems, T-cell responses coincided with treatment efficacy (28–34). As comparable DC populations were identified in humans (35), the concept that similar DC vaccines could be used to treat cancer patients gained favor. Early DC vaccine clinical trials in lymphoma and melanoma were initiated that provided a backdrop for the adoption of DC-based vaccine therapies in a variety of human tumors (36,37), including prostate cancer (38–40), renal cell carcinoma (41,42), NSC lung carcinoma (16), colon cancer (43), and malignant glioma/GBM (13,44–46). As this form of vaccination was increasingly applied clinically, a majority of patients typically exhibited induction of T-cell responses. In contrast, relatively few patients experienced tangible clinical benefits, and such benefits were generally unrelated to T-cell responsiveness (47). This may be due to the ability of tumors to evade host immunity not only by actively suppressing immune induction and/ or effector function, but also through the development of immune resistant tumor variants under immune selection pressure. A complete appreciation of such limitations requires a general knowledge of immune processes and cell types.

THERAPEUTIC CANCER VACCINES AIM TO MOBILIZE ANTIGEN-SPECIFIC T-CELLS

Of the two basic types of immune cells (B and T) capable of adaptive (i.e., memory) responses, only T-cells respond predominantly to cell-derived antigen (Ag; usually peptides). They do so by producing cytokines and/or killing their Ag-expressing target cells. As such, T-cells are most relevant for destruction and long-term protection against tumors. Most vaccine strategies, and DC vaccination in particular, thus seek to mobilize tumor-specific T-cell responses (25).

Molecular and Cellular Interactions in T-Cell Ag Responsiveness

T-cells respond to Ag (such as tumor Ag) through ligation of their Ag receptors (TCRs) by peptide Ag bound to self MHC molecules (designated HLA in humans) on distinct cells (Fig. 1). The TCR is aided in this process by one of two coreceptors, CD4 or CD8, whose mutually exclusive expression defines the two most prevalent types of T-cells. $CD4^+$ and $CD8^+$ T-cells bind distinct types of Ag/MHC (48–50). The CD4 and CD8 glycoproteins themselves act as "coreceptors," binding to non-peptide-binding portions of the same type of peptide/MHC that engages TCR, and juxtaposing critical kinases ($p56^{lck}$ and LAT, for example) close to their TCR-associated signaling (CD3) chain substrates in the process (51–53). In this manner, TCR ligation, signaling, and T-cell activation is facilitated (Fig. 1).

$CD8^+$ T-cells recognize predominantly intracellular peptide Ag bound to ubiquitously expressed MHC class I (MHC I) molecules (HLA-A, B, C in humans), and give rise to (CTL) that can directly kill Ag/MHC I-bearing cells such as tumors (54,55). $CD4^+$ T-cells (helper T-cells, or Th) recognize predominantly endocytosed peptide Ag bound to MHC class II (MHC II) molecules (HLA-DR, DQ, DP, DO in humans) expressed on some myeloid and lymphoid blood cells (55,56). Depending on environmental and/or intercellular signals, Th can differentiate into Th1 and Th2 subtypes (57). Th1 cells secrete a particular array of cytokines (e.g., IL-2, IFN-γ, IL-12) that promote CTL responses. Thus, Th1 and/or CTL responses are most relevant for inducing and monitoring anti-tumor immunity (58).

The importance of T-cells in vaccine-mediated survival benefits is readily apparent in rodent tumor vaccine models, in which increased survival and protection are clearly dependent on the presence of $CD4^+$ or $CD8^+$ T-cells (28–32,59). In many cases, both $CD4^+$ and $CD8^+$ T-cells are essential to transfer therapeutic benefits to naïve hosts. In some intracranial tumor models, however, $CD8^+$ T-cells alone appear to mediate such benefits (29,34). In nearly all rodent tumor vaccine models, increased memory CTL activity correlates with enhanced survival upon vaccination (28–34). The importance of CD8 expression itself in anti-glioma activity is underscored by its specific loss in defective glioma-infiltrating CTL (60,61).

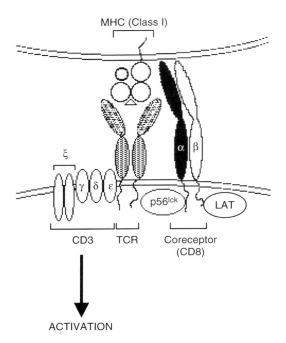

MHC (Class I)

ξ

α β

γ δ ε

p56lck   LAT

CD3   TCR   Coreceptor
(CD8)

ACTIVATION

Figure 1 Molecular interactions in T-cell signaling and activation. Class I or class II major histocompatibility complex (MHC) molecules bind and present peptide antigen (triangle on MHC) to T-cells expressing either CD8 or CD4 coreceptors, respectively. CD4 and CD8 coreceptors can bind to the same MHC molecule as is bound by the T-cell receptor (TCR), and help localize intracellular signaling proteins, such as lck or LAT, to transmembrane signaling proteins (CD3) associated with TCR, thereby potentiating a signaling cascade that ultimately leads to cellular activation.

Activation of Naïve Anti-Tumor T-cells by Dendritic Cells

Although most T-cell responses seen in tumor patients are recall "memory" responses, these can be inefficient and undermined through active suppression and loss of appropriately presented tumor Ag (62–64). Supression of previously activated or tumor-homing T-cells is particularly pronounced in gliomas (see below) (65–67). As a result, tumor vaccine efficacy may be dependent on "naïve" T-cell responses to previously unrecognized tumor Ag (68). Such Ag can induce the activation of naïve T-cells, provided it is presented by DCs, the most potent activators of naïve T-cell responses (26,69). DCs' ability to prime naïve T-cells is in part due to their expression of additional costimulatory molecules (B7, for example) that bind ligands (CD28) on naïve T-cells, providing the additional signal necessary for the naïve T-cell to proliferate and acquire effector function in response to tumor Ag (Fig. 2) (70). DCs are also among the few APCs known to take up Ag endocytically from tumor cells and present it onto their own MHC I molecules as opposed to MHC II; (Fig. 2A) (71–73). DC activity thus represents a means to initiate novel T-cell killing responses against otherwise non-immunogenic tumor cells.

Normally, DCs are present in very small numbers in the circulation. For this reason, and because naïve T-cells reactive to specific Ag may be even more scarce,

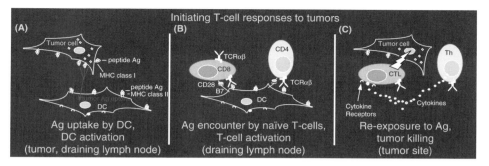

Figure 2 (*See color insert*) Initiating T-cell responses to tumors. (**A**) Dendritic cells (DCs), resident either within the tumor or in draining lymph nodes, take up tumor antigen, fragment it into peptides, and present these peptides on their MHC molecules. (**B**) $CD8^+$ or $CD4^+$ T-cells with receptors (TCRαβ) able to bind these peptide/MHC complexes encounter DCs in draining lymph nodes, where they are activated to become (CTL) or T helper cells (Th), respectively. (**C**) CTL and Th recounter cognate antigen at the tumor site, and collaborate to elicit optimal anti-tumor effector activity.

endogenous anti-tumor immunity may be limited by the rate of encounter between these two cell types. Experimental vaccines that bypass this limitation by administering large numbers of tumor Ag-pulsed, ex vivo-generated DCs to hosts have been extremely successful against many experimental tumors in rodents, including intracranial gliomas (12,27,28,74–76).

When a specific naïve ($CD8^+$) T-cell first encounters Ag usually on DCs in lymphoid tissue such as lymph nodes or spleen; (Fig. 2B), it becomes activated to proliferate, and differentiates to acquire effector function (Fig. 2C). In this process, the T-cells up-regulate proteins that allow them home to, enter into and travel through non-lymphoid tissues, including brain (Fig. 3) (77,78). The blood brain barrier does not prevent the entry of these metabolically active cells (79), that can be triggered to carry out their effector functions (cytokine production, killing) once they re-encounter their antigen within tumor sites (Figs. 2C and 3).

OBSTACLES TO EFFECTIVE ANTI-GLIOMA IMMUNITY

Evidence of Endogenous Immune Suppression

Tumors in general can compromise anti-tumor immunity at the level of T-cell response induction and/or effector function. With respect to gliomas, pioneering work demonstrated that these tumors inhibit T-cell activity (65,66,80–90). Cytokines such as TGF-β, IGF-1, prostaglandin E_2, and IL-6 were eventually implicated, largely from in vitro studies, in the inability to induce anti-tumor T-cell responses (91,92). The release of such immunosuppressive cytokines, as well as other less defined factors (91,93–95), has also been postulated to be a response by the tumor to immune infiltration (92). These potential impediments to glioma anti-tumor immunity serve to "cloak" the tumor from T-cell responsiveness at the level of immune induction. These initial findings fueled suspicion that strong endogenous anti-tumor immune responses were neither possible nor relevant to clinical outcome in glioma patients (96).

It was later shown that T-cells from high-grade glioma patients exhibited intrinsic defects in an array of signaling molecules similar to those seen in other cancer patients

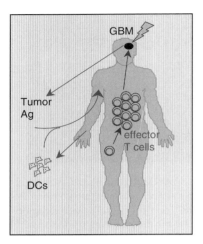

Figure 3 Vaccine-elicited effector T-cell response. Dendritic cell-based (DC) vaccines generate large numbers of tumor antigen-presenting DCs ex vivo, bypassing a potential limitation to endogenous immune activation in patients. Re-administration of tumor antigen-pulsed DCs as vaccine aims to elicit expansion and anti-tumor effector functions in tumor-reactive T-cells, which can then migrate to and kill tumors in situ.

(66,97–100). Importantly, the severity of these T-cell defects was correlated with glioma size, consistent with notions that a glioma-derived factor elicited the defects (66), and/or that dysfunctional immune effectors exacerbated glioma progression. Although a tumor-derived factor responsible for T-cell defectiveness in glioma patients has not yet been definitively identified, alternative mechanisms generating T-cell defects that also exacerbate tumor progression have now been validated in glioma-bearing mice (61). This suggests that host T-cell competence could have some bearing on glioma outcome in patients.

At the level of immune effector cell survival, FasL expression on glioma vasculature, which could lead to infiltrating T-cell apoptosis, has been correlated with the preponderance of CD4$^+$ helper over CD8$^+$ killer T-cells infiltrating patients' gliomas (101). This is consistent with the differential susceptibility to fas-mediated cell death among CD4$^+$ and CD8$^+$T-cells, as well as a skewing of local anti-glioma immunity away from CTL promotion. In addition, thymic production of nascent CD8$^+$T-cells (recent thymic emigrants, or RTEs), which may be particularly important in countering glioma progression (102), is dramatically diminished due to intrinsic apoptosis in response to experimental glioma growth in rats (103). Finally, non-neoplastic normal astrocytes themselves have been reported to suppress both T-cell activation and effector function through upregulation of CTLA-4, a negative regulatory molecule that binds competitively to CD28 on T-cells (104). This illustrates a mechanism that potentially contributes to the generally refractory nature of the brain with respect to protective T-cell responses (96), and further highlights the formidable obstacles to mounting and sustaining such responses to malignant gliomas. Defects in glioma-associated antigen-presenting cells have also been described, including the down-regulation of MHC class I, and class II, B7, and other costimulatory molecules (95,105). Taken together, these findings raise the possibility that the depressed T-cell induction as well as reduced effector function associated with gliomas contributes to their dismal clinical outcome.

EVIDENCE OF EFFECTIVE ANTI-GLIOMA IMMUNITY

Evidence of Endogenous Immune Benefits in Glioma Patients

Despite the evidence that T-cell immunity is reduced and that such reduction may worsen clinical outcome in malignant glioma patients, recent indirect evidence also suggests that endogenous immunity may effectively combat glioma growth. Patients with allergies, autoimmune conditions (i.e., pathologic anti-self cellular immune responses), and especially both, for example, were found to be at low risk for developing gliomas, including GBM (106,107). In addition, the case for gliomas eliciting endogenous immune responses against specific antigens was recently substantiated by a report that up to a third of GBM patients harbor IgG antibodies to the transcription factor SOX6, which is highly overexpressed on glioma tissue, whereas healthy individuals and other cancer patients do not (108). Taken together with data on T-cell defects and glioma outcome, these recent studies underscore the possibility that endogenous T-cell immunity remains intact, and may have a positive bearing on glioma clinical manifestation and/or outcome.

Immune Induction in Glioma Vaccine Trials

The evidence that endogenous cellular immune suppression might worsen glioma progression does not necessarily mean that bolstering cellular immunity through vaccination can improve clinical outcomes in glioma patients. In addition, the ability of DCs or any other means to activate anti-tumor T-cells in potentially immune-suppressed glioma patients is by no means a foregone conclusion, regardless of the relevance of analogous endogenous processes. It is necessary to demonstrate induction of anti-tumor T-cell responses and to monitor associated clinical outcomes in GBM patients in this regard. These have been explicit goals of therapeutic DC vaccine trials.

Yu et al. conducted the first phase I clinical vaccine trial, which utilized MHC I-eluted peptides from cultured autologous tumor cells pulsed to immature (DCs) (13). Vaccine was administered in three semi-weekly courses to nine newly-diagnosed high-grade glioma (2 anaplastic astrocytoma, seven GBM) patients, all of whom had undergone image-complete resection and radiotherapy. Due to the lack of radiographically detectable tumor tissue resulting from image-complete resections in this study, radiographic responses could not be informatively monitored. Four of seven patients tested exhibited positive CTL response induction. In addition, post-vaccine infiltration of tumor by memory and CD8$^+$ T-cells was observed in two of four re-resected patients, and these two appeared to survive longer than their counterparts without CD8$^+$ infiltration during the reported time span. Moreover, although the population size and diversity within this trial precluded the acquisition of statistically significant survival data, there appeared to be a modest improvement in survival compared with historical controls. No serious adverse effects were observed.

Kikuchi et al. conducted a phase I trial in eight recurrent malignant glioma (1 anaplastic oligodendroglioma, two anaplastic astrocytoma, five GBM) patients, which utilized DC fused to glioma cells (44). This strategy potentially minimizes activation of T-cell responses to normal brain antigens that could increase the risk of autoimmunity. Vaccine was administered in 3–7 courses every 3 weeks. Increased anti-glioma responsiveness that in two patients appeared specific to autologous tumor cells was observed after vaccination in six patients analyzed. Two "partial" radiographic responses, in which either one portion of tumor regressed while another progressed, or tumor-associated brain edema but not tumor itself was diminished, were seen. No serious adverse effects were observed.

Yamanaka et al. conducted a phase I/II trial in 10 recurrent high-grade glioma (one non-descript, one mixed, one analplastic oligodendroglioma, seven GBM) patients (45). Five patients received 2–6 intradermal vaccinations with tumor lysate-pulsed DC, and five patients received 1–10 intradermal vaccinations as well as 1–7 intratumoral administrations via Ommaya reservoir of lysate-pulsed DC, at 3 week intervals. Three of eight patients tested exhibited increased immunological responsiveness to tumor lysate following vaccination. Two partial radiographic responses were observed, in which contrast enhanced tumor images, but not necessarily other tumor regions, were diminished. In addition, no serious adverse effects were observed.

A phase II trial reported by Yu et al. targeted 12 recurrent (three anaplastic astrocytoma, one GBM) and two newly-diagnosed (one anaplastic astrocytoma, one GBM) patients, and administered four tumor lysate-pulsed DC vaccinations every two week (46). As in the first glioma DC vaccine trial, image-complete resections precluded informative monitoring of radiographic responses in this trial. In vitro responses against autologous tumor lysate were induced following vaccination in six of 10 patients analyzed, and in vivo responses against known tumor antigens were observed in four of nine patients analyzed. In addition, evidence consistent with post-vaccine CD8$^+$ memory cell infiltration into tumors was provided. Finally, vaccinated patients appeared to enjoy markedly prolonged survival relative to historical controls in this non-randomized trial (Fig. 4). This apparent survival enhancement is remarkable, because vaccination of newly-diagnosed GBM patients in the earlier phase I trial from this same institution exhibited only modestly enhanced survival (13). The phase II trial, on the other hand, utilized 25-fold greater numbers of antigen-pulsed DCs than the original, highlighting the possibility of dose-limited vaccine-enhanced T-cell responsiveness.

In this last DC therapy trial, it was not possible for the authors to rule out a selection bias favoring inherently longer survival of vaccinated versus control patients independent

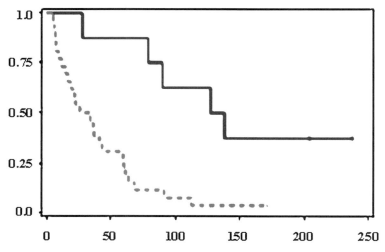

Figure 4 Kaplan-Meier survival curve of DC vaccinated study group ($n = 10$; solid line), and control group ($n = 51$; dashed line) of patients with recurrent GBM from time of sec craniotomy. The median survival for the study and control groups were 132 and 30 weeks, respectively, for recurrent patients. The Mantel COX log-rank test revealed that the survival curves for the two groups were significantly different, ($p = 0.003$). Of note, 3 patients have survived over 200 weeks. *Source*: From Ref. 46.

of their treatment status, particularly as the relevant group of patients was treated at a later point in their disease than patients in an earlier vaccine trial from this same group. This would tend to bias the test population toward inherently longer survival, a common confounding issue in the interpretation of non-randomized clinical trials. In this context, empirical pre-treatment tumor recurrence data have recently been employed to support a likely absence of selection bias among non-randomized vaccinated glioma patient populations, and to validate treatment-related affects (109). Similar post hoc empirical analysis, which might complement techniques that group glioma patients into outcome categories based purely on statistical trends to minimize selection bias (3), could help resolve whether apparent changes in DC vaccine clinical outcomes are related to actual treatment.

Although differing widely in design, these clinical vaccine trials demonstrate that T-cell responses can indeed be induced in high-grade glioma patients, despite concerns over T-cell suppression. They also provided fallible evidence that is nonetheless consistent with improved clinical outcomes in the highest-grade glioma (GBM) patients due to such responses.

IMPROVING GLIOMA VACCINES

Identifying the cells capable of slowing or halting tumor progression in cancer patients, identifying the critical effector functions of the immune system in counteracting human tumor progression, or both, is required to improve clinical cancer vaccines. While such a cellular basis of beneficial immunity is readily apparent in experimental animals upon successful transfer of protective immunity by $CD8^+$ and/or $CD4^+$ T-cells, the failure of a variety of T-cell indices to correlate with clinical benefits in vaccine trials makes this a much more daunting task in patients (47). Similarly, administration of DC vaccines to cancer patients has failed to elicit the relatively dramatic affects expected of this therapy based on early animal studies, revealing that antigen-pulsed DC administration is not likely to constitute the sole limitation to clinically effective anti-tumor immunity in patients, as it so often does in experimental rodents (17). The conclusion that arises is that tumor Ag-pulsed DC therapy is sufficient to counteract tumor growth in animal models, but that additional parameters critically limit the ability of human T-cells to elicit net tumor destruction.

Autoimmune sequelae have also been observed in cancer patients treated with some forms of immunotherapy (110), raising particular concerns for vaccines for tumors in vital tissues such as the brain. Thus, major challenges facing DC vaccine therapy for cancer patients in general and glioma patients in particular, include diminishing the risk of pathologic autoimmunity, identifying the cellular basis of beneficial anti-tumor immunity, and increasing the proportion of patients experiencing such benefits. Recently developed molecular assays for identifying and quantifying nascent T-cell subpopulations and T-cell recognition of tumor antigens have proven invaluable in advancing knowledge along these lines.

Safety and Autoimmunity

Although no autoimmune sequelae were evident in DC glioma vaccinated glioma patients, their design allows T-cell responses against unidentified antigens that could be expressed on normal brain cells. Coupled with the brain's vital nature, this emphasizes concern over potential pathologic autoimmune reactions against normal brain components following DC therapy in glioma patients. Thus, the need to move toward greater specificity when designing future generations of glioma vaccines is recognized. Progress in this regard has now been realized through analysis of known tumor antigen epitopes on glioma tissue.

The characterization of tumor antigens on gliomas was initially intended as a means to target toxic moieties to tumors using specific antibody-toxin conjugates. A mutant form of EGFR (vIII) expressed on up to 50% of human GBM has been the most vigorously pursued glioma-associated antigen in this regard (111,112). Attempts to identify and incorporate peptide epitopes from EGFRvIII into therapeutic vaccines for gliomas are also in development (113). An alternative approach, identifying antigens expressed by gliomas that have already been linked to immune responses and/or regression in distinct human tumors (i.e., melanoma), may increase the likelihood of achieving beneficial immune responses in the context of DC vaccination, and has recently been undertaken.

Examining the expression of melanoma antigen genes on primary cell lines from GBM patients was originally performed to provide evidence of tumor status, and, hence, suitability of such lines as sources of tumor antigen for DC vaccines (13). The first antigens examined, gp100, MAGE-1, and TRP-2, were originally identified in non-glioma tumors, representing two subclasses of tumor antigens: differentiation antigens and cancer/testis antigens (24,25). More recent studies show that GBM patients vaccinated with autologous tumor lysate-pulsed DCs can mount responses directed against epitopes of TRP-2, a melanoma antigen also expressed by gliomas (114), as well as those against distinct classes of tumor antigens such as Her-2 (46,102) and AIM-2 (115), in addition to gp100 and MAGE-1 (Fig. 5) (46). Together with studies on SOX6 (108), this analysis further demonstrates intact cellular as well as T-dependent humoral immunity in glioma patients, and identifies tumor-selective epitopes that could be useful in increasing glioma vaccine specificity, monitoring immunological endpoints after vaccination, or both. The development of DC vaccines that target these specific epitopes in glioma patients, while potentially increasing the risk of immune resistance due to tumor epitope loss following

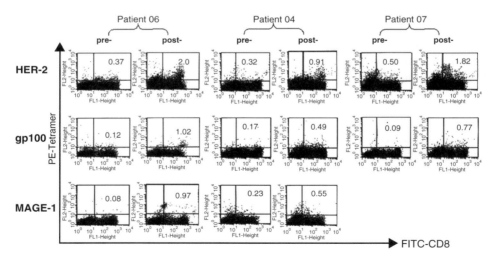

Figure 5 Identification of tumor associated antigen specific T-cells in PBMC from four pre- and post-vaccinations. PBMC were stained with HLA-A2 restricted tetramers for HER-2, gp100, and MAGE-1 (*y*-axis), then cells were stained for the CD8 (*x*-axis). The number shown in the plots indicate the percentage of TAA specific T-cells in whole PBMC population. *Source*: From Ref. 46.

vaccination (62,64), should substantially reduce the risk of vaccine-induced autoimmunity against normal brain components. Empirical assessment of the relative impact of these competing risks on glioma vaccine efficacy will determine the practicality of incorporating such epitopes into therapeutic vaccines.

Fundamental Limitations to Beneficial Cellular Immunity in Glioma Patients

In glioma DC vaccine trials, as in distinct cancer vaccine trials, vaccination is insufficient to elicit net tumor destruction in a majority of treated patients, and radiological decreases in tumor is either not evident, somewhat subjective, or partial in nature. As a rational approach to improving therapeutic DC vaccines against glioma, a broad consideration of parameters limiting tumor destruction by T-cells, built upon recent studies of endogenous and vaccine-induced immunity in glioma patients, is useful. Since animal tumor models may be inaccurate in this regard (17), the nature of such parameters limiting beneficial anti-tumor immunity might best be appreciated from more successful immunotherapeutic approaches in cancer patients. For gliomas, successful therapies of any sort are very rare, and the administration of cytokines or receptor-specific antibodies has generally failed to elicit net glioma destruction (116). A recent clinical trial, on the other hand, has revealed surprising evidence of glioma destruction following adoptive T-cell therapy (117).

It has been argued that adoptive transfer of Ag-reactive T-cells is consistently more clinically beneficial than DC vaccination in cancer patients (118). This argument gained further credibility when one Dudley et al. found that a majority of melanoma patients enjoyed objective clinical responses following adoptive transfer of ex vivo-cultured, tumor-reactive T-cells derived from the patients' tumors (110). A series of clinical trials performed previously by this same group, including several DC therapy trials for similar melanoma patients, failed to reach this degree of success (25). The unique success of adoptive T-cell therapy was dependent on the pre-existence of a starting population of highly tumor-reactive T-cells in cultures, on the number of such cells adoptively transferred, and on chemo-ablation of hosts to facilitate homeostatic expansion of the transferred cells (110). These findings parallel the recent glioma adoptive T-cell trial, which documents impressive and long-term objective tumor regression by serial imaging studies in up to a third of patients treated with 10^7–10^8 adoptively transferred, tumor-reactive T-cells (117).

Unfortunately, the inefficiency of generating the huge numbers of highly tumor-reactive cultured T-cells required for adoptive therapy currently precludes its wider application in glioma patients. In addition, and acknowledging caveats of interpreting clinical outcomes in non-randomized clinical trials, it seems that only DC vaccination has hinted of improved patient survival in high-grade glioma/GBM patients (13,46), a therapy that can be universally applied to patients with surgically accessible tumors. Consequently, the apparent success of adoptive T-cell therapy in eliciting net destruction of gliomas in situ may be most useful in defining critical limitations to beneficial anti-glioma immunity. In this respect, the dependence of immune tumor destruction on the presence of highly glioma-reactive T-cells in the host is inferred. In addition, the constraint of peripheral expansion and/or peak numbers of adoptively transferred T-cells in vivo appears to critically limit their clinical efficacy. A critical limitation to beneficial anti-tumor immunity in human cancer patients therefore exists at the level of tumor-reactive T-cells. Since tumor reactivity of T-cells per se does not appear to be unique in humans, this implies that an associated characteristic - one that perhaps defines a particular group of T-cells—critically limits beneficial anti-glioma immunity.

Based on these considerations, beneficial anti-tumor T-cells as a group are expected to possess intrinsically high tumor-reactivity, to be limited in number prior to vaccination in cancer patients, and ample in rodents used for tumor studies. Moreover, these cells are expected to confer clinical benefits according to both their pre-vaccine numbers and the degree to which they expand in vivo post-vaccination. While perhaps obvious, these points provide a template guiding the analysis of discrete T-cell populations that may dominantly mediate beneficial anti-tumor responses.

The Thymus and Anti-Tumor Immunity

The first hints as to the nature of a discrete group of T-cells that might critically limit beneficial anti-glioma immunity followed from the appreciation that numbers of highly tumor-reactive T-cells, like other antigen-specific T-cells, depend upon randomly-generated T-cell receptor (TCR) specificities. Since each T-cell is normally capable of recognizing and responding to one or a limited set of related antigenic epitopes, the existence of an antigen-specific T-cell is therefore dependent upon a fairly high level of T-cell (TCR repertoire) diversity. Hence, the level of T-cells specific for all tumor epitopes should also be dependent on a certain level of TCR repertoire diversity, with greater repertoire diversity conferring greater capacity to respond to multiple unrelated tumor epitopes.

The production and emigration of nascent, thymus-derived T-cells (recent thymic emigrants, or RTEs) is critical to the maintenance of TCR repertoire diversity in most vertebrates, and T-cell diversity declines dramatically as thymus production of RTEs declines later in life (119–121). Thus, T-cells from older patients, being relatively deficient in RTEs, would have decreased capacity to respond to tumor epitopes. This expected (and actual) decline in RTE production with age closely parallels the strongly age-dependent progression of high-grade gliomas, including GBM (102,122). In addition, RTEs themselves are expected to be less subject to immune suppression due to their nascent status. RTE survival signaling and homeostatic expansion is also uniquely exempt from competitive interference by other T-cells (123), potentially minimizing constraints on the in vivo expansion of RTEs similar to those impeding the expansion of adoptively transferred T-cells. This exemption could also conceivably minimize susceptibility of RTEs to signaling molecule defects as well, since such defects appear to follow from limited local access to T-cell survival ligands (61). The possibility that RTEs might represent a unique pre-tolerized T-cell subpopulation that might be uniquely reactivity to tumor antigens was also considered. Finally, recent studies suggest that RTE levels, particularly those of $CD8^+$ RTEs, may be 10-fold lower in healthy human subjects relative to experimental rodents (124,125). Such speculative considerations tend to favor the view that RTEs may be uniquely competent to initiate or sustain anti-tumor responses in patients, and thus encouraged the hypothesis that RTEs play a significant dose-limiting role in beneficial anti-glioma immunity in patients.

The notion that RTEs are significantly involved in beneficial anti-glioma immunity ceased to be speculative when $CD8^+$ RTEs were found to be specifically enriched within tumor-infiltrating T-cells, as thymic activity and peripheral RTEs decreased, in rats bearing either of two intracranial gliomas (103,126). While no guarantee of meaningfully representing immune trends in human cancer patients (17), this added weight to the notion that $CD8^+$ RTEs as a group are dominantly involved in beneficial anti-glioma immunity. Peripheral levels of $CD8^+$ RTEs also uniquely correlate with levels of $CD8^+$ T-cells infiltrating human GBM (r = 0.92; $P < 0.03$) whereas total peripheral $CD8^+$ T-cells do not

($r = 0.15$; $P > 0.7$), suggesting that CD8$^+$ RTEs are similarly relevant in GBM patients (CJ Wheeler, KL Black, unpublished data).

CD8$^+$ RTE Activity and Dominance

Based on the above considerations, tumor antigen reactivity, pre-existing RTE levels and post-vaccine responses were quantified in glioma patients, and tested for the ability to predict clinical outcomes in GBM patients. Using molecular as well as phenotypic markers for RTEs (121,127), the presence and post-vaccine responsiveness of CD8$^+$ RTEs was found to not only accurately predict age-dependent clinical outcome in GBM patients generally, but to largely account for the influence of age, the strongest established prognostic factor, on such outcome (Fig. 6) (102). In addition, glioma-bearing mice specifically deficient in thymic production of CD8$^+$ RTEs, but not peripheral CD8$^+$ T-cell activity, exhibited the decreased age-dependent survival and strong correlation between thymic cell production and clinical outcome observed in human GBM patients (Fig. 7). This suggests that CD8$^+$ RTE production critically influences age-dependent

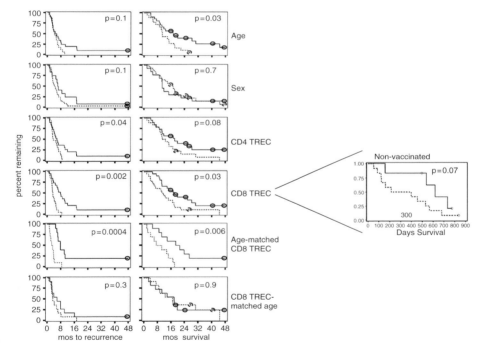

Figure 6 TRECs within purified T-cells, a molecular parameter quantifying RTE levels, account for age-dependent GBM outcome. Patients were separated for analyses by the indicated parameters above or below their median values in the entire population, in CD8 TREC-matched cohorts, or in age-matched cohorts as indicated, and Kaplan-Meier analysis was performed. Open circles reflect censured clinical outcome data. Each cohort patient was matched for either age (36–66 year range in each cohort; $n = 10$/cohort; $P = 0.96$) or CD8$^+$ TRECs (1.5–4309.5 and 0.6–5530.4 ranges in old and young cohorts, respectively; $n = 11$/cohort; $P = 0.86$), to a counterpart with distinct CD8$^+$ TRECs ($P < 0.05$) or age ($P < 0.008$), respectively. Expansion to right depicts contribution of non-vaccinated patient subgroup to ability of CD8 TRECs to predict survival. 2-tailed Mann-Whitney log-rank tests for disease-free and overall survival were calculated with SAS software. *Source:* Modified from Ref. 102.

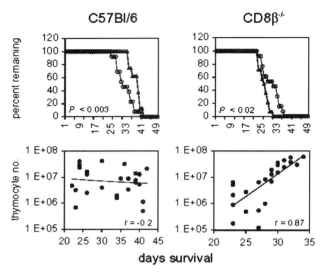

Figure 7 Decreased thymic $CD8^+$ T-cell production in $CD8\beta^{-/-}$ mice limits glioma progression in an age-dependent manner. $CD8\beta^{-/-}$ mice are specifically deficient in thymic production, but not peripheral activity, of $CD8^+$ T-cells. *Top row*: Intracranial tumor cell implantation into younger (*open circles*) and older (*solid triangles*) wild-type C57Bl/6 or $CD8\beta^{-/-}$ mice reveals uniquely decreased survival in older $CD8\beta^{-/-}$ mice ($P<0.02$; Mantel-Cox log rank). *Bottom row*: Thymocyte numbers were determined in all glioma-bearing wild-type C57Bl/6 or $CD8\beta^{-/-}$ mice, and correlated (Pearson's coefficients) with survival time. Strong correlation similar to that observed between $CD8^+$ RTEs and GBM patient clinical outcome ($r=0.86$; $P<0.001$ in both cases) was observed exclusively in $CD8\beta^{-/-}$ mice. *Source*: From Ref. 102.

glioma host survival in human patients and in mice deficient in their generation, but not in wild-type mice typically used for experimental tumor studies (102). The level of $CD8^+$ RTE proliferation and/or migration in patients' peripheral blood also correlated strongly ($r=0.96$) with type I cytokine response in vitro in DC-vaccinated GBM patients (102). Moreover, the vast majority of T-cells binding any of four distinct tumor Ag/HLA multimers exhibited a $CD8^+$ RTE phenotype, and related activated cells were specifically expanded in vivo upon vaccination. Finally, calculated numbers of $CD8^+$ RTEs responding in vivo uniquely predicted both disease-free and overall GBM patient survival following DC vaccination.

Taken together, these findings suggest that the $CD8^+$ RTE subpopulation possess intrinsically high tumor reactivity, that their levels are limited prior to vaccination in many GBM patients, and that the number of these cells responding in vivo determines the degree to which they account for clinical outcome in vaccinated GBM patients. Thus, these cells appear to both directly mediate and critically limit beneficial anti-glioma immune responses, and appear to dominate over other responding T-cells in this regard upon DC vaccination. This knowledge affords extraordinary opportunities to both rationally improve existing DC-based therapies, as well as to probe immune influences on established glioma characteristics in patients.

We propose that existing DC-based vaccine therapies for glioma can be rationally improved by increasing the production of normally rare $CD8^+$ RTEs in patients. Alternatively, determining the salient features of $CD8^+$ RTEs that afford them the apparent ability to dominantly influence glioma progression may allow the transfer of greater tumor-destructive capacity onto more readily available T-cells. In this context, the salient feature of CD8$^+$ RTEs that affords these cells apparently greater responsiveness to tumor antigens appears to be evident at the level of tumor antigen/HLA recognition, as evidenced by their dominant role in binding tumor antigen/HLA multimers (102). This points to possible modifications of antigen/HLA receptors (i.e., TCR and/or CD8) on CD8$^+$ RTEs that may render them more cognitive of and reactive to tumor antigens. These putative modifications are also expected to diminish with the further maturation of CD8$^+$ RTEs in the periphery. Indeed, we have detected temporally restricted modifications specific to both human and murine CD8$^+$ RTEs (CJ Wheeler, unpublished data). Examining these critical modifications on CD8$^+$ RTEs may provide an increased understanding of tumor antigen responsiveness by T-cells, how to increase such responsiveness in more abundant T-cells, and of critical tumor-immune interactions generally.

Immunoediting and Glioma Immune Susceptibility

Active suppression of immunity in tumor hosts may afford the tumor a critical growth advantage under a wide variety of conditions. From one perspective, the goal of immunotherapy is to break free from or overwhelm such suppressive mechanisms to substantially destroy tumor cells in situ. Tumors such as malignant gliomas are highly genetically plastic, however, and as such may be able to evade immune destruction by altering expression of their own intrinsic immune susceptibility genes. This mode of immune evasion was first realized clinically when vaccinated lymphoma patients experiencing long post-vaccine remissions, suffered recurrence by tumors devoid of immunizing antigen, of antigen processing machinery, or of appropriate HLA restriction elements (62–64). Later, it was also shown that the immune effector cells and molecules collaborate to stably alter tumor malignant behavior in rodents (128,129). Such evasiveness is distinguished from active immune suppression in that it does not impair the inherent ability of immune cells to carry out their effector functions. This distinction is important, because focusing on active immune suppression encourages strategies to enhance immune function, whereas focusing on tumor immune evasion encourages the very different strategy of bypassing or exploiting the tumor's ability to adapt to immune selective pressure. Conceivably, immune enhancement could even speed the development of immune-resistant tumor variants, a possibility that could worsen clinical outcome in tumor patients. In this regard, documenting, and understanding the development of resistance to immune-mediated destruction of tumors may be a key to successful immunotherapy for cancer.

Concepts pertaining to the interaction between tumor and immunity have recently been overhauled, and a discussion of these changes helps contextualize recent work in vaccinated glioma patients pursuant to using T-cell indices to probe immune influences on gliomas, as well as to understanding the development of immune resistance in tumors. The immunoediting model put forth by Schreiber and colleagues (130) updates the earlier concept of immune surveillance, wherein host immunity prevents the development of nascent tumors, and thereafter becomes irrelevant (131). This new model, substantiated by a growing body of experimental evidence (129,130,132), holds that tumors experience three distinct phases of interactions with host immunity: elimination, equilibrium, and escape (Fig. 8). Elimination refers to the complete immune-mediated destruction of nascent tumor cells prior to their establishment, essentially embodying the original immune surveillance hypothesis (129,131). Equilibrium refers to a further latent phase of tumor establishment wherein immune activity effectively kills off the most immune-sensitive

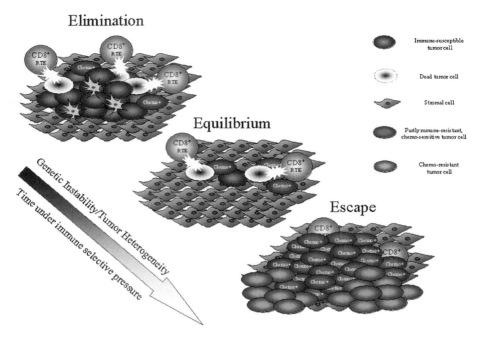

Figure 8 (*See color insert*) The immunoediting model in the context of glioma-immune dynamics. Tumor cells susceptible to destruction (*blue*) by immune cells (activated CD8$^+$ RTE progeny, *green*) initially grow interspersed with normal cells in the brain, leading to antigen uptake by nearby antigen-presenting cells (*yellow-orange*) and distal activation of CD8$^+$ RTEs. Activated progeny of CD8$^+$ RTEs then localize to the tumor site and eradicate most tumor cells in the elimination phase. To the extent that this process is not absolutely successful, tumor cells may enter the equilibrium phase, wherein immune-resistant tumor cells are selected to produce a new population of tumor variants in the equilibrium phase. The elimination, and possibly the equilibrium phase likely precede clinical tumor presentation. Immune-resistant tumor cells whose growth rate exceeds that of immune-mediated tumor cells destruction become clinically detectable in the escape phase. These immune-selected tumor cells are proposed to be rare or absent in the initial glioma cell population, uniquely chemosensitive, and possessing a growth advantage over other tumor variants specifically under conditions of strong anti-tumor immunity. Chemo-resistant tumor variants (*orange*), with unknown susceptibility to immune attack, would be similarly selected following inefficient chemotherapeutic tumor destruction. *Source*: Adapted from Ref. 130.

tumor cells, while failing to similarly eradicate less susceptible tumor subpopulations. This dynamic leads to the eventual selection of tumors that are immune resistant, whose growth outstrips immune constraints in the escape phase. The strong influence of CD8$^+$ RTEs on GBM clinical outcome suggests that these tumors may generally exist in a transitory phase between equilibrium and escape. Thus, hope that continued improvement in bolstering anti-glioma immunity will result in ever-increased slowing of glioma progression is tempered by the likelihood that such slowing will quickly reach an asymptotic limit due to the selection of immune-resistant tumor variants.

The concept that glioma progression may be slowed below a finite level of T-cell immunity, yet potentially exacerbated by hastening the development of immune resistant tumors above that level is consistent with our recent findings. GBM patient groups that, on average, experience lower levels of immune response enhancement following vaccination also appear to enjoy significantly prolonged survival, whereas patients exhibiting greater average immune responses after vaccination fail to exhibit prolonged survival (CJ Wheeler, KL Black, unpublished data). Resolution of this conundrum can only come from understanding how immune selective forces fundamentally alter gliomas. Based on such understanding, the restoration of immune susceptibility by reversing immune-induced changes could be attempted. Alternatively, an attempt could be made to determine whether CTL responses that do not result in net tumor destruction nevertheless constrain glioma cells in ways that are therapeutically exploitable. Although little direct evidence exists to suggest such a possibility, one recent study whose results are outlined below may afford a unique opportunity to gain insight into, and possibly exploit, glioma immune resistance in just such a manner.

Bypassing Immune Limitations in Glioma Patients: Post-Vaccine Chemosensitization

A critical property of clinically effective anti-tumor immune effector cells is the ability to reproducibly alter large proportions of tumor cells in situ. Ideally, this would involve the wholesale destruction of tumor cells, but net tumor growth may also be constrained in less obvious ways. For example, recent evidence suggests that GBM tumors recurring after vaccination may be more sensitive to conventional chemotherapy than recurrent tumors in non-vaccinated patients (109).

Although originating from distinct clinical studies not designed to address synergy between vaccination and chemotherapy, empirical validation allowed a comparison among three patient groups treated with either vaccine or chemotherapy alone, or with chemotherapy after vaccination (109). Vaccinated patients receiving subsequent chemotherapy exhibited significantly delayed tumor progression and longer survival relative to those receiving vaccinations without subsequent chemotherapy or to those receiving chemotherapy alone (Fig. 9). Multiple patients also exhibited objective ($>50\%$) regression of tumor burden, an extremely rare phenomenon in GBM (Fig. 9). Improved clinical outcome appeared dependent on the specific combination of therapeutic vaccination followed by chemotherapy, suggesting a substantial therapeutic slowing of GBM progression and extension of overall patient survival that appeared to markedly surpass that in previous vaccine as well as chemotherapy studies in high-grade glioma patients (8). Although both glioma clinical outcome and chemotherapeutic responsiveness are age-dependent, a stronger correlation existed between $CD8^+$ RTEs and chemotherapeutic responsiveness than between age and chemotherapeutic responsiveness, and $CD8^+$ RTE levels predicted a significant increase in such responsiveness (Fig. 10).

This study suggests that T-cell immune activity, mediated predominantly by $CD8^+$ RTEs, appears insufficient to eradicate gliomas in situ, but also confers enhanced sensitivity of the glioma to genotoxic agents (i.e., various forms of chemotherapy). An additional study describes GBM regression following post-vaccine chemotherapy. Evidence consistent with tumor recurrence after vaccination in this study, however, was interpreted as inflammatory response, leading to the conclusion that subsequent tumor regression after chemotherapy was elicited by vaccination alone (133). We suspect that GBM regression in this study, which utilizes IL-4-expressing glioma cells rather than antigen-pulsed DCs as vaccine, is also due to post-vaccine chemotherapy rather than vaccination alone. This alternate interpretation is more consistent with the notion that immune-selected GBM cells, regardless of the means of initiating immune selection, are particularly chemo-sensitive. We propose that the dominant cellular mediators of such selection are $CD8^+$ RTEs, the affects of which on glioma composition can be easily visualized in the context of the immunoediting model (Fig. 8). Because chemosensitivity

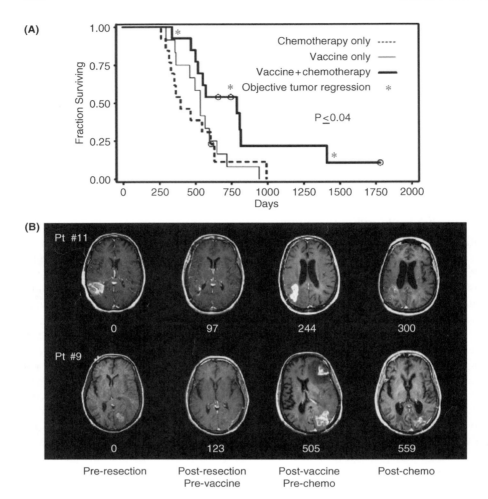

Figure 9 (**A**) Overall survival in patients receiving vaccine, chemotherapy, or vaccine + chemotherapy. Overall survival was defined as the time from first diagnosis of brain tumor (de novo GBM in all cases) to death due to tumor progression. Kaplan-Meyer survival plots with censored values in open circles are shown for each group. Survival of the vaccine group was identical to that of chemotherapy group ($p = 0.7$, log-rank). Survival of vaccine + chemotherapy group was significantly greater relative to survival in the other two groups together ($p = 0.048$, log-rank), greater than survival in the chemotherapy group alone ($p = 0.028$, log-rank), and greater than survival in the vaccine group alone ($p = 0.048$, log-rank). (**B**) Tumor regression following post-vaccine chemotherapy. Days after diagnosis are represented by numbers under individual MRI scans, with individual patients' scans in each row. All scans except the pre-resection scan for patient #2 were performed post-contrast enhancement with gadolinium. *Source*: From Ref. 109.

of gliomas, including GBM, has been linked to tumor genetics (134), superimposition of these data onto the immunoediting model suggests that immune selection may drive in situ glioma evolution away from a chemo-resistant genotype, and toward a chemosensitive one (Fig. 8). An equally valid alternative notion, that post-vaccine chemotherapy enhances anti-tumor immune responses by selectively killing suppressor T-cells, is inconsistent with recent data that suggests the induction of genetic abnormalities associated with glioma chemosensitivity after DC vaccination (CJ Wheeler, KL Black, unpublished data).

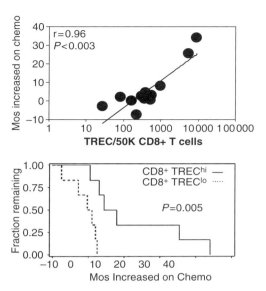

Figure 10 Levels of nascent CD8$^+$T-cells (CD8$^+$ recent thymic emigrants, or CD8$^+$ RTEs) are strongly associated with chemotherapeutic responses following vaccination. TRECs, a molecular measure of RTEs, within purified CD8$^+$T-cells collected at the time of surgery were correlated with the increase in time to tumor progression [time to recurrence after chemotherapy minus time to recurrence after vaccination in the same patient (*top*)]. Patients were subdivided based on median CD8$^+$ TREC level, and Kaplan-Meier survival analyses conducted (*bottom*). Data were derived from all vaccinated de novo and secondary GBM patients for whom chemotherapeutic response and TREC results were available ($n = 12$). Correlations with and predictive power of patient age or IFN-γ response magnitude were not statistically significant. *Source*: From Ref. 109.

The result of combining therapeutic vaccination with genotoxic therapies may be to increase the proportion of patients experiencing clinical vaccine benefits, in addition to increasing the apparent magnitude of such benefits. Since age is the single most dominant factor influencing the outcome of most human tumors, it will be additionally important to determine whether cellular immune processes similarly influence clinical outcome and chemotherapeutic efficacy in distinct human tumors. If so, the clinical expectations associated with immune-based cancer therapies would be substantially broadened.

SUMMARY AND CONCLUSIONS

The field of cancer vaccination has witnessed substantial progress in the past 5 years. Clinical cancer vaccines in general, including those for GBM and other high-grade gliomas, have progressed to the point that they consistently elicit tumor-specific CTL expansion in a majority of recipients (13,44–46). Impressive clinical responses have been observed, but in general these still occur in small subgroups of patients (16,37,42,109). In addition, and unlike in rodent tumor vaccine models, clinical improvement in vaccinated cancer patients does not generally coincide well with anti-tumor memory T-cell responses (47). These observations suggest that vaccination is sufficient to elicit substantial tumor-destructive T-cells in rodents, but that additional factors limit their tumor-destructive activity in vaccinated human patients (17). In the past 5 years, glioma research has not only culminated in the successful launching of multiple clinical vaccine trials, but has also contributed significant milestones toward the goals of identifying and overcoming such obstacles to more effective therapeutic cancer vaccines.

We now know that the induction of T-cell responses against autologous tumors is possible through the administration of unfractionated antigen-pulsed or tumor-fused DCs in high-grade glioma patients, including GBM, and that this proceeds without serious autoimmune sequelae given the current natural histories of these cancers. This validates evidence that endogenous immunity is intact, potentially protective, and can be enhanced in glioma patients, while opening the door to the development of more specific and optimized glioma vaccines. A number of candidate antigens expressed by gliomas that could be useful in this regard have now been characterized, including EGFRvIII, Her-2, MAGE-1, TRP-2, gp100, AIM-2, and SOX6. Clinical application of epitopes derived from these antigens will follow demonstration of their efficacy in animal vaccine models.

A discrete group of T-cells involved in beneficial anti-glioma immunity has now been identified. This has allowed greater focus on the induction of T-cell responses relevant to clinical outcome in the monitoring of DC vaccine trials for GBM patients, and thereby promises to link immunological with clinical endpoints in vaccine trials. In addition, this identification has revealed evidence that a specific subgroup of T-cells (CD8$^+$ RTEs) is unusually responsive to tumor antigens in general. Clearly, the further development of animal models that accurately reflect human glioma-CD8$^+$ RTE interaction dynamics is necessary to address potential therapeutic applications of CD8$^+$ RTEs in the context of adaptive or adoptive immunotherapy. Such models should also allow definitive examination of the potential impact of CD8$^+$ RTEs on other forms of cancer as well. In addition, elucidating molecular and cellular mechanisms for the apparent dominance of human CD8$^+$ RTEs in anti-glioma immunity, as well as salient effector mechanisms afforded by the activated progeny of these cells, may facilitate the enhancement of anti-tumor reactivity in less rare or otherwise suppressed T-cells. Such efforts may also lead to improved clinical efficacy in glioma therapy.

In the past year, evidence has been presented that vaccination, while ineffective alone in de novo GBM patients, may afford increased tumor sensitization to chemotherapy. This is particularly significant for GBM patients, in whom novel regressions of large tumor masses are now observed following post-vaccine chemotherapy. Definitive substantiation of post-vaccine glioma chemosensitization awaits the development of suitable animal models. In addition, the apparent success of combining DC vaccination and chemotherapy, which is linked to tumor genetics in glioma, justifies further examination of how human glioma genotypes may be globally altered by anti-tumor immunity. This kind of genetic analysis may allow the identification of discrete genes/proteins mediating post-vaccine chemo-sensitivity in gliomas, as well as provide useful surrogates for the realization of post-vaccine chemosensitization in the clinic. Additionally, analysis of global vaccine-induced alteration of gliomas may provide further insight as to how gliomas evade immunity, and how such evasion may be successfully exploited therapeutically.

To be sure, general issues that hamper objective interpretation of clinical vaccine success in cancer patients require much attention as well. Universally optimized standards for the design or monitoring of DC therapy and other vaccines have not been established. These shortcomings are expected of a therapeutic modality still in development, and measures discouraging this situation should be adopted as outcomes from cancer vaccine trials improve. In this respect, the study of glioma patient immunity and immunotherapy will necessarily follow trends set in more extensively investigated tumor systems. On another level, however, the rapid progression and short clinical histories of high-grade gliomas, their relatively confined, non-metastatic nature, and the existence of clear demographic predictors of disease outcome have allowed the study of these tumors—and particularly that of GBM—to contribute uniquely to our knowledge of beneficial immunity in cancer patients. These properties should continue to favor the analysis of tumor-immune interaction dynamics in gliomas, the results of which promise to improve therapies for malignant glioma and other cancer patients.

REFERENCES

1. DeAngelis LM. Medical progress: brain tumors. N Engl J Med 2001; 344:114.
2. Davis FG, Kupelian V, Freels S, McCarthy B, Surawicz T. Prevalence estimates for primary brain tumors in the United States by behavior and major histology groups. Neuro-Oncol 2001; 3:152.
3. Curran WJJ, Scott CB, Horton J, et al. Recursive partitioning analysis of prognostic factors in three Radiation Therapy Oncology Group malignant glioma trials. J Natl Cancer Inst 1993; 85:690.
4. Kreth FW, Warnke PC, Scheremet R, Ostertag CB. Surgical resection and radiation therapy versus biopsy and radiation therapy in the treatment of glioblastoma multiforme. J Neurosurg 1993; 78:762.
5. Quigley MR, Flores N, Maroon JC, Sargent B, Lang S, Elrifai A. Value of surgical intervention in the treatment of glioma. Stereotact Funct Neurosurg 1995; 65:171.
6. Hentschel SJ, Lang FF. Current surgical management of glioblastoma. Cancer J 2003; 9:113.
7. Reavey-Cantwell JF, Haroun RI, Zahurak M, et al. The prognostic value of tumor markers in patients with glioblastoma multiforme: analysis of 32 patients and review of the literature. J Neurooncol 2001; 55:195.
8. Stupp R, Hegi ME. Recent developments in the management of malignant glioma. J Clin Oncol 2003; 779:1091–1118.
9. Fine HA, Dear KBG, Loeffler JS. Meta-analysis of radiation therapy with and without adjuvant chemotherapy for malignant gliomas in adults. Cancer 1993; 71:2585.
10. Diete S, Treuheit T, Dietzmann K, Schmidt U, Wallesch CW. Sex differences in length of survival with malignant astrocytoma, but not with glioblastoma. J Neurooncol 2001; 53:47.
11. Glick RP, Lichtor T, Mogharbel A, Taylor CA, Cohen EP. Intracerebral versus subcutaneous immunization with allogeneic fibroblasts genetically engineered to secrete interleukin-2 in the treatment of central nervous system glioma and melanoma. Neurosurgery 1997; 41:898.
12. Liau LM, Black KL, Prins RM, et al. Treatment of intracranial gliomas with bone marrow-derived dendritic cells pulsed with tumor antigens. J Neurosurg 1999; 90:1115.
13. Yu JS, Wheeler CJ, Zeltzer PM, et al. Vaccination of malignant glioma patients with peptide-pused dendritic cells elicits systemic cytotoxicity and intracranial T-cell infiltration. Cancer Res 2001; 61:842.
14. Rosenberg SA, Yang JC, Schwartzentruber DJ, et al. Immunologic and therapeutic evaluation of a synthetic peptide vaccine for the treatment of patients with metastatic melanoma. Nat Med 1998; 4:321.
15. Lee KH, Wang E, Nielsen MB, et al. Increased vaccine-specific T-cell frequency after peptide-based vaccination correlates with increased susceptibility to in vitro stimulation but does not lead to tumor regression. J Immunol 1999; 163:6292.
16. Fong L, Hou Y, Rivas A, et al. Altered peptide ligand vaccination with Flt3 ligand expanded dendritic cells for tumor immunotherapy. Proc Natl Acad Sci USA 2001; 98:8809.
17. Bodey B, Bodey BJ, Siegel SE, Kaiser HE. Failure of cancer vaccines: the significant limitations of this approach to immunotherapy. Anticancer Res 2000; 20:2665.
18. Jensen CO. Centralb Bakt Parasitenk Infektionskrankh 1903; 34:28.
19. Haldane JBS. The genetics of cancer. Nature 1933; 132:265.
20. Gorer PA. The antigenic basis of tumour transplantation. J Pathol Bacteriol 1938; 44:691.

21. Zinkernagel RM, Doherty PC. MHC-restricted cytotoxic T-cells: studies on the biological role of polymorphic major transplantation antigens determining T-cell restriction-specificity, function, and responsiveness. Adv Immunol 1979; 27:51.

22. Van Pel A, Boon T. Protection against a nonimmunogenic mouse leukemia by an immunogenic variant obtained by mutagenesis. Proc Natl Acad Sci USA 1982; 79:4718.

23. van den Bruggen P, Traversari C, Chomez P, et al. A gene encoding an antigen recognized by cytolytic T lymphocytes on human melanoma. Science 1991; 254:1643.

24. Boon T, Cerottini JC, Van den Eynde B, Van der Bruggen P, Van Pel A. Tumor antigens recognized by T lymphocytes. Annu Rev Immunol 1994; 12:337.

25. Rosenberg SA. Cancer vaccines based on the identification of genes encoding cancer regression antigens. Immunol Today 1997; 18:175.

26. Inaba K, Metlay JP, Crowley MT, Steinman RM. Dendritic cells pulsed with protein antigens in vitro can prime antigen-specific, MHC-restricted T-cells in situ. J Exp Med 1990; 172:631.

27. Mayordomo JI, Zorina T, Storkus WJ, et al. Bone marrow-derived dendritic cells pulsed with synthetic tumour peptides elicit protective and therapeutic anti-tumour immunity. Nat Med 1995; 1:1297.

28. Zitvogel L, Mayordomo JI, Tjandrawan T, et al. Therapy of murine tumors with tumor peptide-pulsed dendritic cells: dependence on T-cells, B7 costimulation, and T helper cell 1-associated cytokines. J Exp Med 1996; 183:87.

29. Sampson JH, Archer GE, Ashley DM, et al. Subcutaneous vaccination with irradiated, cytokine-producing tumor cells stimulates CD8+ cell-mediated immunity against tumors located in the "immunologically privileged" central nervous system. Proc Natl Acad Sci USA 1996; 93:10399.

30. Gong J, Chen D, Kashiwaba M, Kufe D. Induction of antitumor activity by immunization with fusions of dendritic and carcinoma cells. Nat Med 1997; 3:558.

31. Wang J, Saffold S, Cao X, Krauss J, Chen W. Eliciting T-cell immunity against poorly immunogenic tumors by immunization with dendritic cell-tumor fusion vaccines. J Immunol 1998; 161:5516.

32. Okada H, Tahara H, Shurin MR, et al. Bone marrow-derived dendritic cells pulsed with a tumor-specific peptide elicit effective anti-tumor immunity against intracranial neoplasms. Int J Cancer 1998; 78:196.

33. Matsui S, Ahlers JD, Vortmeyer AO, et al. A model for CD8+ CTL tumor immunosurveillance and regulation of tumor escape by CD4 T-cells through an effect on quality of CTL. J Immunol 1999; 163:184.

34. Walker PR, Calzascia T, Schnuriger V, et al. The brain parenchyma is permissive for full antitumor CTL effector function, even in the absence of CD4 T-cells. J Immunol 2000; 165:3128.

35. Romani N, Gruner S, Brang D, et al. Proliferating dendritic cell progenitors in human blood. J Exp Med 1994; 180:83.

36. Hsu FJ, Benike C, Fagnoni F, et al. Vaccination of patients with B-cell lymphoma using autologous antigen-pulsed dendritic cells. Nat Med 1996; 2:52.

37. Nestle FO, Alijagic S, Gilliet M, et al. Vaccination of melanoma patients with peptide- or tumor lysate-pulsed dendritic cells. Nat Med 1998; 4:328.

38. Murphy GP, Tjoa BA, Simmons SJ, et al. Infusion of dendritic cells pulsed with HLA-A2-specific prostate-specific membrane antigen peptides: a phase II prostate cancer vaccine trial involving patients with hormone-refractory metastatic disease. Prostate 1999; 38:73.

39. Murphy GP, Tjoa BA, Simmons SJ, et al. Phase II prostate cancer vaccine trial: report of a study involving 37 patients with disease recurrence following primary treatment. Prostate 1999; 39:54.

40. Fong L, Brockstedt D, Benike C, Wu L, Engleman EG. Dendritic cells injected via different routes induce immunity in cancer patients. J Immunol 2001; 166:4254.

41. Holtl L, Rieser C, Papesh C, et al. Cellular and humoral immune responses in patients with metastatic renal cell carcinoma after vaccination with antigen pulsed dendritic cells. J Urol 1999; 161:777.

42. Kugler A, Stuhler G, Walden P, et al. Regression of human metastatic renal cell carcinoma after vaccination with tumor cell-dendritic cell hybrids. Nat Med 2000; 6:332.

43. Morse MA, Nair S, Fernandez-Casal M, et al. Peroperative mobilization of circulating dendritic cells by Flt3 ligand administration to patients with metastatic colon cancer. J Clin Oncol 2000; 18:3883.

44. Kikuchi T, Akasaki Y, Irie M, Homma S, Abe T, Ohno T. Results of a phase I clinical trial of vaccination of glioma patients with fusions of dendritic and glioma cells. Cancer Immunol Immunother 2001; 50:337.

45. Yamanaka R, Abe T, Yajima N, et al. Vaccination of recurrent glioma patients with tumour lysate-pulsed dendritic cells elicits immune responses: results of a clinical phase I/II trial. Br J Cancer 2003; 89:1172.

46. Yu JS, Liu G, Ying H, Yong WH, Black KL, Wheeler CJ. Vaccination with tumor lysate-pulsed dendritic cells elicits antigen-specific cytotoxic T-cells in patients with malignant glioma. Cancer Res 2004; 64:4973.

47. Panelli MC, Wunderlich J, Jeffries J, et al. Phase 1 study in patients with metastatic melanoma of immunization with dendritic cells presenting epitopes derived from the melanoma-associated antigens MART-1 and gp100. J Immunother 2000; 23:487.

48. Norment AM, Salter RD, Parham P, Engelhard VH, Littman DR. Cell-cell adhesion mediated by CD8 and MHC class I molecules. Nature 1988; 336:79.

49. Salter RD, Benjamin RJ, Wesley PK, et al. A binding site for the T-cell co-receptor CD8 on the alpha 3 domain of HLA-A2. Nature 1990; 345:41.

50. Konig R, Huang LY, Germain RN. MHC class II interaction with CD4 mediated by a region analogous to the MHC class I binding site for CD8. Nature 1992; 356:796.

51. Letourneur F, Gabert J, Cosson P, Blanc D, Davoust J, Malissen B. A signaling role for the cytoplasmic segment of the CD8 alpha chain detected under limiting stimulatory conditions. Proc Natl Acad Sci USA 1990; 87:2339.

52. Miceli MC, von Hoegen P, Parnes JR. Adhesion versus coreceptor function of CD4 and CD8: role of the cytoplasmic tail in coreceptor activity. Proc Natl Acad Sci USA 1991; 88:2623.

53. Abraham N, Miceli MC, Parnes JR, Veillette A. Enhancement of T-cell responsiveness by the lymphocyte-specific tyrosine protein kinase p56lck. Nature 1991; 350:62.

54. Sweetser MT, Morrison LA, Braciale VL, Braciale TJ. Recognition of pre-processed endogenous antigen by class I but not class II MHC-restricted T-cells. Nature 1989; 342:180.

55. Braciale TJ, Morrison LA, Sweetser MT, Sambrook J, Gething MJ, Braciale VL. Antigen presentation pathways to class I and class II MHC-restricted T lymphocytes. Immunol Rev 1987; 98:95.

56. Adorini L, Ullrich SJ, Appella E, Fuchs S. Inhibition by brefeldin A of presentation of exogenous protein antigens to MHC class II-restricted T-cells. Nature 1990; 346:63.

57. Seder RA, Paul WE. Acquisition of lymphokine-producing phenotype by CD4+T-cells. Annu Rev Immunol 1994; 12:635.

58. Surman DR, Dudley ME, Overwijk WW, Restifo NP. Cutting edge: CD4+T-cell control of CD8+T-cell reactivity to a model tumor antigen. J Immunol 2000; 164:562.

59. Dranoff G, Jaffee E, Lazenby A, et al. Vaccination with irradiated tumor cells engineered to secrete murine granulocyte-macrophage colony-stimulating factor stimulates potent, specific, and long-lasting anti-tumor immunity. Proc Natl Acad Sci USA 1993; 90:3539.

60. Prins RM, Graf MR, Merchant RE. Cytotoxic T-cells infiltrating a glioma express an aberrant phenotype that is associated with decreased function and apoptosis. Cancer Immunol Immunother 2001; 50:285.

61. Prins RM, Incardona F, Lau R, et al. Characterization of defective CD4-CD8- T-cells in murine tumors generated independent of antigen specificity. J Immunol 2004; 172:1602.

62. Jager E, Ringhoffer M, Karbach J, Arand M, Oesch F, Knuth A. Inverse relationship of melanocyte differentiation antigen expression in melanoma tissues and CD8+ cytotoxic-T-cell

responses: evidence for immunoselection of antigen-loss variants in vivo. Int J Cancer 1996; 66:470.

63. Jager E, Ringhoffer M, Altmannsberger M, et al. Immunoselection in vivo: independent loss of MHC class I and melanocyte differentiation antigen expression in metastatic melanoma. Int J Cancer 1997; 71:142.

64. Ohnmacht GA, Wang E, Mocellin S, et al. Short-term kinetics of tumor antigen expression in response to vaccination. J Immunol 2001; 167:1809.

65. Mahaley MS, Jr., Brooks WH, Roszman TL, Bigner DD, Dudka L, Richardson S. Immunobiology of primary intracranial tumors. Part 1: studies of the cellular and humoral general immune competence of brain-tumor patients. J Neurosurg 1977; 46:467.

66. Morford LA, Elliott LH, Carlson SL, Brooks WH, Roszman TL. T-cell receptor-mediated signaling is defective in T-cells obtained from patients with primary intracranial tumors. J Immunol 1997; 159:4415.

67. Morford LA, Dix AR, Brooks WH, Roszman TL. Apoptotic elimination of peripheral T lymphocytes in patients with primary intracranial tumors. J Neurosurg 1999; 91:935.

68. Schweighoffer T, Schmidt W, Buschle M, Birnstiel ML. Depletion of naive T-cells of the peripheral lymph nodes abrogates systemic antitumor protection conferred by IL-2 secreting cancer vaccines. Gene Ther 1996; 3:819.

69. Croft M, Duncan DD, Swain SL. Response of naive antigen-specific CD4+T-cells in vitro: characteristics and antigen-presenting cell requirements. J Exp Med 1992; 176:1431.

70. Schlom J, Hodge JW. The diversity of T-cell co-stimulation in the induction of antitumor immunity. Immunol Rev 1999; 170.

71. Singh-Jasuja H, Toes RE, Spee P, et al. Cross-presentation of glycoprotein 96-associated antigens on major histocompatibility complex class I molecules requires receptor-mediated endocytosis. J Exp Med 2000; 191:1965–1974.

72. den Haan JM, Lehar SM, Bevan MJ. CD8(+) but not CD8(−) dendritic cells cross-prime cytotoxic T-cells in vivo. J Exp Med 2000; 192:1685.

73. Subklewe M, Paludan C, Tsang ML, Mahnke K, Steinman RM, Munz C. Dendritic cells cross-present latency gene products from Epstein-Barr virus-transformed B cells and expand tumor-reactive CD8(+) killer T-cells. J Exp Med 2001; 193:405.

74. Siesjo P, Visse E, Sjogren HO. Cure of established, intracerebral rat gliomas induced by therapeutic immunizations with tumor cells and purified APC or adjuvant IFN-gamma treatment. J Immunother Emphasis Tumor Immunol 1996; 19:334.

75. Toes REM, van der Voort EIH, Schoenberger SP, et al. Enhancement of tumor outgrowth through CTL tolerization after peptide vaccination is avoided by peptide presentation of dendritic cells. J Immunol 1998; 160:4449.

76. Ni HT, Spellman SR, Jean WC, Hall WA, Low WC. Immunization with dendritic cells pulsed with tumor extract increases survival of mice bearing intracranial gliomas. J Neurooncol 2001; 51:1.

77. Jalkanen S, Reichert RA, Gallatin WM, Bargatze RF, Weissman IL, Butcher EC. Homing receptors and the control of lymphocyte migration. Immunol Rev 1986; 91:39.

78. Lampson LA. Beyond inflammation: site directed immunotherapy. Immunol Today 1998; 19:17.

79. Hickey WF. Leukocyte traffic in the central nervous system: the participants and their roles. Semin Immunol 1999; 11:125.

80. Brooks WH, Roszman TL, Rogers AS. Impairment of rosette-forming T lymphocytes in patients with primary intracranial tumors. Cancer 1976; 37:1869.

81. Woosley RE, Mahaley MSJ, Mahaley JL, Miller GM, Brooks WH. Immunobiology of primary intracranial tumors. Part 3: Microcytotoxicity assays of specific immune responses of brain tumor patients. J Neurosurg 1977; 47:871.

82. Menzies CB, Gunar M, Thomas DG, Behan PO. Impaired thymus-derived lymphocyte function in patients with malignant brain tumour. Clin Neurol Neurosurg 1980; 82:157.

83. Brooks WH, Latta RB, Mahaley MS, Roszman TL, Dudka L, Skaggs C. Immunobiology of primary intracranial tumors. Part 5: Correlation of a lymphocyte index and clinical status. J Neurosurg 1981; 54:331.

84. Gately MK, Glaser M, McCarron RM, et al. Mechanisms by which human gliomas may escape cellular immune attack. Acta Neurochir (Wien) 1982; 64:175.

85. Wood GW, Morantz RA. Depressed T lymphocyte function in brain tumor patients: monocytes as suppressor cells. J Neurooncol 1983; 1:87.

86. Elliott LH, Brooks WH, Roszman TL. Cytokinetic basis for the impaired activation of lymphocytes from patients with primary intracranial tumors. J Immunol 1984; 132:1208.

87. Ausiello C, Maleci A, Spagnoli GC, Antonelli G, Cassone A. Cell-mediated cytotoxicity in glioma-bearing patients: differential responses of peripheral blood mononuclear cells to stimulation with interleukin-2 and microbial antigen. J Neurooncol 1988; 6:329.

88. Ausiello CM, Palma C, Maleci A, et al. Cell mediated cytotoxicity and cytokine production in peripheral blood mononuclear cells of glioma patients. Eur J Cancer 1991; 27:646.

89. McVicar DW, Davis DF, Merchant RE. In vitro analysis of the proliferative potential of T-cells from patients with brain tumor: glioma-associated immunosuppression unrelated to intrinsic cellular defect. J Neurosurg 1992; 76:251.

90. Brooks WH, Roszman TL, Mahaley MS, Woosley RE. Immunobiology of primary intracranial tumours. II Analysis of lymphocyte subpopulations in patients with primary brain tumours. Clin Exp Immunol 1977; 29:61.

91. Bodmer S, Strommer K, Frei K, et al. Immunosuppression and transforming growth factor-beta in glioblastoma. Preferential production of transforming growth factor-beta 2. J Immunol 1989; 143:3222.

92. Black KL, Chen K, Becker DP, Merrill JE. Inflammatory leukocytes associated with increased immunosuppression by glioblastoma. J Neurosurg 1992; 77:120.

93. Kuppner MC, Hamou MF, Sawamura Y, Bodmer S, de Tribolet N. Inhibition of lymphocyte function by glioblastoma-derived transforming growth factor beta 2. J Neurosurg 1989; 71:211.

94. Lafarge-Frayssinet C, Duc HT, Frayssinet C, et al. Antisense insulin-like growth factor I transferred into a rat hepatoma cell line inhibits tumorigenesis by modulating major histocompatibility complex I cell surface expression. Cancer Gene Ther 1997; 4:276.

95. Parney IF, Farr-Jones MA, Chang LJ, Petruk KC. Human glioma immunobiology in vitro: implications for immunogene therapy. Neurosurgery 2000; 46:1169.

96. Weller M, Fontana A. The failure of current immunotherapy for malignant glioma. Tumor-derived TGF-beta, T-cell apoptosis, and the immune privilege of the brain. Brain Res Brain Res Rev 1995; 21:128.

97. Matsuda M, Petersson M, Lenkei R, et al. Alterations in the signal-transducing molecules of T-cells and NK cells in colorectal tumor-infiltrating, gut mucosal and peripheral lymphocytes: correlation with the stage of the disease. Int J Cancer 1995; 61:765.

98. Reichert TE, Rabinowich H, Johnson JT, Whiteside TL. Mechanisms responsible for signaling and functional defects. J Immunother 1998; 21:295.

99. Lai P, Rabinowich H, Crowley-Nowick PA, Bell MC, Mantovani G, Whiteside TL. Alteration in expression and function of signal transducing proteins in tumor-associated T and NK cells in patients with ovarian carcinoma. Clin Cancer Res 1996; 2:161.

100. Rabinowich H, Suminami K, Reichert T, et al. Expression of cytokine genes or proteins and signaling molecules in lymphocytes associated with human ovarian carcinoma. Int J Cancer 1996; 68:276.

101. Yu JS, Lee PK, Ehtesham M, Samoto K, Black KL, Wheeler CJ. Intratumoral T-cell subset ratios and fas ligand expression on brain tumor endothelium. J Neuro-Oncol 2003; 64:55.

102. Wheeler CJ, Black KL, Liu G, et al. Thymic CD8 + T-cell production strongly influences tumor antigen recognition and age-dependent glioma mortality. J Immunol 2003; 171:4927.

103. Prins RM, Graf MR, Merchant RE, Black KL, Wheeler CJ. Deficits in thymic function and output of recent thymic emigrant T-cells during intracranial glioma progression. J Neuro-Oncol 2003; 64:45.

104. Gimsa U, ORen A, Pandiyan P, et al. Astrocytes protect the CNS: antigen-specific T helper cell responses are inhibited by astrocyte-induced upregulation of CTLA-4 (CD152). J Mol Med 2004; 82:364.

105. Badie B, Bartley B, Schartner J. Differential expression of MHC class II and B7 costimulatory molecules by microglia in rodent gliomas. J Neuroimmunol 2002; 133:39.

106. Wiemels JL, Wiencke JK, Sison JD, Miike R, McMillan A, Wrensch M. History of allergies among adults with glioma and controls. Int J Cancer 2002; 98:609.

107. Brenner AV, Linet MS, Fine HA, et al. History of allergies and autoimmune diseases and risk of brain tumors in adults. Int J Cancer 2002; 99:252.

108. Ueda R, Iizuka Y, Yoshida K, Kawase T, Kawakami Y, Toda M. Identification of a human glioma antigen: SOX6, recognized by patients' sera. Oncogene 2004; 23:1420.

109. Wheeler CJ, Das A, Liu G, Yu JS, Black KL. Clinical responsiveness of glioblastoma multiform to chemotherapy after vaccination. Clin Cancer Res 2004; 10:5316.

110. Dudley ME, Wunderlich JR, Robbins PF, et al. Cancer regression and autoimmunity in patients after clonal repopulation with antitumor lymphocytes. Science 2002; 298:850.

111. Wikstrand CJ, Hale LP, Batra SK, et al. Monoclonal antibodies against EGFRvIII are tumor specific and react with breast and lung carcinomas and malignant gliomas. Cancer Res 1995; 55:3140.

112. Sampson JH, Crotty IE, Lee S, et al. Unarmed, tumor-specific monoclonal antibody effectively treats brain tumors. Proc Natl Acad Sci USA 2000; 97:7503.

113. Moscatello DK, Ramirez G, Wong AJ. A naturally occurring mutant human epidermal growth factor receptor as a target for peptide vaccine immunotherapy of tumors. Cancer Res 1997; 57:1419.

114. Liu G, Khong HT, Wheeler CJ, Yu JS, Black KL, Ying H. Molecular and functional analysis of tyrosinase-related protein (TRP)-2 as a cytotoxic T lymphocyte target in patients with malignant glioma. J Immunother 2003; 26:301.

115. Liu G, Yu JS, Zeng G, et al. AIM-2: a novel tumor antigen is expressed and presented by human glioma cells. J Immunother 2004; 27:220.

116. Ehtesham M, Black KL, Yu JS. Recent progress in immunotherapy for malignant glioma: treatment strategies and results from clinical trials. Cancer Control 2004; 11:192.

117. Plautz GE, Miller DW, Barnett GH, et al. T-cell adoptive immunotherapy of newly diagnosed gliomas. Clin Cancer Res 2000; 6:2209.

118. Kessels HW, Wolkers MC, Schumacher TN. Adoptive transfer of T-cell immunity. Trends Immunol 2002; 23:264.

119. Mackall CL, Gress RE. Thymic aging and T-cell regeneration. Immunol Rev 1997; 160:91.

120. Berzins SP, Boyd RL, Miller JF. The role of the thymus and recent thymic migrants in the maintenance of the adult peripheral lymphocyte poo. J Exp Med 1998; 187:1839.

121. Douek DC, McFarland RD, Keiser PH, et al. Changes in thymic function with age and during the treatment of HIV infection. Nature 1998; 396:690.

122. Burger PC, Vogel FS, Green SB, Strike TA. Glioblastoma multiforme and anaplastic astrocytoma. Pathologic criteria and prognostic implications. Cancer 1985; 56:1106.

123. Berzins SP, Godfrey DI, Miller JFAP, Boyd RL. A central role for thymic emigrants in peripheral T-cell homeostasis. Proc Natl Acad Sci USA 1999; 96:9787.

124. Steffens CM, Al-Harthi L, Shott S, Yogev R, Landay A. Evaluation of thymopoiesis using T-cell receptor excision circles (TRECs): differential correlation between adult and pediatric TRECs and naive phenotypes. Clin Immunol 2000; 97:95.

125. Sempowski GD, Gooding ME, Liao HX, Le PT, Haynes BF. T-cell receptor excision circle assessment of thymopoiesis in aging mice. Mol Immunol 2002; 38:841.

126. Wheeler CJ, Yu J, Black KL. Cellular immunity in the treatment of brain tumors. Clin Neurosurgery 2004; 51:132.

127. McFarland RD, Douek DC, Koup RA, Picker LJ. Identification of a human recent thymic emigrant phenotype. Proc Natl Acad Sci USA 2000; 97:4215.

128. Shankaran V, Ikeda H, Bruce AT, et al. IFNgamma and lymphocytes prevent primary tumour development and shape tumour immunogenicity. Nature 2001; 410:1107.

129. Dunn GP, Old LJ, Schreiber RD. The immunobiology of cancer immunosurvaillance and immunoediting. Immunity 2004; 21:137.

130. Dunn GP, Bruce AT, Ikeda H, Old LJ, Schreiber RD. Cancer immunoediting: from immuno-surveillance to tumor escape. Nat Immunol 2002; 3:991.

131. Burnet FM. The concept of immunological surveillance. Prog Exp Tumor Res 1970; 13:1.

132. Smyth MJ, Godfrey DI, Trapani JA. A fresh look at tumor immunosurveillance and immunotherapy. Nat Immunol 2001; 2:293.

133. Okada H, Lieberman FS, Edington HD, et al. Autologous glioma cell vaccine admixed with interleukin-4 gene transfected fibroblasts in the treatment of recurrent glioblastoma: preliminary observations in a patient with a favorable response to therapy. J Neuro-Oncol 2003; 64:13.

134. Leuraud P, Taillandier L, Medioni J, et al. Distinct responses of xenografted gliomas to different alkylating agents are related to histology and genetic alterations. Cancer Res 2004; 64:4648.

15

Replicating Viruses for Brain Tumor Treatment

Hong Jiang
Department of Neuro-Oncology, University of Texas M. D. Anderson Cancer Center, Houston, Texas, U.S.A.

Frank McCormick
Cancer Center/Cancer Research Institute, University of California at San Francisco, San Francisco, California, U.S.A.

Candelaria Gomez-Manzano
Department of Neuro-Oncology, University of Texas M. D. Anderson Cancer Center, Houston, Texas, U.S.A.

David T. Curiel
Med-Division of Human Gene Therapy, University of Alabama at Birmingham, Birmingham, Alabama, U.S.A.

Frederick F. Lang
Department of Neurosurgery, University of Texas M. D. Anderson Cancer Center, Houston, Texas, U.S.A.

W. K. Alfred Yung and Juan Fueyo
Department of Neuro-Oncology, University of Texas M. D. Anderson Cancer Center, Houston, Texas, U.S.A.

INTRODUCTION

Brain tumors pose a significant therapeutic challenge. This is especially true of glioblastoma multiforme (GBM), the most malignant type of brain tumor, which accounts for one-third of all brain tumors. The prognosis of patients diagnosed with GBM is grim. Most die within one year and even the most intricate combinations of therapies generally fail (1,2). This conundrum is compounded by the fact that malignant glioma cells are extremely resistant to apoptosis so that chemotherapy alone has not been a sufficiently effective treatment. Because gliomas generally localize within the central nervous system, local treatment strategies have traditionally been utilized. The standard treatment approach of surgical removal followed by external beam irradiation has often led to delayed progression and prolonged survival (3). Unfortunately, tumor recidivism followed

293

by unstoppable progression is the rule. Despite the explosive growth of knowledge in the field of cancer biology and extraordinary improvements in the treatment of many common human cancers, therapies for malignant glioma have improved little during the past several decades (4). Today's challenge is to develop more rational and efficacious therapies to target the specific genetic anomalies of brain tumors.

As the genetic basis underlying the genesis of brain tumors has been delineated, numerous genetic defects have been tagged as promising therapeutic targets. Brain tumors are considered to be amenable to local therapies, such as gene therapy, because in contrast to many other types of cancer, gliomas rarely metastasize and their recurrence typically results from a failure of local control. History has shown, however, that targeting only one gene at a time may not be an efficacious approach when facing the complicated process of gliomagenesis, during which numerous genes involved in regulating cell proliferation, differentiation, and death are abnormal. Gene targeting has also been limited by the lack of availability of an efficient system for delivering therapeutic agents to the bulk of the tumor (5,6). Therefore a recent goal has been to develop strategies to target the ultimate phenotype of cancer cells—uncontrolled explosion of the cancer cell population—and to utilize reagents whose killing power can be expanded in a population of cancer cells by self-replication (Fig. 1). Replicating oncolytic viruses are therefore viewed as attractive agents for implementing these strategies.

A virus should meet most of the following requirements if it is to become an oncolytic agent. It must recognize cellular receptors in the target tissue, have the ability to infect dividing and quiescent tumor cells, be only mildly pathogenic in normal human cells, have a high oncolytic capacity, have the ability to amplify an initial low dose of

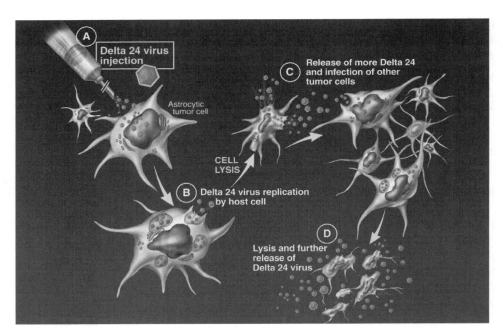

Figure 1 (*See color insert*) Inoculation and spread of oncolytic adenoviruses, such as Delta-24, in cancer cells. After lysis of the infected cell, viral progenies spread and infect other cancer cells. The explosion of viral population will eventually wipe out the tumor cells. Normal cells surrounding the tumor will be spared because Delta-24 encompasses a deletion in E1A gene that restricts the viral replication only in cancer cells.

inoculum by replication, be genetically stable, be susceptible to genetic manipulation, and finally, be amenable to high-titer production and purification. While other selectively replicating viruses meet some of these requirements and have been used as oncolytic agents, human group C adenoviruses (Ad) meet all of these criteria (7).

Viral therapy against cancer made its debut approximately fifty years ago after observations of occasional tumor regression in cancer patients with viral infections or in those who had been vaccinated (8). Although cancer treatment using Ad induced a short-term response in most of the patients treated, it did not prevent tumor progression and produced toxicity (9). Currently, Ad are being modified to improve target specificity and anticancer potency. The primary paradigm of this approach is an adenoviral system with genomic modifications that allow it to use abnormally expressed cell receptors to exclusively infect cancer cells and replicate preferentially in cells with abnormal tumor suppressor pathways or in cells with overexpressed cancer-related proteins.

In this review, we dissect the concepts underlying the use of oncolytic (or conditionally replicative) Ad, including the main strategies currently used to restrict adenoviral replication and the infectivity of tumor cells (Table 1). We discuss safety measures involving the control of adenoviral replication with conventional drugs and the insertion of suicide genes in the adenoviral genome to produce a bystander effect and to incapacitate the adenovirus in case a runaway infection occurs, applying oncolytic Ad as delivery vectors for pro-drug strategies, siRNA, and non-invasive molecular imaging systems and the feasibility of combining them with chemotherapy and radiotherapy. We end this chapter with a brief description of other oncolytic viruses that could potentially be

Table 1 Potential Strategies and Targets for Oncolytic Adenoviral Therapy

Strategies	Targets	Nature of the targets	Status of the targets in glioma cells	Cellular localization of the targets
Functional deletions				
Deletion in E1B-55 kD	p53 pathway	pro-apoptosis	Aberrant	Nucleus
Deletion in E1A	Rb pathway	Negative cell-cycle regulator	Aberrant	Nucleus
Transcription regulation of early genes with TSPs				
E2F-1 promoter	E2F-1	Cell-cycle modulator	Overexpressed	Nucleus
hTERT promoter	Telomerase	Telomere maintenance	Overexpressed	Nucleus
HIF-1α promoter	HIF-1α	Hypoxia-inducible	Overexpressed	Nucleus
Nestin second intron	Nestin	Neural progenitor marker	Overexpressed	Nucleus
GFAP enhancer	GFAP	Glial cell marker	Overexpressed	Nucleus
Modification of viral tropism				
RGD motif in fiber	Integrins	Adhesion-related protein	Overexpressed	Cell surface
Bispecific adapter	EGFR	Growth factor receptor	Overexpressed	Cell surface
Bispecific adapter	FGFR	Growth factor receptor	Overexpressed	Cell surface
Bifunctional PEG	uPAR	Invasion-related protein	Overexpressed	Cell surface

Abbreviations: RGD, Arg-Gly-Asp; PEG, polyethylene glycol.

developed as anti-glioma tools, and offer some future directions for the development and application of oncolytic viral strategies.

THE UNDERLYING PRINCIPLE OF ONCOLYTIC VIRUSES—CANCER SELECTIVITY

Wild-type Ad induce cell death by replicating in and lysing infected cells. This inherent cytotoxicity, together with the efficiency by which viruses can spread from one cell to another, inspired the notion that replication-competent viruses could be one solution for addressing the delivery problem (aptly expressed as "vector gap") in cancer gene therapy. An oncolytic or conditionally replicative adenovirus (CRAd) is a genetically modified adenovirus that, given specific circumstances, is unable to dominate cellular division machinery, and has attenuated activity in normal cells, but retains the ability to efficiently lyse tumor cells. Selective killing is especially critical for brain tumors because tumor cells that infiltrate far from the solid tumor mass are typically intermingled with normal supportive cells (astrocytes) and functioning neurons, the loss of which results in neurologic deficits. Indeed, most therapies for brain tumors fail because of their inability to selectively kill invading tumor cells without damaging the normal infiltrated adjacent brain. Advances in understanding the biology of Ad and cancer have given scientists working in this field the ability to modify the viral genome to target viruses specifically to cancer cells.

Functional Deletion in Critical Viral Genes

Because Ad lack the enzymes required for replication, they rely on the enzymatic machinery of the host cell to replicate the adenoviral genome. To overtake the host cell DNA replication machinery, the adenovirus expresses a series of genes immediately after infection. Called *early genes*, they encode proteins that bind and inactivate cellular protein regulators of cell cycle progression and apoptosis. Studying the interactions between adenoviral and critical cellular proteins led to the discovery of important tumor suppressor genes. The first adenoviral gene expressed after infection is called E1A (E designates early). The E1A products bind to and inactivate retinoblastoma protein (Rb), propelling the cell into unscheduled DNA synthesis, which creates a favorable environment for replication. Forced entry into S phase may trigger p53-mediated apoptosis during the early stage of viral infection, aborting the process of adenoviral replication. To abrogate the p53-induced apoptotic response, Ad encode E1B-55kD, which binds to and inactivates p53, resulting in a prolonged cell life that facilitates the propagation of viral particles. Biologic logic thus inspired the design of replication-competent Ad that do not interact with critical cell proteins while successfully inducing selective lysis in cancer cells, and that are unable to acquire a replication phenotype in normal cells.

Abrogating E1B-55kD/p53 Binding—ONYX-015 (dl1520)

In a seminal work and with basis on the knowledge of virus-host cell interactions, a team lead by Frank McCormick constructed and tested an adenovirus that was unable to express the p53-antagonical E1B-55kD protein (10). The idea behind this strategy was to construct a replication-competent adenovirus that would not replicate in wild-type p53 cells but that was capable of acquiring a completely developed replication phenotype in mutant p53 cells. To suppress p53 induction, Ad of group C types 2 and 5 produce a 55K protein from the E1B region. This protein binds directly to p53 and targets it or degradation, through a complex that includes E4orf6 and cellular proteins involved in proteasome-mediated degradation. Mutants of E1B-55kD that do not bind p53 efficiently are defective for replication in normal cells. In view of the fact that nearly of all tumors harbor a p53-dysfunction, their preconditioned environment likely favors adenoviral replication. Furthermore, disabling E1B-55kD would prevent viral propagation in normal, non-cancerous cells, which initiated the hypothesis that Ad would be able to selectively replicate in tumor cells. This concept was initially bolstered by the observation that the mutant virus *dl*1520 (a double mutant adenovirus that was unable to synthesize the E1B-55kD protein) was extremely deficient in its ability to transform rat embryo fibroblast cells (11). A similar virus, ONYX-015 (*dl*1520), which is a chimeric human group C (Ad2 and Ad5) adenovirus, was the first CRAd to demonstrate preferential replication as well as antitumor efficacy in some p53-deficient human tumor cells (10,12).

ONYX-015 lacks E1B-55kD protein, as a result of a deletion in the gene. It is defective for replication in normal epithelial cells. In normal cells, ONYX-015 induces E1a-mediated S-phase at rates that exceed that of wild type adenovirus, and viral DNA replication is initiated, but virus production is not complete and many cells die through E1a-triggered p53-dependent apoptosis. In cells infected with wild type adenovirus, E1a expression is down regulated as infection proceeds because translation of its mRNA is shut down, along with other capped mRNAs, as part of the switch to the late phase of replication. This switch depends on E1B-55kD and is therefore defective in normal cells. Failure to shut off host protein synthesis contributes to attenuation of ONYX-015 in normal cells. Indeed, p53-dependent attenuation depends on this failure: if ONYX-015 shut down translation of host mRNAs, p53-dependent genes would not be translated (13) (Oshea, Johnson, She, McCormick, in preparation).

Initially, it was assumed that p53 status conditioned the ability of ONYX-015 to replicate in cancer cells, but this assumption was later shown to be incorrect. In fact, variable replication is due to varying degrees to which each cell complements functions of E1B-55kD unrelated to p53. McCormick and collaborators are currently investigating the molecular basis of other functions of E1B-55kD that are complemented in some cancer cells but not in others.

ONYX-015 is the prototype of oncolytic Ad, has undergone extensive testing in the clinic, and has proven safe with promising signs of efficacy. Importantly, no clinically emergent signs of liver toxicity were observed: in most cases, elevated liver markers preceded ONYX-015 treatment and were not significantly increased following infusion. ONYX-015 is therefore safe at these doses, and indeed, a maximally tolerated dose was not achieved. Lack of detectable effects on normal liver tissue is remarkable, particularly since mouse models suggested viruses of this type could cause direct damage through infection of hepatocytes. However, more recent data suggests that human liver cells are poorly infectable in vivo, although they are readily infectable in cell culture. This may be because the receptor for adenovirus is engaged in tight cell:cell junctions in healthy cells and cannot be accessed efficiently by incoming virus particles. Patients with head and neck cancer who were treated by direct injection of such viruses into their tumor masses underwent limited clinical responses (14), and more encouraging results of a phase II trial in combination with 5-fluorouracil and cysplatin have been reported (15). ONYX-015 has also been recently tested in patients with malignant gliomas. In this regard, The NABTT CNS Consortium conducted a dose-escalation trial of intracerebral injections of ONYX-015 (16). Cohorts of six patients at each dose level received doses of vector from 10^7 plaque-forming units (pfu) to 10^{10} pfu into a total of 10 sites within the resected glioma cavity. None of the 24 patients experienced serious adverse events related to

ONYX-015. The maximum tolerated dose was not reached at 10^{10} pfu. The median time to progression after treatment with ONYX-015 was 46 days (range 13 to $452+$ days). The median survival time was 6.2 months (range 1.3 to $28.0+$ months). One patient has not progressed and 1 patient showed regression of interval-increased enhancement. With more than 19 months of follow-up, 1/6 recipients at a dose of 10^9 and 2/6 at a dose of 10^{10} pfu remain alive. The authors conclude that injection of ONYX-015 into glioma cavities is well tolerated at doses up to 10^{10} pfu.

McCormick's group is working in approaches with which effectiveness of ONYX-015 could be improved in the future. In parallel, efforts are underway to develop second generation viruses that may be more potent, but maintain ONYX-015s excellent safety profile.

In addition to E1B-55kD mutants, virologists have tested the anticancer effect of E1B-19kD mutants. In one study, an E1b-19kD-deleted viral mutant (Ad337) was more efficient than wild-type adenovirus in suppressing tumor growth in established flank tumors of a murine model (17).

Attenuating the E1A/Rb Interaction—E1A Mutants

Rb protein is a prototypic tumor suppressor gene product and the master regulator of the G1 checkpoint in the cell cycle. In its hypophosphorylated state, Rb negatively controls the G1/S transition. Rb exerts its function by binding E2F transcription factors, which are the primary positive force underlying the transcription of genes needed for the G1 to S phase transition. Once Rb is hyperphosphorylated by upstream cyclin-dependent kinases, it is disabled and releases E2Fs, thereby allowing the transition to S phase to occur (18). The Rb pathway is frequently inactivated in various cancers and abnormalities of Rb regulators have been characterized in most high-grade gliomas, resulting in the release of E2F transcription factors from Rb which equals the effect of E1A binding with pRb (19–21). Importantly, the physical interaction between E1A and Rb requires the presence of two noncontiguous regions of amino acids (aa) 30 to 60 and 122 to 129 (19).

We previously tested an oncolytic adenovirus with a mutant E1A protein that is unable to bind Rb protein. To disrupt the E1A protein / Rb binding function, a deletion was made in its conserved region 2 (CR2). The mutant adenovirus has a deletion of aa 122 to 129 comprising a 24-bp region and for that reason, was named Delta-24 (22). Immunoprecipitation analyses verified that after this deletion Delta-24 is unable to bind Rb protein. However, titration experiments in 293 cells demonstrated that the Delta-24 adenovirus could replicate in and lyse cancer cells with great efficiency (Fig. 2). Lysis of most human glioma cells was observed within 10 days after infection with Delta-24 at 10 PFU/cell. In vivo, a single dose of the Delta-24 virus induced a dramatic inhibition of tumor growth in nude mice (Fig. 3). However, normal fibroblasts or cancer cells with restored Rb activity were resistant to the Delta-24 adenovirus. These results suggest that the E1A-mutant Delta-24 adenovirus may be clinically and therapeutically useful against gliomas and possibly other cancers with a disrupted Rb pathway (22). After this report on the Delta-24 strategy, Delta-24 was tested in a different laboratory (23) and it is being used as platform for the development of combined tumor-selective replication and tumor-targeting approaches (24,25).

Simultaneously Targeting Aberrant p53 and Rb Pathways

In addition to strategies targeting either abnormal p53 or Rb pathways in cancer cells, adenovirus can be designed to simultaneously target both tumor suppressors. One oncolytic virus, O1/PEME, has been reported to have increased selectivity for cells with

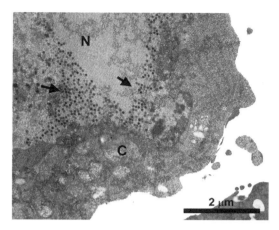

Figure 2 Transmission electron micrograph of Delta-24 adenovirus in an infected glioma cell. Pellets from U-251 MG cells infected with Delta-24 were fixed in 2% glutaraldehyde and post-fixed for 1 hour in 1% osmium tetroxide. Samples were counterstained with uranyl acetate and lead citrate. The viral particles (*arrows*) are assembled and tend to accumulate in the nucleus, forming inclusion bodies. There may be as many as 10,000 virions propagated in one cell. *Abbreviations*: C, cytoplasm; N, nucleus.

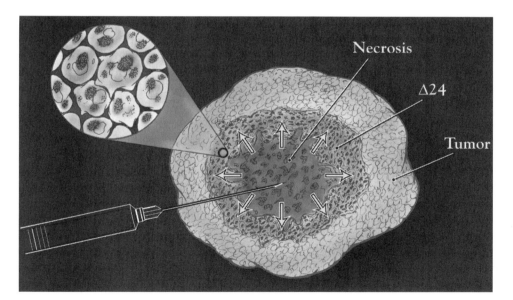

Figure 3 (*See color insert*) Schematic illustration of the predicted spread pattern of Delta-24 within treated gliomas. After intratumoral injection of Delta-24, the viruses infect and lyse the cancer cells, and spread to the vicinity of the injection site, forming three distinct and concentric tumor zones: an innermost central core of necrosis and cellular debris; a middle zone that consists of large numbers of tumor cells with prominent viral inclusions intermixed with apparently intact tumor cells (close up); and a peripheral zone of intact tumor cells with few scattered cells with signs of infection. This "three zone" pattern could be used to characterize the oncolytic effect in gliomas during clinical trials. Arrows indicate the direction of the viral wave.

p53 defects (26). This virus contains a p53-regulated promoter that is placed upstream of a cDNA for an antagonist of the E2F transcription factor, the product of which blocks E2F and late viral gene transcription. This work demonstrated that alterations to viral genomes, such as eliminating the redundant effects of viral gene products on cellular factors, led to more efficient and more selective oncolytic replication. Adenoviral strains with modifications to the p300/CBP binding domain of E1A that interfere with p53 function, and overexpression of the adenoviral death protein E3-11.6 kDa (27) have been shown to increase the replication of the virus in tumor cells, compared to ONYX-015. Another strategy used to target p53 and Rb was combining ONYX-015 and Delta-24 deletions in the same construct. In this regard, a novel replication-selective adenovirus (CB1) incorporating a double deletion of a 24 bp Rb-binding region in the *E1A* gene, and a 903 bp deleted region in the *E1b* gene that abrogates the expression of a p53-binding E1B-55 kDa protein exerted a potent anticancer effect in vitro in human glioma cell lines but acquired a highly attenuated replicative phenotype in both serum-starved and proliferating normal human astrocytes. In vivo experiments using intracranially implanted glioma xenografts in nude mice showed that a single dose of CB1 ($1.5 \times 10(8)$ PFU/tumor) significantly improved survival (28).

E1-Deleted Oncolytic Adenoviruses

In addition to minimal deletions, an E1 deletion can still allow adenoviral replication under favorable conditions. Thus, a complete deletion of E1 can be complemented by factors that are expressed by tumor cells, thereby allowing for selective replication—albeit at low levels (29,30). These mutant viruses prevent cell-cycle progression by inducing arrest at the G2/M checkpoint in cancer cells. Because virus infection, uptake and replication in cells is more efficient during S and G2/M phases, lysis that is mediated by an *E1*-deleted virus can occur more frequently in cells that are progressing through the cell cycle, such as tumor cells. Knowing that *E1*-deleted adenovirus replication can occur in tumor cells led to the development of new tactics to obtain tumor-specific transgene expression. Recently developed viral vectors include not only an *E1* deletion, which allows the virus to replicate its DNA only in tumor cells, but also a genomic rearrangement that during DNA replication places a reporter or a suicide transgene downstream of a constitutive promoter. In the absence of adenoviral DNA replication and genome rearrangement, the transgene exists in an antisense direction (31).

In addition to the above modifications, rather than deleting viral inhibitors of cell death, such as E1b-19kDa, one could seek to enhance the mechanism by which Ad promote cell death. Preserving the adenovirus E3-11.6kDa death protein in a CRAd has been shown to enhance the release of viral progeny and oncolytic potency (27,32). Proteolysis of keratins by L3-23kDa and inhibition of cell translation by L4-100kDa also promote cell lysis and the release of progeny (33). The dependence of the oncolytic potency of CRAds on these viral functions remains to be studied. Finally, adenovirus mutants defective in other arenas such as intracellular trafficking, nuclear import of the viral genome, RNA splicing, nuclear export of RNA, or protein translation are potential CRAd candidates.

Using Tumor or Tissue-Specific Promoters to Restrict the Expression of Essential Viral Genes

Another strategy that can be used to improve the specificity of oncolytic viruses is to limit their replication through transcriptionally targeting viral genes that are essential for replication using tumor-and/or tissue-specific promoters (TSP). This is usually accomplished by inserting the promoter upstream of E1A or other early genes, restricting viral replication and propagation within the tumor and/or to a specific type of tissue. Controlling the dissemination of the virus in this manner can greatly improve the specificity and safety of an oncolytic therapy. Paul Hallenbeck (Genetic Therapy–Novartis; Gaithersburg, MD) and Daniel R. Henderson (Calydon; Sunnyvale, CA) have pioneered this avenue of research using alfa-fetoprotein (AFP) and prostate-specific antigen (PSA) promoters to drive the adenovirus *E1A* gene to treat hepatocellular and prostate carcinomas, respectively (34–36).

Tumor-Specific Promoters

The Rb tumor suppressor protein pathway is dysregulated in most human cancers, resulting in an excess of "free" E2F in the cells. E2F-responsive promoters, such as the E2F-1 promoter, should thus be more active in cancer cells than in normal cells. Based on this prediction, adenoviral vectors containing transgenes driven by the E2F-1 promoter were constructed. These vectors produced tumor-selective gene expression in gliomas in vivo (37). Recently, replication-competent Ad were constructed by inserting the human E2F-1 promoter element upstream of E1A or E4 genes. This manipulation caused extensive cell death in a panel of tumor cells but not in non-proliferating normal cells in vitro (38–40). In another study, a human adenovirus, ONYX-411, that selectively replicates in human tumor cells, but not normal cells, depending upon the status of their retinoblastoma tumor suppressor protein (pRb) pathway. Early and late viral gene expression as well as DNA replication were significantly reduced in a functional pRb-pathway-dependent manner, resulting in a restricted replication profile similar to that of nonreplicating Ad in normal cells both in vitro and in vivo. In contrast, the viral life cycle and tumor cell killing activity of ONYX-411 was comparable to that of wild-type adenovirus following infection of human tumor cells in vitro as well as after systemic administration in tumor-bearing animals. This strategy could be applied to glioma therapy.

Human telomerase reverse transcriptase (hTERT) is the catalytic subunit of telomerase. More than 90% of all human tumors reactivate telomerase, suggesting its requirement for the viability of cancer cells. As a consequence, telomerase is universally recognized as a tumor marker and an attractive target for gene therapy strategies (41). An approach that used the telomerase promoter to control the expression of E1A, E1B, and E4 genes produced selective replication in human cancer cells, but not in normal cells such as human fibroblasts (40,42–45). However, the use of a wild-type hTERT promoter is limited by its inability to induce the high level of cancer cell-specific expression necessary for targeted gene therapy to be effective. To improve cancer cell specificity and the strength of the hTERT promoter, one strategy involved reinforcing the hTERT promoter by incorporating additional copies of c-Myc and Sp1 binding sites adjacent to the promoter. Used to control E1A expression, the modified promoter enhanced viral replication and induced a cytopathic effect only in cancer cells (46). Malignant gliomas in particular are one of the best candidates for telomerase-targeted therapy because glioma cells are predominantly telomerase-positive, whereas normal brain tissues do not express telomerase (47).

Solid tumors with areas of hypoxia are the most aggressive and resistant to radiotherapy and chemotherapy and hypoxia is a major factor in treatment failure. The cellular response to hypoxia is controlled by the hypoxia-inducible factor-1 (HIF-1) transcription factor. HIF-1 consists of an oxygen-regulated alpha subunit and a constitutively expressed beta subunit, which bind each other and translocate to the nucleus. There they activate the transcription of various genes involved in glycolysis, inhibiting apoptosis, and promoting angiogenesis and metastasis (48). The activity of the HIF-1 complex is controlled primarily by levels of the alpha subunit and a series of mechanisms that control HIF-1 pathway activation. HIF-1α is overexpressed in many human tumors where its upregulation correlates with a poor prognosis and treatment failure. HIF-1 is, therefore, another potentially important target for cancer chemotherapy (48,49). To target HIF-1 in cancer cells, new oncolytic Ad were developed. In them, E1A or E4 genes under the control of an optimized minimal promoter containing HIF recognition elements demonstrated that the induction of the E1A gene, as well as viral replication and cytolysis depend on HIF activity. As a consequence, these viruses efficiently kill HIF-1α-activated cells in vitro and in vivo, as well as cells grown under hypoxic conditions (40,50,51). This therapeutic approach can be used to treat all solid tumors that develop hypoxia, regardless of their tissue of origin or specific underlying genetic alterations. Additionally, the expression of suicide genes under the control of a hypoxia-responsive element (HRE) can be activated through HIF-1 in brain tumor cells (52).

In another approach, Tcf binding sites were inserted into E1A, E1B, E2, and E4 promoters to improve viral selectivity aimed at cells with activated wnt signaling pathways (53), the potential significance of which is that the Tcf responsive element has a putative role in the development of gliomas (54). The Cox-2 promoter was also placed upstream of the E1A gene to improve viral selectivity for carcinomas (55,56). The importance of this approach is that the two most common types of human brain tumors, gliomas and meningiomas, aberrantly overexpress eicosanoid-producing enzymes, such as the cyclooxygenases (COX-1 and COX-2). The resulting release of a spectrum of eicosanoids may promote tumorigenesis and the development of peritumorous brain edema, as shown by the killing of glioma and meningioma cells in vitro and animal models after exposure to COX-2 inhibitors (57).

Tissue-Specific Promoters

Some tumors overexpress proteins that reflect their tissue origin. These proteins can be used to localize the CRAd to a specific type of tissue, although their expression is not exclusive to tumor tissue. In the developing brain the 38-kDa intermediate filament protein nestin is expressed specifically in neuroepithelial stem cells and neuronal precursors. However nestin is not expressed in the adult brain. Importantly for targeting strategies, nestin is upregulated in human malignant gliomas (58,59). In an elegant study, Kurihara and colleagues utilized a nestin regulatory element whose activity was evaluated by the *lacZ* reporter gene. The authors of this work constructed a nestin gene regulator by placing nestin's second intron before the 5′ upstream region (2iNP). To obtain enhanced expression of this tissue-specific regulator, Kurihara and collaborators utilized the adenovirus double-infection method with a Cre-loxP on/off switching system in seven human glioma cell lines. The authors found X-gal staining and high nestin regulator-promoted beta-galactosidase activities in four of the seven glioma/glioblastoma cell lines. LacZ expression was nearly undetectable in the non-glioma and HeLa cell lines, and it was negligible in COS-7 cells (59).

The enhancer region of the glial fibrillary acidic protein (GFAP) is another glioma-related gene-regulating element that can be used for conditional transcription. It contributes to a high level of reporter gene expression in cells of glial origin, whereas its expression in nonglial cells is undetectable (60). A replication-competent adenovirus with a GFAP promoter placed upstream of E1A could be restricted to acquire a replication phenotype in glioma cells. In an attempt to limit toxic effects on normal tissues, Vandier and collaborators constructed a recombinant adenoviral vector, Adgfa2TK, in which the HSV-TK gene is driven by the GFP promoter (61). Infection with Adgfa2TK of glial cell lines followed by GCV treatment revealed a high level of toxicity in glial cell lines, but little or no toxicity in non-glial cell lines. In vivo, injection of Adgfa2TK into C6 tumors grown in nude mice followed by intraperitoneal GCV treatment significantly repressed tumor growth compared with the controls (61). In another study (60), a replication-incompetent (E1-deleted) adenovirus 5 vector was modified by the addition of three tandem repeats of a 300- bp fragment enhancer region of the GFAP gene coupled to a minimal promoter sequence from human cytomegalovirus to drive a tetracycline-controlled transactivator. Using beta-galactosidase as a reporter gene, this study demonstrated a high level of expression in cells of glial origin (including cell lines derived from GBM) but no detectable expression in non-glial cells (neuroblastoma or fibroblasts). Furthermore, expression was tightly regulated by anhydrous tetracycline. This strategy appears to be the first gene therapy delivery system that is glial-cell specific and also allows for the repression of ectopic gene expression. A most dramatic demonstration of the use of specific promoters to target glial cells occurred during the systemic administration of adenovirus. In one of the most interesting of such studies, Morelli and collaborators utilized recombinant replication-defective adenovirus vectors encoding an apotosis-related molecule under the control of the astrocyte-specific GFAP promoter (62). The cell type-specific expression of FasL was first demonstrated in vitro in glial cells. Furthermore, the authors showed that GFAP-mediated transgene expression was not detected in fibroblastic or epithelial cell lines. As a final test of the stringency of transgene-specific expression, the Ad were injected directly into the bloodstream of mice. Control Ad encoding the therapeutic gene under the control of a non-cell-type-specific promoter induced acute generalized liver hemorrhage with hepatocyte apoptosis, while the Ad containing the GFAP promoter sequences were completely non-toxic. This study demonstrates the specificity of transgene expression, enhanced safety during systemic administration, and tightly regulated control of transgene expression of highly cytotoxic gene products encoded within transcriptionally targeted Ad.

TSP can limit viral replication within a certain tissue type, but viral replication exclusively in cancer cells cannot be expected. Thus, combining the TSP approach with other targeting systems should be used to improve replication selectivity and the safety of the oncolytic viral system. If promoter fidelity in the viral context can be improved, promoter regulation is attractive because it has an advantage, compared with E1A mutants, in that the absence of E1A expression in normal cells may decrease E1A-associated toxicity.

Modifying the Tropism of the Adenovirus—Targeting the Glioma Cell Surface

The entry of adenovirus into cells is initiated when the knob portion of its fiber protein binds with the coxsackie and adenovirus receptor (CAR) on cell surface (63,64). Binding is strengthened by the interaction between the RGD tripeptide amino acid sequence (located at the adenoviral penton base) with $\alpha_v\beta_3$ and $\alpha_v\beta_5$ integrins of the cell (65,66). The native virus receptor CAR is expressed by most normal cell types (67), but is heterogeneous in cancer cells (68). In fact, cancer cells are characterized as a paucity of CAR expression (68). Therefore, modifications in adenovirus are required to limit the tropism to CAR and to redirect the virus to cancer cells. Currently, the use of targeted viral vectors to localize gene transfer to specific cell types is possible and has shown many advantages over conventional, non-targeted vectors in gene therapy strategies for cancer. The resulting improvements from the targeted adenovirus vectors are likely to increase safety and efficacy, reduce immunogenicity and toxicity, and enable the systemic administration of these vectors for multiple indications including cancer.

Compared to a vector with intact native receptor binding interactions, gene expression of the targeted adenoviral vectors in the liver and other organs is substantially reduced following systemic administration of a vector containing mutations that ablate CAR and integrin binding, suggesting that these receptor interactions are important for in vivo gene transfer (69). Similarly, ablation of CAR and integrin binding also results in large reductions in gene transfer following direct adenoviral injection into muscle and brain (70). Although ablation of CAR and integrin binding greatly reduced gene expression in the liver and other organs compared to vectors with an intact native binding mechanism, the vector particles are still rapidly taken up by the liver after intravenous administration (71,72). It thus appears that other interactions are responsible for adenoviral uptake in the liver as well. In addition, ablation of CAR binding alone has not been found to markedly reduce liver gene transfer (73–75), suggesting that the standard two-step model of attachment via the CAR and entry by means of integrins does not apply to in vivo gene transfer to the liver. To target oncolytic Ad to glioma cells, two things are necessary: (1) knock out the native receptor interactions and (2) redirect the vector to a glioma related receptor. Thus, the retargeted Ad will selectively infect glioma cells but not normal cells, including liver cells.

Two general approaches have been used to achieve these basic requirements. The first approach is a one-component system in which the virus particle is genetically modified to ablate native receptor interactions and redirect the virus to a novel receptor. A second general approach is a two-component system in which Ad is complexed with other molecules to redirect binding alone or to both block CAR binding and redirect binding (Table 2) (76).

Table 2 Strategies for Retargeting Adenovirus Tropism to Cancer Cells

Strategies	Ligands	Vectors	Reference
One-component targeting			
Fiber protein HI loop	RGD	Ad5LucRGD, Delta-24-RGD[a]	(77,25)
	HA	AdZ.F2K(HA)	(73)
Fiber protein C-terminus	RGD	AdZ.F(RGD)	(72)
	K20	F/K20-Adv	(90)
Hexon protein	RGD	AE57	(78)
T4 fibritin	CD40L	Ad5LucFF/CD40L	(81)
Protein IX C-terminus	Flag octapeptide	AdLucIXflag	(79)
Two-component targeting			
Bispecific adapter	EGF	AdΔ24-425S11[a]	(99)
Bispecific adapter	FGF	AdCMVLuc + FGF2-Fab	(102)
Bifunctional PEG	uPA	Ad/PEGu7-peptide	(106)

[a] Oncolytic adenovirus.
Abbreviations: HA, hemagglutinin; K20, 20 lysine residues.

One-Component Targeting

In the "one-component" approach, the adenovirus is genetically modified to ablate native receptor interactions and a novel ligand is genetically incorporated into one of the adenovirus coat proteins. However, genetically modifying fiber and other capsid proteins is complicated by the complexity of the adenoviral genome and the viral assembly function of capsid protein. When modifying the genome to improve the specificity of viral infection, the replication and assembly machinery of the virus should be maintained to preserve the potency required for an efficacious oncolytic agent. Hence, the size, position and posttranslational modification of the targeting ligands are critical in determining if a contemplated strategy will be compatible with an oncolytic adenovirus. Inserting ligands into the hexon protein, fiber protein HI loop, C-terminus of fiber protein, C-terminus of capsid protein IX (74,75,77–79), and partially substituting fiber knob protein for phage T4 fibritin (80,81), are among the best examined genetic modifications of the adenovirus capsid.

One of the first successful and encouraging effort made to genetically modify adenoviral tropism was the insertion of the RGD motif (Arg-Gly-Asp) into the hexon protein, HI loop or C-terminal of the viral fiber protein (74,75,77,78). This strategy improved adenoviral entry into cells independently from the expression of CAR. The RGD-retargeted vector increased gene delivery to endothelial and smooth muscle cells expressing αv integrins (74,82).

The expression of CAR is generally minimal in glioma cells (22), which could be explained by CAR's potential role as a tumor suppressor in glioma cells (25,83–85). However, $\alpha_v\beta_3$ and $\alpha_v\beta_5$ integrins are both expressed in glioma cells and in the tumor's vasculature (86). Integrin expression generally correlates with the histologic grade of the tumor. For example, $\alpha_v\beta_3$ expression is prominent in astrocytic tumors. $\alpha_v\beta_3$ and $\alpha_v\beta_5$ integrins are markers of tumor vascularization, particularly endothelial proliferation, which suggests that they have roles in glioma-associated angiogenesis. The $\alpha_v\beta_3$ integrin also participates in neoangiogenesis and cell migration at the periphery of high-grade gliomas (86). Because the cell-receptor scenario in glioma cells consists of low levels of CAR and high levels of RGD-related integrins (83,84), Ad retargeted to bind integrins should be able to circumvent the lack of CAR expression on the glioma cell surface, thus improving viral entry into cancer cells while diminishing the ability of the targeted construct to infect normal brain cells.

In the first report of an oncolytic adenovirus (Delta-24) modified by the genetic introduction of an RGD sequence in the fiber knob domain of a CRAd, the authors showed that the fiber knob protein modification fostered CAR-independent transduction (Fig. 4), enhancing viral propagation and an oncolytic effect in vitro and in vivo in prostate and lung cancers (87). When this RGD-modified vector was later tested in gliomas, it was more cytopathic to both low-and high-CAR-expressing glioma lines than Delta-24, and it replicated more efficiently in both types of cell lines. In glioma xenografted mice, intratumoral injection of Delta-24-RGD was associated with complete regression of the glioma xenografts and longer survival than intratumoral injection of Delta-24 (Fig. 5). Furthermore, 60% of Delta-24-RGD-treated mice but only 15% of Delta-24-treated mice survived longer than 4 months. The antitumor activity of Delta-24-RGD suggests that it has the potential to be an effective agent in the treatment of gliomas (25).

In another attempt to target gliomas via selective infectivity, Yoshida and colleagues generated a fiber-mutant adenovirus vector, F/K20, that encompasses a stretch of 20 lysine residues added at the C terminus of the fiber (88). By using Adv carrying a

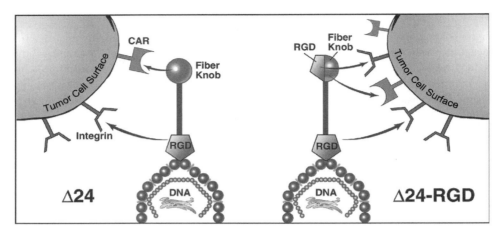

Figure 4 (*See color insert*) CAR-independent infection by Delta-24-RGD. An adenovirus, such as Delta-24, initiates infection by fiber knob-CAR binding that is subsequently strengthened by integrin binding with RGD motif in the penton base. Delta-24-RGD encompasses an ectopic RGD-motif in the knob portion of the fiber. This genomic modification results in CAR-independent infection. This type of tropism modification enhances the oncolytic potency of Delta-24, especially in cancer cells (such as glioma cells) with low CAR but high RGD-related integrin expression on the cell surface.

reporter lacZ gene (AxCAZ2) with either F/K20 or wild-type fiber (F/wt), the authors examined the transduction efficiency of F/K20-Adv. No significant difference in the transduction efficiency between F/K20 and F/wt-Adv was observed in a human fibroblast line or various tumor cell lines, including melanoma, prostate, esophageal, and pancreatic cancer lines. In clear contrast, F/K20-Adv demonstrated a remarkably enhanced efficiency in the genetic transduction of human glioma cells (88). The authors used the mutant adenovirus to transfer therapeutic genes, but a similar system could be utilized to generate replication-competent oncolytic Ad.

In general, one-component systems offer advantages for producing a manufacturable therapeutic adenovirus and for completely ablating all native adenovirus-receptor interactions (76).

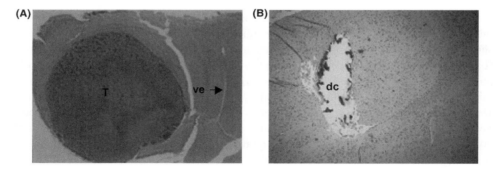

Figure 5 (*See color insert*) Histopathologic examination of the brains of Delta-24-RGD-treated mice. (**A**) Gross morphologic features of a representative tumor. Shown is a hematoxylin-and-eosin-stained coronal section of the brain of a mouse treated with UV-inactivated Delta-24-RGD that died 19 days after implantation of U-87 MG cells. (**B**) Cavity of the dystrophic calcification (dc) is apparent in the basal ganglia implantation site (hematoxylin-and-eosin staining, ×100). T: tumor; ve: lateral ventricle (*arrow*).

Two-Component Targeting

In the "two-component" approach, a bispecific molecule is complexed with the adenovirus. The bispecific component simultaneously blocks native receptor binding and redirects virus binding to a tumor-or tissue-specific receptor, involving a bifunctional adaptor or bridging molecule that binds to the vector and to a target receptor. Some potential targets have been implemented by a "two-component" approach to redirect oncolytic Ad to glioma cells, including, but not limited to, epidermal growth factor receptor (EGFR), fibroblast growth factor receptor (FGFR), and urokinase-type plasminogen activator (uPA).

As many as 90% of high-grade astrocytic gliomas express EGFR, which is associated with EGFR gene amplification in 40% to 50% of GBMs (89–91). EGFR protein overexpression without gene amplification has been reported in 12% to 38% of GBMs (91–93). To take advantage of the fact that EGFR expression is higher in glioma cells than in postmitotic glia and neurons, Delta-24 was directed to EGFR with adapter molecule, resulting in higher infection efficiency and oncolytic replication in CAR-deficient cancer cells and augmented lateral spread in CAR-deficient 3-D tumor spheroids in vitro. Compared to the parental control with native tropism, the new CRAd exhibited a similar level of cytotoxicity in CAR-positive cancer cells, but up to1000-fold enhanced oncolytic potency in CAR-deficient, EGFR-positive cancer cells. In addition, the EGFR-targeted CRAd primary killed human CAR-deficient brain tumor specimens that were refractory to effects from the control virus (94).

Fibroblast growth factors (FGFs) and the FGF signaling pathway likely play significant roles in tumor development and progression (95) and FGF is produced in more than 90% of human glioma and meningioma tissues (96). To target adenovirus to FGF receptor, FGF2 is chemically conjugated to a neutralizing anti-adenoviral antibody to ablate normal viral tropism and confer FGF2 receptor specificity (97). FGF2-retargeted vectors transduced cells at higher levels than non-retargeted vectors. Furthermore, when adenoviral vectors encoding therapeutic transgenes were administered to tumor-bearing animals, the clinical benefit of enhanced transduction was demonstrated by significantly improved survival rates in groups treated with retargeted FGF2 compared to non-retargeted vectors (98).

Because uPAR is overexpressed on the malignant glioma cell surface (99,100), an uPA-retargeted adenovirus would specifically and potently transduce adenovirus into gliomas. A recent report provided support for this hypothesis. A 7-residue peptide derived from uPA (u7-peptide) was coupled to an adenovirus with bifunctional polyethylene glycol (PEG). This retargeted virus transferred the gene more efficiently into human airway epithelial cells that express uPAR (101). Therefore, the EGFR, FGFR, and uPAR could be excellent targets for producing an efficacious adenovirus-mediate therapy for gliomas.

Compared to one-component retargeting, the advantage of two-component approach is that it does not impose serious constraints on the sizes or types of ligands that can be used and offers great flexibility in rapidly validating the feasibility of targeting via a particular receptor. However, this technology is currently limited by the difficulty of applying it to replication-competent Ad. The reason for this is because although delivery can be accomplished by conjugating the virus to ligands, intratumoral spread requires the genetic incorporation of capsid modifications so that they are present in the progeny. Another potential disadvantage is that including the additional protein adaptor increases the number of hurdles to overcome when translating two-component systems into clinical and commercial applications.

PHARMACOLOGICALLY REGULATABLE
ONCOLYTIC ADENOVIRUSES

The safe use of oncolytic Ad in humans could be considerably improved if after injection into the patient, further regulation or inhibition of viral replication outside of the patient was possible. One promising approach appears to be the use of oncolytic adenoviuruses that carry pharmacologically regulatable promoters in addition to the tumor-specific features of conventional replication-competent constructs. This latter feature offers a way to control adenoviral replication temporally and externally. To this end, it has been shown that adenoviral replication can be regulated by controlling E1A gene expression with a mouse mammary tumor virus (MMTV) promoter through the addition of dexamethasone or its antagonist RU486. While the virus with E1A under the control of the human cytomegalovirus immediate early promoter produced constitutively high levels of E1A, a second virus, with E1A expression regulated by the glucocorticoid-responsive MMTV promoter produced E1A expression in a dose-dependent manner upon dexamethasone treatment. Efficient growth of this virus also required the presence of dexamethasone (102).

The E1A and E4 promoters in other oncolytic Ad, have been replaced by a small portion of the pS2 promoter containing two estrogen-responsive elements, or by a minimal dual-specific promoter that responds to estrogen and hypoxia, both for the treatment of estrogen receptor-positive breast cancer (40,103). Furthermore, cytotoxicity was modulated by anti-estrogen treatment in the latter study. Another study found that addition of ganciclovir to an AdV expressing the herpes simplex virus thymide kinase (HSV-*tk*) from an E1B-deleted adenovirus inhibits adenoviral replication in vivo (104).

Other investigators developed a system to control the replication of adenovirus temporally based on the small-molecule dimerizer rapamycin (105). In this system, one adenoviral vector, AdC4, expresses transcription factors whose activity is regulated by the non-immunosuppressive rapamycin analog AP21967. A second vector, Ad(Z12-I-E1aE1b19k), contains E1 genes placed downstream of binding sites for the regulated transcription factor. Co-infection of several cell lines by the vector pair leads to dimerizer-dependent E1 expression and increased viral replication. Furthermore, expression of a reporter gene from a replication-defective vector, Ad-GM-CSF, was augmented by up to 18-fold by co-infection with the pair of conditionally replicating vectors in the presence of dimerizer. Similar results are obtained when the vectors are directly injected into subcutaneous HT1080 xenograft tumors in nude mice.

More recently, Fechner and colleagues developed a novel system allowing external pharmacologic control of adenovirus replication (106). The authors showed that a tumor-selective E1B-deleted oncolytic adenovirus was tightly regulated by doxycycline-controlled adenoviral E1A gene expression, and therefore by vector replication. Oncolytic adenovirus replication was switched on by addition and switched off by withdrawing doxycycline. The system resulted in efficient tumor cell killing after induction by doxycycline, whereas cells were unaffected by the uninduced system. It was also employed for efficient external control of transgene expression from cotransfected replication-deficient adenovectors. Furthermore, a liver cell-specific human alpha-1-antitrypsin-promoter driving a tetracycline-controlled transcriptional silencer allowed specific protection of cells with alpha-1-antitrypsin-promoter activity in the absence of doxycycline in vitro and in vivo (106). This report is the first to delineate a new principle of "tissue protective" gene therapy. The concept of using externally controlled oncolytic Ad has great potential to improve the safety of cancer gene therapy.

ONCOLYTIC ADENOVIRUS AS DELIVERY VEHICLES

Sufficient vector delivery to tumor may be the crux of efficacious gene therapy. Regardless of a vector's potential therapeutic ability, its activity is essentially dependent upon, and limited by the delivery system used. A phase I clinic trial of a replication-deficient adenoviral vector, Ad-p53, demonstrated a disappointing level of delivery in gliomas. An assessment of transduction efficiency demonstrated that p53 was distributed no further than 5–8 mm beyond the catheter with either low or high concentrations of the vector (107). To capitalize on their greater efficiency at disseminating in tumor than replication-deficient vectors, oncolytic viruses have been used to transport genes to enhance anticancer efficacy.

Delivering Therapeutic Genes

The expression of therapeutic genes by oncolytic viruses is a promising strategy that can be used to improve viral oncolysis, augment gene transfer compared with a nonreplicating adenoviral vector, or combine virotherapy and gene therapy.

In animal model experiments, tumor cells transduced with the cytokine interleukin-4 (IL-4) inhibited in vivo tumor growth by stimulating local inflammatory and/or immune responses (108,109). In contrast, interleukin-10 (IL-10) did not cause localized tumor killing or generate host immunity (110). When murine genes encoding IL-4 or IL-10 were delivered via oncolytic herpes simplex viruses (HSV) into intracranial gliomas in immunocompetent mice, IL-4 HSV significantly prolonged the survival of the tumor-bearing mice. Conversely, tumor-bearing mice that received IL-10 HSV had an identical median survival to the saline-treated controls (111). A similar strategy delivers a human interferon consensus gene into tumors using an adenovirus. Complete regression of breast cancer in a mouse xenograft model demonstrated the validity of this approach (112). A new CRAd, AdΔ24-p53, was constructed to express functional p53 while replicating in cancer cells. It exhibited enhanced oncolytic potency in 80% of tested human cancer cell lines with various tissue origins and different p53 statuses. CRAd potency was increased up to >100-fold with the expression of p53 (113). Recently, one group reported on a hTERT-targeted replicative adenovirus expressing mouse endostatin that was used to inhibit neoangiogenesis. This vector suppressed xenografts in nude mice compared to the vector without the transgene (114). Another strategy used the endogenous adenoviral gene expression machinery (promoter, splicing, polyadenylation) to drive transgene expression in the multi-gene E3 transcription unit of a replicating human adenovirus. Superior transgene expression levels were achieved compared to those generated from a replication-deficient virus (115).

Oncolytic viruses have also been used to transport genes to enhance anticancer efficacy by activating prodrugs. The enzyme/prodrug systems delivered by replicating Ad include herpes simplex virus thymidine kinase/ganciclovir (HSV-tk/GCV), cytosine deaminase/5-fluorocytosine (CD/5-FC), and rat cytochrome P450 2B1/cyclophosphamide (CYP2B1/CPA) (116,117). It has been reported that the intrinsic oncolytic effects of E1B-55kD-deleted Ad could be significantly enhanced in several solid xenograft tumor models when followed by the use of a HSV-tk/GVC system, alone or in combination with a CD/5-FC protocol (116,118,119). A shortcoming of this approach is that because activated prodrugs like GCV and 5-FC interfere with DNA metabolism, they can also cause antiviral activity and antagonize viral propagation and cell lysis (120,121). Further research is necessary to assess the replicative potential of the virus/prodrug and the optimal schedule for drug administration to improve the oncolytic effect of the system used. In contrast with the HSVptk/GCV and CD/5-FU paradigms, the CYP2B1/CPA (cyclophosphamide) suicide system does not significantly inhibit viral replication, and the addition of CPA was shown to enhance the oncolytic effects of the virus (116,122). A phase I study of replication-competent adenovirus-mediated double suicide gene therapy for the treatment of locally recurrent prostate cancer demonstrated that intraprostatic administration of the replication-competent Ad5-CD/TKrep virus followed by 2 weeks of 5-FC and GCV prodrug therapy can be safely applied to humans and produces beneficial biologic activity (123,124).

Delivering Therapeutic Small Interfering RNAs (siRNAs)

Posttranscriptional gene silencing (PTGS) or RNA interference (RNAi) are powerful tools for silencing gene expression. This mechanism was initially considered as an aberrant phenomenon limited to few plant species. It has become clear that PTGS occurs in both plants and animals and has roles in viral defense and transposon silencing mechanisms (125). The use of RNAi triggered by the introduction of small double-stranded RNA (dsRNA or siRNA) into mammalian cells as a device to diminish the expression of specific genes can potentially selectively inhibit the expression of disease-associated genes in humans. Among the most dynamic and exciting applications of siRNA are in cancer research and therapy. However, the lack of an efficient delivery system limits its application (126). Because tumor-selective replication-competent viruses are especially suited to efficiently delivering anticancer genes to tumors, they might successfully address this stumbling block. Their intrinsic capacity to kill cancer cells also makes these viruses promising anticancer agents by themselves.

The development of a replication-competent retroviral vector expressing small hairpin RNA (shRNA) under the control of the human H1 promoter was recently reported. The vector-mediated delivery of shRNA targeted against glyceraldehyde-3-phosphate dehydrogenase (GAPDH) specifically reduced GAPDH expression in mammalian cells (127). Moreover, CRAds based on the Delta-24 prototype were constructed by encoding shRNAs targeted against firefly luciferase driven by the RNA polymerase III U6 promoter. These replicating viruses specifically silenced the expression of the target gene in human cancer cells to 30% of control viral levels. This finding shows the promise of using RNAi's in the context of cancer gene therapy via delivery by oncolytic viruses (128).

Delivering Molecules for Monitoring the Kinetics of Viral Infection by Imaging

Noninvasive localization of gene expression (molecular imaging) relies on the transduction of marker genes that encode enzymes or receptors that lead to a regional accumulation of radiolabelled or paramagnetic marker substrates or receptor binding compounds. These substrates or compounds can then be detected by radionuclide or magnetic-resonance imaging (MRI). In addition, I-124-labeled 5-iodo-2′-fluoro-2′deoxy-1-beta-D-arabinofuranosyluracil (FIAU), a specific substrate for HSV-1 thymidine kinase (HSV-1-*tk*), and positron-emission tomography (PET) have been successfully used for the noninvasive localization of retroviral (129), adenoviral (130), and herpes viral (131) vector-mediated HSV-1-*tk* gene expression in rodent models.

When oncolytic Ad are used for cancer research and therapy, it is essential to monitor the kinetics and the expansion of the viruses. When the agents are applied to cancer patients, repeated biopsies for this purpose are an intrusively aggressive way of obtaining information or an impossible approach for those with inaccessible tumors, such as brain tumors. The ability to use oncolytic Ad to transport molecules that could be tracked by imaging would provide a wealth of information to clinicians in the future, and also spare patients numerous long and painful procedures.

Several studies have been already performed in preclinical settings and one, at least, has been performed in the context of a phaseI/II clinical trial in patients with malignant gliomas. An interesting study was conducted using the replication-conditional HSV-1 vector in a nude rat glioma xenograft model. To study vector replication, spread and HSV-1-tk and lacZ gene coexpression in vivo, the accumulation rate of FIAU was measured with PET and coexpressed lacZ gene activity was examined. The investigators found that recombinant HSV-1 vector-mediated HSV-1-tk gene expression can be noninvasively monitored by PET. The temporal and spatial relationships between HSV-1-tk and lacZ gene coexpression in culture and in vivo were also examined. The results showed that indirect in vivo imaging of therapeutic gene expression has potential applicability to tumor tissue infected with any recombinant HSV-1 vector where a therapeutic gene is substituted for the lacZ gene (131). Subsequently, a novel replication-competent adenoviral vector with the HSV1-tk gene in E3 driven by the natural E3 promoter was tested in mice with human glioma xenografts via the radioactive tracer 123I-labeled FIRU. Gamma camera imaging and direct measurement of radioactivity in the tumors revealed increased uptake of tracer with a greater I.U. number and also demonstrated increased accumulation of tracer in the tumors treated with the replication-competent adenoviral vector (132). Importantly, Jacobs and coworkers used PET with [124I]-FIAU, to identify the location, magnitude, and extent of vector-mediated HSV-1-tk gene expression in a phase I/II clinical trial of gene therapy for recurrent glioblastoma in five patients (131). The extent of HSV-1-tk gene expression seemed to predict the therapeutic response. This study dramatically showed that the expression of an exogenous gene introduced by gene therapy into patients with gliomas can be monitored noninvasively by PET.

In another study, the imaging technology used was developed with the human sodium iodide symporter (hNIS), which permits noninvasive monitoring of adenoviral vectors and quantification of gene expression. Measuring vector volume within the tumor was used to optimize adenovirus-mediated suicide gene therapy for prostate cancer. A replication-competent adenovirus (Ad5-yCD/mutTK(SR39)rep-hNIS) coexpressing a therapeutic yeast cytosine deaminase (yCD)/mutant herpes simplex virus thymidine kinase (mutTK(SR39)) fusion gene and the hNIS gene was constructed. Ad5-yCD/mutTK(SR39)rep-hNIS and a replication-defective hNIS adenovirus (rAd-CMV-FLhNIS) were injected into the contralateral lobes of canine prostate tissue and hNIS activity was monitored in live animals following administration of sodium pertechnetate (Na(99m)TcO(4)) using gamma camera scintigraphy. High-resolution autoradiography of prostate sections coupled with 3D reconstruction of gene expression demonstrated that the magnitude and volume of gene expression could be quantified with submillimeter resolution (133).

In addition, a hTERT targeted replication-competent adenovirus co-infected with a replication-deficient adenovirus expressing green fluorescent protein (GFP) revealed fluorescence in cancer cells but not in normal cells in an in vitro study. Established subcutaneous tumors could be visualized by a three-chip color cooled, charged-coupled camera after intratumoral injection of both vectors. Intrathoracic administration of the vectors was used to visualize disseminated tumor nodules in mice after intrathoracic implantation (45).

These preliminary findings in pre-clinical models and a small patient group show that in vivo imaging of gene expression and adenoviral replication is feasible and that vector-mediated gene expression may predict the therapeutic effect. Noninvasive monitoring of the distribution of transgene expression or adenoviral replication over time is highly desirable and will have a critical impact on the development of standardized gene therapy protocols and on efficient and safe vector applications in human beings.

COMBINATION OF ONCOLYSIS AND CHEMOTHERAPY

Combination therapy with agents that act through different mechanisms will hopefully make the emergence of treatment-resistant disease less likely. Ideally, the toxicities associated with the agents used would be nonoverlapping, thereby creating safe combinations for treatment (134). Clinical studies have already shown that viral therapy is well suited for combination with chemotherapy, although the rationale for combining Ad with chemotherapy has not been completely established. The additive synergistic mechanisms of combined therapies that have been observed in the clinical setting are also not yet entirely understood. One hypothesis is that the induction of S phase by E1A adenoviral protein may be responsible for cell cycle-mediated chemosensitivity. In fact, Ad are able to induce a significant number of cells to enter the S phase. An E1A-mutant adenovirus that is unable to bind the Rb protein also produces similar results in cancer cells (22). Overrepresentation of the S phase cell population may augment the effect of concurrently used chemotherapeutic agents and also dramatically improve the anticancer effect of S phase-specific agents such as topoisomerase inhibitors.

Intratumoral adenoviral replication results in the expression of pro-apoptotic molecules, including tumor necrosis factor (135). The presence of tumor necrosis factor in the tumor milieu may improve the efficacy of pro-apoptotic drugs because of its synergistic action with some chemotherapeutic drugs in inducing apoptosis (136,137). The specific ability of Ad to infect and kill arrested cancer cells should improve the anticancer effect of many chemotherapeutic agents that are most effective in actively dividing cells. Also, the adenovirus could target a population of cells that are normally "resistant" to chemotherapeutic drugs. Further investigation is needed to identify the mechanisms underlying the potential synergy between replication-competent adenoviral agents and chemotherapy.

Preclinical murine tumor model studies demonstrated that *dl*1520 can be safely and effectively combined with cisplatin and 5-FU and that efficient viral replication can still occur (12,138). More importantly, evidence of favorable effects from combining adenoviral therapy and chemotherapy has been obtained in multiple trials. Promising clinical data have been obtained from patients with recurrent head and neck cancer treated with intratumoral *dl*1520 and intravenous cisplatin and 5-FU (134,139). Of the 37 patients treated in one study, 19 responded to the therapy, a response rate that compares favorably with chemotherapy alone in previous trials (30% to 40%). Cooperation between the virus and drug was further demonstrated when patients were used as their own controls. Patients with more than one tumor mass had a single tumor injected with *dl*1520, but their remaining masses were not injected with adenovirus. When the treated and untreated masses were exposed to chemotherapy, the effect of adding viral therapy to chemotherapy could be assessed. The *dl*1520-injected tumors had a significantly better response rate and were less likely to progress than the non-injected tumors. Some of the non-injected control tumors that progressed after patients were treated with chemotherapy alone were next treated with *dl*1520. Two of the four injected tumors completely regressed (134).

A pilot trial was conducted to determine the safety and feasibility of treatment with intravenously delivered ONYX-015 in patients with advanced malignancies. The study showed that *dl*1520 could be administered safely in combination with Irinotecan (CPT-11), 5-FU or low-dose IL-2 and was able to access malignant tissue following intravenous infusion (140).

In addition to studies in which Ad were intratumorally and intravenously injected, a phase I/II trial of *dl*1520 administered by hepatic artery infusion in combination with intravenous 5-FU and leukovorin has been performed ($n = 33$ total). Following phase I dose escalation, 15 patients with colorectal carcinoma were treated with combination therapy after failing to respond to either *dl*1520 or chemotherapy alone. One patient had a partial response and 10 patients demonstrated stable disease (134). Because the combined data illustrate the potential value of combining adenoviral therapy with chemotherapeutic interventions, further investigation is warranted.

COMBINATION OF ONCOLYSIS AND RADIOTHERAPY

Radiation therapy is an effective treatment for some localized tumors, although radiotherapy alone is not always successful. Oncolytic Ad that can replicate in cancer cells, force the cells into unscheduled DNA synthesis. It is expected that an increased number of cancer cells in S phase should result in sensitization to radiotherapy. Combining oncolytic Ad and radiotherapy could thus yield a broader therapeutic index. In fact, in vitro studies showed that oncolytic Ad sensitized cancer cells to irradiation (118,141). The viruses potentiated radiation therapy in cervical carcinoma, prostate cancer, lung adenocarcinoma, and malignant glioma animal models (142–146). The same group is currently investigating the replication-competent PSA-selective oncolytic virus CV706 to treat recurrent organ-confined prostate cancer in clinical trials and demonstrated that CV706-mediated cytotoxicity is synergistic with radiation. When radiation therapy was combined with CV706, cytotoxicity was synergistically augmented in the LNCaP human prostate cancer cell line and its animal xenografts. A significant increase of virus burst size, with no reduction in specificity of CV706-based cytopathogenicity in vitro and in vivo was also demonstrated (147). In addition, a phase I study showed that replication-competent adenovirus-mediated double-suicide gene therapy can be combined safely with conventional-dose three-dimensional conformal radiation therapy (3D-CRT) in patients with intermediate-to high-risk prostate cancer (124).

Because preclinical evaluations and clinical trials of replication-competent viruses have produced more promising results when combined with conventional therapeutics, Lamfers and coworkers assessed the effects of Delta-24-RGD in combination with radiotherapy (145). These authors showed that low-dose irradiation before Delta-24-RGD infection decreased the viability of glioma cells more effectively than Delta-24-RGD alone, with effects ranging from additive to supra-additive. In addition, although Delta-24-RGD induced significant tumor growth delay compared with untreated controls and led to long-term survival in 6 of 9 mice, when viral treatment was combined with irradiation, tumor regression occurred in all mice, resulting in long-term survival without evidence of tumor regrowth in all cases. This study thus provided evidence that Delta-24-RGD antitumor activity in malignant glioma can be enhanced by irradiation. These results strongly support further clinical development of Delta-24-RGD in combination with radiation therapy for the treatment of malignant gliomas.

OTHER ONCOLYTIC VIRUSES

In addition to Ad several oncolytic viruses target tumor cells through different avenues. Although there is a wealth of information on HSV used as oncolytic agents (148), we will mention only those strategies that have been translated to the clinical setting. G207 is an attenuated replication-competent HSV1 with defects of both *UL39* and *ICP34.5* expression (149). Loss of *UL39* expression restricts replication of the virus to cells with elevated ribonucleotide reductase activity, presumably because of p16 tumor-suppressor dysfunction. Defects in ICP34.5 function might restrict replication to cells that possess decreased PKR activity (150)—possibly due to expression of a constitutively active form of RAS (151). G207 has been tested in a phase I trial in patients with recurrent malignant glioma (152). Administration was carried out by direct stereotactic injection into the tumor. Doses of up to 3×10^9 infectious units were well tolerated and a maximum tolerated dose was not achieved. This trial showed that inoculation of an attenuated HSV, the wild-type counterpart's main pathogenic effect of which is encephalitis, remained relatively safe in a human brain. The 1716 is an HSV1 mutant with a disruption in the 34.5 gene, which encodes the PKR inhibitor ICP34.5 (153). This oncolytic virus was also well tolerated at doses of up to 10^5 infectious units after stereotactic injection into recurrent malignant gliomas (154). Analysis of tumor explants revealed viral replication at 4–9 days after injection, and the amount of recovered virus exceeded the input dose in at least some patient samples (155).

Based on its ability to infect and kill cells with an activated RAS signaling pathway, human reovirus has been tested as an oncolytic agent in several different rodent tumor models (156). These studies have confirmed that the virus has potent oncolytic activity against several cancers, including glioma xenografts, Most of these mouse tumor therapy studies have been conducted in the absence of a functional immune system using athymic mice bearing human tumor xenografts. However, efficacy was also demonstrated in immune-competent C3H mice bearing tumors established from syngeneic RAS-transformed fibroblasts. Based on these encouraging preclinical data, human reovirus is currently being tested in human cancer therapy trials.

The Newcastle disease virus strain PV706 was evaluated with systemic intravenous administration as part of a phase I, dose-escalation trial in 79 patients who had various advanced solid malignancies (157). This clinical study provided evidence that systemic, intravenous administration of a Newcastle disease virus was well tolerated in humans.

Vesiculostomatitis virus is a naturally occurring OV that specifically replicates in and lyses tumor cell lines with defects in the IFN-/signaling pathway (158). A vaccinia virus with a deletion in the vaccinia growth factor (*vgf*) gene displays oncolytic properties. Vgf acts as a mitogen that primes neighboring cells for subsequent rounds of viral infection. Vaccinia oncolysis can be increased by also deleting the gene that encodes thymidine kinase. Viruses with mutations in both genes have been shown to have oncolytic specificity (159). It is a promising vector for use in tumor-directed gene therapy, given its enhanced safety profile, tumor selectivity, and the oncolytic effects after systemic delivery (159).

Poliovirus is a neuropathogenic virus that infects and propagates in spinal-cord motor neurons, and causes paralytic effects in humans. The neuropathogenic function of the wild-type virus resides within an internal ribosome entry site (IRES) element in the 5′-nontranslated region. When this element is included in viral vectors, it confers neuron-specific translation of genes that are needed for viral propagation. When this IRES element is substituted with an IRES from human rhinovirus type 2, neuron specificity is lost, the virus cannot propagate in neuronal cells and infection of glial tumor cells is facilitated (160).

Measles virus has also been shown to produce oncolytic effects (161). In fact, in anecdotal reports, measles infection has been associated with regression of Burkitt's lymphoma (162). However, the oncolytic targeting mechanism for this virus remains undetermined. Oncolytic effects of mumps, Sendai, Semliki Forest, and Sindbis viruses have also been reported, but little is known about their targeting mechanisms, oncolytic, or cytotoxic properties (163,164).

FUTURE PERSPECTIVES

The underlying concept of treatment with oncolytic viruses is based on cancer selectivity through restricting either viral replication or infectivity in cancer cells, thus improving the therapeutic index of the virus. To achieve this goal, strategies such as functional deletions, TSPs, and modifying tropism have been tested. To optimize cancer selectivity, the strategies were also combined in one viral genome. However, intensely modifying the viral genome may compromise viral potency. Because the adenovirus has evolved as a perfect adaptable genome, the synergistic interrelation between different adenoviral genes is critical for their efficient reproduction. An expanded understanding of cancer biology and adenoviral biology on viral gene organization, protein function, and virus-host interaction is necessary to provide a greater number of precise guidelines for the research and development of oncolytic Ad. The fundamental principle underlying the success of an oncolytic adenovirus is to design a construct by which small and subtle changes in the viral genome produce optimal cancer selectivity while sparing potency.

Despite the rapid replication and spread of oncolytic Ad in cancer cell lines, a major drawback is their limited dissemination in solid tumor masses. As a consequence, repeated viral injections, at multiple sites and over several days, are required to obtain an efficient response (165,166). One of the factors limiting infectivity is the physical barrier within the tumor. Basement membranes, intermixed normal cells within solid tumors, necrotic regions, and the relatively large size of the virus contribute to limiting the spread of viral particles throughout the entire tumor mass. To overcome the barriers, a fusogenic membrane glycoprotein from the human immunodeficiency virus type 1 was used to facilitate dispersion of adenoviral gene products and viral progeny in a syncytial mass. The success of this strategy, which dramatically improved viral particle spreading suggested that adenoviral dispersion could be increased in a tumor mass (167). Other approaches include degradation of the extracellular matrix by proteases, such as trypsin (167).

Malignant gliomas are aggressive, highly invasive and infiltrating. It has been shown that neural progenitor cells can engraft stably into brain tumors and differentiate along neuronal and glial cell lines. This makes transplanting prodrug-converting neural progenitor cells a feasible strategy for brain tumor therapy (168). Recently, glial-restricted progenitor cells as well as embryonic stem cell-derived neural stem cells were efficiently transduced using an adenoviral vector carrying an EGFP expression cassette. The construct demonstrated tropism for F98 glioma cells, via migration towards a spheroid mass of glioma cells. A tendency to form a barrier around the tumor spheroid was shown in an in vitro tumor confrontation model. In vivo, glioma cell-derived tumor formation in the right striatum resulted in migration of glial as well as neural precursor cells towards the tumor area when cotransplanted in the corpus callosum of the contralateral hemisphere in a murine model. Both cell types surrounded the tumor mass and invaded the experimentally induced tumor. These data suggest that glial-restricted and embryonic stem cell-derived neural precursor cells are good candidates as carriers in an ex vivo gene therapeutic approach to glioma therapy (169). A final consideration regarding the use of stem cells as carriers for oncolytic Ad is to the necessity of restraining viral replication before the cells arrive at tumor sites. If any obstacle is solved, the use of stem cells as carriers for oncolytic adenovirus will have the advantage of targeting glioma cells in the brain while circumventing the early immune response during therapy.

For approximately 100 years the brain has been classified as an "immunologically privileged organ." It is now recognized that the brain possesses immunoreactive potential (170). However, evaluating and managing the immune response during virotherapy remains a challenge. Intratumoral injection followed by intracellular viral replication can xenogenize the host against viral antigens expressed by tumor cells, such as E1A protein, and trigger an inflammatory antitumor reaction involving γ-interferon and TNF-α (171). Because the replication cycle of oncolytic Ad spans 2–3 days, only a few cycles of infection can occur before an immune response is mounted against the infecting agent, which can compromise viral spreading (7). In some studies, immunosuppression has been shown to improve viral oncolysis (172), whereas in others a robust immune response produces an antitumor vaccination effect that also improves viral therapeutic effects (173). The actions of the multiple effector arms of the antiviral immune response might provide an explanation for these discordant findings. The initial infection and propagation phases of the virus within a tumor are met with hyperacute and acute immune responses that probably limit oncolysis. In rats, transient complement and antibody depletion enhance oncolytic effects in the initial phases of the virus-tumor interaction (174–176). Innate immune responses against the viral infection might also increase toxicity to the host because of toxic inflammatory effects of complement activation products, and from elevated cytokine levels, such as IL-6 and TNF-α, as shown in a recent clinical trial (157). As tumors regress, however, and tumor (and viral) antigens are released into the circulation, these antigens can be presented to and activate $CD4^+$ and $CD8^+$ T cells, and lead to the immune destruction of any residual or subsequent tumors (173). Pharmacologic modulation (174,176) or genetic alteration of oncolytic viruses (173) can be used to activate or inhibit different immune mediators. This approach could be used to aid the initial phases of viral infection and propagation within tumors, and to elicit long-lasting immune responses against residual and recurrent tumors.

Neutralizing immunity can limit gene transfer by viral vectors, and this problem has been addressed through various methods. One approach has been to use viral vectors derived from non-human viruses. For example, a simian adenovirus vector has been developed that avoids the preexisting immunity found in humans (177) and could presumably be targeted in a similar manner to human adenovirus vectors. Although this approach offers a means of avoiding preexisting immunity, it does not circumvent the subsequent generation of neutralizing antibodies after initial administration. Another approach to avoid antibody-mediated neutralization as well as clearance mechanisms has been to coat the vector with a polymer such as PEG (178) or poly-[N-(2-hydroxypropyl)methacrylamide] (pHPMA) (179). The polymer may shield the virus from interacting with its native receptor, as well as neutralizing antibodies and may protect the vector from innate clearance mechanisms in the liver subsequent to intravenous injection. Ligands have also been linked to either the PEG or pHPMA polymers to target the vector (180). However, when using PEG as the shielding agent, achieving the proper amount of PEGylation may require some fine-tuning. Also still to be determined are whether targeted gene transfer can be achieved upon systemic delivery and how adaptable the system is for using different types of targeting ligands. Specifically in the case of oncolytic Ad, the lack of suitable animal models for these types of studies requires addressing these problems directly in a clinical setting. Development of accurate syngeneic animal models would be of extraordinary relevance to improve the accuracy of the effectiveness of the replicating competent adenovirus in pre-clinical studies.

In conclusion, oncolytic viruses have opened a new avenue for cancer therapy. With the joint efforts of scientists and clinicians to optimize the modification and application of such agents oncolytic viruses will become important tools in the future therapy of patients with malignant gliomas. In the near future, highly improved oncolytic systems will show that in the fiery battle between genetically modified viruses and cancer cells, the former will prevail.

ACKNOWLEDGMENTS

We thank Joann Aaron (Department of Neuro-Oncology, The University of Texas M. D. Anderson Cancer Center) for editorial assistance.

REFERENCES

1. Kleihues P, Cavenee WK. Pathology and genetics of tumors of the nervous system. Lyon,France: IARC-Press, 2000.
2. Holland EC. Glioblastoma multiforme: the terminator. Proc Natl Acad Sci USA 2000; 97:6242–6244.
3. Giese A, Westphal M. Treatment of malignant glioma: a problem beyond the margins of resection. J Cancer Res Clin Oncol 2001; 127:217–225.
4. Maher EA, Furnari FB, Bachoo RM, et al. Malignant glioma: genetics and biology of a grave matter. Genes Dev 2001; 15:1311–1333.
5. Lang FF, Yung WK, Sawaya R, et al. Adenovirus-mediated p53 gene therapy for human gliomas. Neurosurgery 1999; 45:1093–1104.
6. Lang FF, Bruner JM, Fuller GN, et al. Phase I trial of adenovirus-mediated p53 gene therapy for recurrent glioma: biological and clinical results. J Clin Oncol 2003; 21:2508–2518.
7. Haviv YS, Curiel DT. Engineering regulatory elements for conditionally-replicative adenoviruses. Curr Gene Ther 2003; 3:357–385.
8. Sinkovics J, Horvath J. New developments in the virus therapy of cancer: a historical review. Intervirology 1993; 36:193–214.
9. Kirn D. Replication-selective oncolytic adenoviruses: virotherapy aimed at genetic targets in cancer. Oncogene 2000; 19:6660–6669.
10. Bischoff JR, Kirn DH, Williams A, et al. An adenovirus mutant that replicates selectively in p53-deficient human tumor cells. Science 1996; 274:373–376.
11. Barker DD, Berk AJ. Adenovirus proteins from both E1B reading frames are required for transformation of rodent cells by viral infection and DNA transfection. Virology 1987; 156:107–121.
12. Heise C, Sampson-Johannes A, Williams A, et al. ONYX-015, an E1B gene-attenuated adenovirus, causes tumor-specific cytolysis and antitumoral efficacy that can be augmented by standard chemotherapeutic agents. Nat Med 1997; 3:639–645.
13. McCormick F. Cancer-specific viruses and the development of ONYX-015. Cancer Biol Ther 2003; 2:S157–S160.

14. Nemunaitis J, Khuri F, Ganly I, et al. Phase II trial of intratumoral administration of ONYX-015, a replication-selective adenovirus, in patients with refractory head and neck cancer. J Clin Oncol 2001; 19:289–298.

15. Khuri FR, Nemunaitis J, Ganly I, et al. A controlled trial of intratumoral ONYX-015, a selectively-replicating adenovirus, in combination with cisplatin and 5-fluorouracil in patients with recurrent head and neck cancer. Nat Med 2000; 6:879–885.

16. Chiocca EA, Abbed KM, Tatter S, et al. A phase I open-label, dose-escalation, multi-institutional trial of injection with an E1B-Attenuated adenovirus, ONYX-015, into the peritumoral region of recurrent malignant gliomas, in the adjuvant setting. Mol Ther 2004; 10:958–966.

17. Harrison D, Sauthoff H, Heitner S, et al. Wild-type adenovirus decreases tumor xenograft growth, but despite viral persistence complete tumor responses are rarely achieved—deletion of the viral E1b-19-kD gene increases the viral oncolytic effect. Hum Gene Ther 2001; 12:1323–1332.

18. Sherr CJ. Cancer cell cycles. Science 1996; 274:1672–1677.

19. Whyte P, Williamson NM, Harlow E. Cellular targets for transformation by the adenovirus E1A proteins. Cell 1989; 56:67–75.

20. Putzer BM, Rumpf H, Rega S, et al. E1A 12S and 13S of the transformation-defective adenovirus type 12 strain CS-1 inactivate proteins of the RB family, permitting transactivation of the E2F-dependent promoter. J Virol 1997; 71:9538–9548.

21. Howe JA, Demers GW, Johnson DE, et al. Evaluation of E1-mutant adenoviruses as conditionally replicating agents for cancer therapy. Mol Ther 2000; 2:485–495.

22. Fueyo J, Gomez-Manzano C, Alemany R, et al. A mutant oncolytic adenovirus targeting the Rb pathway produces anti-glioma effect in vivo. Oncogene 2000; 19:2–12.

23. Heise C, Hermiston T, Johnson L, et al. An adenovirus E1A mutant that demonstrates potent and selective systemic anti-tumoral efficacy. Nat Med 2000; 6:1134–1139.

24. Bauerschmitz GJ, Lam JT, Kanerva A, et al. Treatment of ovarian cancer with a tropism modified oncolytic adenovirus. Cancer Res 2002; 62:1266–1270.

25. Fueyo J, Alemany R, Gomez-Manzano C, et al. Preclinical characterization of the antiglioma activity of a tropism-enhanced adenovirus targeted to the retinoblastoma pathway. J Natl Cancer Inst 2003; 95:652–660.

26. Ramachandra M, Rahman A, Zou A, et al. Re-engineering adenovirus regulatory pathways to enhance oncolytic specificity and efficacy. Nat Biotechnol 2001; 19:1035–1041.

27. Tollefson AE, Scaria A, Hermiston TW, et al. The adenovirus death protein (E3-11.6K) is required at very late stages of infection for efficient cell lysis and release of adenovirus from infected cells. J Virol 1996; 70:2296–2306.

28. Gomez-Manzano C, Balague C, Alemany R, et al. A novel E1A-E1B mutant adenovirus induces glioma regression in vivo. Oncogene 2004; 23:1821–1828.

29. Nevins JR. Mechanism of activation of early viral transcription by the adenovirus E1A gene product. Cell 1981; 26:213–220.

30. Steinwaerder DS, Carlson CA, Lieber A. DNA replication of first-generation adenovirus vectors in tumor cells. Hum Gene Ther 2000; 11:1933–1948.

31. Steinwaerder DS, Carlson CA, Otto DL, et al. Tumor-specific gene expression in hepatic metastases by a replication-activated adenovirus vector. Nat Med 2001; 7:240–243.

32. Yu DC, Chen Y, Seng M, et al. The addition of adenovirus type 5 region E3 enables calydon virus 787 to eliminate distant prostate tumor xenografts. Cancer Res 1999; 59:4200–4203.

33. Zhang Y, Schneider RJ. Adenovirus inhibition of cell translation facilitates release of virus particles and enhances degradation of the cytokeratin network. J Virol 1994; 68:2544–2555.

34. Yu DC, Sakamoto GT, Henderson DR. Identification of the transcriptional regulatory sequences of human kallikrein 2 and their use in the construction of calydon virus 764, an attenuated replication competent adenovirus for prostate cancer therapy. Cancer Res 1999; 59:1498–1504.

35. Hallenbeck PL, Chang YN, Hay C, et al. A novel tumor-specific replication-restricted adenoviral vector for gene therapy of hepatocellular carcinoma. Hum Gene Ther 1999; 10:1721–1733.

36. Rodriguez R, Schuur ER, Lim HY, et al. Prostate attenuated replication competent adenovirus (ARCA) CN706: a selective cytotoxic for prostate-specific antigen-positive prostate cancer cells. Cancer Res 1997; 57:2559–2563.

37. Parr MJ, Manome Y, Tanaka T, et al. Tumor-selective transgene expression in vivo mediated by an E2F-responsive adenoviral vector. Nat Med 1997; 3:1145–1149.

38. Tsukuda K, Wiewrodt R, Molnar-Kimber K, et al. An E2F-responsive replication-selective adenovirus targeted to the defective cell cycle in cancer cells: potent antitumoral efficacy but no toxicity to normal cell. Cancer Res 2002; 62:3438–3447.

39. Jakubczak JL, Ryan P, Gorziglia M, et al. An oncolytic adenovirus selective for retinoblastoma tumor suppressor protein pathway-defective tumors: dependence on E1A, the E2F-1 promoter, and viral replication for selectivity and efficacy. Cancer Res 2003; 63:1490–1499.

40. Hernandez-Alcoceba R, Pihalja M, Qian D, et al. New oncolytic adenoviruses with hypoxia- and estrogen receptor-regulated replication. Hum Gene Ther 2002; 13:1737–1750.

41. Blasco MA. Telomeres and cancer: a tale with many endings. Curr Opin Genet Dev 2003; 13:70–76.

42. Huang TG, Savontaus MJ, Shinozaki K, et al. Telomerase-dependent oncolytic adenovirus for cancer treatment. Gene Ther 2003; 10:1241–1247.

43. Zou W, Luo C, Zhang Z, et al. A novel oncolytic adenovirus targeting to telomerase activity in tumor cells with potent. Oncogene 2004; 23:457–464.

44. Kawashima T, Kagawa S, Kobayashi N, et al. Telomerase-specific replication-selective virotherapy for human cancer. Clin Cancer Res 2004; 10:285–292.

45. Umeoka T, Kawashima T, Kagawa S, et al. Visualization of intrathoracically disseminated solid tumors in mice with optical imaging by telomerase-specific amplification of a transferred green fluorescent protein gene. Cancer Res 2004; 64:6259–6265.

46. Kim E, Kim JH, Shin HY, et al. Ad-mTERT-delta19, a conditional replication-competent adenovirus driven by the human telomerase promoter, selectively replicates in and elicits cytopathic effect in a cancer cell-specific manner. Hum Gene Ther 2003; 14:1415–1428.

47. Komata T, Kanzawa T, Kondo Y, et al. Telomerase as a therapeutic target for malignant gliomas. Oncogene 2002; 21:656–663.

48. Giaccia A, Siim BG, Johnson RS. HIF-1 as a target for drug development. Nat Rev Drug Discov 2003; 2:803–811.

49. Welsh SJ, Powis G. Hypoxia inducible factor as a cancer drug target. Curr Cancer Drug Targets 2003; 3:391–405.

50. Cuevas Y, Hernandez-Alcoceba R, Aragones J, et al. Specific oncolytic effect of a new hypoxia-inducible factor-dependent replicative adenovirus on von Hippel-Lindau-defective renal cell carcinomas. Cancer Res 2003; 63:6877–6884.

51. Post DE, Van Meir EG. A novel hypoxia-inducible factor (HIF) activated oncolytic adenovirus for cancer therapy. Oncogene 2003; 22:2065–2072.

52. Ruan H, Wang J, Hu L, et al. Killing of brain tumor cells by hypoxia-responsive element mediated expression of BAX. Neoplasia 1999; 1:431–437.

53. Fuerer C, Iggo R. Adenoviruses with Tcf binding sites in multiple early promoters show enhanced selectivity for tumour cells with constitutive activation of the wnt signalling pathway. Gene Ther 2002; 9:270–281.

54. Xie D, Yin D, Tong X, et al. Cyr61 is overexpressed in gliomas and involved in integrin-linked kinase-mediated Akt and beta-catenin-TCF/Lef signaling pathways. Cancer Res 2004; 64:1987–1996.

55. Yamamoto M, Davydova J, Wang M, et al. Infectivity enhanced, cyclooxygenase-2 promoter-based conditionally replicative adenovirus for pancreatic cancer. Gastroenterology 2003; 125:1203–1218.

56. Davydova J, Le LP, Gavrikova T, et al. Infectivity-enhanced cyclooxygenase-2-based conditionally replicative adenoviruses for esophageal adenocarcinoma treatment. Cancer Res 2004; 64:4319–4327.

57. Nathoo N, Barnett GH, Golubic M. The eicosanoid cascade: possible role in gliomas and meningiomas. J Clin Pathol 2004; 57:6–13.

58. Holland EC. A mouse model for glioma: biology, pathology, and therapeutic opportunities. Toxicol Pathol 2000; 28:171–177.

59. Kurihara H, Zama A, Tamura M, et al. Glioma/glioblastoma-specific adenoviral gene expression using the nestin gene regulator. Gene Ther 2000; 7:686–693.

60. Chen J, Bezdek T, Chang J, et al. A glial-specific, repressible, adenovirus vector for brain tumor gene therapy. Cancer Res 1998; 58:3504–3507.

61. Vandier D, Rixe O, Besnard F, et al. Inhibition of glioma cells in vitro and in vivo using a recombinant adenoviral vector containing an astrocyte-specific promoter. Cancer Gene Ther 2000; 7:1120–1126.

62. Morelli AE, Larregina AT, Smith-Arica J, et al. Neuronal and glial cell type-specific promoters within adenovirus recombinants restrict the expression of the apoptosis-inducing molecule Fas ligand to predetermined brain cell types, and abolish peripheral liver toxicity. J Gen Virol 1999; 80:571–583.

63. Bergelson JM, Cunningham JA, Droguett G, et al. Isolation of a common receptor for Coxsackie B viruses and adenoviruses 2 and 5. Science 1997; 275:1320–1323.

64. Tomko RP, Xu R, Philipson L. HCAR and MCAR:the human and mouse cellular receptors for subgroup C adenoviruses and group B coxsackieviruses. Proc Natl Acad Sci USA 1997; 94:3352–3356.

65. Wickham TJ, Mathias P, Cheresh DA, et al. Integrins alpha v beta 3 and alpha v beta 5 promote adenovirus internalization but not virus attachment. Cell 1993; 73:309–319.

66. Seth P. Adenoviruses: Basic Biology to Gene Therapy. Austin,Texas: R.G. Landes Company, 1999 pp. 31–35.

67. Hitt MM, Addison CL, Graham FL. Human adenovirus vectors for gene transfer into mammalian cells. Adv Pharmacol 1997; 40:137–206.

68. Miller CR, Buchsbaum DJ, Reynolds PN, et al. Differential susceptibility of primary and established human glioma cells to adenovirus infection: targeting via the epidermal growth factor receptor achieves fiber receptor-independent gene transfer. Cancer Res 1998; 58:5738–5748.

69. Einfeld DA, Schroeder R, Roelvink PW, et al. Reducing the native tropism of adenovirus vectors requires removal of both CAR and integrin interactions. J Virol 2001; 75:11284–11291.

70. Thomas CE, Edwards P, Wickham TJ, et al. Adenovirus binding to the coxsackievirus and adenovirus receptor or integrins is not required to elicit brain inflammation but is necessary to transduce specific neural cell types. J Virol 2002; 76:3452–3460.

71. Everett RS, Hodges BL, Ding EY, et al. Liver toxicities typically induced by first-generation adenoviral vectors can be reduced by use of E1, E2b-deleted adenoviral vectors. Hum Gene Ther 2003; 14:1715–1726.

72. Mahasreshti PJ, Kataram M, Wang MH, et al. Intravenous delivery of adenovirus-mediated soluble FLT-1 results in liver toxicity. Clin Cancer Res 2003; 9:2701–2710.

73. Michael SI, Hong JS, Curiel DT, et al. Addition of a short peptide ligand to the adenovirus fiber protein. Gene Ther 1995; 2:660–668.

74. Wickham TJ, Tzeng E, Shears LL, et al. Increased in vitro and in vivo gene transfer by adenovirus vectors containing chimeric fiber proteins. J Virol 1997; 71:8221–8229.

75. Einfeld DA, Brough DE, Roelvink PW, et al. Construction of a pseudoreceptor that mediates transduction by adenoviruses expressing a ligand in fiber or penton base. J Virol 1999; 73:9130–9136.

76. Wickham TJ. Targeting adenovirus. Gene Ther 2000; 7:110–114.

77. Reynolds P, Dmitriev I, Curiel D. Insertion of an RGD motif into the HI loop of adenovirus fiber protein alters the distribution of transgene expression of the systemically administered vector. Gene Ther 1999; 6:1336–1339.

78. Vigne E, Mahfouz I, Dedieu JF, et al. RGD inclusion in the hexon monomer provides adenovirus type 5-based vectors with a fiber knob-independent pathway for infection. J Virol 1999; 73:5156–5161.

79. Dmitriev IP, Kashentseva EA, Curiel DT. Engineering of adenovirus vectors containing heterologous peptide sequences in the C terminus of capsid protein IX. J Virol 2002; 76:6893–6899.

80. Krasnykh V, Belousova N, Korokhov N, et al. Genetic targeting of an adenovirus vector via replacement of the fiber protein with the phage T4 fibritin. J Virol 2001; 75:4176–4183.

81. Belousova N, Korokhov N, Krendelshchikova V, et al. Genetically targeted adenovirus vector directed to CD40-expressing cells. J Virol 2003; 77:11367–11377.

82. McDonald GA, Zhu G, Li Y, et al. Efficient adenoviral gene transfer to kidney cortical vasculature utilizing a fiber modified vector. J Gene Med 1999; 1:103–110.

83. Mori T, Arakawa H, Tokino T, et al. Significant increase of adenovirus infectivity in glioma cell lines by extracellular domain of hCAR. Oncol Res 1999; 11:513–521.

84. Asaoka K, Tada M, Sawamura Y, et al. Dependence of efficient adenoviral gene delivery in malignant glioma cells on the expression levels of the Coxsackievirus and adenovirus receptor. J Neursurg 2000; 92:1002–1008.

85. Kim M, Sumerel LA, Belousova N, et al. The coxsackievirus and adenovirus receptor acts as a tumour suppressor in malignant glioma cells. Br J Cancer 2003; 88:1411–1416.

86. Bello L, Francolini M, Marthyn P, et al. Alpha(v)beta3 and alpha(v)beta5 integrin expression in glioma periphery. Neurosurgery 2001; 49:380–389 discussion 390.

87. Suzuki K, Fueyo J, Krasnykh V, et al. A conditionally replicative adenovirus with enhanced infectivity shows improved oncolytic potency. Clin Cancer Res 2001; 7:120–126.

88. Yoshida Y, Sadata A, Zhang W, et al. Generation of fiber-mutant recombinant adenoviruses for gene therapy of malignant glioma. Hum Gene Ther 1998; 9:2503–2515.

89. Libermann TA, Nusbaum HR, Razon N, et al. Amplification, enhanced expression and possible rearrangement of EGF receptor gene in primary human brain tumours of glial origin. Nature 1985; 313:144–147.

90. McLendon RE, Wikstrand CJ, Matthews MR, et al. Glioma-associated antigen expression in oligodendroglial neoplasms:tenascin and epidermal growth factor receptor. J Histochem Cytochem 2000; 48:1103–1110.

91. Kuan CT, Wikstrand CJ, Bigner DD. EGF mutant receptor vIII as a molecular target in cancer therapy. Endocr Relat Cancer 2001; 8:83–96.

92. Chaffanet M, Chauvin C, Laine M, et al. EGF receptor amplification and expression in human brain tumours. Eur J Cancer 1992; 28:11–17.

93. Tsugu A, Kijima H, Yamazaki H, et al. Localization of aberrant messenger RNA of epidermal growth factor receptor (EGFR) in malignant glioma. Anticancer Res 1997; 17:2225–2232.

94. van Beusechem VW, Mastenbroek DC, van den Doel PB, et al. Conditionally replicative adenovirus expressing a targeting adapter molecule exhibits enhanced oncolytic potency on CAR-deficient tumors. Gene Ther 2003; 10:1982–1991.

95. Powers CJ, McLeskey SW, Wellstein A. Fibroblast growth factors, their receptors and signaling. Endocr Relat Cancer 2000; 7:165–197.

96. Morrison RS. Suppression of basic fibroblast growth factor expression by antisense oligodeoxynucleotides inhibits the growth of transformed human astrocytes. J Biol Chem 1991; 266:728–734.

97. Goldman CK, Rogers BE, Douglas JT, et al. Targeted gene delivery to Kaposi's sarcoma cells via the fibroblast growth factor receptor. Cancer Res 1997; 57:1447–1451.

98. Rancourt C, Rogers BE, Sosnowski BA, et al. Basic fibroblast growth factor enhancement of adenovirus-mediated delivery of the herpes simplex virus thymidine kinase gene results in augmented therapeutic benefit in a murine model of ovarian cancer. Clin Cancer Res 1998; 4:2455–2461.

99. Mignatti P, Rifkin DB. Biology and biochemistry of proteinases in tumor invasion. Physiol Rev 1993; 73:161–195.

100. Murphy G, Atkinson S, Ward R, et al. The role of plasminogen activators in the regulation of connective tissue metalloproteinases. Ann NY Acad Sci 1992; 667:1–12.

101. Drapkin PT, O'Riordan CR, Yi SM, et al. Targeting the urokinase plasminogen activator receptor enhances gene transfer to human airway epithelia. J Clin Invest 2000; 105:589–596.

102. Avvakumov N, Mymryk JS. New tools for the construction of replication-competent adenoviral vectors with altered E1A regulation. J Virol Methods 2002; 103:41–49.

103. Hernandez-Alcoceba R, Pihalja M, Wicha MS, et al. A novel, conditionally replicative adenovirus for the treatment of breast cancer that allows controlled replication of E1a-deleted adenoviral vectors. Hum Gene Ther 2000; 11:2009–2024.

104. Wildner O, Morris JC. The role of the E1B 55 kDa gene product in oncolytic adenoviral vectors expressing herpes simplex virus-tk: assessment of antitumor efficacy and toxicity. Cancer Res 2000; 60:4167–4174.

105. Chong H, Ruchatz A, Clackson T, et al. A system for small-molecule control of conditionally replication-competent adenoviral vectors. Mol Ther 2002; 5:195–203.

106. Fechner H, Wang X, Srour M, et al. A novel tetracycline-controlled transactivator-transrepressor system enables external control of oncolytic adenovirus replication. Gene Ther 2003; 10:1680–1690.

107. Vecil GG, Lang FF. Clinical trials of adenoviruses in brain tumors: a review of Ad-p53 and oncolytic adenoviruses. J Neurooncol 2003; 65:237–246.

108. Tepper RI. Experimental and clinical studies of cytokine gene-modified tumor cells. Hum Gene Ther 1994; 5:153–164.

109. Golumbek PT, Lazenby AJ, Levitsky HI, et al. Treatment of established renal cancer by tumor cells engineered to secrete interleukin-4. Science 1991; 254:713–716.

110. Richter G, Kruger-Krasagakes S, Hein G, et al. Interleukin 10 transfected into Chinese hamster ovary cells prevents tumor growth and macrophage infiltration. Cancer Res 1993; 53:4134–4137.

111. Andreansky S, He B, van Cott J, et al. Treatment of intracranial gliomas in immunocompetent mice using herpes simplex viruses that express murine interleukins. Gene Ther 1998; 5:121–130.

112. Zhang JF, Hu C, Geng Y, et al. Treatment of a human breast cancer xenograft with an adenovirus vector containing an interferon gene results in rapid regression due to viral oncolysis and gene therapy. Proc Natl Acad Sci USA 1996; 93:4513–4518.

113. van Beusechem VW, van den Doel PB, Grill J, et al. Conditionally replicative adenovirus expressing p53 exhibits enhanced oncolytic potency. Cancer Res 2002; 62:6165–6171.

114. Zhang Q, Nie M, Sham J, et al. Effective gene-viral therapy for telomerase-positive cancers by selective replicative-competent adenovirus combining with endostatin gene. Cancer Res 2004; 64:5390–5397.

115. Hawkins LK, Johnson L, Bauzon M, et al. Gene delivery from the E3 region of replicating human adenovirus: evaluation of the 6.7 K/gp19 K region. Gene Ther 2001; 8:1123–1131.

116. Wildner O. Oncolytic viruses as therapeutic agents. Ann Med 2001; 33:291–304.

117. Smith ER, Chiocca EA. Oncolytic viruses as novel anticancer agents: turning one scourge against another. Exp Opin Invest Drugs 2000; 9:311–327.

118. Freytag SO, Rogulski KR, Paielli DL, et al. A novel three-pronged approach to kill cancer cells selectively: concomitant viral, double suicide gene, and radiotherapy. Hum Gene Ther 1998; 9:1323–1333.

119. Wildner O, Morris JC, Vahanian NN, et al. Adenoviral vectors capable of replication improve the efficacy of HSVtk/GCV suicide gene therapy of cancer. Gene Ther 1999; 6:57–62.

120. Carroll NM, Chase M, Chiocca EA, et al. The effect of ganciclovir on herpes simplex virus-mediated oncolysis. J Surg Res 1997; 69:413–417.

121. Todo T, Rabkin SD, Martuza RL. Evaluation of ganciclovir-mediated enhancement of the antitumoral effect in oncolytic, multimutated herpes simplex virus type 1 (G207) therapy of brain tumors. Cancer Gene Ther 2000; 7:939–946.

122. Chase M, Chung RY, Chiocca EA. An oncolytic viral mutant that delivers the CYP2B1 transgene and augments cyclophosphamide chemotherapy. Nat Biotechnol 1998; 16:444–448.

123. Freytag SO, Khil M, Stricker H, et al. Phase I study of replication-competent adenovirus-mediated double suicide gene therapy for the treatment of locally recurrent prostate cancer. Cancer Res 2002; 62:4968–4976.

124. Freytag SO, Stricker H, Pegg J, et al. Phase I study of replication-competent adenovirus-mediated double-suicide gene therapy in combination with conventional-dose three-dimensional conformal radiation therapy for the treatment of newly diagnosed, intermediate- to high-risk prostate cancer. Cancer Res 2003; 63:7497–7506.

125. McManus MT, Sharp PA. Gene silencing in mammals by small interfering RNAs. Nat Rev Genet 2002; 3:737–747.

126. Scherer LJ, Rossi JJ. Approaches for the sequence-specific knockdown of mRNA. Nat Biotechnol 2003; 21:1457–1465.

127. Bromberg-White JL, Webb CP, Patacsil VS, et al. Delivery of short hairpin RNA sequences by using a replication-competent avian retroviral vector. J Virol 2004; 78:4914–4916.

128. Carette JE, Overmeer RM, Schagen FH, et al. Conditionally replicating adenoviruses expressing short hairpin RNAs silence the expression of a target gene in cancer cells. Cancer Res 2004; 64:2663–2667.

129. Tjuvajev JG, Stockhammer G, Desai R, et al. Imaging the expression of transfected genes in vivo. Cancer Res 1995; 55:6126–6132.

130. Gambhir SS, Herschman HR, Cherry SR, et al. Imaging transgene expression with radionuclide imaging technologies. Neoplasia 2000; 2:118–138.

131. Jacobs A, Tjuvajev JG, Dubrovin M, et al. Positron emission tomography-based imaging of transgene expression mediated by replication-conditional, oncolytic herpes simplex virus type 1 mutant vectors in vivo. Cancer Res 2001; 61:2983–2995.

132. Nanda D, de Jong M, Vogels R, et al. Imaging expression of adenoviral HSV1-tk suicide gene transfer using the nucleoside analogue FIRU. Eur J Nucl Med Mol Imaging 2002; 29:939–947.

133. Barton KN, Tyson D, Stricker H, et al. GENIS: gene expression of sodium iodide symporter for noninvasive imaging of gene therapy vectors and quantification of gene expression in vivo. Mol Ther 2003; 8:508–518.

134. Kirn D. Oncolytic virotherapy for cancer with the adenovirus dl1520 (Onyx-015): results of phase I and II trials. Exp Opin Biol Ther 2001; 1:525–538.

135. Rhoades KL, Golub SH, Economou JS. The adenoviral transcription factor, E1A 13S, trans-activates the human tumor necrosis factor-alpha promoter. Virus Res 1996; 40:65–74.

136. Lienard D. High-dose recombinant tumor necrosis factor alpha in combination with interferon gamma and melphalan in isolation perfusion of the limbs for melanoma and sarcoma. J Clin Oncol 1992; 10:52–60.

137. Lejeune FJ, Ruegg C, Lienard D. Clinical applications of TNF-alpha in cancer. Curr Opin Immunol 1998; 10:573–580.

138. Heise C, Lemmon M, Kirn D. Efficacy with a replication-selective adenovirus plus cisplatin-based chemotherapy: dependence on sequencing but not p53 functional status or route of administration. Clin Cancer Res 2000; 6:4908–4914.

139. Biederer C, Ries S, Brandts CH, et al. Replication-selective viruses for cancer therapy. J Mol Med 2002; 80:163–175.

140. Nemunaitis J, Cunningham C, Tong AW, et al. Pilot trial of intravenous infusion of a replication-selective adenovirus (ONYX-015) in combination with chemotherapy or IL-2 treatment in refractory cancer patients. Cancer Gene Ther 2003; 10:341–352.

141. Rogulski KR, Freytag SO, Zhang K, et al. In vivo antitumor activity of ONYX-015 is influenced by p53 status and is augmented by radiotherapy. Cancer Res 2000; 60:1193–1196.

142. Rogulski KR, Wing MS, Paielli DL, et al. Double suicide gene therapy augments the antitumor activity of a replication-competent lytic adenovirus through enhanced cytotoxicity and radiosensitization. Hum Gene Ther 2000; 11:67–76.

143. Freytag SO, Paielli D, Wing M, et al. Efficacy and toxicity of replication-competent adenovirus-mediated double suicide gene therapy in combination with radiation therapy in an orthotopic mouse prostate cancer model. Int J Radiat Oncol Biol Phys 2002; 54:873–885.

144. Toth K, Tarakanova V, Doronin K, et al. Radiation increases the activity of oncolytic adenovirus cancer gene therapy vectors that overexpress the ADP (E3-11.6K) protein. Cancer Gene Ther 2003; 10:193–200.

145. Lamfers ML, Grill J, Dirven CM, et al. Potential of the conditionally replicative adenovirus Ad5-Delta24RGD in the treatment of malignant gliomas and its enhanced effect with radiotherapy. Cancer Res 2002; 62:5736–5742.

146. Geoerger B, Grill J, Opolon P, et al. Potentiation of radiation therapy by the oncolytic adenovirus dl1520 (ONYX-015) in human malignant glioma xenografts. Br J Cancer 2003; 89:577–584.

147. Chen MJ, Chung-Faye GA, Searle PF, et al. Gene therapy for colorectal cancer: therapeutic potential. Biodrugs 2001; 15:357–367.

148. Wakimoto H, Johnson PR, Knipe DM, et al. Effects of innate immunity on herpes simplex virus and its ability to kill tumor cells. Gene Ther 2003; 10:983–990.

149. Mineta T, Rabkin SD, Yazaki T, et al. Attenuated multi-mutated herpes simplex virus-1 for the treatment of malignant gliomas. Nat Med 1995; 1:938–943.

150. Leib DA, Machalek MA, Williams BR, et al. Specific phenotypic restoration of an attenuated virus by knockout of a host resistance gene. Proc Natl Acad Sci USA 2000; 97:6097–6101.

151. Farassati F, Yang AD, Lee PW. Oncogenes in Ras signalling pathway dictate host-cell permissiveness to herpes simplex virus 1. Nat Cell Biol 2001; 3:745–750.

152. Markert JM, Medlock MD, Rabkin SD, et al. Conditionally replicating herpes simplex virus mutant, G207 for the treatment of malignant glioma: results of a phase I trial. Gene Ther 2000; 7:867–874.

153. Kesari S, Randazzo BP, Valyi-Nagy T, et al. Therapy of experimental human brain tumors using a neuroattenuated herpes simplex virus mutant. Lab Invest 1995; 73:636–648.

154. Rampling R, Cruickshank G, Papanastassiou V, et al. Toxicity evaluation of replication-competent herpes simplex virus (ICP 34.5 null mutant 1716) in patients with recurrent malignant glioma. Gene Ther 2000; 7:859–866.

155. Papanastassiou V, Rampling R, Fraser M, et al. The potential for efficacy of the modified (ICP 34.5(-)) herpes simplex virus HSV1716 following intratumoural injection into human malignant glioma: a proof of principle study. Gene Ther 2002; 9:398–406.

156. Russell SJ. RNA viruses as virotherapy agents. Cancer Gene Ther 2002; 9:961–966.

157. Pecora AL, Rizvi N, Cohen GI, et al. Phase I trial of intravenous administration of PV701, an oncolytic virus, in patients with advanced solid cancers. J Clin Oncol 2002; 20:2251–2266 see comment.

158. Stojdl DF, Lichty B, Knowles S, et al. Exploiting tumor-specific defects in the interferon pathway with a previously unknown oncolytic virus. Nat Med 2000; 6:821–825.

159. McCart JA, Ward JM, Lee J, et al. Systemic cancer therapy with a tumor-selective vaccinia virus mutant lacking thymidine kinase and vaccinia growth factor genes. Cancer Res 2001; 61:8751–8757.

160. Gromeier M, Lachmann S, Rosenfeld MR, et al. Intergeneric poliovirus recombinants for the treatment of malignant glioma. Proc Natl Acad Sci USA 2000; 97:6803–6808.

161. Grote D, Russell SJ, Cornu TI, et al. Live attenuated measles virus induces regression of human lymphoma xenografts in immunodeficient mice. Blood 2001; 97:3746–3754.

162. Bluming AZ, Ziegler JL. Regression of Burkitt's lymphoma in association with measles infection. Lancet 1971; 2:105–106.

163. Asada T. Cancer 1974; 34:1907–1928.

164. Wheelock EF, Dingle JH. Observations on the repeated administration of viruses to a patient with acute leukemia. N Engl J Med 1964; 271:645–651.

165. Heise CC, Williams A, Olesch J, et al. Efficacy of a replication-competent adenovirus (ONYX-015) following intratumoral injection: intratumoral spread and distribution effects. Cancer Gene Ther 1999; 6:499–504.

166. Nemunaitis J, Ganly I, Khuri F, et al. Selective replication and oncolysis in p53 mutant tumors with ONYX-015, an E1B-55kD gene-deleted adenovirus, in patients with advanced head and neck cancer: a phase II trial. Cancer Res 2000; 60:6359–6366.

167. Li H, Haviv YS, Derdeyn CA, et al. Human immunodeficiency virus type 1-mediated syncytium formation is compatible with adenovirus replication and facilitates efficient dispersion of viral gene products and de novo-synthesized virus particles. Hum Gene Ther 2001; 12:2155–2165.

168. Barresi V, Belluardo N, Sipione S, et al. Transplantation of prodrug-converting neural progenitor cells for brain tumor therapy. Cancer Gene Ther 2003; 10:396–402.

169. Arnhold S, Hilgers M, Lenartz D, et al. Neural precursor cells as carriers for a gene therapeutical approach in tumor therapy. Cell Transplant 2003; 12:827–837.

170. Harling-Berg CJ, Hallett JJ, Park JT, et al. Hierarchy of immune responses to antigen in the normal brain. Curr Top Microbiol Immunol 2002; 265:1–22.

171. Gooding LR. Regulation of TNF-mediated cell death and inflammation by human adenoviruses. Infect Agents Dis 1994; 3:106–115.

172. Ikeda K, Ichikawa T, Wakimoto H, et al. Oncolytic virus therapy of multiple tumors in the brain requires suppression of innate and elicited antiviral responses. Nat Med 1999; 5:881–887.

173. Todo T, Martuza RL, Rabkin SD, et al. Oncolytic herpes simplex virus vector with enhanced MHC class I presentation and tumor cell killing. Proc Natl Acad Sci USA 2001; 98:6396–6401.

174. Ikeda K, Wakimoto H, Ichikawa T, et al. Complement depletion facilitates the infection of multiple brain tumors by an intravascular, replication-conditional herpes simplex virus mutant. J Virol 2000; 74:4765–4775.

175. Wakimoto H, Ikeda K, Abe T, et al. The complement response against an oncolytic virus is species-specific in its activation pathways. Mol Ther 2002; 5:275–282.

176. Chen Y, Yu DC, Charlton D, et al. Pre-existent adenovirus antibody inhibits systemic toxicity and antitumor activity of CN706 in the nude mouse LNCaP xenograft model: implications and proposals for human therapy. Hum Gene Ther 2000; 11:1553–1567.

177. Xiang Z, Gao G, Reyes-Sandoval A, et al. Novel, chimpanzee serotype 68-based adenoviral vaccine carrier for induction of antibodies to a transgene product. J Virol 2002; 76:2667–2675.

178. Croyle MA, Chirmule N, Zhang Y, et al. "Stealth"adenoviruses blunt cell-mediated and humoral immune responses against the virus and allow for significant gene expression upon readministration in the lung. J Virol 2001; 75:4792–4801.

179. Croyle MA, Yu QC, Wilson JM. Development of a rapid method for the PEGylation of adenoviruses with enhanced transduction and improved stability under harsh storage conditions. Hum Gene Ther 2000; 11:1713–1722.

180. Fisher KD, Stallwood Y, Green NK, et al. Polymer-coated adenovirus permits efficient retargeting and evades neutralising antibodies. Gene Ther 2001; 8:341–348.

16

Adenovirus-Mediated HSV-tk Gene Therapy for Malignant Glioma: Clinical Experience

Kalevi J. Pulkkanen

Department of Molecular Medicine, A. I. Virtanen Institute, University of Kuopio and Department of Oncology, Kuopio University Hospital, Kuopio, Finland

Seppo Yla-Herttuala

Department of Molecular Medicine, A. I. Virtanen Institute, University of Kuopio and Department of Medicine and Gene Therapy Unit, Kuopio University Hospital, Kuopio, Finland

INTRODUCTION

The prevalence of the CNS neoplasms is 1.3 per 10,000 in Western countries. Approximately 60% are gliomas, and half of these are glioblastoma multiforme, which is the most aggressive form of these tumors (1,2). Established treatments for malignant glioma (MG) are surgery, radiotherapy, and chemotherapy. Surgery has a major role in the management of gliomas, but its outcome is often compromised due to a close proximity of vital anatomical structures and the lack of a defined tumor edge in the brain tissue. Radiotherapy is given post-operatively or as the primary treatment in case of a non-resectable tumor. Normal tissues in the CNS can tolerate up to 60 Gy of radiation. However, this may be below the threshold required to kill MG cells, and the risk of residual tumors is high. Chemotherapy is most commonly given post-operatively and/or combined with radiotherapy. Its goal is mainly to control the tumor growth and maintain satisfactory performance for patients as long as possible. The combination of procarbazine, lomustine, and vincristine (PCV) (3,4), and temozolomide (5) have demonstrated a significant prolongation in survival. Generally, no curative treatment for MG exists and long-term control is rarely achieved with current therapy. Established therapies have improved the quality of life and resulted in 3–9 mo prolongation in median survival, which currently is ∼ 12 mo after initial diagnosis (6).

To further improve the prognosis of patients with MG, the development of new treatment modalities has been continuous. After promising results achieved in pre-clinical studies, great expectations were set on gene therapy. The first approach, using either retrovirus- or adenovirus-mediated Herpes simplex virus thymidine kinase (*HSV-tk*) gene therapy, entered into clinical trials in the 1990s, and thus far it has been the most commonly used application. The delivery of the *HSV-tk* gene has been performed by using either stereotactic intratumoral injections or intraoperative injections into the wound bed. In recent years, adenoviruses (Ad) have become the most popular gene transfer vector, and a few of the studies using adenovirus-mediated HSV-tk gene therapy (Ad.HSV-tk) have shown significant efficiency in clinical use.

Other approaches in the treatment of patients with MG have utilized oncolytic viruses (G207, HSV-1 1716, and ONYX-015) (7–9), adenovirus-mediated *p53* tumor suppressor gene restoration (10), cationic liposome-mediated interferon β gene transfer (11), and antisense oligonucleotide directed against insulin-like growth factor type I receptor (12). These small and uncontrolled phase I studies have demonstrated adequate safety and some degree of anti-tumor efficacy with a few long-time survivors.

This chapter (1) highlights the gene therapy-based approaches that are available for the treatment of MG with special focus on the Ad.HSV-tk, and (2) comprehensively reviews the clinical experience of the Ad.HSV-tk gene therapy for MG. The main characteristics, efficacy, and adverse events of the clinical trials are presented in Table 1 and 2.

OVERVIEW OF THE PRECLINICAL GENE THERAPY STRATEGIES FOR MALIGNANT GLIOMA

MG is an attractive target for local gene therapy because of its restricted anatomical location and absence of metastases outside of the CNS. Vectors can be delivered at high concentrations directly to the desired site with only a small risk of systemic toxicity (13,14).

Several strategies have been studied for the treatment of MG. The approaches often converge and can be used in combination to amplify the therapeutic effect (15). HSV-tk (16–18) and cytocine deaminase (CD) (19,20) are the prototypes of cytotoxic suicide gene-based therapies where a two-component system induces cytotoxicity. In a corrective approach, restoration of the function of mutated tumor suppressor genes (21), such as *p53* (22–25), retinoblastoma gene (*Rb*) (26,27), p*16* (28,29), and phosphatase tensin gene (*PTEN*) (30–32) have shown anti-tumor efficacy. Anti-angiogenic gene therapies (33,34) utilizing angiostatin (35–40), endostatin (41–43), anti-VEGF (44–46), and EGFR-targeted (47–49) approaches have demonstrated strongly impaired tumor growth and reduction of VEGF secretion. Immune-gene therapy enhances the immune response against tumors (50) with increased cytokine production (51–56) and tumor-associated antigen presentation (57–61) to stimulate inflammatory reactions and tumor killing cells (62–67). Antisense oligonucleotides can be used to inactivate the expression of a variety of tumor-growth promoting genes (68–72). Oncolytic viruses possessing a targeted competence to replicate in dividing cells (73–76) or in tumor cells deficient for p53 (77,78) and Rb (79) pathways represent a novel treatment platform for MG (80,81). Several of these approaches have been described in detail elsewhere in this book.

ADENOVIRUS-MEDIATED HERPES SIMPLEX VIRUS THYMIDINE KINASE GENE THERAPY

Gene therapy uses nucleic acids, i.e., genes or sequences of DNA as drugs to alter the function of target cells. The delivery of genes demands the use of either viral or non-viral vectors, which optimally should provide effective transduction and expression of the

Table 1 Clinical Adenovirus-Mediated HSV-tk Studies for Malignant Glioma

Authors and phase of study	Number of patients	Ad dose and volume	MTD	Main adverse events[a]	Efficacy and median survival (MS)
Sandmair et al. Phase IIa, 2000	21 (Ad.HSV-tk $n=7$) (Rv.HSV-tk $n=7$) (LacZ $n=7$)	3×10^{10} pfu, 10 ml	Not reached	↑ Anti-Ad Ab and seizures; low-grade fever	↑ Ad.HSV-tk survival time ($p < 0.012$), Ad.HSV-tk 14 mo Rv.HSV-tk 7 mo LacZ 10 mo
Trask et al. Phase I, 2000	13	2×10^9–10^{12} vp, 1 ml	2×10^{11} vp	↑ Confusion and seizures; hyponatremia	3 responders[b], 4 mo
Judy et al. Phase I, 2002	13	2×10^8–10^{11} pfu, volume not given	2×10^{10} pfu	↑ Intracranial pressure	10 mo[c]
Germano et al. Phase I, 2003	11	2.5×10^{11} –9×10^{11} vp, 1 ml	Not reached	None	2 responders[d], 10.4 mo
Smitt et al. Phase I, 2003	14	4.6×10^8 –10^{11} vp, 10 ml	Not reached	None	No anti-tumor response[e], 4 mo
Immonen et al. Phase IIb, 2004	36 (Ad.HSV-tk $n=17$) (Standard therapy $n=19$)	3×10^{10} pfu, 10 ml	Not reached	↑ anti-Ad Ab; local post-operative oedema during GCV treatment	↑ Ad.HSV-tk survival time ($p < 0.0095$), Ad.HSV-tk 14.4 mo Standard therapy 8.8 mo

Some trials are small, prospective, and uncontrolled, and therefore tumor response may not be based on statistical comparison with a control group.

[a] Gene therapy-related.

[b] Minor response in contrast-enhanced MRI, with 3 patients surviving for 25 mo or longer post-gene therapy.

[c] 5 patients alive 12 mo or longer, and 1 patient alive without tumor for 3 yr after Ad.HSV-tk.

[d] Tumor control in contrast-enhanced MRI for more than 12 mo, with 2 patients alive 118 and 227 wk after Ad.HSV-tk.

[e] Progressive disease in contrast-enhanced MRI, but 4 patients alive longer than 1 yr, and 1 patient alive 29 mo after Ad.HSV-tk.

Abbreviations: Ad, adenovirus; MTD, maximum tolerated dose; Rv, retrovirus; pfu, plaque forming unit; ↑, increase; Ab, antibody; vp, virus particle; GCV, ganciclovir; MS, median survival from gene therapy; in case the survival has been given in wk, the conversion to mo has been calculated using the formula as follows: Median survival in mo = median survival in wk / (52 wk/12 mo).

transgene with efficient targeting and sufficient duration. In addition, toxicity to normal cells and tissue should be tolerable.

Adeno- and retroviruses have been the most commonly used gene transfer vectors for MG. The early clinical trials (82–90) were performed using retrovirus-mediated (91–93) HSV-tk gene therapy. Due to a modest anti-tumor effect observed in these early small and

Table 2 Summary of Adverse Events and Their Relationship to the Adenovirus-Mediated HSV-tk Gene Therapy as Reported in the Publications

Gene therapy-related adverse events	Number of events
Short-term fever	6
Increase in seizures	3
Increased intracranial pressure with severe headache	3
Altered mental status	2
Confusion	2
Hyponatremia	2
Lethargy	2
Leukocytosis	2
Local post-operative intracerebral oedema during GCV treatment	2
Increased cerebrospinal fluid protein	1
Hydrocephalus	1
Hypertension	1

Other adverse events	Number of events
Transient elevation in liver enzymes	9
Hemiparesis	5
Cerebrospinal fluid leak	4
Seizures	4
Thrombocytopenia	4
Lethargy	3
Aphasia/dysphasia	2
Hyponatremia	2
Intratumoral hemorrhage	2
Sepsis	2
Urinary tract infection	2
Anemia	1
Deep vein thrombosis	1
Fever	1
Head trauma	1
Phlebitis in arm	1
Proximal weakness (steroids)	1
Rash	1
Vomiting	1

Note: 75 patients in six trials received adenovirus-mediated HSV-tk gene therapy.

uncontrolled trials, reports of low transduction efficiency associated with the retrovirus-mediated vector-producing-cell (VPC) strategy in human clinical situation (94–96), and the results showing no difference in progression-free, median, or 12-mo survival, and safety between the standard treatment and retrovirus-mediated HSV-tk gene therapy arms in a randomized, parallel group, phase III study ($n=248$) by Rainov and co-workers in 2000 (97), the retroviral VPC approach has been largely abandoned.

Adenovirus Vectors

Wild type Ads are non-enveloped double-stranded DNA viruses. The usual clinical manifestation of wild type Ad infection is a common flu or gastroenteritis. So far, approximately fifty human Ad serotypes have been identified. The viral cycle begins with the binding of the Ad to its cell membrane receptor, e.g., human Coxsackie and adenovirus receptor (hCAR) (98), followed by receptor-mediated endocytosis (99). In addition to hCAR, α_v integrins of the target cell membrane play an important role in the virus entry (100). Following internalization, Ads escape endosomes, and virus particles are transported into the nucleus for the viral replication. The Ad genome comprises two major coding regions, early (E1 through E4) and late regions. E1 initiates viral transcription and E2 encodes proteins needed for the replication of the viral genome. The function of E3 is not entirely clear, but it seems to be involved in repression of the host immune system. E4 regulates host gene expression, and transregulates the actions of E2 and late regions. The role of the late regions is mainly to encode proteins responsible for the structure and assembly of the virus particles. The completion of the wild type viral cycle results in a lytic death of the target cell via inhibition of the host cell DNA and protein synthesis, whereafter the progeny of the virion is released (99,101).

Most recombinant Ad vectors are based on serotypes 2 and 5. The first-generation Ads were rendered replication-defective by deleting the E1 and E3 regions from the viral genome. However, low-level transcription of the remaining viral genes elicited significant immune responses in vivo (102–104). Removal of the E2, E3, and E4 regions significantly reduced the host immune response against the second- and third-generation Ads (104–106). Later generation Ads, termed as "gutless," "helper-dependent," or "high capacity" vectors, have been readministered even in the presence of circulating antibodies causing only transient inflammatory responses, but providing an unaffected and long-term transgene expression in the CNS (107–110).

Ads provide several advantages for cancer gene therapy. High titers allow efficient transduction and transgene expression. In case of the first- and second-generation Ads, the expression is fairly short-lived due to the immune responses, and antibody production often prevents repeated administration. However, in the context of most cancer protocols, limited duration of the transgene expression is not considered as a drawback, and the immunogenicity may provide an additional treatment effect. Also, Ads transduce both dividing and non-dividing cells and the potential to cause insertional mutagenesis is highly theoretical (111–114).

Herpes Simplex Virus Thymidine Kinase Gene Therapy

Given the self-renewing nature and genetic redundancy of cancer cells, a direct eradication of tumors is a logical aim for any anti-cancer therapy. Suicide genes (115), especially *HSV-tk* coupled with intravenously administered ganciclovir (GCV) or acyclovir (16–18), and bacterial cytosine deaminase (CD) coupled with 5-fluorocytosine (5-FC) (20) have been the most commonly applied approaches. However, only HSV-tk gene therapy has been used in the clinical trials for MG.

Unlike the endogenous mammalian thymidine kinase, the HSV-tk enzyme expressed by the *HSV-tk* (116) is capable of converting GCV (117) into a monophosphate. Once a monophosphate, it is converted into a GCV-triphosphate by cellular enzymes, which is then incorporated into replicating DNA by cellular DNA polymerases. However, GCV-triphosphates are not compatible substrates for chain elongation, and DNA replication is terminated resulting in cell death (16,115,118).

On the basis of animal experiments $> 10\%$ transduction efficiency is required to achieve a therapeutic effect using HSV-tk gene therapy (119). It has been reported that high-titer Ad results in a sufficient transduction efficiency in clinical situation (94). The killing of the non-transduced tumor cells in vivo is probably significantly augmented by a bystander effect, i.e., diffusion of the toxic triphosphates from the transduced cells via gap junctions (120) into the neighboring cells resulting in the bystander killing (121,122). With different mechanisms, bystander effect occurs also in other enzyme-prodrug systems (115), and may also be mediated via suppression of angiogenesis (123,124), toxicity and contact with dying cells (125), and cytotoxic immune effector cells (118).

CLINICAL TRIALS

In 1996, Eck et al. published a phase I clinical protocol with intention to treat patients with recurrent MG using intratumoral Ad.HSV-tk (126). However, the first completed human Ad.HSV-tk trials were not published until in 2000. Sandmair et al. (2000) (Table 1) enrolled twenty-one patients to study both replication-deficient retrovirus- and adenovirus-HSV-tk gene therapy for primary ($n=8$) and recurrent ($n=13$) MG. All patients underwent tumor resection, and for de novo tumors, post-operative irradiation was given. Seven patients received HSV-tk retroviral VPC (10^9 cells/10 ml), and another seven patients Ad.HSV-tk injections (3×10^{10} plaque forming units) (pfu) intraoperatively into the margins of the tumor cavity, followed by intravenous GCV treatment 5 mg/kg twice a day for 14 days. The medication started 14 or 5 days post-operatively in retrovirus- and adenovirus-treated patients, respectively. As a control group, seven patients received intratumoral adenoviral *LacZ* gene transfer (Ad.*LacZ*) 4–5 days pre-operatively via stereotactic catheter application. Anti-Ad antibodies increased more than 4-fold in three patients in the Ad.HSV-tk group. No serious adverse events were reported, there was no dose limiting toxicity (DLT), and the maximum tolerated dose (MTD) was not reached. The mean survival time in the Ad.HSV-tk group (15 mo) was significantly longer ($p<.012$) than in the retrovirus-mediated HSV-tk (7.4 mo) and Ad.*LacZ* gene transfer (8.3 mo) groups (96).

Trask et al. (phase I, 2000) (Table 1) conducted a non-controlled trial using single stereotactic intratumoral injections of replication-defective Ad.HSV-tk ($2 \times 10^9 - 2 \times 10^{12}$ vector particles) (vp) in thirteen patients with recurrent malignant brain tumors (MG $n=12$). Intravenous GCV was started twenty-four hr after the vector injection using a dose of 5 mg/kg twice daily for 14 days. Adequate safety and feasibility was reported, however, the DLT occurred at the highest dose of Ad.HSV-tk, and these patients exhibited pronounced CNS toxicity. The MTD was reached at 2×10^{11} vp. Post-treatment elevation of anti-Ad antibodies was detected in ten patients. Ten patients died within 10 mo of treatment, and the median survival was 4 mo. However, three patients survived 25 mo or longer showing evidence of extended tumor control (127).

Judy et al. (phase I, 2002) (Table 1) treated thirteen patients with MG (primary $n=2$, recurrent $n=11$), of which twelve patients received stereotactic intratumoral Ad.HSV-tk injections followed by daily intravenous GCV treatment for 6 days. Thereafter these patients underwent tumor resection and received wound bed injections of Ad.HSV-tk to a total dose of $2 \times 10^8 - 2 \times 10^{11}$ pfu followed by 14 days of GCV. One patient received a single stereotactic intratumoral injection of Ad.HSV-tk into an inoperable thalamic tumor followed by 14 days of GCV. The DLT occurred at the highest dose level: these patients experienced transient increased intracranial pressure manifested as severe headache and altered mental status. However, rapid recovery was achieved with adequate medical treatment. The MTD was reached at 2×10^{10} pfu. Data regarding viral shedding was not provided. The median survival was 10 months, five patients were alive at least one year, and one patient showed no recurrence until 3 years after Ad.HSV-tk (128).

Germano et al. (phase I, 2003) (Table 1) treated eleven patients with recurrent MG, divided into three dose-escalating cohorts ($2.5 \times 10^{11} - 9.0 \times 10^{11}$ vp), using intraoperative grid-guided injections of replication-defective Ad.HSV-tk into the wound bed, followed by intravenous GCV treatment starting twenty-four hr post-virus injection at a dose of 5 mg/kg twice daily for 7 days. No signs of systemic or intraparenchymal gene therapy-related toxicity was observed at the reported doses. Serious adverse events were non-gene therapy related. The average and median survival following gene therapy were 13.6 and 10.4 mo, respectively. It was concluded that the favorable safety and efficiency warrants a phase II clinical trial (129).

A dose escalation study for fourteen patients with advanced recurrent high-grade gliomas was conducted by Smitt et al. (2003) (Table 1). Divided into four cohorts, patients received 4.6×10^8–4.6×10^{11} vp of a replication-incompetent Ad vector harboring the *HSV-tk* gene delivered using intraoperative grid-guided wound bed injections. Intravenous GCV treatment was started on the second post-operative day at a dose of 5 mg/kg twice a day for 14 days. The treatment was safe and well tolerated, no DLT occurred, and the MTD was not reached. The overall median survival was 4 months, however, four patients survived longer than one year following gene therapy (130).

The study by Sandmair et al. (see above) was continued by Immonen et al. (phase IIb, 2004) (Table 1) to further assess the efficacy and safety of Ad.HSV-tk in patients with operable primary or recurrent gliomas. Thirty-six patients were randomized to receive either intraoperative Ad.HSV-tk injections (3×10^{10} pfu) into the wound bed, followed by intravenous GCV starting five days post-operatively at a dose of 5 mg/kg twice daily for 14 days ($n = 17$), or standard care comprising radical tumor excision ($n = 19$), followed by radiotherapy in both groups in patients with de novo tumors. The mean survival of patients in Ad.HSV-tk group was significantly better (70.6 wk) than in the standard care group (39 wk) ($p < .0095$). The survival benefit was similar ($p < .0017$) as compared with historical controls from the same unit over two years preceding the study. Anti-Ad antibodies increased more than 4-fold in six patients in the Ad.HSV-tk group. The treatment was well tolerated, and the MTD was not reached. It was concluded that Ad.HSV-tk may provide an effective adjuvant treatment for patients with operable primary or recurrent high-grade gliomas (14).

SAFETY

Safety monitoring is an essential part of every clinical trial performed using virus vectors. Retrovirus-mediated HSV-tk gene therapy for MG has appeared to be safe and well tolerated. Safety has not been a problem in Ad.HSV-tk trials either: reports from the completed trials have uniformly concluded a minimal frequency of serious adverse events, which almost entirely have not been related to the Ad.HSV-tk (Table 2). Initially, one of the major concerns was the potential toxicity of the Ad vectors, which has been observed especially at high doses in non-human primates (131). Viral vectors may also have a potential to create damaging immunological reactions by immune-mediated vector toxicity especially in the presence of circulating antibodies to the virus vectors (107,132) or by triggering autoimmune reactions to self or transgene antigens (133,134). The oncogenic potential of transgenes and vectors is less of a concern because of the mostly quiescent and terminally differentiated cells in the adult CNS. Although a theoretical risk of vector dissemination via vasculature exists, at the present time there is no evidence of germ line modifications or any viral shedding into the body fluids outside CNS. Elevated post-treatment anti-Ad antibodies without any adverse outcomes have been observed in some studies (14,96,127). Based on these six trials, the DLT of Ad seems to occur at doses of $\geq 10^{12}$ vp (127) or $\geq 10^{11}$ pfu (128), while the MTD has been 2×10^{11} vp or 2×10^{10} pfu, or has not been reached at doses of 3×10^{10} pfu (14,96) and $4.6 \times 10^{11} - 9 \times 10^{11}$ vp (129,130). However, caution should be exercised when comparing vp and/or pfu values of different studies (135).

DISCUSSION

The treatment of MG remains a challenge for modern medicine. Implementation of the promising results achieved in pre-clinical gene therapy studies into clinical situation has not been easy, and still appears to be at rather early stages. To eradicate tumors, a treatment must effectively access tumor site and destroy tumor cells. As far as Ad.HSV-tk is concerned, the greatest shortcoming seems to be the limited spatial distribution of the *HSV-tk* forestalling the eradication of tumor cells at a distance from the tumor mass or the margins of the post-resection cavity. The lack of efficiency, at least partly, is due to the treatment execution; direct manual or stereotactic injections of rather small volumes of the vector suspension into the wound bed or into an existing tumor is technically complicated, and estimation of the correct depth of the injections in regard to the extent of parenchyma-invading tumor cells is difficult, not to mention the possible existence of even more distant satellite lesions.

Differences between experimental animal models and human clinical conditions also complicate the translation of gene therapy into clinical use. In pre-clinical models, anti-tumor efficiency has often been demonstrated with a limited number of either non-human or xenogeneic cell lines and transplants with only a short interval between the implantation and therapy. In humans, cancers are usually sporadic, and have been present for months to years resulting in increased heterogeneity, genetic instability and established vasculature. In addition, use of immunodeficient animals is often necessary to test the efficacy of a given approach against tumors of human origin. This may compromise the reliability of the results; when the treatment is applied in a clinical trial, it fails to show effectiveness in patients with normal immune system.

So far, the majority of the completed studies have been early-phase, prospective, and uncontrolled trials with a small number of enrolled patients. Therefore, with a few exceptions, it has been difficult to provide firm evidence for significant anti-tumor responses or prolongation of survival. Several trials have reported one or a few long-term survivors, but this favorable outcome may merely be due to the natural course of the disease rather than a real treatment effect (15). However, with a sufficient number of patients and standard therapy and/or control arms included in the trial design, it is possible to demonstrate whether a candidate therapy is effective (14,96,97).

Optimization and modification of vectors may improve the clinical effectiveness of gene therapy for MG. For most cancer protocols, short-term expression of the transgene and the capability of the vector to elicit an immune response, both characteristic to the first-generation Ads, would be desired properties. However, in the context of MG, the issue is more complex: long-term expression and greater stability of the vector (107–110) might result in a better response against this extremely invasive tumor which often presents as a "whole-brain" disease and has a high rate of recurrence. Oncolytic Herpes simplex virus type 1 vectors (HSV-1 mutants) and conditionally replicating Ads (CRAds) might be capable of reaching distant malignant cells in the brain by resulting in a much higher amount of virus progeny than the input dose of injected viruses at the initial site (76,81,136). Although MG is located in an anatomically restricted site, vectors with the capacity of tumor-specific targeting may add anti-tumor efficacy and reduce toxicity to the normal tissue. In addition to CRAds and HSV-1 mutants, which exploit defective tumor suppressor gene pathways (77,79) or competence to replicate in dividing neuronal cells (73,75), there are multiple ways to engineer Ads to restrict their innate wide tropism to infect a variety of different cell types. Constructs using monoclonal antibodies with a high specificity for the surface proteins of the target cells (transductional targeting) (137), tumor-specific promoters to control viral replication (transcriptional targeting) (138), and capsid modifications (139–142) to overcome variable or absent expression of hCAR (98), have already been tested for MG in pre-clinical models. Also, these targeted (138) or replication-competent (143) vectors could express therapeutic genes to further improve the efficacy. Nevertheless, taken into account all completed gene therapy trials for MG so far, the traditional Ads have demonstrated the best treatment effects (15).

It is unlikely that gene therapy alone will provide cure for MG, at least not in the near future. For safety reasons, but also to increase the efficiency of tumor cell killing, it is common sense to integrate gene therapy with the established treatments. The pursuit to develop new viral and targeting solutions and immune-gene therapies is feverish, and it is difficult to predict, which approach will eventually be the most effective. In the context of MG, even the prolongation of survival for another year beyond current therapies without increased toxicity can be regarded as a genuine success. Today, this has already been achieved in some phase II trials (14,96). However, phase III studies are mandatory to provide firm evidence about the efficacy of gene therapy for the treatment of MG.

ACKNOWLEDGMENTS

This study was supported by Finnish Academy, Kuopio University Hospital (EVO grant 5195), and Ark Therapeutics Ltd.

REFERENCES

1. Annegers JF, Schoenberg BS, Okazaki H, et al. Epidemiologic study of primary intracranial neoplasms. Arch Neurol 1981; 38:217–219.
2. Salcman M. Supratentorial gliomas: clinical features and surgical therapy. In: Wilkins RH, Rengachary SS, eds. Neurosurgery. New York: McGraw-Hill, 1996:777–778.
3. Levin VA, Prados MR, Wara WM, et al. Radiation therapy and bromodeoxyuridine chemotherapy followed by procarbazine, lomustine, and vincristine for the treatment of anaplastic gliomas. Int J Radiat Oncol Biol Phys 1995; 32:75–83.
4. Levin VA, Wara WM, Davis RL, et al. Phase III comparison of BCNU and the combination of procarbazine, CCNU, and vincristine administered after radiotherapy with hydroxyurea for malignant gliomas. J Neurosurg 1985; 63:218–223.
5. Stupp R, Mason WP, van den Bent MJ, et al. Radiation therapy plus concomitant and adjuvant temozolomide for glioblastoma. N Eng J Med 2005; 352:987–996.
6. Fine HA, Dear KB, Loeffler JS, et al. Meta-analysis of radiation therapy with and without adjuvant chemotherapy for malignant gliomas in adults. Cancer 1993; 71:2585–2597.
7. Markert JM, Medlock MD, Rabkin SD, et al. Conditionally replicating herpes simplex virus mutant, G207 for the treatment of malignant glioma: results of a phase I trial. Gene Ther 2000; 7:867–874.
8. Harrow S, Papanastassiou V, Harland J, et al. HSV1716 injection into the brain adjacent to tumour following surgical resection of high-grade glioma: safety data and long-term survival. Gene Therapy 2004; 11:1648–1658.

9. Chiocca EA, Abbed KM, Tatter S, et al. A phase I open-label, dose-escalation, multi-institutional trial of injection with an E1B-Attenuated adenovirus, ONYX-015, into the peritumoral region of recurrent malignant gliomas, in the adjuvant setting. Mol Ther 2004; 10:958–966.

10. Lang FF, Bruner JM, Fuller GN, et al. Phase I trial of adenovirus-mediated p53 gene therapy for recurrent glioma: biological and clinical results. J Clin Oncol 2003; 21:2508–2518.

11. Yoshida J, Mizuno M, Fujii M, et al. Human gene therapy for malignant gliomas (glioblastoma multiforme and anaplastic astrocytoma) by in vivo transduction with human interferon beta gene using cationic liposomes. Hum Gene Ther 2004; 15:77–86.

12. Andrews DW, Resnicoff M, Flanders AE, et al. Results of a pilot study involving the use of an antisense oligodeoxynucleotide directed against the insulin-like growth factor type I receptor in malignant astrocytomas. J Clin Oncol 2001; 19:2189–2200.

13. Yla-Herttuala S. Gene therapy and brain tumors. In: Mikkelsen T, Rosenblum ML, Laerum OD, Bjerkvig R, eds. Brain Tumor Invasion: Biological, Clinical, and Therapeutic Considerations. New York: Wiley-Liss, Inc., 1998:435–445.

14. Immonen A, Vapalahti M, Tyynela K, et al. AdvHSV-tk gene therapy with intravenous ganciclovir improves survival in human malignant glioma: a randomised, controlled study. Mol Ther 2004; 10:967–972.

15. Pulkkanen KJ, Yla-Herttuala S. Gene therapy for malignant glioma: current clinical status. Mol Ther 2005; 4:585–598.

16. Moolten FL. Drug sensitivity ("suicide") genes for selective cancer chemotherapy. Cancer Gene Ther 1994; 1:279–287.

17. Culver KW, Ram Z, Wallbridge S, et al. In vivo gene transfer with retroviral vector-producer cells for treatment of experimental brain tumors. Science 1992; 256:1550–1552.

18. Chen SH, Shine HD, Goodman JC, et al. Gene therapy for brain tumors: regression of experimental gliomas by adenovirus-mediated gene transfer in vivo. Proc Natl Acad Sci USA 1994; 91:3054–3057.

19. Dong Y, Wen P, Manome Y, et al. In vivo replication-deficient adenovirus vector-mediated transduction of the cytosine deaminase gene sensitizes glioma cells to 5-fluorocytosine. Hum Gene Ther 1996; 7:713–720.

20. Mullen CA, Kilstrup M, Blaese RM. Transfer of the bacterial gene for cytosine deaminase to mammalian cells confers lethal sensitivity to 5-fluorocytosine: a negative selection system. Proc Natl Acad Sci USA 1992; 89:33–37.

21. Merlo A. Genes and pathways driving glioblastomas in humans and murine disease models. Neurosurg Rev 2003; 26:145–158.

22. Bogler O, Huang HJ, Kleihues P, et al. The p53 gene and its role in human brain tumors. Glia 1995; 15:308–327.

23. Lang FF, Yung WK, Sawaya R, et al. Adenovirus-mediated p53 gene therapy for human gliomas. Neurosurgery 1999; 45:1093–1104.

24. Li H, Alonso-Vanegas M, Colicos MA, et al. Intracerebral adenovirus-mediated p53 tumor suppressor gene therapy for experimental human glioma. Clin Cancer Res 1999; 5:637–642.

25. Gomez-Manzano C, Fueyo J, Kyritsis AP, et al. Adenovirus-mediated transfer of the p53 gene produces rapid and generalized death of human glioma cells via apoptosis. Cancer Res 1996; 56:694–699.

26. He J, Olson JJ, James CD. Lack of p16INK4 or retinoblastoma protein (pRb), or amplification-associated overexpression of cdk4 is observed in distinct subsets of malignant glial tumors and cell lines. Cancer Res 1995; 55:4833–4836.

27. Fueyo J, Gomez-Manzano C, Yung WK, et al. Suppression of human glioma growth by adenovirus-mediated Rb gene transfer. Neurology 1998; 50:1307–1315.

28. Serrano M, Hannon GJ, Beach D. A new regulatory motif in cell-cycle control causing specific inhibition of cyclin D/CDK4. Nature 1993; 366:704–707.

29. Fueyo J, Gomez-Manzano C, Yung WK, et al. The functional role of tumor suppressor genes in gliomas: clues for future therapeutic strategies. Neurology 1998; 51:1250–1255.

30. Rasheed BK, Stenzel TT, McLendon RE, et al. PTEN gene mutations are seen in high-grade but not in low-grade gliomas. Cancer Res 1997; 57:4187–4190.

31. Furnari FB, Huang HJ, Cavenee WK. The phosphoinositol phosphatase activity of PTEN mediates a serum-sensitive G1 growth arrest in glioma cells. Cancer Res 1998; 58:5002–5008.

32. Cheney IW, Johnson DE, Vaillancourt MT, et al. Suppression of tumorigenicity of glioblastoma cells by adenovirus-mediated MMAC1/PTEN gene transfer. Cancer Res 1998; 58:2331–2334.

33. Folkman J. Fighting cancer by attacking its blood supply. Sci Am 1996; 275:150–154.

34. Carmeliet P, Jain RK. Angiogenesis in cancer and other diseases. Nature 2000; 407:249–257.

35. O'Reilly MS, Holmgren L, Chen C, et al. Angiostatin induces and sustains dormancy of human primary tumors in mice. Nat Med 1996; 2:689–692.

36. Griscelli F, Li H, Bennaceur-Griscelli A, et al. Angiostatin gene transfer: inhibition of tumor growth in vivo by blockage of endothelial cell proliferation associated with a mitosis arrest. Proc Natl Acad Sci USA 1998; 95:6367–6372.

37. Griscelli F, Li H, Cheong C, et al. Combined effects of radiotherapy and angiostatin gene therapy in glioma tumor model. Proc Natl Acad Sci USA 2000; 97:6698–6703.

38. De Bouard S, Guillamo JS, Christov C, et al. Antiangiogenic therapy against experimental glioblastoma using genetically engineered cells producing interferon-alpha, angiostatin, or endostatin. Hum Gene Ther 2003; 14:883–895.

39. Tanaka T, Cao Y, Folkman J, et al. Viral vector-targeted antiangiogenic gene therapy utilizing an angiostatin complementary DNA. Cancer Res 1998; 58:3362–3369.

40. Ma HI, Guo P, Li J, et al. Suppression of intracranial human glioma growth after intramuscular administration of an adeno-associated viral vector expressing angiostatin. Cancer Res 2002; 62:756–763.

41. O'Reilly MS, Boehm T, Shing Y, et al. Endostatin: an endogenous inhibitor of angiogenesis and tumor growth. Cell 1997; 88:277–285.

42. Peroulis I, Jonas N, Saleh M. Antiangiogenic activity of endostatin inhibits C6 glioma growth. Int J Cancer 2002; 6:839–845.

43. Read TA, Sorensen DR, Mahesparan R, et al. Local endostatin treatment of gliomas administered by microencapsulated producer cells. Nat Biotechno 2001; 19:29–34.

44. Plate KH, Breier G, Weich HA, et al. Vascular endothelial growth factor is a potential tumour angiogenesis factor in human gliomas in vivo. Nature 1992; 359:845–848.

45. Saleh M, Stacker SA, Wilks AF. Inhibition of growth of C6 glioma cells in vivo by expression of antisense vascular endothelial growth factor sequence. Cancer Res 1996; 56:393–401.

46. Ciafre SA, Niola F, Wannenes F, et al. An anti-VEGF ribozyme embedded within the adenoviral VAI sequence inhibits glioblastoma cell angiogenic potential in vitro. J Vasc Res 2004; 41:220–228.

47. Maruno M, Kovach JS, Kelly PJ, et al. Transforming growth factor-alpha, epidermal growth factor receptor, and proliferating potential in benign and malignant gliomas. J Neurosurg 1991; 75:97–102.

48. Hoi SU, Espiritu OD, Kelley PY, et al. The role of the epidermal growth factor receptor in human gliomas: I The control of cell growth. J Neurosurg 1995; 82:841–846.

49. van Beusechem VW, Grill J, Mastenbroek DC, et al. Efficient and selective gene transfer into primary human brain tumors by using single-chain antibody-targeted adenoviral vectors with native tropism abolished. J Virol 2002; 76:2753–2762.

50. Lowenstein PR. Immunology of viral-vector-mediated gene transfer into the brain: an evolutionary and developmental perspective. Trends Immunol 2002; 23:23–30.

51. Book AA, Fielding KE, Kundu N, et al. IL-10 gene transfer to intracranial 9L glioma: tumor inhibition and cooperation with IL-2. J Neuroimmunol 1998; 92:50–59.

52. Saleh M, Wiegmans A, Malone Q, et al. Effect of in situ retroviral interleukin-4 transfer on established intracranial tumors. J Natl Cancer Inst 1999; 91:438–445.

53. Kikuchi T, Joki T, Saitoh S, et al. Anti-tumor activity of interleukin-2-producing tumor cells and recombinant interleukin 12 against mouse glioma cells located in the central nervous system. Int J Cancer 1999; 80:425–430.

54. Kominsky S, Johnson HM, Bryan G, et al. IFNgamma inhibition of cell growth in glioblastomas correlates with increased levels of the cyclin dependent kinase inhibitor p21WAF1/CIP1. Oncogene 1998; 17:2973–2979.
55. Natsume A, Mizuno M, Ryuke Y, et al. Antitumor effect and cellular immunity activation by murine interferon-beta gene transfer against intracerebral glioma in mouse. Gene Ther 1999; 6:1626–1633.
56. Natsume A, Tsujimura K, Mizuno M, et al. IFN-beta gene therapy induces systemic antitumor immunity against malignant glioma. J Neurooncol 2000; 47:117–124.
57. Sharpe AH, Freeman GJ. The B7-CD28 superfamily. Nat Rev Immunol 2002; 2:116–126.
58. Huang AY, Golumbek P, Ahmadzadeh M, et al. Role of bone marrow-derived cells in presenting MHC class I-restricted tumor antigens. Science 1994; 264:961–965.
59. Parney IF, Petruk KC, Zhang C, et al. Granulocyte-macrophage colony-stimulating factor and B7-2 combination immunogene therapy in an allogeneic Hu-PBL-SCID/beige mouse-human glioblastoma multiforme model. Hum Gene Ther 1997; 8:1073–1085.
60. Melcher A, Todryk S, Bateman A, et al. Adoptive transfer of immature dendritic cells with autologous or allogeneic tumor cells generates systemic antitumor immunity. Cancer Res. 1999; 59:2802–2805.
61. Joki T, Kikuchi T, Akasaki Y, et al. Induction of effective antitumor immunity in a mouse brain tumor model using B7-1 (CD80) and intercellular adhesive molecule 1 (ICAM-1; CD54) transfection and recombinant interleukin 12. Int J Cancer 1999; 82:714–720.
62. Wang RF, Wang X, Rosenberg SA, et al. Identification of a novel major histocompatibility complex class II-restricted tumor antigen resulting from a chromosomal rearrangement recognized by CD4(+) T cells. J Exp Med 1999; 189:1659–1668.
63. Wang RF, Wang X, Atwood AC, et al. Cloning genes encoding MHC class II-restricted antigens: mutated CDC27 as a tumor antigen. Science 1999; 284:1351–1354.
64. Albert ML, Sauter B, Bhardwaj N. Dendritic cells acquire antigen from apoptotic cells and induce class I-restricted CTLs. Nature 1998; 392:86–89.
65. Banchereau J, Steinman RM. Dendritic cells and the control of immunity. Nature 1998; 392:245–252.
66. Pardoll DM. Inducing autoimmune disease to treat cancer. Proc Natl Acad Sci USA 1999; 96:5340–5342.
67. Aoki H, Mizuno M, Natsume A, et al. Dendritic cells pulsed with tumor extract-cationic liposome complex increase the induction of cytotoxic T lymphocytes in mouse brain tumor. Cancer Immunol Immunother 2001; 50:463–468.
68. Chin L, Tam A, Pomerantz J, et al. Essential role for oncogenic Ras in tumour maintenance. Nature 1999; 400:468–472.
69. Galderisi U, Cascino A, Giordano A. Antisense oligonucleotides as therapeutic agents. J Cell Physiol 1999; 181:251–257.
70. Khazenzon NM, Ljubimov AV, Lakhter AJ, et al. Antisense inhibition of laminin-8 expression reduces invasion of human gliomas in vitro. Mol Cancer Ther 2003; 2:985–994.
71. Lee Y, Vassilakos A, Feng N, et al. GTI-2040, an antisense agent targeting the small subunit component (R2) of human ribonucleotide reductase, shows potent antitumor activity against a variety of tumors. Cancer Res 2003; 63:2802–2811.
72. Resnicoff M, Tjuvajev J, Rotman HL, et al. Regression of C6 rat brain tumors by cells expressing an antisense insulin-like growth factor I receptor RNA. J Exp Ther Oncol 1996; 1:385–389.
73. Mineta T, Rabkin SD, Yazaki T, et al. Attenuated multi-mutated herpes simplex virus-1 for the treatment of malignant gliomas. Nat Med 1995; 1:938–943.
74. McKie EA, Brown SM, MacLean AR, et al. Histopathological responses in the CNS following inoculation with a non-neurovirulent mutant (1716) of herpes simplex virus type 1 (HSV 1): relevance for gene and cancer therapy. Neuropathol Appl Neurobiol 1998; 24:367–372.
75. McKie EA, MacLean AR, Lewis AD, et al. Selective in vitro replication of herpes simplex virus type 1 (HSV-1) ICP34.5 null mutants in primary human CNS tumours—evaluation of a potentially effective clinical therapy. Br J Cancer 1996; 74:745–752.

76. Jacobs A, Breakefield XO, Fraefel C. HSV-1-based vectors for gene therapy of neurological diseases and brain tumors: part II. Vector systems and applications. Neoplasia 1999; 1:402–416.

77. Bischoff JR, Kirn DH, Williams A, et al. An adenovirus mutant that replicates selectively in p53-deficient human tumor cells. Science 1996; 274:373–376.

78. Ries S, Korn WM. ONYX-015: mechanisms of action and clinical potential of a replication-selective adenovirus. Br J Cancer 2002; 86:5–11.

79. Fueyo J, Gomez-Manzano C, Alemany R, et al. A mutant oncolytic adenovirus targeting the Rb pathway produces anti-glioma effect in vivo. Oncogene 2000; 19:2–12.

80. Kirn D, Martuza RL, Zwiebel J. Replication-selective virotherapy for cancer: Biological principles, risk management and future directions. Nat Med 2001; 7:781–787.

81. Shah AC, Benos D, Gillespie GY, et al. Oncolytic viruses: clinical applications as vectors for the treatment of malignant gliomas. J Neurooncol 2003; 65:203–226.

82. Ram Z, Culver KW, Oshiro EM, et al. Therapy of malignant brain tumors by intratumoral implantation of retroviral vector-producing cells. Nat Med 1997; 3:1354–1361.

83. Klatzmann D, Valery CA, Bensimon G, et al. A phase I/II study of herpes simplex virus type 1 thymidine kinase "suicide" gene therapy for recurrent glioblastoma. Study Group on Gene Therapy for Glioblastoma. Hum Gene Ther 1998; 9:2595–2604.

84. Shand N, Weber F, Mariani L, et al. A phase 1–2 clinical trial of gene therapy for recurrent glioblastoma multiforme by tumor transduction with the herpes simplex thymidine kinase gene followed by ganciclovir. GLI328 European-Canadian Study Group. Hum Gene Ther 1999; 10:2325–2335.

85. Valery CA, Seilhean D, Boyer O, et al. Long-term survival after gene therapy for a recurrent glioblastoma. Neurology 2002; 58:1109–1112.

86. Izquierdo M, Martin V, de Felipe P, et al. Human malignant brain tumor response to herpes simplex thymidine kinase (HSVtk)/ganciclovir gene therapy. Gene Ther 1996; 3:491–495.

87. Izquierdo M, Cortes ML, Martin V, et al. Gene therapy in brain tumours: implications of the size of glioblastoma on its curability. Acta Neurochir Suppl 1997; 68:111–117.

88. Packer RJ, Raffel C, Villablanca JG, et al. Treatment of progressive or recurrent pediatric malignant supratentorial brain tumors with herpes simplex virus thymidine kinase gene vector-producer cells followed by intravenous ganciclovir administration. J Neurosurg 2000; 92:249–254.

89. Palu G, Cavaggioni A, Calvi P, et al. Gene therapy of glioblastoma multiforme via combined expression of suicide and cytokine genes: a pilot study in humans. Gene Ther 1999; 6:330–337.

90. Prados MD, McDermott M, Chang SM, et al. Treatment of progressive or recurrent glioblastoma multiforme in adults with herpes simplex virus thymidine kinase gene vector-producer cells followed by intravenous ganciclovir administration: a phase I/II multi-institutional trial. J Neurooncol 2003; 65:269–278.

91. Miller AD. Retroviral Vectors. Current Topics in Microbiology and Immunology. Berlin-Heidelberg: Springer, 1992:1-24.

92. Miller AD, Buttimore C. Redesign of retrovirus packaging cell lines to avoid recombination leading to helper virus production. Mol Cell Biol 1986; 6:2895–2902.

93. Vile RG, Russell SJ. Retroviruses as vectors. Br Med Bull 1995; 51:12–30.

94. Puumalainen AM, Vapalahti M, Agrawal RS, et al. Beta-galactosidase gene transfer to human malignant glioma in vivo using replication-deficient retroviruses and adenoviruses. Hum Gene Ther 1998; 9:1769–1774.

95. Harsh GR, Deisboeck TS, Louis DN, et al. Thymidine kinase activation of ganciclovir in recurrent malignant gliomas: a gene-marking and neuropathological study. J Neurosurg 2000; 92:804–811.

96. Sandmair AM, Loimas S, Puranen P, et al. Thymidine kinase gene therapy for human malignant glioma, using replication-deficient retroviruses or adenoviruses. Hum Gene Ther 2000; 11:2197–2205.

97. Rainov NG. A phase III clinical evaluation of herpes simplex virus type 1 thymidine kinase and ganciclovir gene therapy as an adjuvant to surgical resection and radiation in adults with previously untreated glioblastoma multiforme. Hum Gene Ther 2000; 11:2389–2401.

98. Bergelson JM, Cunningham JA, Droguett G, et al. Isolation of a common receptor for Coxsackie B viruses and adenoviruses 2 and 5. Science 1997; 275:1320–1323.

99. Shenk T. Adenoviridae: The viruses and their replication. In: Fields BN, Knipe DM, eds. Fields Virology. New York: Raven Press, 1996:2111–2148.

100. Wickham TJ. Targeting adenovirus. Gene Ther 2000; 7:110–114.

101. Kremer EJ, Perricaudet M. Adenovirus and adeno-associated virus mediated gene transfer. Br Med Bull 1995; 51:31–44.

102. Kozarsky KF, Wilson JM. Gene therapy: adenovirus vectors. Curr Opin Genet Dev 1993; 3:499–503.

103. Danthinne X, Imperiale MJ. Production of first generation adenovirus vectors: a review. Gene Ther 2000; 7:1707–1714.

104. Kay MA, Glorioso JC, Naldini L. Viral vectors for gene therapy: the art of turning infectious agents into vehicles of therapeutics. Nat Med 2001; 7:33–40.

105. Romano G, Michell P, Pacilio C, et al. Latest developments in gene transfer technology: achievements, perspectives, and controversies over therapeutic applications. Stem Cells 2000; 18:19–39.

106. Wang Q, Finer MH. Second-generation adenovirus vectors. Nat Med 1996; 2:714–716.

107. Thomas CE, Schiedner G, Kochanek S, et al. Peripheral infection with adenovirus causes unexpected long-term brain inflammation in animals injected intracranially with first-generation, but not with high-capacity, adenovirus vectors: toward realistic long-term neurological gene therapy for chronic diseases. Proc Natl Acad Sci USA 2000; 97:7482–7487.

108. Thomas CE, Schiedner G, Kochanek S, et al. Preexisting antiadenoviral immunity is not a barrier to efficient and stable transduction of the brain, mediated by novel high-capacity adenovirus vectors. Hum Gene Ther 2001; 12:839–846.

109. Zou L, Zhou H, Pastore L, et al. Prolonged transgene expression mediated by a helper-dependent adenoviral vector (hdAd) in the central nervous system. Mol Ther 2000; 2:105–113.

110. Zou L, Yuan X, Zhou H, et al. Helper-dependent adenoviral vector-mediated gene transfer in aged rat brain. Hum Gene Ther 2001; 12:181–191.

111. Mountain A. Gene therapy: the first decade. Trends Biotechnol 2000; 18:119–128.

112. Vile RG, Russell SJ, Lemoine NR. Cancer gene therapy: hard lessons and new courses. Gene Ther 2000; 7:2–8.

113. Yang Y, Nunes FA, Berencsi K, et al. Cellular immunity to viral antigens limits E1-deleted adenoviruses for gene therapy. Proc Natl Acad Sci USA 1994; 91:4407–4411.

114. Umana P, Gerdes CA, Stone D, et al. Efficient FLPe recombinase enables scalable production of helper-dependent adenoviral vectors with negligible helper-virus contamination. Nat Biotechnol 2001; 19:582–585.

115. Aghi M, Hochberg F, Breakefield XO. Prodrug activation enzymes in cancer gene therapy. J Gene Med 2000; 2:148–164.

116. McKnight SL. The nucleotide sequence and transcript map of the herpes simplex virus thymidine kinase gene. Nucleic Acids Res 1980; 8:5949–5964.

117. Faulds D, Heel RC. Ganciclovir. A review of its antiviral activity, pharmacokinetic properties and therapeutic efficacy in cytomegalovirus infections. Drugs 1990; 39:597–638.

118. Ramesh R, Marrogi AJ, Freeman SM. Tumor killing using the HSV-tk suicide gene. In: Boulikas T, ed. Gene Therapy and Molecular Biology. Palo Alto, California: Gene Therapy Press, 1998:253–263.

119. Sandmair AM, Turunen M, Tyynela K, et al. Herpes simplex virus thymidine kinase gene therapy in experimental rat BT4C glioma model: effect of the percentage of thymidine kinase-positive glioma cells on treatment effect, survival time, and tissue reactions. Cancer Gene Ther 2000; 7:413–421.

120. Mesnil M, Piccoli C, Tiraby G, et al. Bystander killing of cancer cells by herpes simplex virus thymidine kinase gene is mediated by connexins. Proc Natl Acad Sci USA 1996; 93:1831–1835.

121. Freeman SM, Abboud CN, Whartenby KA, et al. The "bystander effect": tumor regression when a fraction of the tumor mass is genetically modified. Cancer Res 1993; 53:5274–5283.

122. Vrionis FD, Wu JK, Qi P, et al. The bystander effect exerted by tumor cells expressing the herpes simplex virus thymidine kinase (HSVtk) gene is dependent on connexin expression and cell communication via gap junctions. Gene Ther 1997; 4:577–585.

123. Bouvet M, Ellis LM, Nishizaki M, et al. Adenovirus-mediated wild-type p53 gene transfer down-regulates vascular endothelial growth factor expression and inhibits angiogenesis in human colon cancer. Cancer Res 1998; 58:2288–2292.

124. Liu Y, Thor A, Shtivelman E, et al. Systemic gene delivery expands the repertoire of effective antiangiogenic agents. J Biol Chem 1999; 274:13338–13344.

125. Frank DK, Frederick MJ, Liu TJ, et al. Bystander effect in the adenovirus-mediated wild-type p53 gene therapy model of human squamous cell carcinoma of the head and neck. Clin Cancer Res 1998; 4:2521–2528.

126. Eck SL, Alavi JB, Alavi A, et al. Treatment of advanced CNS malignancies with the recombinant adenovirus H5.010RSVTK: a phase I trial. Hum Gene Ther 1996; 7:1465–1482.

127. Trask TW, Trask RP, Aguilar-Cordova E, et al. Phase I study of adenoviral delivery of the HSV-tk gene and ganciclovir administration in patients with current malignant brain tumors. Mol Ther 2000; 1:195–203.

128. Judy KD, Eck SL. The use of suicide gene therapy for the treatment of malignancies of the brain. In: Lattime EC, Stanton LC, eds. Gene therapy of cancer. San Diego: Academic Press, 2002:505–512.

129. Germano IM, Fable J, Gultekin SH, et al. Adenovirus/herpes simplex-thymidine kinase/ganciclovir complex: preliminary results of a phase I trial in patients with recurrent malignant gliomas. J Neurooncol 2003; 65:279–289.

130. Smitt PS, Driesse M, Wolbers J, et al. Treatment of relapsed malignant glioma with an adenoviral vector containing the herpes simplex thymidine kinase gene followed by ganciclovir. Mol Ther 2003; 7:851–858.

131. Nunes FA, Furth EE, Wilson JM, et al. Gene transfer into the liver of nonhuman primates with E1-deleted recombinant adenoviral vectors: safety of readministration. Hum Gene Ther 1999; 10:2515–2526.

132. Byrnes AP, Rusby JE, Wood MJ, et al. Adenovirus gene transfer causes inflammation in the brain. Neuroscience 1995; 66:1015–1024.

133. Dewey RA, Morrissey G, Cowsill CM, et al. Chronic brain inflammation and persistent herpes simplex virus 1 thymidine kinase expression in survivors of syngeneic glioma treated by adenovirus-mediated gene therapy: implications for clinical trials. Nat Med 1999; 5:1256–1263.

134. Zermansky AJ, Bolognani F, Stone D, et al. Towards global and long-term neurological gene therapy: unexpected transgene dependent, high-level, and widespread distribution of HSV-1 thymidine kinase throughout the CNS. Mol Ther 2001; 4:490–498.

135. Nyberg-Hoffman C, Shabram P, Li W, et al. Sensitivity and reproducibility in adenoviral infectious titer determination. Nat Med 1997; 3:808–811.

136. Alemany R, Balague C, Curiel DT. Replicative adenoviruses for cancer therapy. Nat Biotechnol 2000; 18:723–727.

137. Grill J, van Beusechem VW, van der Valk P, et al. Combined targeting of adenoviruses to integrins and epidermal growth factor receptors increases gene transfer into primary glioma cells and spheroids. Clin Cancer Res 2001; 3:641–650.

138. Vandier D, Rixe O, Besnard F, et al. Inhibition of glioma cells in vitro and in vivo using a recombinant adenoviral vector containing an astrocyte-specific promoter. Cancer Gene Ther 2000; 7:1120–1126.

139. Shinoura N, Yoshida Y, Tsunoda R, et al. Highly augmented cytopathic effect of a fiber-mutant E1B-defective adenovirus for gene therapy of gliomas. Cancer Res 1999; 59:3411–3416.

140. Dmitriev I, Krasnykh V, Miller CR, et al. An adenovirus vector with genetically modified fibers demonstrates expanded tropism via utilization of a coxsackievirus and adenovirus receptor-independent cell entry mechanism. J Virol 1998; 72:9706–9713.

141. Kanerva A, Wang M, Bauerschmitz GJ, et al. Gene transfer to ovarian cancer versus normal tissues with fiber-modified adenoviruses. Mol Ther 2002; 5:695–704.

142. van Beusechem VW, Mastenbroek DC, van den Doel PB, et al. Conditionally replicative adenovirus expressing a targeting adapter molecule exhibits enhanced oncolytic potency on CAR-deficient tumors. Gene Ther 2003; 10:1982–1991.

143. Nanda D, Vogels R, Havenga M, et al. Treatment of malignant gliomas with a replicating adenoviral vector expressing herpes simplex virus-thymidine kinase. Cancer Res 2001; 61:8743–8750.

Index